MW00838061

EVALUATION AND TREATMENT OF MYOPATHIES

Second Edition

SERIES EDITOR
Sid Gilman, MD, FRCP
William J. Herdman Distinguished University Professor of Neurology
University of Michigan

Contemporary Neurology Series

EVALUATION AND TREATMENT OF MYOPATHIES

Second Edition

Edited By

Emma Ciafaloni, MD
Associate Professor of Neurology and Pediatrics
University of Rochester School of Medicine and Dentistry
Department of Neurology
Rochester, New York

Patrick F. Chinnery, FRCP, FMedSci
Director, Institute of Genetic Medicine
Newcastle University
Newcastle upon Tyne, UK

Robert C. Griggs, MD
Professor of Neurology, Medicine, Pediatrics, Pathology
and Laboratory Medicine, Center for Human Experimental Therapeutics
University of Rochester School of Medicine and Dentistry
Department of Neurology
Rochester, New York

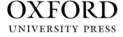

OXFORD
UNIVERSITY PRESS

OXFORD
UNIVERSITY PRESS

Oxford University Press is a department of the University of Oxford.
It furthers the University's objective of excellence in research, scholarship,
and education by publishing worldwide.

Oxford   New York
Auckland   Cape Town   Dar es Salaam   Hong Kong   Karachi
Kuala Lumpur   Madrid   Melbourne   Mexico City   Nairobi
New Delhi   Shanghai   Taipei   Toronto

With offices in
Argentina   Austria   Brazil   Chile   Czech Republic   France   Greece
Guatemala   Hungary   Italy   Japan   Poland   Portugal   Singapore
South Korea   Switzerland   Thailand   Turkey   Ukraine   Vietnam

Oxford is a registered trademark of Oxford University Press
in the UK and certain other countries.

Published in the United States of America by
Oxford University Press
198 Madison Avenue, New York, NY 10016

© Oxford University Press 2014

All rights reserved. No part of this publication may be reproduced, stored in a
retrieval system, or transmitted, in any form or by any means, without the prior
permission in writing of Oxford University Press, or as expressly permitted by law,
by license, or under terms agreed with the appropriate reproduction rights organization.
Inquiries concerning reproduction outside the scope of the above should be sent to the
Rights Department, Oxford University Press, at the address above.

You must not circulate this work in any other form
and you must impose this same condition on any acquirer.

Library of Congress Cataloging-in-Publication Data
Evaluation and treatment of myopathies / edited by Robert C. Griggs,
Emma Ciafaloni, Patrick F. Chinnery. — Second edition.
    p. ; cm.
Preceded by Evaluation and treatment of myopathies / Robert C. Griggs, Jerry R. Mendell, Robert G. Miller. c1995.
Includes bibliographical references and index.
ISBN 978–0–19–987393–7 (alk. paper)
I. Griggs, Robert C., 1939– editor of compilation.   II. Ciafaloni, Emma, editor of compilation.
III. Chinnery, Patrick F., editor of compilation.   IV. Griggs, Robert C., 1939– Evaluation and
treatment of myopathies. Preceded by (work):
[DNLM: 1. Muscular Diseases—diagnosis.   2. Muscular Diseases—therapy. WE 550]
RC925
616.7′44—dc23
2013039999

The science of medicine is a rapidly changing field. As new research and clinical experience broaden our knowledge,
changes in treatment and drug therapy occur. The author and publisher of this work have checked with sources believed
to be reliable in their efforts to provide information that is accurate and complete, and in accordance with the standards
accepted at the time of publication. However, in light of the possibility of human error or changes in the practice
of medicine, neither the author, nor the publisher, nor any other party who has been involved in the preparation or
publication of this work warrants that the information contained herein is in every respect accurate or complete. Readers
are encouraged to confirm the information contained herein with other reliable sources, and are strongly advised to check
the product information sheet provided by the pharmaceutical company for each drug they plan to administer.

9 8 7 6 5 4 3 2 1
Printed in China
on acid-free paper

Emma Ciafaloni would like to dedicate this book to Nicholas.
And to her patients, who teach her every day, not only about muscle diseases, but about life.
Patrick Chinnery dedicates this textbook to Rachel, Sarah, Catherine, Lucy, James, Arthur and Jasper.
Berch Griggs dedicates the textbook to his wife Rosalyne.

Contents

SECTION 2   SPECIFIC MYOPATHIES

Foreword

The authors asked me to write a foreword to this book, a request as surprising as it was flattering. Frequently, a foreword consists of vapid comments on the excellence of the authors, the timeliness of the information or the necessity of including yet another volume on the student's groaning bookshelf. So many books are published, so few have a lasting impact. Those that do, shape the behavior and attitudes of those in the field for decades. Duchenne's monograph, Adams, Denny Brown and Pearson's "Diseases of Muscle," Walton's "Disorders of Voluntary muscle," Coers and Woolf's "The Innervation of Muscle." There may be more recent examples but egos are easily bruised and I shall cite none. What, then is the common thread of such texts?

First, the author is speaking from personal experience and saying 'This is what I believe'—or, after the first half of the 20th century, 'This is what we believe.' Belief is easy for the young, more difficult for the old. Statements by those who have been tempered by years of disappointment are more credible than any made in the flush of the first success. On the other hand, the opinions of the elderly sometimes become ossified and should be avoided. Compromise is necessary.

Horatius on the bridge over the Tiber comes to mind. In Macaulay's epic poem there is an apt stanza. The giant Tuscan army facing Horatius and his two comrades on the bridge wavered:

'But those behind cried "Forward!"

And those before cried "Back!"'

So it is with science. More senior members look fondly on old familiar theories and askance at 'newfangled' ideas. More junior members are often unaware of what has been done by their predecessors and espouse each new research finding with an enthusiasm that is sometimes (not always) misplaced. The uncomfortable fact that the Tuscan army did not actually get anywhere should be ignored for the purpose of this simile.

The second feature of these influential texts is that, while providing a comprehensive review, they leave out extraneous material. Otherwise, reading is more soporific than instructive. I am not interested in the color of the chicken when I am boiling an egg. I am sure there are journals devoted to the niceties of chicken tinting and, if I become interested, I shall read them.

Turning from the general to the specific, how does this book measure up? I have read it, not all of it but more than just skimming through the references to see if my name was mentioned. I found it easy to read and full of useful information. Past, present and, sometimes, future work is referenced in a way that provides an excellent balance. Significant aspects of neuromuscular disease are fully discussed but the reader is not burdened with irrelevances. There is a far more important aspect to the book which has to do with the authors themselves. To say that they are eminent in their field is to understate the case. They have the quality that I mentioned above of bridging the gap between the old and new. More than that, they have the perspective to be able to tell us, not only what is true and important today but what is likely to remain true in the next decade. I do not know if this book will become a 'classic' but I do know that if I wanted to learn more about neuromuscular disease the first people that I would consult are the authors of this book.

Michael Brooke
http://www.mhbrooke.org/ underneath

Preface

This second edition of *Evaluation and Treatment of Myopathies* cannot really be viewed as a sequel to the first edition written by Griggs, Mendell and Miller and published in 1995. The majority of the diseases considered in this new edition had not been identified 18 years ago and although many chapter headings are similar, the only information that has evolved as opposed to being replaced is the still-crucial clinical approach to patients and the clinical neurophysiology of neuromuscular diseases. Virtually everything else is new. In the process of dealing with the wealth of new material of clinical importance, we realized that our readership would be best served by asking new authors expert in their sub-subspecialty to author chapters. Myopathies, and even subgroups of myopathies, are now too diverse and have too much known about pathogenesis for a single myologist to be an authority on our entire field.

This book is not intended to be encyclopedic but instead, to focus on what the clinician seeing the patient with myopathy *must* know to make a diagnosis and plan appropriate treatment. The book presents diseases as they present to a clinician. Although the experimental therapeutics of myopathies is in its infancy, much can be done to prevent complication and maintain normal activities. Major advances in treatment are on the drawing board for most myopathies. We point out where these developments are likely to come from and stress what must be done in the interval.

Emma Ciafaloni, M.D.
Patrick F. Chinnery, FRCP FMedSci
Robert C. Griggs, M.D., F.A.A.N.

Contributors

Anthony A. Amato, MD
Vice-chairman, Department of Neurology
Brigham and Women's Hospital
Professor of Neurology
Harvard Medical School
Boston, MA

Patrick Gordon, FRCP, PhD, MBBS
Consultant Rheumatologist and Honorary
 Senior Lecturer
Department of Rheumatology
King's College Hospital
London, UK

Gráinne S. Gorman, MRCP
Wellcome Trust Centre for Mitochondrial
 Research,
Institute for Ageing and Health, Newcastle
 University
Newcastle upon Tyne, UK

Michael K. Hehir, MD
Assistant Professor of Neurological Sciences
University of Vermont
Burlington, VT

**Heinz Jungbluth, MD, PhD,
 MRCP, MRCPCH**
Senior Lecturer and Consultant in Paediatric
 Neurology
Department of Paediatric Neurology—
 Neuromuscular Service
Evelina Children's Hospital
St Thomas' Hospital, and
Department of Clinical Neurosciences
Institute of Psychiatry
King's College
London, UK

Wendy M. King, PT
Associate Professor
Department of Neurology
Neuromuscular Disease Center
Wexner Medical Center, The Ohio State
 University
Columbus, OH

Andrew Mammen, MD, PhD
Co-director, Johns Hopkins Myositis Center
Associate Professor of Neurology and Medicine
Johns Hopkins University School of Medicine
Baltimore, MD

Francesco Muntoni, FRCPCH, FMedSci
Dubowitz Neuromuscular Centre and MRC
 Centre for Neuromuscular Diseases
UCL Institute of Child Health and
 Great Ormond Street Hospital for
 Children (GOSH)
Department of Developmental Neuroscience
London, UK

Gerald Pfeffer, MD, CM, FRCPC
Institute of Genetic Medicine
Newcastle University
Newcastle upon Tyne, UK

Araya Puwanant, MD
Instructor of Neurology
University of Rochester School of Medicine
 and Dentistry
Department of Neurology
Rochester, NY

Michael R. Rose, BSc, MD, FRCP
Consultant Neurologist and Honorary Senior
  Lecturer
King's College Hospital and King's College
  London, UK

Duygu Selcen, MD
Associate Professor of Neurology and
  Pediatrics
Department of Neurology
Mayo Clinic Children's Center
Rochester, MN

Caroline Sewry, PhD, FRCPath
Professor of Muscle Pathology
Dubowitz Neuromuscular Centre
Institute of Child Health and Great Ormond
  Street Hospital
London, and
Wolfson Centre for Inherited Neuromuscular
  Diseases
The Robert Jones and Agnes Hunt
  Orthopaedic Hospital
Oswestry, UK

EVALUATION AND TREATMENT OF MYOPATHIES

Second Edition

Approach to the Patient With Muscle Disease

Chapter 1

Structure and Function of Normal Muscle

Robert C. Griggs

THE MOTOR UNIT

The concept of *the motor unit* was developed by Charles Sherrington.[1] A knowledge of the normal motor unit is essential to understanding the pathophysiology of all neuromuscular diseases and interpreting muscle pathology and clinical neurophysiology.

The motor unit is the final common pathway for motor activity and muscle is the final effector of the motor unit. The motor unit (Figure 1–1) is composed of the anterior horn cell, its peripheral axon, the axon's terminal branches, the associated neuromuscular junctions, and the muscle fibers they innervate. In normal subjects, muscle fibers from a single motor unit are spatially dispersed throughout as much as 30% of the muscle[2] and only a few fibers innervated by the same anterior horn cell are contiguous.

The number of motor units varies greatly between muscles, from 100 in the intrinsic muscles of the hands to approximately 1,000 in certain leg muscles.[3] The number of muscle fibers per motor unit varies from as few as 10 in the extraocular muscles, to nearly 2,000 in leg muscles such as the gastrocnemius.[4] The

3

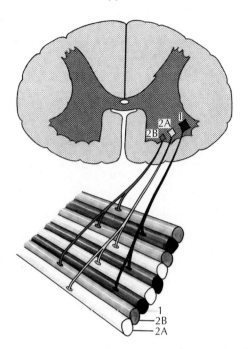

Figure 1–1. Diagram of a cross section of the spinal cord showing three motor neurons and their motor units. Type 1 motor units are slow-twitch oxidative and are innervated by the largest motor neurons, type 2A motor units are fast-twitch oxidative glycolytic and have intermediate-size motor neurons, and type 2B motor units are fast-twitch glycolytic and have the smallest motor neurons. Each motor unit is composed of the same muscle fiber types (1, 2A, 2B). The muscle fibers appear as they would in ATPase stain pH 4.6.

total number of muscle fibers per muscle varies more than 1,000-fold, from 1,000 fibers in the extraocular muscles, to more than one million in large thigh muscles.

MUSCLE FIBER TYPES

Motor units differ not only in size but also in the biochemical and physiologic properties of their muscle fibers. A number of biochemical, histochemical, and physiologic classifications have been proposed.[3,4,8,32] Figure 1–2 gives a classification useful in the interpretation of muscle pathology. On the basis of histochemistry, muscle fibers can be divided into three major types, which correlate with physiologic properties: type 1 (slow-twitch oxidative), type 2A (fast-twitch oxidative glycolytic), and type 2B (fast-twitch glycolytic). A motor unit is composed of a uniform muscle fiber type,

corresponding to type 1, 2A, or 2B motor units. The histochemical profile of normal human muscle is illustrated in Figures 1–2 and 1–3. The adenosine triphosphatase (ATPase) stain is most reliable in differentiating fiber types, and the three fiber types can be best demonstrated with preincubation at pH 4.6. Under these conditions type 1 fibers appear dark, type 2A are light, and type 2B are intermediate. With preincubation at pH 4.3, another fiber type appears, the 2C fibers, which are thought to be undifferentiated. In development they precede the appearance of types 2A and 2B and are believed to differentiate into one of these types. Motor units are never composed of only type 2C fibers.

Oxidative enzymes and lipid content correspond to the physiologic properties. Type 1 fibers are richest in lipid and oxidative enzymes, type 2A are intermediate, and type 2B have the least (Figure 1–2).

Analysis of histochemical fiber type is useful in the interpretation of muscle pathology. Preferential abnormalities of a single fiber type occur in certain muscle disorders: for example, type 2B fibers atrophy in cachexia, disuse, and corticosteroid atrophy. In myotonia congenita, type 2B fibers may be absent,[9] and in myotonic dystrophy, type 1 fibers may be preferentially atrophied.[5]

Neural Control of Muscle Fiber Type

Experimental studies in animals and clinical observations in humans indicate that the anterior horn cell determines the characteristics of the muscle fibers it supplies.[6] All muscle fibers within the same motor unit are identical in histochemical and physiologic type. This determination of muscle characteristics by motor nerve can be demonstrated using cross-innervation experiments in animals. For example, if the nerve to the pure type 1 soleus muscle of a guinea pig is exchanged with a nerve innervating a muscle of mixed fiber type (cross-innervation), subsequent examination of the soleus muscle demonstrates a mixture of muscle fiber types.[6] Although no human muscles are composed of only one fiber type, these experiments are relevant to the interpretation of human muscle biopsies, because reinnervation of muscle often follows denervation, leading to *type grouping* (large areas of muscle composed of fibers of the same type). The exact means by which individual

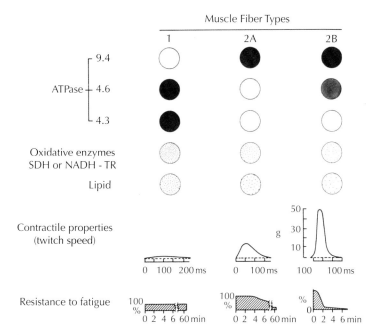

Figure 1–2. Histochemical and physiologic properties of muscle fibers: type 1 (slow-twitch oxidative), type 2A (fast-twitch oxidative glycolytic), and type 2B (fast-twitch glycolytic). The upper portion shows the staining properties in ATPase at pH 9.4, 4.6, and 4.3. Type 1 fibers show more oxidative enzymes and lipid, type 2A fibers show intermediate amounts, and type 2B fibers show the least amounts. The lower portion demonstrates greater force generation but also greater fatigability in type 2B fibers and low force but excellent fatigue resistance in type 1 fibers. Type 2A fibers are intermediate in these properties.

nerve fibers determine muscle fiber type is not clear, but the pattern of firing of the neuron is probably a major factor. Experiments in animals have demonstrated that different patterns of electrical stimulation can change the biochemical and physiologic properties of muscle fibers.[7,8]

Activation of Motor Units According to Muscle Fiber Type

With each body movement, the central nervous system selectively activates motor units having muscle fiber characteristics best suited to perform the required task. Motor units with type 1, slow-twitch, slowly fatiguing muscle fibers are designed for continuous and prolonged activity. Their energy supply for ATP generation is derived from substrate metabolism through the oxidative pathways of mitochondria.[9] Motor neurons innervating type 1 muscle fibers are small in diameter; recruitment occurs with low-intensity exertion or contraction (Figure 1–4).[19] To perform higher intensity effort, such as lifting a heavy weight, larger, higher threshold, more

rapidly conducting motor neurons are recruited. These large neurons innervate type 2A fast-twitch, oxidative glycolytic muscle fibers.[19] With very high intensity exercise or maximal exertion of the muscle, the neurons innervating the type 2B, fast-twitch, rapidly fatiguing, glycolytic fibers are recruited.[9]

SEQUENTIAL RECRUITMENT OF MOTOR UNITS

The physiologic properties of motor units and their response to voluntary contraction are such that each muscle possesses a stereotyped pattern of recruiting and an orderly sequence for the activation of its motor units.[29] Low intensity or endurance activity depends primarily on type 1 fibers. Type 2 motor units are activated only with rapid or forceful contraction.[19] This fact partly underlies the ability of muscles to gain size and strength with repeated heavy exertion. An increase in the myofibril content of muscle fibers, and possibly a small increase in the number of muscle fibers, occur with repeated heavy exertion.[10,18] By contrast,

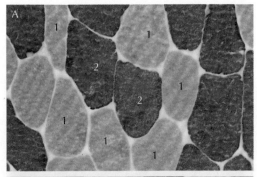

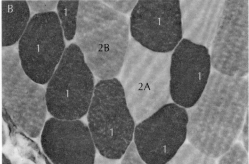

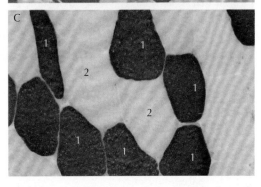

Figure 1–3. Serial sections of normal skeletal muscle showing the same muscle fibers in ATPase stains at different pH. (A) At pH 9.4, two fiber types are seen: type 1 (light) and type 2 (dark). (B) At pH 4.6, three fiber types are seen: type 1 (dark), type 2A (light), and type 2B (intermediate). (C) At pH 4.3. the reversal of fiber types is complete. demonstrating only two types: type 1 (dark) and type 2 (light).

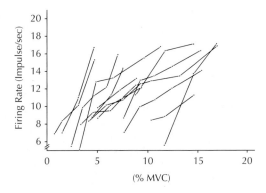

Figure 1–4. Representative curves from normal first dorsal interosseous muscle of single-motor-unit firing rates at different levels of voluntary contraction. MVC = maximum voluntary contraction strength.

unit pools.[12] A predominance of slow-twitch fibers is found in athletes trained for endurance events, and the number of fast-twitch fibers is greater in weight lifters than in untrained people.[12] The distribution of fiber type in sedentary individuals did not change after a period of exercise training, however.[12] It appears that the motor unit pool may vary considerably from individual to individual but that this variation is largely determined by genetic differences. It remains possible that exercise training during growth and development may significantly influence the motor unit pool of an adult. A lack of activation of some motor units may underlie the weakness common in many sedentary persons and in disabled or hospitalized patients.[13]

VOLUNTARY CONTROL OF MOTOR UNIT ACTIVITY

Relationship of Size to the Recruitment of Single Motor Units

According to the so-called size principle, the larger the cell body of the motor neuron, the higher the conduction velocity of its axon and the stronger the muscular contraction produced when it is stimulated.[14] Larger motor neurons are also *recruited* into activity at higher thresholds during reflex action, and with intracellular electrical stimulation.[15] Both indirect and direct evidence demonstrates that small (type 1) motor units are recruited before larger (type 2) units and that the sequence of motor unit recruitment is the same with each voluntary contraction.[16]

endurance training increases capillary density and the size and numbers of mitochondria.[10]

EFFECT OF TRAINING ON HUMAN MOTOR UNITS

Several attempts have been made to change contractile properties of motor units in humans, but most studies have not demonstrated significant conversion of fiber type.[11] On the other hand, a comparison of sedentary individuals with athletes of various types has yielded differences in motor

Firing Rates of Single Motor Units

Two mechanisms increase the force of voluntary contractions in human muscle: Either inactive motor units may be recruited, or the firing rate of already active units may be increased[17] (see Figure 1–4). The electrical behavior of single muscle fibers during moderate contraction of human muscles is the same as that of the corresponding nerve fiber, and the gradual increase in the strength of contraction is associated with an increase in firing frequency of the active motor units.[15] Frequency modulation, an increase or decrease in motor unit firing, has been suggested as the most important factor in fine control of muscle contraction.[18] The order of recruitment and relative roles of the two types of motor units are adapted both to the speed and to the strength of contraction.

Impaired Voluntary Control of Motor Units

A patient who is malingering or cannot exert full effort because of pain will have a ratchet-like and "give way" quality on muscle testing. This "give way" weakness results from the normal, rapid derecruitment of motor units that occurs with sudden relaxation; the patient then reinitiates voluntary effort, giving a ratchet-like quality to the contraction as the examiner tests strength. Patients with central nervous system disorders are often weak and characteristically fatigue easily. Such patients may demonstrate marked slowing of rapid movements, as well as spasticity and hyperreflexia. Patients with upper motor neuron disease have great difficulty in both initiating and maintaining motor unit recruitment, so that they exhibit symptoms that result from disordered motor control and impairment of fine movements.[19] Muscle power often increases with encouragement during examination, as the patient slowly recruits additional motor units.

MUSCLE STRUCTURE AND FUNCTION

Advances in the understanding of muscle structure and function have led to corresponding advances in understanding the hereditary diseases of muscle that arise from mutations of muscle proteins. The discovery of mutations by "reverse genetics," in which positional cloning of mutated genes has defined the cause of diseases in advance of knowledge about the involved proteins, has rapidly accelerated understanding of muscle structure and function.[20] The discovery of dystrophin, mutations of which cause Duchenne muscular dystrophy, was the first example and has led to the discovery of other muscle proteins abnormalities that cause other muscular dystrophies and many other myopathies.[21] These myopathies can be categorized by the location and function of the affected protein within the muscle fiber or cell:

- Sarcolemma
- Basement membrane
- Contractile apparatus and associated sarcomeric structure
- Cytoskeleton
- Sarcoplasm
- Lysosomes
- Dystrophin-associated protein complex
- Nucleus
- Mitochondria
- Sarcoplasmic reticulum

The *sarcolemma*, the cell membrane of the muscle fiber, includes the surface of myofiber, the T-tubular network, and the neuromuscular and myotendinous junctions. Ion channels are present within the sarcolemmal structures and their mutations result in diseases called "channelopathies" (Box 1.1) discussed in chapter 9. The sarcolemma limits and facilitates movement of protein and lipids through the cell membrane, and defects in the trafficking of both result in a range of myopathies[22] (Box 1.1): dysferlinopathies, caveolinopathies, myotubular myopathies, and centronuclear myopathy; and carnitine transporter deficiencies (chapters 4, 6, and 7).[23,24,25,26]

The basement membrane surrounds the muscle fiber and is made up of the basal lamina and the fibrillar reticular lamina. These structures serve to link the cytoskeleton and sarcolemma of the muscle fibers. They also play a role in myofiber development and regeneration as well as in synaptogenesis. The basement membrane is made up of collagen, laminins, perlecan, and agrin, each of which are important in myopathies (Box 1.2).[27,28,29,30,31]

Box 1.1 Disorders of the Sarcolemma

Channelopathies (sodium, chloride, potassium, and calcium)

Periodic paralysis (Ca^{++}, Na$^+$, K$^+$)
Nondystrophic myotonias (Na$^+$ and Cl$^-$)
Malignant hyperthermia (Ca^{++})

Membrane trafficking

dysferlinopathies (distal, limb-girdle muscular dystrophies)
calveolin-3 disorders (rippling muscle disease, limb-girdle muscular dystrophies, distal myopathy)
myotubularin (congenital myopathy, centronuclear myopathy)
dynamin (centromuclear myopathy)
amphiphysin-2 (centronuclear myopathy)
carnitine transporter (carnitine deficiency myopathy)

Box 1.2 Disorders of Proteins of the Basement Membrane

Collagen VI (congenital muscular dystrophy, Bethlem myopathy)
Laminin-α2 (congenital muscular dystrophy, Emery-Dreifuss muscular dystrophy)
Perlecan (Schwartz-Jampel syndrome)
Carnitine transporter (primary carnitine deficiency)

The *contractile* apparatus consists of the proteins of the sarcomere (Figure 1–5). Each muscle cell, or fiber, contains bundles of myofibrils each of which are made up of sarcomeres. The sarcomere is the basic unit of contraction and consists of thin filaments (made up of actin, tropomyosin, troponins, and nebulin) and thick filaments (made up of myosin). Actin and myosin are cross-linked at the Z-disk, which contains a network of other proteins (ZASP, telethonin, myotilin, γ-filamin), and at the M-line, which contains titin and myomesin. Mutations in each of the proteins of the sarcomere cause specific myopathies (Box 1.3).[32,33,34,35,36,37]

The *cytoskeleton* links adjacent bundles of myofibrils with each other and with the sarcolemma and basement membrane, and is made up of microtubules, intermediate filaments, and actin filaments. The cytoskeleton is also important in the integration of the Golgi complex and other organelles of the myofiber. The cytoskeleton links with the contractile apparatus at the X-disk and includes the proteins desmin, α B-cystrallin, plectin, myotilin, filamin C, and Zasp (Box 1.4).

The separation of the various disorders based on their postulated subcellular location fails to accurately characterize the dystrophin-associated protein complex, which includes components of the muscle fiber extracellular matrix, sarcolemmas, and cytoskeleton (Box 1.5 and chapter 4, Figure 4-2). This

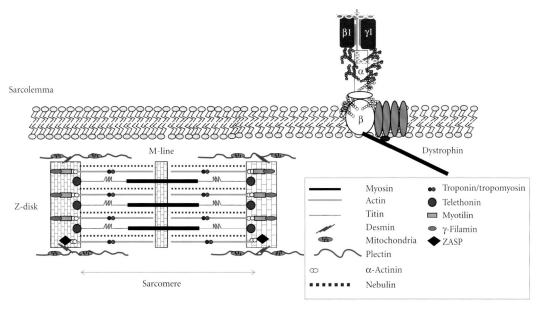

Figure 1–5. The major protein components of the sarcomere. The thin filaments consist of actin, tropomyosin, troponins, and nebulin, and the thick filaments are composed of myosin. Tropomyosin locates to the groove formed between actin strands and spans many actin monomers. Troponin associates with each molecule of tropomyosin. Actin and myosin are cross-linked at the Z-disk and M-band. Myosin filaments in the M-band are cross-linked by a protein network composed of titin and myomesin. Titin and nebulin are two giant proteins attributed with a role in myofibril alignment and elasticity. The N-terminus of titin is embedded in the Z-disk and extends to the M-line. Nebulin has its C-terminus anchored in the Z-line and extends into the I-band. The Z-disk forms a tetragonal network over the actin filament ends from two adjacent sarcomeres. (Modified from Karpati et al., *Disorders of Voluntary Muscle*, 8th ed., Cambridge, 2010, 59.)

Box 1.3 Disorders of Contractile Apparatus Proteins

Actin (nemaline myopathy, congenital fiber-type-disproportion)
Myosin (hyaline body myopathy, Laing myopathy, hereditary inclusion body myopathy, myosin storage myopathy)
Troponin (nemaline myopathy, distal myopathy, congenital fiber-type-disproportion, cardiomyopathy, arthrogryposis)
Nebulin (nemaline myopathy, distal myopathy)
Titin (tibial muscular dystrophy, limb-girdle muscular dystrophy, cardiac/skeletal myopathy)
FLH1 (reducing body myopathy, scapuloperoneal dystrophy)
Telethonin (limb-girdle muscular dystrophy)

complex of proteins is important in cell development, cell-signaling, and maintaining structural integrity of the muscle fiber. Mutations in the proteins of the complex cause of a wide spectrum of muscular dystrophies (Box 1.5).

The *sarcoplasm* contains the mitochondria, *Golgi apparatus*, glycogen, ribosomes, lipid droplets, and lipofuscin as well as the T-tubulae and sarcoplasmic reticulum. Disorders of the mitochondria are considered in chapter 8 and

Box 1.4 Disorders of Cytoskeletal Proteins

Desmin (myofibrillar myopathy)
α B-crystallin (myofibrillar myopathy)
Plectin (muscular dystrophy with epidermal bullosa simplex)
Myotilin (limb-girdle muscular dystrophy, myofibrillar myopathy, spheroid-body myopathy)
Filamin C (limb-girdle muscular dystrophy, myofibrillar myopathy)
ZASP (distal myopathy/myofibrillar myopathy)

Box 1.5 Disorders Caused by Mutations of Proteins in the Dystrophin-Associated Protein Complex

Dystroglycan complex

α-dystroglycan (congenital myopathy, limb-girdle muscular dystrophy): Fukutin and Fukintin-related protein; muscle-eye-brain disease)

Sarcoglycan–sarcospan complex

α-sarcoglycan: limb-girdle muscular dystrophy 2D
β-sarcoglycan: limb-girdle muscular dystrophy 2E
γ-sarcoglycan: limb-girdle muscular dystrophy 2C
δ-sarcoglycan: limb-girdle muscular dystrophy 2F

Dystrophin

Duchenne muscular dystrophy
Becker muscular dystrophy
Cardiomyopathy
HyperCKemia

Integrin α-7—congenital myopathy

disorders of glycogen and lipid metabolism in chapter 7. The *sarcoplasmic reticulum* regulates calcium release and uptake, disorders of which relate to the ryanodine receptor, SERCA1, and selenoproteins (Box 1.6).[38,39,40] The lysosomes of the myofiber accumulate digested cellular organelles and proteins. *Lysosomes* contain the products of digestion within autophagic vacuoles. Both hereditary and acquired diseases demonstrate pathologic accumulations of autophagic vacuoles (Box 1.7).[41,42,43]

The nucleus containing DNA and RNA is integral to myofiber development, growth, and repair. Since all of the myofiber's genes (except those of mitochondrial DNA) the nucleus is the site of the genetic mutations

---

Box 1.6 Disorders of Sarcoplasma Reticular Proteins

Ryanodine receptor

> Central core disease
> Multi/mini core disease
> Centronuclear myopathy
> Malignant hyperthermia

SERCA 1—Brody disease

Selenoprotein

> Rigid spine syndrome
> Multi/mini-core disease
> Congenital fiber type disproportion

Mallory body myopathy

Box 1.7 Diseases Characterized by Lysosomal Autophagic Vacuoles

Hereditary
> Pompe's disease (acid maltase deficiency)
> Danon's disease (LAMP 2 mutation)
> X-linked vacuolar myopathy with excessive autophagy (XMEA; cause unknown)
> Distal myopathy
> Toxic—Chloroquine myopathy
> Inclusion-body myositis/myopathies

---

of the rest of the cell. Those are mutations of DNA that produce their pathogenetic influences at the level of the DNA and RNA itself. These include myotonic dystrophy (DM1 and DM2), discussed in chapter 4.[44] It is also likely that facioscapulohumeral muscular dystrophy is a disorder in which failure of repression of a gene within nuclear heterochromatin is responsible for both FSHD1 and FSHD2 (chapter 4).[45]

The nucleus is surrounded by the nuclear envelope, which includes the so-called LEM proteins (named for laminin, emerin, and MAN1).

Mutations of lamin A cause both a limb-girdle muscular dystrophy and Emery-Dreifuss muscular dystrophy. Mutations of emerin causes the disease from which it was named: Emery-Dreifuss muscular dystrophy (chapter 4).[46,47,48]

REFERENCES

1. Lidell E, Sherrington C: Recruitment and some other features of reflex inhibition. Proc Royal Soc London, 1925;97B:488–518.
2. Burke RE, Levine DN, Tsairis P, Zajac FE III: Physiological types and histochemical profiles in

motor units of the cat gastrocnemius. J Physiol (Lond), 1973;234:723.

3. Brooke MH, Kaiser KK: Muscle fiber types: how many and what kind? Arch Neuro, 1970; Oct;23(4):369–379.

4. Crews J, Kaiser KK, Brooke MH: Muscle pathology of myotonia congenita. J Neurol Sci, 1976;28:449.

5. Engel WK: Selective and nonselective susceptibility of muscle fiber types. A new approach to Human neuromuscular diseases. Arch Neurol, 1970;22:97.

6. Samaha FJ, Guth L, Albers RW: The neural regulation of gene expression in the muscle cell. Exp Neurol, 1970;27:276.

7. Buller AJ, Eccles JC, Eccles RM: Interactions between motoneurons and muscles in respect of the characteristic speeds of their responses. J Physiol (Lond), 1960;150:417.

8. Salmons S, Vrbova G: The influence of activity on some contractile characteristics of mammalian fast and slow muscles. J Physiol (Lond), 1969;201:535.

9. Peter JB, Barnard RJ, Edgerton VR, Gillespie CA, Stempel KE: Metabolic profiles of three fiber types of skeletal muscle in guinea pigs and rabbits. Biochemistry 1972;11:2627.

10. Jones DA, Rutherford OM, Parker DF: Physiological changes in skeletal muscle as a result of strength training. Q J Exp Psychol 1989;74:233.

11. Edstrom L, Grimby L: Effect of exercise on the motor unit. Muscle Nerve, 1986;9:104–126.

12. Saltin B, Gollnick PD: Skeletal muscle adaptability: Significance for metabolism and performance. In Peachey LD, Adrian RH, and Geiger SR (eds): Handbook of Physiology. American Physiological Society, Bethesda, MD, 1983, p 555.

13. Hainaut K, Duchateau J: Muscle fatigue. effects of training and disuse. Muscle Nerve, 1989;12:660.

14. Stuart DG, Enoka RM: Motoneurons, motor units, and the size principle. In Rosenberg RN (ed): The Clinical Neurosciences. Vol 5. Churchill Livingstone, New York, 1983, p 471.

15. Burke RE: Motor units in mammalian muscle. In Sumner AJ (ed): The Physiology of Peripheral Nerve Disease. WB Saunders, Philadelphia, 1980, p 133.

16. Milner-Brown HS, Stein RB, Yemm R: The orderly recruitment of human motor units during voluntary isometric contractions. J Physiol (Lond), 1973;230:359.

17. Miller RG, Sherratt M: Firing rates of human motor units in partially denervated muscle. Neurology, 1978;28:1241.

18. Milner-Brown HS, Stein RB, Yemm R: Changes in firing rate of human motor units during linearly changing voluntary contractions. J Physiol (Lond), 1973;230:371.

19. Shahani BT (Ed): Electromyography in CNS Disorders: Central EMG. Butterworth. Boston. 1984.

20. Blake DJ, Weir A, Newey SE, Davies KE: Function and genetics of dystrophin and dystrophin-related proteins in muscle. Physiol Rev, 2002;82:2, 291–329.

21. Cohn D, Campbell KP: Molecular basis of muscular dystrophies. Muscle Nerve, 2000;23:10, 1456–1471.

22. Dowling JJ, Gibbs EM, Feldman EL: Membrane traffic and muscle: lessons from human disease. Traffic, 2008;9:7, 1035–1043.

23. Han R, Campbell KP: Dysferlin and muscle membrane repair. Curro Opin Cell Biol, 2007;19:4, 409–416.

24. Matsuda C, Hayashi YK, Ogawa M, Aoki M, Murayama K, et al: The sarcolemmal proteins dysferlin and caveolin-3 interact in skeletal muscle. Hum Mol Genet, 2001;10:17, 1761–1766.

25. Minetti C, Sotgia F, Bruno C, Scartezzini P, Broda P, Bado M, et al: Mutations in the caveolin-3 gene cause autosomal dominant limb-girdle muscular dystrophy. Nat Genet, 1998;18:4, 365–368.

26. Selcen D, Stilling G, Engel AG: The earliest pathologic alterations in dysferlinopathy. Neurology, 2001;56:11, 1472–1481.

27. Lampe AK, Bushby KM: Collagen VI related muscle disorders. J Med Gene, 2005; 42:9, 673–685.

28. Pepe G, Giusti B, Bertini E, Brunelli T, Saitta B, Comeglio P, et al: A heterozygous splice site mutation in COL6A1 leading to an in-frame deletion of the alpha1(VI) collagen chain in an Italian family affected by Bethlem myopathy. Biochem Biophys Res Commun, 1999;258:3, 802–807.

29. Baker NL, Morgelin M, Pace RA, Peat RA, Adams NE, Gardner RJ, et al: Molecular consequences of dominant Bethlem myopathy collagen VI mutations. Ann Neurol, 2007;62:4, 390–405.

30. Yurchenco PD, Cheng YS, Campbell K, Li S: Loss of basement membrane, receptor and cytoskeletal lattices in a laminin-deficient muscular dystrophy. J Cell Sci, 2004;117(Pt 5), 735–742.

31. Sturm M, Girard E, Bangratz M, Bernard V, Herbin M, Vignaud A, et al: Evidence of a dosage effect and a physiological endplate acetylcholinesterase deficiency in the first mouse models mimicking Schwartz-Jampel syndrome neuromyotonia. Hum Mol Genet, 2008; 17:20, 165–181.

32. Paulin D, Li Z: Desmin: a major intermediate filament protein essential for the structural integrity and function of muscle. Exp Cell Res, 2004;301:1,1–7.

33. Claeys KG, Fardeau M, Schroder R, Suominen T, Tolksdorf K, Behin A, et al: Electron microscopy in myofibrillar myopathies reveals clues to the mutated gene. Neuromuscul Disord, 2008,18:8, 656–666.

34. McMillan JR, Akiyama M, Rouan F, Mellerio JE, Lane EB, Leigh IM, et al: Plectin defects in epidermolysis bullosa simplex with muscular dystrophy. Muscle Nerve, 2007;35:1, 24–35.

35. Foroud T, Pankratz N, Batchman AP, Pauciulo MW, Vidal R, Miravalle L, et al: A mutation in myotilin causes spheroid body myopathy. Neurology, 2005;65:12, 1936–1940.

36. Selcen D, Ohno K, Engel AG: Myofibrillar myopathy: clinical, morphological and genetic studies in 63 patients. Brain, 2004;127:Pt 2, 439–451.

37. Selcen D, Engel AG: Mutations in ZASP define a novel form of muscular dystrophy in humans. Ann Neurol, 2005;57:2, 269–276.

38. Jungbluth H, Muller CR, Halliger-Keller B, Brockington M, Brown SC, Feng L, et al: Autosomal recessive inheritance of RYR1 mutations in a congenital myopathy with cores. Neurology, 202;59:2, 284–287.

39. Davis MR, Haan E, Jungbluth H, Sewry C, North K, Muntoni F, et al: Principal mutation hotspot for central core disease and related myopathies in the C-tenninal transmembrane region of the RYR1 gene. Neuromuscul Disord, 2003;13:2, 151–157.

40. Treves S, Jungbluth H, Muntoni F, Zorzato F: Congenital muscle disorders with cores: the ryanodine receptor calcium channel paradigm. Curro Opin Pharmacol, 2008;8:3, 319–326.
41. Malicdan MC, Noguchi S, Nonaka J, Saftig P Nishino I: Lysosomal myopathies: an excessive build-up in autophagosomes is too much to handle. Neuromuscul Disord, 2008;18:7, 521–529.
42. Kimura N, Kumamoto T, Kawamura Y, Himeno T, Nakamura KI, Ueyama H, et al: Expression of autophagy-associated genes in skeletal muscle: an experimental model of chloroquine-induced myopathy. Pathobiology, 2007;74:3,169–176.
43. Tanaka Y, Guhde G, Suter A, Eskelinen EI, Hartmann D, Lullmann-Rauch R, et al: Accumulation of autophagic vacuoles and cardiomyopathy in LAMP-2-deficient mice. Nature, 2000;406:6798, 902–906.
44. Nakamori M, Thornton CA. Epigenetic changes and non-coding expanded repeats. Neurobiology of Disease 2010;39, 21–27

45. Lemmers RJ, Tawil R, Petek LM, Balog J, Block GJ, Santen GW, et al: Digenic inheritance of an SMCHD1 mutation and an FSHD-permissive D4Z4 allele causes facioscapulohumeral muscular dystrophy type 2. Nat Genet, 2012;Dec;44:12, 1370–1374.
46. Manilal S, Nguyen TM, Sewry CA, Morris GE: The Emery-Dreifuss muscular dystrophy protein, emerin, is a nuclear membrane protein. Hum. Mol. Genet, 1996;5:6, 801–808.
47. Lammerding J, Schulze PC, Takahashi T, Kozlov S, Sullivan T, Kamm RD, et al: Lamin A/C deficiency causes defective nuclear mechanics and mechanotransduction. J Clin Invest, 2004;113:3, 370–378.
48. van Engelen BG, Muchir A, Hutchison CJ, van der Kooi VJ, Bonne G, Lammens M: The lethal phenotype of a homozygous nonsense mutation in the lamin A/C gene. Neurology, 2005;64:2, 374–376.

Chapter 2

Evaluation of the Patient With Myopathy

Robert C. Griggs
Emma Ciafaloni

INTRODUCTION

Most patients with muscle symptoms do not have an identifiable disease of muscle. Paradoxically, patients who complain of weakness and tiredness usually have normal strength. On the other hand, many patients with objective weakness, particularly when it develops slowly, do not report weakness as a symptom. Patients who have symptoms but no known or definable disease are hard to discuss and hard to care for. Chapter 12 reviews the current state of knowledge about normal fatigue and muscle pain and suggests diagnostic and management strategies useful for these patients.

Although advances in molecular genetics have defined the genetic lesion in many myopathies, there is much about molecularly defined diseases that we do not yet understand. For example, we now know that a protein (dystrophin) is missing in all muscles of patients with Duchenne dystrophy. However, many muscles are normal early in life and some (such as extraocular muscles) never become weak. Why? Moreover, dystrophin is present in all mammalian species' muscle, but in some mammals (e.g., mice) it can be genetically absent, and the animals still have virtually normal strength.

Among the many unanswered questions concerning muscle disease are:

1. What accounts for the selective and at times asymmetrical involvement of individual muscles—particularly the proximal > distal predilection?
2. Why do genetic defects of muscle have their onset at different ages and progress at different rates?
3. What environmental factors and what additional genetic influences contribute to intersubject variability.

DEFINITION OF MYOPATHY

By convention, the neuromuscular diseases are classified into four categories, subdividing the two cells of the motor unit—the neuron and the muscle cell—into disorders of (1) anterior horn cell, (2) peripheral nerve, (3) neuromuscular junction, and (4) muscle. Certain clinical and laboratory criteria have been used to defend this subdivision (Boxes 2.1 and 2.2).

Box 2.1   Definition of Myopathy: Clinical Criteria

Clinical Features Suggestive of Myopathy

Distribution of weakness: proximal, symmetric
Muscle bulk: relatively preserved or enlarged
Muscle palpation (unreliable: indurated, tender)
Muscle percussion: diminished muscle contraction; myotonia, rippling
Reflexes: parallel muscle strength

Clinical Features Contravening Myopathy

Distal weakness
Fasciculations: suggest anterior horn cell disease
Tongue atrophy
Tremor: suggests peripheral neuropathy, anterior horn cell disease, or CNS disease
Sensory signs (or symptoms): suggest peripheral neuropathy or CNS disease
Pathologic fatigue:[a] suggests neuromuscular junction defect
Early absence of reflexes

[a]Demonstrable weakness with successive testing of strength

Box 2.2 Laboratory Findings Suggestive of Myopathy

Serum Enzymes

Elevations of creatine kinase (> four-fold)

Electromyography

Potentials: brief, low-voltage, polyphasic
Recruitment: increased
Interference pattern: full in weak muscles
Fasciculations: absent

Nerve Conduction

Normal sensory responses; normal motor conduction velocity and distal latency;
CMAP may be low. No decrement of CMAP on repetitive nerve stimulation

Muscle Biopsy

Muscle fiber necrosis and regeneration; central nuclei
Hypertrophy, abnormally round muscle fibers

Increase in Endomysial Connective Tissue

However, diseases currently believed to be exclusively in muscle may eventually prove to result, in part, from an abnormality of the neuron. For example, corticosteroid "myopathy" merits the name chiefly because weakness predominates in proximal muscles. Many other criteria, however, belie the term: serum levels of creatine kinase, the muscle enzyme, are usually normal, and muscle morphology shows only atrophy, rather than traditional indications of a myopathy, such as muscle necrosis (see chapter 11). Although electromyography (EMG) may show a myopathic pattern with small, numerous action potentials, such abnormalities are not specific for myopathy and can be found in other disorders in which a primary defect in muscle is not implicated, such as neuromuscular junction diseases (e.g., myasthenia gravis and the Lambert-Eaton syndrome). The pathogenesis of corticosteroid-induced weakness ultimately is related to elevated steroid levels and is probably mediated by direct effects on muscle. Whether corticosteroids also alter neuronal firing pattern, the neuromuscular junction, muscle hormone receptors, or still other factors is unclear. Thus, the term *corticosteroid myopathy* is widely accepted even though the pathophysiology of the disorder remains uncertain.

Similarly, in acid maltase deficiency, biochemical analysis can identify a specific deficiency of enzyme activity in muscle, and the morphologic and biochemical alterations can be reproduced in cultured muscle.[1] Nevertheless, coexisting disease is present in anterior horn cells and peripheral nerve, and various features of the muscle biopsy and of electromyography suggest that denervation contributes to the clinical picture.[2] As in many disorders in which the pathogenesis of weakness is not yet known, clinical and laboratory findings in these patients do not adequately define the site of pathology—but the weight of evidence favors myopathy.

The Hereditary Myopathies

Lacking a satisfactory scientific definition of myopathy, this text includes the gamut of hereditary disorders implicating muscle dysfunction, including

1. the muscular dystrophies, with caveats concerning their pathogenesis;
2. disorders whose biochemical abnormalities are expressed in muscle;
3. disorders with distinctive morphologic alterations in muscle; and
4. disorders characterized by abnormalities of the muscle membrane.

Gene-mapping studies have confirmed that the genetic defects of muscular dystrophy are present in somatic cells other than muscle. Many of these inherited disorders fulfill our definition of myopathy if muscle weakness is a major feature of the illness. In some disorders, however, although muscle is clearly involved, myopathy is overshadowed by more evident disease in other tissues (Box 2.3). If myopathy can dominate the picture, failing to classify the disease first and foremost as a myopathy may simply be the result of another specialty claiming it first. Thus, carnitine deficiency is usually classified with the myopathies, but it also can present as an encephalopathy or as a primary cardiomyopathy (see chapter 7).

Box 2.3 Some Inherited Disorders with Frequent Subclinical or Slight Muscle Involvement

Ataxia-Telangiectasia (Louis-Bar Syndrome)

Spinocerebellar Degeneration

Friedreich's ataxia
Refsum's disease

Lipoprotein Disorders

An-alphalipoproteinemia (Tangier disease)
A-betalipoproteinemia (Bassen-Kornzweig syndrome)

Hematologic Disorders

Hemoglobinopathies
Acanthocytosis
McLeod syndrome

Connective Tissue Disease

Marfan's syndrome
Ehlers-Danlos syndrome

Mucopolysaccharidoses

Sphingolipidoses

Dysmorphic Syndromes

Noonan's syndrome
Cornelia de Lange syndrome

Prader-Willi Syndrome

The Inflammatory Myopathies

This text includes both primary and secondary inflammatory myopathies. The categorization of one disease as an inflammatory myopathy (such as dermatomyositis) can be arbitrary, because inflammation is often lacking, whereas inflammation can be present in a hereditary diseases such as facioscapulohumeral muscular dystrophy and the dysferlinopathies (chapter 4). Historical classifications will persist until the pathogenesis of each myopathy is fully understood.

Myopathies Due to Systemic Diseases

Chapter 11 summarizes these conditions. These disorders occur in two broad categories. The first includes disorders with impressive muscle pathology but little clinical evidence in terms of symptoms and signs to support myopathy. Sarcoidosis, polyarteritis, amyloidosis, parasitic infections, and neoplasms may be recognized in the muscle of patients without muscle weakness. A substantial number of metabolic defects such as the leukodystrophies, lipoprotein disorders, and hereditary ataxias (see Box 2.3) also may produce muscle pathology, but they rarely present with symptomatic myopathy.

The second category encompasses disorders with symptoms and signs of muscle disease caused by a disorder of systems other than muscle. Endocrinopathies, metabolic derangements, infections, and various toxins and drugs are frequent causes of such muscle disease. Particularly common is muscle wasting associated with aging, inactivity, pain, malnutrition, and cardiopulmonary failure. Recognizing a coexisting, distinct primary myopathy in such patients demands great clinical acumen.

CLINICAL EVALUATION

To diagnose and treat the patient with weakness due to neuromuscular disease, the lesion must be localized to the appropriate portion of the motor unit. Systematic clinical evaluation is needed to localize disease to the anterior horn cell, peripheral nerve, neuromuscular junction, or muscle. Some neuromuscular disorders have distinctive symptoms and physical findings that suggest the diagnosis. Box 2.1 lists abnormalities on examination that occur singly or in various combinations in different myopathies.

In most patients with myopathies, the major problem is weakness; less commonly, muscle pain or cramping appear first. Patients with prominent complaints of pain often have disease of joint, bone, or nerve rather than of muscle. Patients with depression, anemia, or systemic illness may also complain of weakness, although they usually mean a generalized sense of *asthenia*. Through a careful examination and history, the true nature of the patient's problem usually can be determined.

History

WEAKNESS

In most cases, motor signs precede motor symptoms. Athletes and other very strong individuals may notice a loss of strength before it is apparent to the examiner. In taking the history, the clinician must ask the patient about his or her ability to perform a specific activity, because patients often are able to ignore slowly progressive weakness by unconsciously compensating for loss of strength. Often only an acute or abrupt change will prompt a complaint of muscle weakness; patients may avoid medical attention until they encounter difficulty carrying out specific tasks. In addition, historical features can help to define the regional distribution of weakness (Table 2–1), and the loss of a specific ability such as climbing stairs, getting up from the floor, or opening jars can document the evolution and course of a disease.

FATIGUE

The "fatigue" that occurs in healthy persons *must be distinguished from pathologic fatigability* resulting from a defect in neuromuscular transmission, from a defect in muscle metabolism, or from upper motor neuron dysfunction.[10,20] The symptom of fatigue must also be separated into *pathologic fatigability* characterized by loss of *function,* and *asthenia* characterized by loss of *"energy."* Examples of

Table 2–1 **Signs and Symptoms of Muscle Weakness**

Location	Signs and Symptoms
Ocular	Ptosis, double vision, dysconjugate or limited eye movements
Facial	Sclera visible while sleeping or during eyelid closure; inability to "bury the eyelashes," smile, whistle
Palatal	Nasal escape of liquids, nasal speech
Pharyngeal	Weight loss, difficulty swallowing, recurrent pneumonias secondary to aspiration of liquid or food, cough or dyspnea during meals
Trunk	Accentuated lumbar lordosis, scoliosis, protuberant abdomen, difficulty sitting up from supine
Shoulder and arms	Winging of scapulae, difficulty lifting objects above the head, inability to do push-ups
Forearm and hand	Finger or wrist drop, inability to make a tight fist and blanch the knuckles, inability to prevent escape from hand grip
Pelvic	Waddling gait, difficulty stepping up onto a chair, rising from squat (with one or both legs), rising from a chair (with or without using hand support)
Leg and foot	Inability to hop or walk on toes, walk on heels, or spread or curl toes

pathologic fatigability include dysconjugate eye movements, ptosis, dysphagia, and dysarthria, which occur particularly in myasthenia gravis and related conditions. In contrast, patients with asthenia may require bed rest, need frequent naps, and complain that they have no energy, but they rarely report loss of strength of specific muscle groups.

Fatigability due to a failure of neuromuscular junction transmission can often be demonstrated electrophysiologically by repetitive nerve stimulation of selected muscles (see section on Repetitive Nerve Stimulation). Fatigue resulting from impaired muscle metabolism often requires provocative exercise testing (see Chapters 7 and 9). Fatigue of other components of motor function such as suprasegmental control (the upper motor neuron) or the muscle contractile apparatus is difficult to evaluate clinically and is particularly troublesome to distinguish from volitional and motivational factors; some techniques (interpolated twitch, intermittent tetanic stimulation) can help with these issues.[3] In upper motor neuron dysfunction, fatigability occurs rapidly when the patient attempts to maintain a maximum muscular contraction. EMG recordings have demonstrated a concomitant decrease in the total number and the firing rate of recruited motor unit potentials.[4] Thus electrophysiologic studies may help to reveal whether fatigability results from an abnormality in neuromuscular transmission or in suprasegmental control of the firing of the anterior horn cell.

MUSCLE PAIN, CRAMPS, AND STIFFNESS

Myalgias in association with acute viral illness and postexertional muscle pain are part of everyday experience. Muscle discomfort in these instances is usually self-limited and differs from the complaints of muscle pain that result from a hereditary or acquired abnormality of muscle metabolism, from an inflammatory myopathy, or from a toxic myopathy (Box 2.4). Components other than muscle fibers, including connective tissue, blood vessels, nerves, and tendons, often are responsible for muscle pain. Still more commonly, joint pain may be referred to adjacent muscles. Joint diseases such as polymyalgia rheumatica, rheumatoid arthritis, or lupus erythematosus often present with muscle pain and stiffness. Patients use subjective terms to describe muscle pain; words such as "cramp," "charley horse," "spasm," "seizing up," "lameness," "rheumatism," or "leaders" often tell more about a patient's cultural heritage than about his or her muscle function. Many patients with muscle pain turn out to have a definable disease of muscle, but many do not. In fact, most patients with myopathies have little or no muscle pain.

Fibrositis or *fibromyalgia* is a common but poorly understood disorder. Patients complain bitterly of muscle pain and tenderness and often can identify specific areas of tender muscle or skin (trigger points), but muscle biopsy

Box 2.4 Major Causes of Muscle Pain, Cramps, and Stiffness

The most common causes of muscular pain are other than primary muscle disease:

Circulatory insufficiency
Joint disease
Bone disease
Neuropathy
Anterior horn cell disease
Fasciitis
Fibromyalgia

Muscle disorders are often painless. Those with pain include:

Inflammatory myopathies: dermatomyositis; polymyositis; myositis with collagen vascular disease; viral, bacterial, and parasitic myositis
Substrate-utilization defects: glycogenolysis, glycolysis, fatty-acid oxidation, purine nucleotide cycle
Toxic myopathies: alcohol, narcotics, clofibrate, zidovudine
Endocrinopathies: hypothyroidism, hyperthyroidism, hypoparathyroidism, hyperparathyroidism
Metabolic disorders: lowered sodium, potassium, calcium, magnesium, phosphate; elevated sodium, calcium

Myotonia (occasionally painful): DM2, myotonia congenita

---

fails to demonstrate specific abnormalities. As discussed further in chapter 12, sleep disturbances are frequent in such patients.

A *muscle cramp* is associated with involuntary, high-frequency discharge of many motor units and is promptly relieved by stretching the affected muscle.[5] Muscle cramp must be differentiated from a muscle *contracture,* which is related to defects in carbohydrate metabolism. Although associated with painful shortening of the muscle belly and sustained contraction of the muscle, contractures are electrically silent when studied by electromyography.[6]

Muscle cramps are frequent in diseases of the anterior horn cell, such as amyotrophic lateral sclerosis (ALS), and in disorders of the peripheral nerve, if the axon is affected. Less common diseases that can result in muscle cramps include the *stiff-man syndrome,* where cramps originate in the anterior horn cells, and *Isaac's syndrome,* a disorder in which continuous firing of muscle fibers is associated with

muscle stiffness and hyperhidrosis, and in which cramps originate in the distal peripheral nerves. Cramps of neurogenic origin can be blocked by pharmacologic agents. Quinine, which stabilizes the muscle membrane, is sometimes helpful, but agents that prevent repetitive nerve discharges, such as carbamazepine or phenytoin, are more frequently effective (chapter 12).

Two well-characterized metabolic glycolytic defects of skeletal muscle that are associated with painful contractures are muscle phosphorylase deficiency (McArdle's disease) and phosphofructokinase deficiency. In both of these disorders, failure of energy production results from an enzyme deficiency that blocks glycogen or glucose metabolism. These patients develop a painful, hard, contracted muscle during vigorous exercise (see chapter 7). In carnitine palmitoyltransferase (CPT) deficiency, oxidation of long-chain fatty acids is impaired, and many of these patients experience muscle pain and discomfort, usually described as a "tightness" rather than a muscle cramp (see chapter 7).

In normal individuals, muscle cramps are commonly encountered during swimming and at night. Swimmers are particularly prone to develop cramping of the calf muscles which appears to be related to a passive shortening of the gastrocnemius muscle during swimming with the ankle plantar flexed. Neural input superimposed on this passively shortened muscle without concomitant resistance or tension to limit the contractile response produces a painful muscle cramp. A similar mechanism is thought to produce nocturnal leg cramps, in which the muscle once again is passively shortened because of ankle plantar flexion. During normal muscle activity, an inhibitory feedback input to the spinal cord from the Golgi tendon organ protects against a muscle cramp.[5]

Dehydration with decreased plasma volume may be a cause of cramps, although the exact mechanism of their origin is unknown.[7]

Paresthesias and Dysesthesias

Paresthesias and dysesthesias are characteristic of peripheral nerve or central nervous system disease; their occurrence in a weak patient either points away from a diagnosis of myopathy or suggests that both neuropathy and myopathy are present.

Examination

DEMONSTRATION AND QUANTIFICATION OF WEAKNESS

Muscle strength can be tested by manual testing and from observation of functional activity (see Table 2–4). Functional assessment is particularly useful in children unable to cooperate with individual muscle testing. On the other hand, manual muscle testing can be used to quantify muscle strength by applying a grading system. The most widely used system is the 0-to-5 scale developed by the Medical Research Council (MRC) of Great Britain (Table 2–2).[50] One major problem inherent in this scale is that grade 4 ("opposing some resistance"), together with grade 5 (normal strength), often encompass 80% to 90% of the range of muscle strength.[12] The scale has

Table 2–2 Medical Research Council (MRC) Manual Muscle Testing Scale[8]

MRC Grade	Degree of Strength
5	Normal
4	Able to oppose resistance
3	Able to oppose gravity
2	Able to move with gravity eliminated
1	Trace movement
0	No movement

been modified to address this problem by adding pluses and minuses (Table 2–3); this useful change subdivides the large range of grade 4 strength.[28]

Devices for Quantification of Strength

The need to quantify strength or document a change with therapy has led to the use of a variety of myometers.[21,47] Most clinicians do not use these devices, as most require the physician to undergo rigorous training before precise, reproducible measurements can be

Table 2–3 Expanded MRC Scale for Manual Muscle Testing

Modified MRC Grade	Degree of Strength
5	Normal strength
5–	Equivocal, barely detectable weakness
4+	Definite but slight weakness
4	Able to move the joint against combination of gravity and some resistance[a]
4–	Capable of minimal resistance
3+	Capable of transient resistance but collapses abruptly
3	Able to move through full range against gravity without resistance to the movement
3–	Able to move against gravity but not through full range
2	Able to move with gravity eliminated
1	Flicker of movement
0	No movement

[a]The subdivisions 4S (a strong 4), 4 (a moderate 4), and 4W (a weaker 4) are often useful.

Table 2–4 Testing of Muscle Function in Young Children

Muscle Group	Sign or Symptom
Ocular	Limitation in eye movements, ptosis
Bulbar function	Cry, speech, suck, tongue
Neck flexion	Head control (Figure 2–7)
Shoulder girdle	Suspension
Hip and trunk	Gait, jumping and running ability
Trunk and proximal leg	Gowers' sign (Figure 2–1)
Respiratory	Use of accessory muscles; paradoxical diaphragm movement

obtained, and patient motivation has a marked and variable effect on testing. One exception is the hand dynamometer, which requires little training for accurate use. For example, the JAMAR hand dynamometer (Asimow Engineering Company, Santa Monica, CA), was found reliable in measuring hand grip strength when tests were compared between different observers.[31]

Strength Testing in Young Children

Children less than 5 years of age often are unable to cooperate with testing. Moreover, strength testing in childhood may be difficult because of the lack of criteria for what constitutes normal strength. In young children, function testing can provide a reproducible means of assessing muscle function (Table 2–4). Careful analysis of gait on either running or walking, watching a child getting up from the floor (Gowers' sign; Figure 2–1), flexing the neck on the chest in a supine position (Figure 2–2), and elevating the arms to see if winging occurs (Figure 2–3) are all helpful approaches. Lifting the child with the examiner's hands in the axillae detects shoulder girdle weakness if the patient's shoulder girdle rises upward. Whereas the normal child involuntarily exerts downward pressure against the examiner's hands, the weak child will "fall through on suspension." Abnormal findings on these tests are not specific for myopathy, however; patients with other causes of proximal weakness show identical signs.

Strength Testing in Infants

The recognition of congenital and early onset infantile weakness from neuromuscular disease is especially challenging. Because congenital myopathies and indeed all neuromuscular diseases are rare, central nervous system disease is much more commonly associated with motor system disease. Infants with both central and neuromuscular causes of motor system disease are often termed *floppy babies* (Figures 2–4

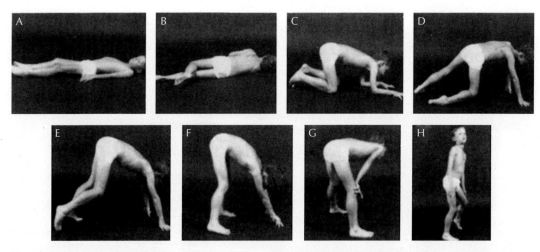

Figure 2–1. Gowers' sign. A patient with Duchenne dystrophy is shown rising from the floor. The most common cause of weakness in young boys is Duchenne dystrophy, but Gowers' sign is present in any disorder characterized by proximal weakness. To stand, the patient must roll from supine to prone (A and B), push off the floor (C–E), lock his knees (F), and then "climb up on his legs" (G and H).

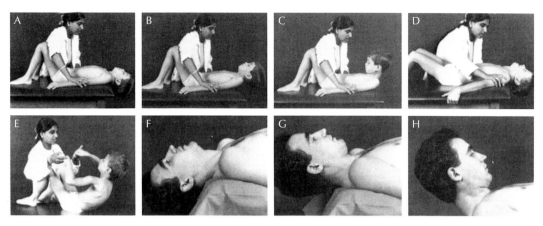

Figure 2–2. Testing neck flexion. (A–C) Normal child. (D) Neck flexor weakness in Duchenne dystrophy. The patient is unable to lift his head against gravity. It is important to fix the shoulders on the examining table. (E) Severe neck flexor weakness (grade 2 MRC) is present even from infancy in patients with Duchenne dystrophy. (F–H) Whereas the patient with Duchenne dystrophy is able to hold the head up only if gravity is partially eliminated, the patient with Becker dystrophy can lift his head against gravity.

to 2–7). Distinguishing between central and neuromuscular cause requires careful attention to the history evaluating babies for CNS injuries: hypoxia, hemorrhage, or severe developmental disease. Most infants with a CNS cause for being floppy have preserved reflexes and are often lethargic. Infants with neuromuscular disease are generally alert and areflexic.

MUSCLE BULK

Muscle Atrophy

Atrophy and hypertrophy of muscle are difficult to quantify because of the marked variation among normals. Atrophy is particularly difficult to estimate in children because of overlying adipose tissue. A visual judgment of muscle bulk is more reliable than measurements, because the circumference of the limbs, chest, and abdomen do not accurately assess the adiposity of the patient. Atrophy is easier to appreciate when it is asymmetric. Small muscles are not necessarily abnormal unless the patient is weak; this is especially true in elderly patients. Such an appearance occurs frequently in normal children or in adults who have "down weighted" to achieve greater speed in long-distance running and other endurance sports.

Myopathies characteristically produce less atrophy than neuropathies when degrees of

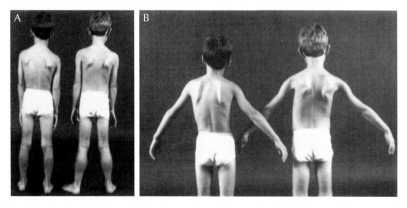

Figure 2–3. Scapular winging. Brothers with Duchenne dystrophy are elevating their arms. Protrusion of the scapulae is present bilaterally.

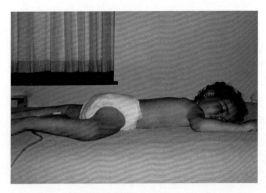

Figure 2–4. Hypotonic, quadriparetic child: Centronuclear myopathy.

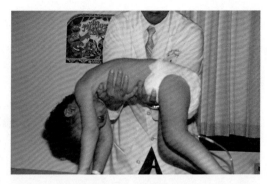

Figure 2–6. "Floppy" child: Hypotonia with suspension.

weakness are comparable. This preservation of muscle bulk in myopathies may reflect damaged muscle fibers that generate little or no force, as well as replacement of muscle fibers by connective tissue and fat.

Muscle Enlargement

An isolated or symmetric increase in the size of an individual muscle or a group of muscles may occur with exercise. Abnormal enlargement

may result from increased spontaneous activity such as occurs with myotonia (Box 2.5). This results in true hypertrophy of muscle fibers. Enlargement reflecting an increase in fat and connective tissue may produce pseudohypertrophy, although the pseudohypertrophy in Duchenne dystrophy is not exclusively the result of fat and connective tissue replacement, because some muscle fibers are truly hypertrophied in this condition. Muscle enlargement is usually recognized as abnormal only when selected individual muscles are enlarged in comparison with other normal or atrophied muscles; for example, the calves in Duchenne dystrophy, or the extensor digitorum brevis (EDB) muscle in limb-girdle and other muscular dystrophies (Figures 4–4, 4–5, 4–20). Muscles also can enlarge from infiltration by amyloid or parasites.

Several disorders other than primary myopathies can produce focal enlargement and masses in muscle. Such swelling can accompany

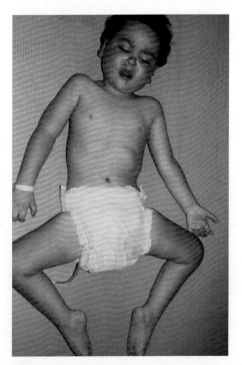

Figure 2–5. "Floppy," hypotonic child with congenital myopathy.

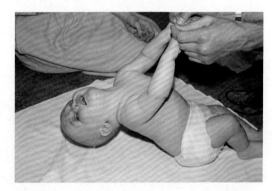

Figure 2–7. Head lag in a floppy baby with congenital myopathy.

Box 2.5 Causes of Generalized or Focal Muscle Enlargement

Muscle Fibers Histologically Normal

Exercise
Spasticity (especially with high cervical spinal cord disease)
Myotonic disorders: myotonia congenita, paramyotonia congenita, hyperkalemic periodic paralysis
Flier's syndrome (acanthosis nigricans, insulin resistance)

Muscle Fibers Histologically Abnormal

Muscular dystrophy: Duchenne, Becker, limb-girdle
Spinal muscular atrophy: Kugelberg-Welander disease
Radiculopathies
Glycogen storage disease: adult acid maltase
Endocrinopathies: hypothyroidism, acromegaly

Infiltration With Pathologic Material

Connective tissue and fat: muscular dystrophy
Parasitic infestations: e.g., cysticercosis, schistosomiasis
Amyloidosis
Sarcoidosis

Focal Enlargement or Masses

Myositis
Granulomas (esp. sarcoidosis)
Ectopic ossification
Calcinosis
Ruptured tendons

Neoplasms

generalized muscle disease due to inflammatory infiltrates or calcium deposits. Single or multiple muscle masses in the absence of weakness can reflect neoplastic involvement, focal myositis, infection, ectopic ossification, or tendon rupture.

MUSCLE PALPATION

Palpation of weak, stiff, painful, or enlarged (or symptomatic) muscles may provide diagnostic clues. Calcium deposits are usually discrete and may be separable from surrounding tissues. Neoplasms and inflammatory lesions may also be defined. On the other hand, the texture of muscle, often described as "fibrotic," "doughy," or "flabby," is usually not diagnostic. Muscle tenderness is not a specific sign, and it rarely accompanies inflammation confined to the muscle unless there is extension into the overlying fascia. Pitting edema confined to the muscle is uncommon, but in dermatomyositis (particularly the childhood form), edema of the subcutaneous tissue involving the arms is a valuable sign.

FATIGUE

Pathologic fatigue is the hallmark of neuromuscular junction disease, but as noted earlier (section on Fatigue), some degree of fatigue is normal. Fatigue may also be the result of limited effort. Useful, objective clinical signs that are not likely to result from poor motivation include worsening of ptosis, the development of dysconjugate eye movements, the peek sign (lid opening after initial closure during a Bell's phenomenon),[9] and the development of rhinolalia (nasal speech). Patients cannot mimic these abnormalities by decreased effort, and voluntary efforts cannot simulate ptosis.

MYOTONIA

In some myopathies, myotonia may be the only clinical sign that indicates an underlying muscle disease. Myotonia is the sustained contraction of muscle caused by spontaneous repetitive depolarization of the muscle membrane. The phenomenon arises directly from the muscle membrane and persists in the absence of nerve supply (see chapter 9). Myotonia is clinically and electrophysiologically distinct from a true muscle cramp or from the unusual neuromyotonia, which requires intact innervations by the peripheral nerve. True muscle cramps, which result from spontaneous discharge of motor nerves, occur either when the muscle is at rest or after muscular contraction and can occasionally be provoked by strong muscular contraction in strength testing. They produce a firm mounding-up of the muscle which is promptly eliminated by stretching it. Such cramps are usually intensely painful, whereas myotonia is usually painless. (For exceptions see chapter 9). Neuromyotonia (previously known as neurotonia and Isaac's syndrome) manifests as continuous muscle rippling and stiffness at rest. It results from bursts of very high frequency discharges of peripheral nerve. Eyelid action myotonia can be elicited as shown in Figure 9–1A & B (chapter 9). Myotonia can also be elicited either by having the patient forcefully contract a muscle, such as eye closure (see chapter 9, Figure 9–10A–C) or clenched fist (*action myotonia*),[2] or by tapping a muscle (*percussion myotonia;* see chapter 9, Figure 9–9A & B). To elicit percussion myotonia, the muscle belly is struck sharply with a soft device such as a reflex hammer. In the normal patient, percussion of the finger extensors produces extension that lasts less than half a second. In the patient with myotonia, the fingers remain partially extended and then gradually fall. Similarly, percussion of the tongue (by tapping a tongue blade; see chapter 4, Figure 4–9A & B) or thenar

eminence can produce a sustained contraction that results in a local depression. This depression in the tongue is termed the "napkin-ring sign" and elsewhere is termed "dimpling."

Myotonia is usually more prominent in the cold or after prolonged rest with the body in a fixed posture. Myotonia typically diminishes or "warms up" with repeated exercise. If myotonia worsens with repeated activity, it is termed *paradoxical myotonia*. The myotonic phenomenon can arise from a number of genetically distinct muscle membrane disorders (see chapter 9).

Percussion myotonia must be distinguished from the normal *muscle percussion response* and *myoedema*. When percussed with a reflex hammer, the muscle is briefly depolarized and contracts, resembling a muscle stretch reflex. This contraction may be confusing in patients with neuropathies, who usually have hypoactive reflexes, because the muscle percussion response remains brisk,[10] presumably because denervated muscle fibers continue to be subject to mechanical depolarization.

MYODEMA AFTER PERCUSSION

Myoedema is a localized, persistent, electrically silent swelling after percussion that reflects a local contraction induced by the release of calcium ions from the sarcoplasmic reticulum.[11] It is not pathologically significant but must be distinguished from myotonia: Myoedema produces swelling whereas myotonia produces dimpling. Myoedema was once considered a sign of malnutrition, but this misattribution was likely based on its prominence in subjects with little overlying subcutaneous tissue.

SPONTANEOUS MOVEMENTS OF MUSCLE

None of the spontaneous movements discussed in this are signs of myopathy. Muscle twitches or *fasciculations* may be an important sign of neuromuscular disease and may also be a presenting symptom. They result from the spontaneous contraction of muscle fibers within a motor unit and arise from ectopic electrical activity, usually in the distal axon.[12] Fasciculations most frequently accompany motor neuron disease and, less commonly, peripheral nerve disorders. They are diagnostically significant when they accompany weakness but they occur in many normal individuals, particularly in tense individuals or following exercise (so-called benign or contraction fasciculations).[13] They also can accompany certain metabolic disorders such as hyperparathyroidism, hyperthyroidism, and hypomagnesemia and may also occur with toxic effects of drugs, including theophylline, caffeine, terbutaline, lithium, and anticholinesterase agents.

Fasciculations may be obscured by overlying adipose tissue but they are readily seen in the tongue (unprotruded) and the interosseous muscles. Fasciculations are rarely an early complaint in most neuromuscular diseases; in fact, many patients with severe weakness are surprisingly unaware of their presence. It is the exceptional patient with motor neuron disease who presents with florid fasciculations preceding the onset of weakness.

Myokymia, a pattern of muscle contraction that produces a "writhing" or rippling appearance in the involved area, is the result of spontaneous discharge of large motor units. Myokymia indicates neuronal disease[14]; denervation is followed by sprouting from adjacent neurons, with enlargement of the motor unit territory.

Minipolymyoclonus results from the spontaneous contraction of enlarged motor units (see section on Electromyography) in patients with motor neuron disease and produces small amplitude movements of fingers and toes when an extremity is at rest.[15] Similar but accentuated movements occur when patients hold

their hands in the outstretched position. *Tremor,* attributed to weakness,[16] is almost invariably present in patients with symptomatic weakness due to nerve disease. This tremor is probably an exaggeration of the normal physiologic tremor that results from the synchronized discharge of enlarged motor units in patients who have a reduced number of surviving motor neurons.[17]

General Examination

Neuromuscular diseases should be suspected in individuals with various skeletal abnormalities including narrow facies, high-arched palate, pectus deformities of the chest, scoliosis, pes cavus or pes planus, and hammer toes. Associated cardiac and pulmonary abnormalities are discussed in chapter 13. Primary muscular diseases, except for the myotonic dystrophies, are associated with remarkably few nonmuscular problems. The inflammatory myopathy dermatomyositis is also associated with involvement of not only skin but also lungs, gastrointestinal, and other organs. Vascular inflammation and occlusion occur; these can be visualized clinically by careful examination of the fingernails (Figure 2–8).

FACIAL APPEARANCE

Certain facies are diagnostically distinctive. For example, the facial appearance of adult-onset

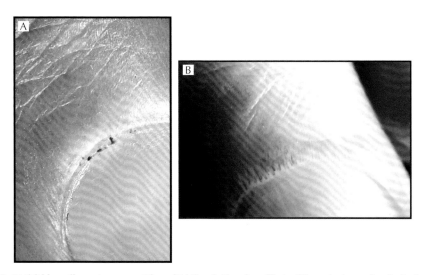

Figure 2–8. Nail fold capillary microscopy: Thrombi (A) and dilated capillaries (B) can be imaged at the bedside with the 20-diopter lens of an ophthalmoscope (using an immersion oil to prevent back-reflection).

(chapter 4, Figure 4–8) or congenital (chapter 4, Figure 4–10) myotonic dystrophy is typical and important to recognize, the narrow atrophic or "hatchet" face may be present when other manifestations of the disease are minimal or absent. A somewhat similar facial appearance, however, can occur in centronuclear (myotubular) myopathy and nemaline (rod) myopathy. In contrast, in myotonia congenita (chapter 9, Figure 9–12) or paramyotonia congenita, muscle contraction and possibly masseter muscle hypertrophy produce an abnormal appearance that is particularly apparent during cold exposure. Facial weakness in facioscapulohumeral muscular dystrophy produces a glum appearance (chapter 4, Figure 4–11), in which the sclera is frequently visible during gentle lid closure, although the sclera may also be exposed in other disorders with facial weakness.

Ptosis produces a characteristic facial appearance especially if accompanied by frontalis muscle contracture and redundancy of the upper eyelids. Ptosis is usually present in oculopharyngeal muscular dystrophy (chapter 4, Figure 4–14), Kearns-Sayre syndrome, and familial progressive ophthalmoplegia. Patients with myasthenia gravis may present a similar appearance but typically they also display lower facial weakness that produces a "snarling" appearance. Efforts to smile accentuate the effect because the initial normal upturn of the corners of the mouth is followed rapidly by a downturn as facial muscles fatigue.

THE TONGUE

Inspecting lingual muscles for atrophy and fasciculations is important. Normal variations that may be confusing include the scrotal or geographic tongue, as well as prominent rugations or deep clefts that can be confused with atrophy. Also, tremblings in a normal, incompletely relaxed tongue often resemble fasciculations. Nevertheless, tongue atrophy is easily detected in patients with ALS and other motor neuron diseases. A distinctive, triple-furrowed tongue can also be a useful sign of tongue muscle atrophy and is found in severe myasthenia gravis and in myotonic dystrophy. Enlargement of the tongue is frequent in late stages of Duchenne dystrophy and occasionally occurs in acid maltase deficiency. It is also noted occasionally in myopathies of systemic illness such as amyloidosis, hypothyroidism, and acromegaly.

GAIT

Walking reveals weakness of hip-stabilizing and trunk musculature. Compensation for truncal weakness results in a lordotic posture. A waddling gait is caused by an inability to prevent hip drop or hip dip as the leg swings through. When quadriceps weakness is severe, the patient keeps the leg fully extended to prevent the knee from buckling. This maneuver becomes obvious when the patient demonstrates "back kneeing" or a genu recurvatum. Quadriceps weakness is also associated with "toe walking," which permits the stabilizing action of the gastrocnemius muscle. This muscle can act to extend the knee while producing plantar flexion. This "toe walking" is accompanied by shortening of the Achilles tendon. Some muscle conditions such as myotonic dystrophy, distal myopathy, or facioscapulohumeral dystrophy, all of which can cause early foot drop, result in a steppage gait identical to that observed in peripheral neuropathies. If severe proximal and distal weakness coexist, the patient takes short, circumducting steps with the knee held in an extended (locked) position to prevent catching the toes on the floor.

The position of the hands during gait testing is often indicative of proximal weakness (chapter 4, Figure 4–5) Weakness of shoulder girdle muscles results in the dorsum of the hands facing forward.

REFLEXES

Muscle stretch reflexes may be preserved in myopathies until there is profound loss of strength (see Box 2.1). Myotonic dystrophy, especially DM1, is an exception. These patients are hyporeflexic or areflexic when muscles are still relatively strong, raising the possibility of an associated neural component. Patients with congenital myotonic dystrophy may have a spastic diplegia due to central nervous system disease (see chapter 4).

DIFFERENTIAL DIAGNOSIS

The myopathies have a relatively small number of distinct clinical presentations, each of which has a defined list of likely diagnoses. The following sections describe these presentations and indicate clinical features useful in establishing that a patient has, in fact, a primary muscle disease.

Disorders Presenting at Birth With Hypotonia

Although all neuromuscular causes combined account for far fewer floppy infants than do central nervous system causes, spinal muscular atrophy, congenital myopathies, congenital muscular dystrophy, congenital myasthenia gravis, and rare forms of peripheral neuropathies must all be considered (Box 2.6). As a rule, myopathy and other neuromuscular diseases are suggested if the patient appears alert but has hypoactive or absent tendon reflexes. Skeletal abnormalities such as pes cavus, high-arched palate, pectus excavatum, and joint contractures also suggest a neuromuscular basis for hypotonia. Rarely, superimposed anoxic brain damage in a patient with a myopathy that produces respiratory failure may cause hyperreflexia.

Disorders Presenting in Infancy

Spinal muscular atrophy (Werdnig-Hoffman disease) is the most common neuromuscular disease presenting in infancy. It varies in severity and may start prior to birth or at any time in the first months of life. The cases with earliest onset are the most severe and usually culminate in respiratory failure. Fasciculations of the tongue and limb muscles help establish the diagnosis, although limb fasciculations may be obscured by overlying adipose tissue. Spinal muscular atrophy is not treatable and does not improve.

Some conditions presenting in infancy that either remit spontaneously or improve

---

Box 2.6 Disorders Presenting at Birth with Hypotonia (The Floppy Infant)

Central Hypotonia (most common cause of hypotonia at birth)[a,b]

Myopathies

Congenital myotonic dystrophy[a]
Centronuclear (myotubular) myopathy[a]
Muscular dystrophies-congenital
Congenital fiber-type disproportion[a]
Central core disease
Nemaline (rod) myopathy
Glycogen storage diseases (acid maltase and phosphorylase deficiencies)
Lipid storage diseases (carnitine deficiency)

Other Neuromuscular Diseases

Spinal muscular atrophy (Werdnig-Hoffman disease)
Congenital and infantile myasthenia gravis
Congenital amyelinating and hypomyelinating neuropathies
Hereditary motor and sensory neuropathies

Arthropathies

[a]Frequently present with respiratory difficulties. [b]Central nervous system disorders of many types.

with treatment include infantile botulism, congenital myotonic dystrophy, cytochrome oxidase deficiency, congenital myasthenias, or infantile myasthenia gravis. Rare forms of acquired, treatable, inflammatory demyelinating neuropathies in infancy have also been reported.[18]

Disorders Presenting in Childhood With Progressive Proximal Weakness

Duchenne dystrophy is the commonest cause of progressive weakness in boys. In girls, spinal muscular atrophy, a limb-girdle dystrophy,

and dermatomyositis are the most commonly encountered (Box 2.7). Spinal muscular atrophy is distinguishable from a myopathy by the presence of tremor, minipolymyoclonus, or fasciculations.

Disorders Presenting in Adulthood

PROGRESSIVE PROXIMAL WEAKNESS

Acute weakness that evolves over a matter of hours is rarely a myopathy; much more frequently, it results from neuromuscular junction or peripheral nerve disease (Box 2.8). The major exception is the muscle dysfunction

---

Box 2.7 Neuromuscular Diseases Presenting as Progressive Weakness in Childhood

Myopathies

Muscular dystrophy: Duchenne, Becker, Emery-Dreifuss, facioscapulohumeral, limb-girdle, congenital
Inflammatory myopathies: dermatomyositis, polymyositis, inclusion body myositis[a]
Lipid storage myopathy: carnitine deficiency
Glycogen-storage disease
Acid maltase deficiency
Endocrine-metabolic disorders: hypokalemia, hypocalcemia, hypercalcemia
Central core disease
Nemaline myopathy
Centronuclear myopathy
Mitochondial myopathies

Spinal Muscular Atrophy

Kugelberg-Welander disease

Neuromuscular Junction Disorder

Botulism
Myasthenia gravis
Lambert-Eaton syndrome[a]

Neuropathy

Chronic inflammatory demyelinating polyneuropathy
Hereditary motor and sensory neuropathies

[a]Rarely presents in childhood.

Box 2.8 Neuromuscular Diseases Causing Rapidly Progressive Weakness

Myopathies

Inflammatory
Idiopathic: polymyositis, dermatomyositis; paroxysmal rhabdomyolysis
Toxic: colchicine, cholesterol lowering agents (CLAM)
Viral: influenza, Coxsackie B
Parasitic: trichinosis
Protozoal: toxoplasmosis
Metabolic: glycogen and lipid disorders, especially carnitine palmitoyltransferase deficiency
Endocrinopathies: hyperthyroidism, corticosteroid related
Electrolyte imbalance: hypokalemia and hyperkalemia, hypocalcemia and hypercalcemia, hypophosphatemia, hypermagnesemia
Periodic paralysis

Neuromuscular Junction

Myasthenia gravis
Congenital myasthenias
Lambert-Eaton syndrome
Botulism
Hypermagnesemia

Neuropathy

Guillian-Barré syndrome
Porphyria
Diphtheria
Proximal diabetic neuropathy

Anterior Horn Cell

Poliomyelitis
West Nile virus
Rabies
Amyotrophic lateral sclerosis (rarely progresses rapidly)

Radiculopathy

Cytomegalovirus polyradiculopathy

produced by electrolyte or metabolic derangements (chapter 11). Myopathy produced by infectious and inflammatory diseases often causes acute muscle pain, resulting in apparent weakness. Slowly progressive proximal weakness in adults is usually due to myopathy (Box 2.9). This fact leads to the erroneous, circular argument that all proximal weakness results from myopathy, as opposed to other forms of neuromuscular disease. This, of course, is not true, and it is misleading to describe proximal weakness using the term *proximal myopathy.* Neurogenic disease can cause proximal weakness; of the slowly

Box 2.9 Causes of Slowly Progressive Proximal Weakness in Adulthood

Myopathies

> Muscular dystrophies: limb-girdle, facioscapulohumeral, Becker, Emery-Dreifuss, myotonic dystrophy (DM2 > DM1)
> Inflammatory: polymyositis, dermatomyositis, inclusion body myositis, viral (HIV)
> Metabolic: acid-maltase deficiency, lipid storage, mitochondrial
> Endocrine: thyroid, parathyroid, adrenal, pituitary disorders
> Toxic: alcohol, corticosteroids, local injections of narcotics; colchicine, chloroquine

Neuromuscular Junction

> Myasthenia gravis
> Congenital myasthenic syndromes
> Lambert-Eaton syndrome

Neuropathy

> Chronic inflammatory demyelinating polyradiculoneuropathy
> Proximal diabetic neuropathy

Anterior Horn Cell

> Spinal muscular atrophy

Amyotrophic lateral sclerosis

progressive neuropathies, chronic inflammatory demyelinating polyneuropathy is the best example. Hyporeflexia and sensory involvement usually distinguish this disorder from myopathies. Patients with generalized myasthenia gravis also have proximal weakness, but fatigue is conspicuous, and most also have involvement of ocular and bulbar muscles. The less common myasthenic syndrome (Lambert-Eaton), frequently characterized by fatigue and autonomic symptoms as well as proximal weakness, is often mistakenly diagnosed as a myopathy. The anterior horn cell disorders, ALS and spinal muscular atrophy, may present with proximal weakness, although the weakness in ALS is often asymmetric. The presence of fasciculations and, for ALS, hyperreflexia (as well as other signs of upper motor-neuron involvement) help to distinguish these conditions from myopathy.

PROGRESSIVE DISTAL WEAKNESS

Distal weakness (Box 2.10) is usually caused by peripheral neuropathy or anterior horn cell disease. The most common myopathy presenting with distal weakness is myotonic dystrophy. More rare causes of distal muscle weakness due to primary muscle disease include inclusion body myositis, Distal myopathies, scapuloperoneal and facioscapulohumeral dystrophies, centronuclear (myotubular) myopathy, and nemaline myopathy. Selective bilateral weakness of the gastrocnemius and soleus muscles strongly suggests the autosomal-recessive, distal myopathy of Miyoshi (chapter 4). In this condition, and in some other causes of distal myopathic weakness (such as scapuloperoneal dystrophy), the EDB muscle is hypertrophied (chapter 4, Figure 4–20), a sign seldom seen in neurogenic disease. Virtually none of

---

Box 2.10 Causes of Progressive Distal Weakness in Adulthood

Myopathies

> Myotonic dystrophy (DM1 >> DM2)
> Distal myopathies (many)
> Facioscapulohumeral dystrophy
> Inclusion body myositis
> Nemaline myopathy
> Centronuclear myopathy

Metabolic Disorders

> Debrancher deficiency
> Phosphorylase b kinase deficiency
> Lipid storage myopathy (usually proximal)

Anterior Horn Cell

> Spinal muscular atrophy
> Amyotrophic lateral sclerosis

---

the myopathies associated with systemic disease (chapter 11) present primarily with distal weakness.

PROGRESSIVE OCULAR MUSCLE OR BULBAR WEAKNESS

The reasons for the remarkable sparing of ocular muscles in most myopathies remain a mystery. On the other hand, certain muscle disorders primarily affect the ocular muscles (Box 2.11). Ptosis alone is seen in myotonic dystrophy, whereas ptosis plus extraocular muscle involvement occurs in mitochondrial myopathies, oculopharyngeal muscular dystrophy, and centronuclear myopathy. Because their dysconjugate gaze is long-standing, these patients seldom complain of double vision (although it may be present on direct questioning). Double vision is a frequent complaint of those with recent-onset myasthenia gravis and other neuromuscular junction disorders.

The extraocular muscles are seldom weak in most peripheral neuropathies or in ALS. The reason they are spared is unknown, although it may be partially explained in peripheral neuropathy by the relatively short length of the axons that innervate them. The sparing of the eye muscles in motor neuron disease is accounted for less easily; weakness of extraocular muscles may develop in patients with motor neuron disease who live for many years with chronic ventilator support.

Bulbar weakness, including difficulty swallowing, coughing, and speaking, is unusual in most myopathies but does occur in inclusion body myositis, polymyositis, and dermatomyositis and is prominent in oculopharyngeal dystrophy and myotonic dystrophy. Bulbar weakness may be seen in certain other myopathies but is more characteristic of neuromuscular junction and motor neuron disorders (Box 2.12).

OTHER PRESENTATIONS OF MYOPATHIES

Myopathies may also present with episodic weakness, myoglobinuria, muscle pain, or myotonia. Unexplained respiratory failure is the first sign of several myopathies (see chapter 13).

Box 2.11 Neuromuscular Diseases Causing Progressive Ocular Muscle Weakness

Myopathies

Progressive external ophtalmoplegia with ragged red fibers, Kearns-Sayre syndrome, other mitochondrial myopathies
Oculopharyngeal muscular dystrophy
Oculopharyngealdistal dystrophy
Myotonic dystrophy (uncommonly)
Centronuclear (myotubular) myopathy
Hyperthyroidism

Neuromuscular Junction

Myasthenia gravis
Lambert-Eaton syndrome (uncommon presentation)
Congenital myasthenias
Infantile botulism

Box 2.12 Neuromuscular Diseases Causing Progressive Bulbar Weakness

Myopathies

Oculopharyngeal muscular dystrophy
Oculopharyngoaldistal dystrophy
Myotonic dystrophy
Inflammatory myopathy
Polymyositis
Dermatomyositis
Inclusion body myositis
Mitochondrial syndromes
Hyperthyroidism (rare)

Neuromuscular Junction

Myasthenia gravis
Congenital myasthenias
Lambert-Eaton syndrome

Peripheral Neuropathies

Chronic inflammatory demyelinating polyneuropathy (rare)
Diphtheritic polyneuropathy

(continued)

Anterior Horn Cell

Amyotrophic lateral sclerosis
Progressive bulbar or pseudobulbar palsyX-linked bulbospinal muscular atrophy (Kennedy syndrome)

LABORATORY EVALUATION

Blood Studies

CREATINE KINASE

The serum creatine kinase (CK), previously termed *creatine phosphokinase*, is the single most useful blood enzyme study for the evaluation of patients with neuromuscular disease. CK catalyzes the reversible reaction of adenosine-5'-triphosphate (ATP) and creatine to form adenosine diphosphate (ADP) and phosphocreatine. It is elevated in the majority of patients with myopathies but may be normal in slowly progressive muscle disorders. In progressive disorders such as Duchenne dystrophy the CK falls toward normal late in the course, as muscle mass diminishes. The CK level may be helpful in distinguishing different forms of muscular dystrophy. For example, the ambulatory patient with Duchenne muscular dystrophy invariably has a CK value at least 10 times (and often up to 100 times) normal, whereas in most other myopathies, such as limb-girdle muscular dystrophy, there are lesser elevations (chapter 4).

Many times the CK will rise modestly (usually to less than 10 times normal) in neuromuscular diseases of neuropathic cause. Examples include the spinal muscular atrophies and ALS. The elevation probably reflects damage to muscle fibers that are injured by the increased demands placed on weak muscles.

Elevations in CK can occur with minor muscle trauma, viral illnesses, or strenuous exercise and on a hereditary basis.[19] The CK is higher in Black individuals (Box 2.13). *In a patient without muscle weakness or pain it is unusual for a slightly (threefold or less) elevated CK to be caused by an unsuspected* or *developing myopathy.* The most common cause of abnormally high CK blood levels (hyperCKemia) in asymptomatic persons is recent exercise or injury. We repeat the CK determination after 5 days of rest without vigorous exercise, and pursue further evaluation only if the CK elevation

---

Box 2.13 Causes of Sustained Elevations of Creatine Kinase without Clinical Neuromuscular Disease

Exercise (acute or chronic)

Black race
Enlarged muscles (weight lifters)
Muscle trauma: frequent falls, injections, EMG needles
Active psychosis or delirium
Drug use: alcohol, narcotics, and others
Endocrine disorders: hypothyroidism, hypoparathyroidism
Presymptomatic myopathies: muscular dystrophy (all forms), polymyositis, McArdle's disease
Carrier state: Duchenne and Becker dystrophies
Malignant hyperthermia
Hereditary hyperCKemia

persists. If the CK elevation is less than two to three times normal, evaluation is frequently unrewarding, but if the level is increased more than fivefold, subjects often prove to have an underlying myopathy that has not yet emerged clinically.

CK occurs as three isozymes: MM, the principal form in cardiac and skeletal muscle; MB, occurring in a higher proportion than normal in regenerating cardiac and skeletal muscle; and BB, occurring predominantly in the brain. The relatively higher amount of CK-MB in diseased heart muscle once led to the hope that one might recognize coexisting cardiac disease within the myopathies by an elevation of CK-MB, but elevated CK-MB is found within the skeletal muscle—and consequently in the serum—of patients with active myopathy or even with chronic strenuous exercise,[20] so that it is an unreliable indicator.

The CK level may not be elevated in some myopathies or may even be *lowered* by a number of factors, as indicated in Box 2.14. Occasionally, benign elevations of CK appear on a genetic basis.[21]

Serum tests for other muscle enzymes are considerably less valuable than determining the level of CK. The aspartate aminotransferase and lactate dehydrogenase levels, although less markedly elevated than CK, are often obtained more routinely, and if found to be elevated, may provide an early clue to possible myopathy. Similarly, alanine aminotransferase and aldolase levels may be slightly elevated. All four of these other enzymes, however, are present in liver and other tissues at levels equal to or greater than those in muscle and consequently have little or no value in the evaluation and follow-up of patients with neuromuscular disease. Gamma-glutamyl transferase (GGT), which is found at low levels or is absent in normal muscle, is usually normal in patients with neuromuscular disease. Because GGT is elevated in patients with hepatocellular disease, its determination can be helpful in evaluating the patient with an elevated CK for the presence of coincidental liver disease, although GGT is elevated in patients with myotonic dystrophy who show no clinical or other laboratory evidence of liver disease.[22]

SERUM CREATININE

Patients with severe muscle wasting from any cause, including myopathy, have serum creatinine values below normal. Levels of 0.1 to 0.4 mg/100 ml (normal = 0.8–1.2 mg/100 ml) are frequent and can lead to an underestimation of the severity of coincidental renal disease. Occasionally, depressed serum creatinine values provide a clue that muscle wasting is more profound and long-standing than the clinical findings suggest.

OTHER BLOOD STUDIES

Abnormal serum potassium or calcium levels should prompt consideration of a related endocrinopathy or malignancy or of an acquired metabolic disorder (see chapter 11).

Box 2.14 Causes of Normal Creatine Kinase Level in the Presence of Active Myopathy

Profound muscle wasting

Corticosteroid administration[a]
Hereditary factors[a]
Collagen diseases[a]
Alcoholism[a]
Hyperthyroidism[a]

[a]It is likely that muscle wasting is the cause of lowered CK in each of the conditions listed.

Complications of myopathies may occasionally cause alterations in the results of routine blood studies. For instance, respiratory insufficiency may lead to hypoxia and hypercapnia, which in turn cause an elevated hematocrit and serum bicarbonate level.

Urine Studies

Serum and urine may contain myoglobin as an accompaniment to muscle breakdown, particularly in metabolic disorders of muscle (chapter 6). When large quantities are excreted, urine tests for blood are positive. Smaller increases in serum or urine myoglobin may be detected in slowly progressive muscle diseases and even in the carrier state for disorders such as Duchenne dystrophy.

Measurement of the 24-hour urinary creatinine excretion provides a convenient estimate of skeletal muscle mass.[23] Precise and accurate measurements of creatinine excretion depend on consuming a diet free of animal flesh prior to and during the period of urine collection and on a careful 24-hour urine collection.[23] Creatine, the precursor of creatinine, is made by the kidney and other organs and then taken up by muscle, where it is used to synthesize creatine phosphate. Creatine phosphate and creatine are in turn broken down to creatinine, which is then excreted in the urine. Creatine excretion depends even more than does creatinine on dietary intake of meats and is of little value in the clinical setting.[23] Only when a patient receives a meat-free diet for three days prior to and during an inpatient evaluation can one make reliable measurements of creatinine and creatine excretion. For this reason dual-energy X-ray absorptiometry (DEXA scanning) has become a more standard way of assessing muscle mass in longitudinal studies.[24]

Muscle Imaging Procedures

Roentgenography of muscle can define mass lesions in muscle and identify calcium, fat, and tumors but is of no value for diagnosis of myopathies. Similarly, ultrasound and computed tomography are of limited value. Magnetic resonance imaging has become valuable in both diagnosis and serial study of muscle diseases. The diagnostic use of MRI depend on the identification of distinctive patterns of muscle involvement: atrophy, inflammation, replacement with fat or connective tissue, and water content. The major limitations of MRI include its high cost; the difficulty of performing MRI in children or other subjects unable to maintain a position during imaging; and limitations posed by implanted ferromagnetic materials. The rapidly declining cost of molecular genetic testing makes it likely that such testing will preempt MRI (and most other diagnostic methods) for diagnosis. Serial imaging of muscle, where great attention is paid to standardization of technique, holds great promise for the quantitative assessment of treatment benefit.[25]

DEMONSTRATING PATTERNS OF MUSCLE INVOLVEMENT

MRI can extend the sensitivity of the clinical examination by objective evidence of selective, specific involvement of particular muscles that characterize a myopathy.[26,32] Thus, in facioscapulohumeral muscular dystrophy both the distribution of the weakness as well as its asymmetry can be visualized. Similarly in Emery-Dreifuss muscular dystrophy there is selective thigh muscle involvement (vastus) with sparing of the rectus femoris. Such selective involvement is difficult to detect clinically (Figure 2–9). In the distal myopathies, Finnish investigators have carefully categorized MRI

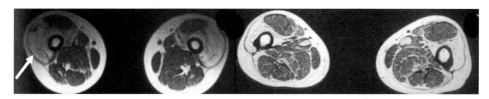

Figure 2–9. Transverse T_1-weighted images through thigh muscles in two patients with autosomal-dominant Emery-Dreifuss muscular dystrophy with *LMNA* gene mutations. Note the striking selective involvement of the vastus muscles with sparing of the rectus femoris that shows remarkable hypertrophy.

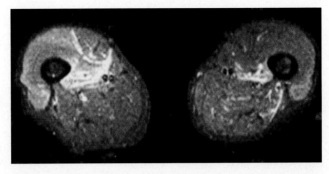

Figure 2–10. Short T_1 inversion recovery MRI image of upper leg of adult patient with dermatomyositis showing hyperintensity of the vastus medialis muscles, predominantly on the right.

abnormalities that permit prediction of genotype[27,28] (Figures 2–9 and 2–10). Similar helpful distinctions can be made among the congenital myopathies and muscular dystrophies.[29]

DETECTING MUSCLE INFLAMMATION, REPLACEMENT, AND OTHER PATHOLOGY

Keeping in mind the axiom that "neuroradiologists are not neuropathologists," it is nonetheless possible to detect helpful changes that distinguish inflammatory from noninflammatory myopathies (Figure 2–11).[30] Similarly the distinctive MRI indications of fatty infiltration

of muscle can point to preclinical evidence of disease in dysferlinopathy and to specific diagnosis in both sporadic and hereditary inclusion body myositis/myopathy.[31]

QUANTIFICATION OF MUSCLE MASS

The search for biomarkers that can be used for the early detection of response to treatment have prompted longitudinal studies of MRI undermining the precision of MRI measurements as well as the longitudinal progression. Both Duchenne muscular dystrophy[9] and inclusion body myositis[1,2] have been studied.

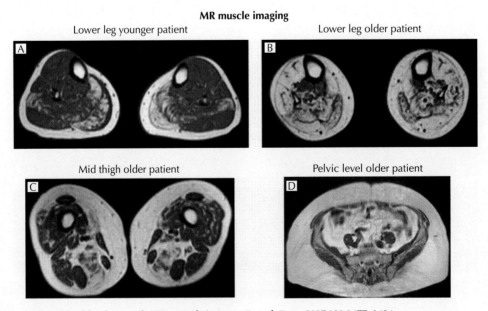

Figure 2–11. MRI of distal myopathy (Zaspopathy). Griggs R et al. Brain 2007;130:1477–1484.

ELECTRODIAGNOSIS

In general the major value of electrodiagnostic testing is to shed further light on the pathophysiology of weakness and fatigability. Whether the weakness is of a neurogenic or myogenic origin or is due to a defect in neuromuscular transmission, or is the result of an upper motor-neuron lesion can be clarified by needle electromyography and nerve stimulation studies. The findings are generally not specific, however, and must always be used in the context of other clinical findings to arrive at a specific diagnosis. Here we focus on the electrodiagnostic findings of myopathies.

The Technique of Electromyography

A concentric or monopolar needle electrode is used to record electromyographic activity. Disposable concentric needle electrodes are reliable and are well tolerated by patients because they are very sharp and have no risk of transmitting infection to the patient. The electrical activity of the muscle is amplified and displayed for visual analysis on an oscilloscope. An auditory signal accompanies the visual record. The patient lies relaxed and is periodically asked to contract the muscle under study. The needle electrode is moved into numerous sites in each muscle. Muscle should be chosen based on clinical examination and distribution of weakness. In each muscle the electrical activity is evaluated in three steps:

1. with the muscle totally relaxed, to evaluate insertional activity and spontaneous activity;
2. while the patient voluntarily contracts the muscle slightly, to evaluate the characteristics of individual motor *unit potentials* (amplitude, duration, and phases); and
3. while the patient is asked to contract the muscle maximally, to evaluate *recruitment pattern*.

Abnormal Spontaneous Activity

Spontaneous activity arising from the endplate is associated with some discomfort for the patient. The shape and discharge frequency help to differentiate endplate spikes from fibrillations and positive sharp waves (PSWs). Normal spontaneous endplate activity (Figure 2–12) is initially negative (upgoing), often discharges profusely at high frequencies, and rapidly attenuates upon needle movement away from the endplate.

Fibrillations (Figure 2–13A) are spontaneous electrical discharges generated from muscle fibers. They are initially positive, very brief in duration (1–3 ms) and low in amplitude (less than 600 μV) *Fibrillations are easily recognized by their sound similar to "raindrops on a thin roof."*

PSWs (Figure 2–13B) exhibit a different shape with a marked initial positive deflection and gradual repolarization and slow hyperpolarization phases. PSWs have the same pathophysiologic significance as fibrillations and

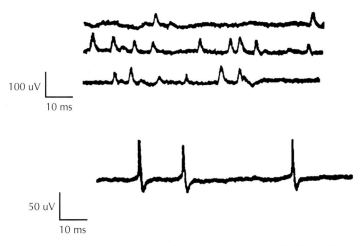

Figure 2–12. Two types of normal endplate activity, recorded with a concentric needle electrode: initially negative diphasic potentials (bottom) and negative spikes (top).

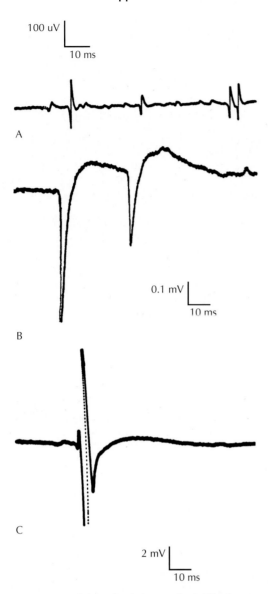

Figure 2–13. (A) Needle EMG recording of fibrillations. (B) Positive sharp waves. (C) Fasciculation.

represent the spontaneous discharge of an injured muscle fiber. Discharge patterns are similar to those of fibrillations.

Fibrillations and PSWs, although common in neurogenic disorders, are also present in virtually any muscle disease and indeed even in neuromuscular junction disorders (such as botulism). Their presence in a muscle disorder implies that the muscle fiber has been disconnected from its nerve supply. This can follow segmental necrosis when a part of the fiber

downstream from the necrotic area becomes isolated from the endplate region of the fiber. In general, fibrillations and PSWs are numerous in active disease and inconspicuous in disorders that are very slowly progressive or indolent. This point may be particularly useful in evaluating, for example, a patient with inflammatory myopathy, in whom the presence of profuse fibrillations and PSWs suggests active disease.

Fasciculation potentials (Figure 2–13C) represent the spontaneous discharge of one or more motor units and are most common in chronic neurogenic disorders. Fasciculations typically discharge singly, or slowly at a rate between one and five per second, and they are larger in amplitude and longer in duration than fibrillations. Fasciculations are the result of irritability of the neuronal cell body or axon. They may be benign, as in patients with benign fasciculations, or can be a sign of serious underlying neuronal disease, particularly motor neuron disease.

Complex repetitive discharges (CRDs) are particularly common in patients with inflammatory myopathy but may be found in many other chronic disorders. Both the onset and cessation are abrupt and the shape is usually complex and polyphasic, consisting of action potentials from groups of muscle fibers firing at high frequencies and in near synchrony (Figure 2–14A). The presence of large numbers of CRDs indicates active disease. CRDs should not be misinterpreted as myotonia.

Cramp potentials are the high-frequency discharge of many motor unit potentials and are usually associated with intense muscular pain. The electromyogram of a cramp shows a full recruitment pattern on the oscilloscope screen (Figure 2–14B). The cramp is usually abolished by muscle stretch, with abrupt cessation of motor unit discharges.

Myotonia (see chapter 9) occurs both with insertion or movement of the needle electrode and when muscle is percussed or voluntarily contracted. Myotonic discharges are high-frequency discharges of single muscle fibers, which wax and wane in both amplitude and frequency (Figure 2–14C). The discharges appear as either positive sharp waves or brief (< 5 ms) spikes and vary in frequency from 40 to 80 Hz. Myotonia is almost always a sign of primary muscle disease and appears in myotonic

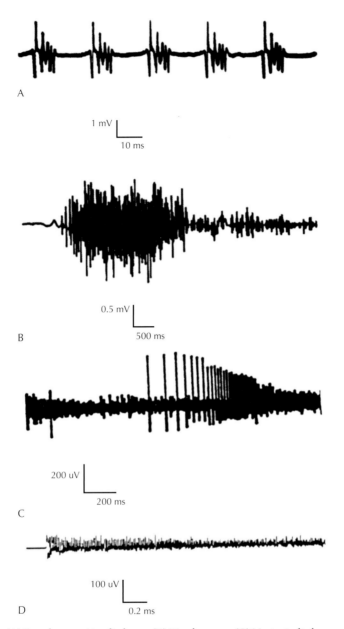

Figure 2–14. (A) Complex repetitive discharge. (B) Muscle cramp. (C) Myotonic discharges. (D) Neuromyotonia.

dystrophy type 1 and 2, the nondystrophic myotonias, acid maltase deficiency, and less frequently in myositis, toxic myopathies, and hypothyroidism. Myotonic discharges may be found in any of these conditions even without clinical evidence of myotonia.

Neuromyotonia appears in the clinical disorder of continuous muscle fiber activity (Isaac's syndrome; see chapter 9), where there is continuous muscle rippling and stiffness; neuromyotonia also occurs in tetany. Neuromyotonic discharges are single muscle fiber potentials that fire at rates of 150 to 300 Hz (Figure 2–14D); because of the very high rate of firing, these potentials often decrease in amplitude during the long, continuous runs of activity. The discharges are not affected by voluntary activity of the muscle.

Voluntary Activity

THE NORMAL MOTOR UNIT

The *motor unit potential (MUP)* is the sum of the action potentials of the individual muscle fibers in the activated motor unit that lie within the field of the recording electrode. Normally, no more than 10 to 30 fibers contribute to the shape of the MUP, and it is likely that only 3 to 8 fibers contribute to the high-amplitude, negative phase seen during a typical clinical EMG study (Figure 2–15, top). The configuration of a MUP may be monophasic, diphasic, triphasic, or polyphasic (four or more phases). The shape of the MUP in normal individuals is influenced by the person's age, the muscle being studied, and the type of electrode used.

Activation of motor units during weak voluntary muscle contraction permits the analysis of motor unit morphology: duration, amplitude, and number of phases, by visual inspection of the screen. In neurogenic weakness, MUPs are enlarged in amplitude and duration; chronic or very chronic disorders will have a decreased number of phases, while in more acute to subacute disorders the number of phases may be increased. (Figure 2–15, bottom); they can be identified by a louder sound on the auditory output (thunk). Short-duration MUPs are found in diseases with either anatomic or physiologic loss of muscle fibers from the motor unit territory or atrophy of individual muscle fibers (Figure 2–15, middle).

SHORT-DURATION MOTOR UNITS

In primary muscle disease, MUPs are brief in duration and reduced in amplitude. (These are termed "myopathic" potentials, with the caveat that follows.) All forms of muscular dystrophy, inflammatory myopathy, and congenital myopathy usually feature "myopathic" MUPs, but short-duration and low-amplitude MUPs also may occur in neuromuscular junction disorders (e.g., botulinin intoxication, the myasthenic Lambert-Eaton syndrome, and myasthenia gravis) and during early reinnervation after nerve injury. On the other hand, not all disorders of muscle have abnormal motor unit configuration; for example, the MUPs may be normal in both amplitude and duration in patients with disuse atrophy of muscle or thyrotoxic myopathy (chapter 11).

Polyphasic motor unit potentials (Figure 2–16A) have, by definition, five or more phases and can be seen in either myopathic or neurogenic disorders. The important difference is in the duration, which is short in polyphasic myopathic units, and prolonged in neurogenic/

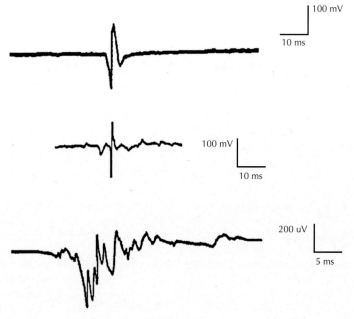

Figure 2–15. Top: Normal motor unit potential. Middle: Myopathic motor unit potential. Bottom: Neurogenic motor unit potential.

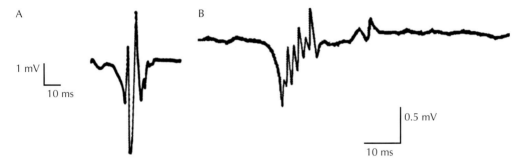

Figure 2–16. (A) Polyphasic motor unit potential. (B) Long-duration motor unit potential.

reinnervated polyphasic units and in nascent units (early reinnervation).

LONG-DURATION MOTOR UNITS

Long-duration motor units (Figure 2–16B) are frequently seen in patients with chronic myopathy as well as in chronic neurogenic disorders. Fiber splitting and reinnervation presumably lead to the increased duration of motor units in long-standing myopathy. Satellite potentials, small and delayed components of the motor unit that are frequently time-locked to its main component, may be very long in duration. These long-duration motor units occur in conditions such as chronic polymyositis, recurrent myoglobinuria, Emery-Dreifuss muscular dystrophy, and inclusion body myositis. Thus, electrodiagnostic findings of long-duration motor units make differentiation between a chronic, severe primary muscle disease and neuropathy sometimes difficult. This confusion is particularly characteristic of inclusion body myositis,

where long-duration motor units are accompanied by marked fibrillations, a reduced recruitment pattern in weak muscles, increased fiber density, and increased jitter.[23]

Quantitative Electromyography

Quantitative EMG measures the configurations of the MUP and the recruitment pattern.[33] The duration and peak-to-peak amplitude (Figure 2–17) of at least 20 different MUPs are usually obtained in seven to nine insertions and are measured at a gain of 0.1 mV/cm. Measurements are usually made with a concentric needle electrode while the patient gives a weak contraction. The mean duration is determined both for potentials of simple shape and for those exhibiting polyphasia. The incidence of polyphasic potentials is determined and compared with the 95% confidence limits for age-matched normal subjects. Abnormality is defined by a duration of MUPs differing from

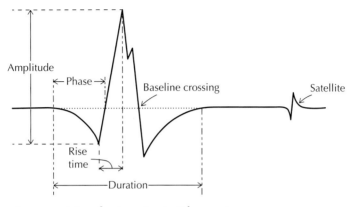

Figure 2–17. Schematic representation of motor unit potential parameters.

the normal mean by more than 20% or by an amplitude differing by more than 40%.[13] More than 12% polyphasia is abnormal. In addition, the pattern of recruitment is recorded at full effort using a continuous, direct-writing strip chart (Figure 2–18, top); the amplitude of the total electrical activity, termed "the envelope" (disregarding solitary high peaks), is measured. In subjects over 15 years old, values less than 2 mV suggest myopathy.

In patients with myopathy (Figure 2–18, middle), the average duration of the MUP is shortened by 20% to 60%, reflecting loss of fibers. In more advanced weakness, the shortening of the duration results from the loss of the slow initial component and the terminal component of the MUP because of the reduced fiber density in the periphery of the motor unit. Alterations in motor unit amplitude have less diagnostic significance because this measurement depends on the distance between the generator and the needle electrode. A reduced

amplitude may be seen as often in neuropathy as in myopathy.

The amplitude of the recruitment pattern developed at full effort parallels the changes in duration and amplitude of individual motor units and is reduced in muscular dystrophy and other myopathies. *In general, however, a full pattern of recruitment (MUPs filling the oscilloscope screen) in a weak muscle indicates early recruitment and strongly suggests myopathy* (see Figure 2–18, middle). In long-standing neurogenic weakness seen with a chronic neuropathy, the recruitment pattern is that of individual motor units even at maximum effort (Figure 2–18, bottom).

The electrodiagnostic evaluation of a patient with rapidly evolving muscle weakness is often difficult. When weakness is acute and severe and MUPs are obviously reduced in duration and amplitude with early recruitment, the diagnosis of myopathy is highly likely. In patients with less marked weakness, where the changes in MUP are more subtle, or in those with a more protracted illness and some long-duration motor units, the use of quantitative techniques is especially applicable. Although these techniques take more time, computer-assisted measurement of MUPs can now be used to facilitate their application.

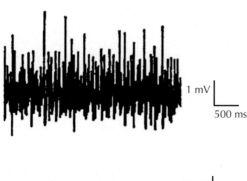

1 mV

500 ms

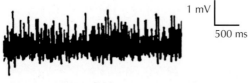

1 mV

500 ms

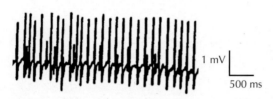

1 mV

500 ms

Figure 2–18. Maximum voluntary contraction of normal tibialis anterior (top), early recruitment in myopathy (middle), and reduced recruitment with high discharge frequencies in neuropathy (bottom).

Electrical Stimulation Tests: Nerve Conduction Studies

Because neurogenic disorders may produce weakness that mimics the clinical features of a muscle disease, ruling them out by evaluating motor and sensory nerve conduction is important. In particular, acquired demyelinating neuropathies such as the Guillain-Barré syndrome and chronic inflammatory demyelinating polyneuropathy may be mistaken for myopathies clinically, but will usually show slowing of nerve conduction velocity (Figure 2–19). In myopathies, on the other hand, nerve conduction studies are generally normal. These studies are also important in differentiating demyelinating from axonal neuropathies.

Factors that contribute to nerve conduction slowing in normal subjects include reduced limb temperature, age over 65 years or age less than 5 years, and submaximal stimulation.[36] Temperature is an extremely important

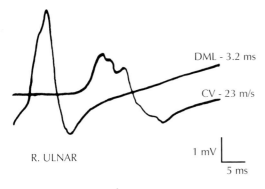

DML - 3.2 ms

CV - 23 m/s

R. ULNAR

1 mV

5 ms

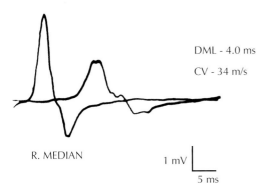

DML - 4.0 ms

CV - 34 m/s

R. MEDIAN

1 mV

5 ms

Figure 2–19. Motor nerve conduction studies in a patient with chronic inflammatory polyradiculoneuropathy, illustrating dispersion and slowing secondary to demyelination. DML = distal motor latency; CV—conduction velocity

factor that is commonly ignored. Reduced temperature of an extremity decreases nerve conduction velocity in normal nerves. In patients with cool limbs, especially those with arterial insufficiency or muscle wasting and loss of normal insulating tissue, velocity decreases 2.5 m/sec for each degree that skin temperature falls below 34° C.[36] Age-related changes must be considered in infants and elderly patients.

MOTOR NERVE CONDUCTION

Technique of Testing

Stimulating electrodes are either handheld or securely taped on clean skin over the nerve at the point of stimulation. An electrical stimulus is applied to the nerve at an intensity approximately 25% greater than that required to produce a maximum response of the muscle. The compound muscle action potential (CMAP) is recorded, amplified, and displayed on a cathode ray oscilloscope (Figure 2–20). A stimulus artifact appears on the record at the moment of stimulation of the nerve; after several milliseconds, the action potential of the muscle begins. The delay between the stimulus and the muscle action potential is the time for impulse conduction from the point of stimulation of the nerve, including time across the neuromuscular junction. The CMAP of the muscle is the summation of the potentials of all the muscle fibers that respond to nerve stimulation. The response is normally a biphasic potential with an initial negative (upgoing) phase. The latency of the muscle potential is measured from the onset of the stimulus artifact to the onset of the negative phase. A stimulus is then given more proximally along the course of the nerve. The difference in latency between the two points of nerve stimulation permits calculation of the conduction velocity of the most rapidly conducting nerve fibers in that segment (see Figure 2–20A–D). The amplitude of the CMAP, usually measured from baseline to negative peak, is expressed in millivolts. The size of the evoked muscle action potential is proportional to the number and size of responsive muscle fibers.

Changes in the amplitude of the CMAP can be followed over time to estimate the amount of functioning muscle tissue. Table 2–5 gives normal data for the most commonly studied peripheral nerves.

Abnormalities of Motor Nerve Conduction

There are two major categories of motor nerve conduction abnormalities:

1. Normal or slightly slowed conduction velocity with reduced CMAP amplitude, a pattern typical of axonal neuropathies but also seen in some severe myopathies.
2. Marked slowing of nerve conduction velocity (less than 70% of the lower limit of normal), often with a relatively normal CMAP amplitude in response to distal simulation but a small or desynchronized response to proximal stimulation. This finding suggests a primary demyelinating neuropathy. Reduced CMAP amplitude with normal conduction velocity may also reflect abnormal neuromuscular transmission (especially Lambert-Eaton syndrome or botulism) or

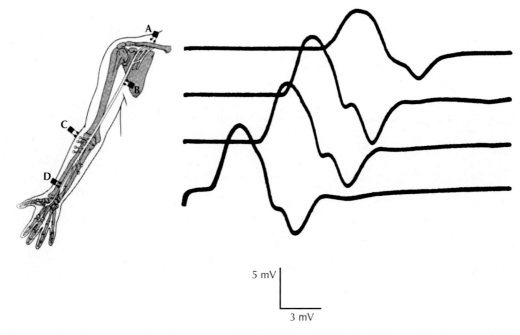

5 mV

3 mV

Figure 2–20. Evoked compound muscle action potentials (CMAPs) recorded over the abductor pollicis brevis muscle (left). The median nerve was stimulated at four different sites (A-D), producing similar CMAPs (right) after different latencies.

abnormal muscle membrane function, such as myotonic disorders or periodic paralysis. *These abnormalities are useful diagnostically but will be missed without careful attention to CMAP amplitude.* The technique and clinical relevance of this form of testing are discussed hereafter in "Repetitive Nerve Stimulation" and in chapter 9.

SENSORY NERVE CONDUCTION

Technique of Testing

The compound sensory nerve action potential (SNAP) is recorded with surface electrodes placed over the cutaneous sensory nerve or with needle electrodes placed subcutaneously near the nerve. A maximal stimulus is applied,

Table 2–5 Normal Values—Nerve Conduction Studies

MOTOR NERVES

	Amplitude[a]	Distal Latency[b]	Conduction Velocity[c]
Median	5	4.5	50
Ulnar	6	3.4	50
Peroneal	2	6.5	41
Tibial	4	7.0	41

SENSORY NERVES

	Amplitude[a]	Distal Latency[d]
Median	20	3.7
Ulnar	15	3.4
Sural	7	4.3

[a]Lower limit of normal amplitude of the evoked action potential measured from baseline to negative peak (motor, median nerve; sensory, ulnar nerve). [b]Upper limits of normal latency to onset of the evoked response (in ms) from stimulation at the second wrist crease or the ankle. [c]Lower limit of normal conduction velocity between elbow and wrist, or knee and ankle (in ms). [d]Upper limits of normal latency (in ms) to peak stimulation of digital nerves, recording at second wrist crease for median and ulnar sensory nerves. Stimulation at calf, 14 cm proximal to recording site at lateral malleolus for sural nerve.

which in normal individuals produces a low-amplitude (usually less than 50–60µV), triphasic response; an initial, small positive phase is followed by a much larger negative phase and another small positive phase. The shape of this potential results from the summation of the nerve action potentials of the large myelinated sensory nerve fibers. The sural nerve and cutaneous nerves such as the digital branches of the median and ulnar nerves are routinely studied (see Table 2–5). Sensory potentials can be recorded from the digital nerves using ring electrodes around the fingers. The potential is recorded over more proximal portions of the nerve (antidromic conduction), or they can be recorded over the mixed nerve with stimulation of the sensory fibers of the digital nerves (orthodromic conduction). The latency of the sensory response is measured from the stimulus artifact to either the onset of the response (from which a conduction velocity of the fastest fibers may be estimated) or, more frequently, to the peak of the negative phase.

Abnormalities of Sensory Nerve Conduction

Abnormalities include (1) a reduction in the amplitude of the sensory action potential, (2) a prolongation of duration, (3) a slowing of conduction velocity or prolonged distal latency, or (4) the absence of, or inability to record, the SNAP. An abnormality of the nerve action potential indicates neuropathy. The sensory action potential is normal in myopathies, diseases of the neuromuscular junction, abnormalities of the muscle membrane, diseases of the anterior horn cell, and (in sensory nerves) lesions proximal to the dorsal root ganglion. Virtually all of the conditions discussed in this book are associated with normal sensory nerve conduction studies.

Repetitive Nerve Stimulation

Repetitive nerve stimulation is valuable in the diagnosis of disorders of neuromuscular transmission, either presynaptic or postsynaptic. It is also helpful in evaluating disorders of the muscle membrane. In neuromuscular transmission disorders, muscle weakness is the result of failure of endplate potentials to reach the threshold necessary to trigger muscle action potentials. Muscle fibers then fail to contract, and patients experience both weakness and

fatigue. For the endplate potential to exceed the threshold and for depolarization to produce a muscle action potential, it is necessary to have (1) a sufficient release of acetylcholine from nerve terminals and (2) a normal number and sensitivity of postsynaptic acetylcholine receptors. Patients with an abnormality of either type will experience pathologic fatigue and weakness. Repetitive nerve stimulation at low rates in such patients usually produces a decrement >10% in the amplitude of the CMAP amplitude during the first few stimuli. The progressive decline in amplitude of the CMAP reflects the loss of individual muscle fiber action potentials that contribute to the larger potential at the start of repetitive stimulation. Different patterns of response are obtained in presynaptic and postsynaptic disorders, as well as in defects of muscle membrane excitation, as discussed in section on The Abnormalities.

Technique of Testing

The examiner selects preferably a weak muscle for recording the CMAP and applies a series of supramaximal stimuli (usually 5–10) to the motor nerve supplying that muscle, at a rate of 2 to 3 Hz. The muscles selected usually include the intrinsic hand muscles, trapezius, deltoid, biceps brachii, tibialis anterior, and facial muscles. Several technical factors must be considered to avoid false-positive and false-negative results. False negatives may result from cold temperature (warming to skin temperature of 37° C greatly increases test sensitivity) or ingestion of anticholinesterase medication, which should be avoided for 12 hours if it is safe to do so. False positives result from movement of electrodes, submaximal stimulation, or failure to immobilize the limb. A true decremental response is quite reproducible. High-frequency stimulation also may result in false-positive results. This type of stimulation, which is painful and produces artifactual movement, should rarely be necessary.

Abnormalities of Repetitive Nerve Stimulation

Myasthenia Gravis. Myasthenia gravis results from a reduced number of available acetylcholine receptors in the postsynaptic muscle membrane. Muscle fibers may fail to fire after either low or high rates of nerve discharge or electrical stimulation. In many patients, the first noted

CMAP is almost always normal, followed by a decrement (>10%) with either 2 or 3 Hz stimulation (compare Figures 2–21A & B). The decrement is usually maximal between the first and fourth responses, without much further decline by the fourth or fifth potential. Normal subjects show a transient slight (<20%) increase in the amplitude of the CMAP (facilitation) immediately following brief exercise (either voluntary or by involuntary tetanic contraction). This is thought to be related to increased mobilization of acetylcholine vesicles. In myasthenia gravis, facilitation immediately following exercise often results in an increase of as much as 40% in the amplitude of the first response compared with that obtained at rest. This increase is accompanied by a lessening of the decrement observed prior to exercise (repair). A few minutes after exercise, the amplitude of the first potential declines, and the decremental response compared with the pre-exercise response increases. This postactivation exhaustion reflects a reduced output of acetylcholine from the nerve terminal after a period of titanic muscle contraction. In normal individuals the reduced acetylcholine

output will have little effect because of the abundance of acetylcholine receptors on each muscle fiber. In myasthenia gravis, however, the reduction in the number of acetylcholine receptors diminishes the safety factor.

Single-fiber electromyography (SFEMG) is a highly sensitive means of detecting neuromuscular transmission dysfunction in patients with excessive fatigue.[34] If repetitive nerve stimulation studies are negative (which occurs in 30% of patients with generalized myasthenia gravis), SFEMG is very useful. The variability of discharge between two muscle fibers in the same motor unit (jitter; Figure 2–22) provides a quantitative measure of abnormal neuromuscular transmission. The main disadvantage of the technique is that it may be abnormal in many neuromuscular diseases; however, a normal finding in a patient with limb fatigue casts strong doubt on the diagnosis of myasthenia.

Lambert-Eaton Myasthenic Syndrome and Other Presynaptic Abnormalities. In contrast to myasthenia gravis, the CMAP in the

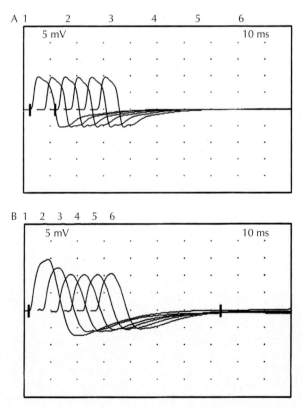

Figure 2–21. (A) Normal response to repetitive stimuli (3 Hz). (B) Decremental response to repetitive stimuli (3 Hz) in myasthenia gravis.

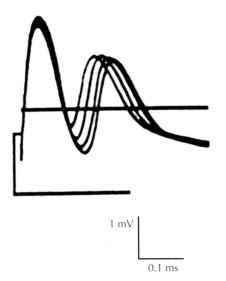

1 mV

0.1 ms

Figure 2–22. Single-fiber EMG recording of two muscle fiber action potentials. The variability of the second fiber with respect to the first is the basis for calculating jitter.

pronounced enhancement of postactivation facilitation (compare Figures 2–23A & B).

The Lambert-Eaton myasthenic syndrome caused by decreased Ca influx in the nerve terminal, resulting in inadequate release of acetylcholine. Other disorders that impair function of the nerve terminal are listed in Box 2.15. Pronounced facilitation of the CMAP and improved strength are produced in all of these conditions in response to high rates of repetitive nerve stimulation or a strong voluntary contraction. The high firing frequencies lead to an increased concentration of calcium in the region of the nerve terminal, and this in turn stimulates a greater but short lasting release of quanta of acetylcholine. In most of these conditions, there is also a decremental response to 2 or 3 Hz stimulation, which may be more conspicuous after exercise-induced postactivation facilitation.

MUSCLE BIOPSY

Indications for Biopsy

Lambert-Eaton myasthenic syndrome is markedly reduced in amplitude. Immediately following brief 10 second exercise (or tetanic nerve stimulation), however, the CMAP amplitude increases by 100% or more because of

If the clinical features and the laboratory and EMG results suggest muscle disease, and the clinical evaluation does not lead to specific

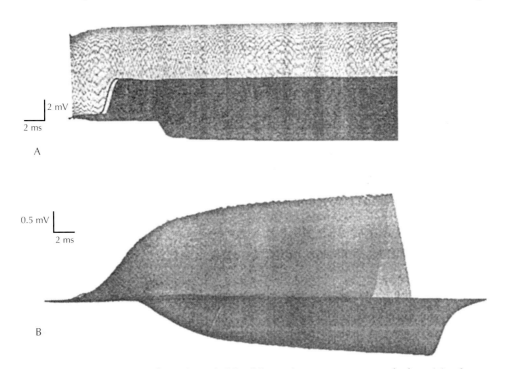

2 mV

2 ms

A

0.5 mV

2 ms

B

Figure 2–23. Repetitive nerve stimulation (50 Hz) of the abductor digiti minimi in a normal subject (A) and in a patient with Lambert-Eaton syndrome (B).

Box 2.15 Presynaptic Neuromuscular Junction Disorders

Botulism

Lambert-Eaton Syndrome

Black widow spider bite

Metabolic disturbances

> Hypermagnesemia
> Hypocalcemia

Medication

> Aminoglycoside antibiotics
> Streptomycin
> Neomycin
> Gentamicin
> Tobramycin
> Amikacin
> Polymyxins
> Anticonvulsants
> Phenytoin
> Trimethadione
> Antiarrhythmics
> Quinidine
> Procainamide
> Lithium

---

molecular diagnostic studies, a muscle biopsy may be appropriate. On the other hand, if clinical and laboratory features indicate a neurogenic cause for weakness, the muscle biopsy is rarely diagnostic. A muscle biopsy cannot differentiate anterior horn cell from peripheral nerve disease or a demyelinating from an axonal neuropathy. These distinctions are usually made by electrophysiologic testing or possibly nerve biopsy.

Selection of Biopsy Sites

The choice of muscle on which to perform the biopsy must be carefully determined by the clinical features of each patient. For practical purposes, in the upper extremities the muscles of choice are either the deltoid or biceps muscles; in the lower extremities, the quadriceps (usually vastus lateralis) is preferable. Moderately affected muscles (MRC grade 4) are chosen over those severely involved (MRC grade 0–2) because of the possibility of obtaining samples too late in the course of the illness to demonstrate the distinguishing features of a specific disorder. It is important to avoid muscles that may be damaged by unrelated conditions. This is particularly true for sites of recent muscle trauma (including EMG needle studies), local injections, or known circulatory disturbances. A biopsy of certain muscle groups in which the tendon insertion extends throughout the muscle (so-called pinnate muscles, including the gastrocnemius) may give rise to confusion, because inadvertent sampling of a myotendinous junction causes difficulty in interpretation (see section on Histologic Features of Myopathy).

Tissue Removal and Preparation

NEEDLE BIOPSY

The indications for needle biopsy versus open muscle biopsy are not universally agreed on. Both have advocates, and to a great extent the experience of the clinician and the expertise of the laboratory processing the tissue will favor one technique over the other. Advantages of needle biopsy include the lack of a scar and the possibility of sampling from more than one muscle, as well as from multiple sites in a muscle, and performing serial biopsies if necessary. The disadvantages include a smaller and difficult-to-orient sample and a specimen less satisfactory for electron microscopy. A larger incision is needed for an open biopsy, but the overall discomfort is probably similar with both procedures. The size of a needle biopsy (100–300 mg of muscle) is suitable for most histologic and biochemical studies.

OPEN BIOPSY

Open biopsies permit the taking of larger specimens, which may be necessary for the biochemical study of muscles; a larger specimen also increases the likelihood of demonstrating focal disease such as vasculitis and decreases sampling errors. Open biopsies allow a sample of muscle to be fixed at the in situ length, either in a clamp or fastened to a stick, prior to plunging into fixative (buffered glutaraldehyde) for ultrastructural examination. Open biopsies generally yield samples about 8 to 10 mm in length and about 4 to 5 mm in cross-sectional diameter (cylindrical in shape).

The fresh tissue sample is mounted on a chuck, usually held in place by gum tragacanth, and plunged for at least 10 to 15 seconds into isopentane cooled to –160° C. For best tissue sampling, the frozen muscle should extend out of the gum tragacanth so that sections will not be surrounded by embedding media. Sections measuring 8 to 10 microns in thickness are used for a battery of histologic and histochemical stains, which permit most of the subcellular organelles and several of the enzyme systems to be systematically analyzed for specific abnormalities (Table 2–6).

Histologic Techniques

For general histology, hematoxylin and eosin (H&E) and a modified Gomori trichrome are most useful. The latter particularly allows visualization of mitochondria and the tubular system of muscle, which is highlighted by red staining. The ATPase stain done with preincubation at pH 9.4, 4.6, and 4.3 allows a thorough evaluation of histochemistry fiber types (see Figure 1–3). The NADH tetrazolium reductase (NADH-TR) highlights sarcoplasmic reticulum, T-tubules, and mitochondria. The mitochondria can be selectively stained with a succinic dehydrogenase (SDH) reaction or

Table 2–6 Battery of Stains and Histochemical Reactions

Stains and Histochemical Reactions	Usefulness
H&E, modified trichrome	General histology and cellular detail
ATPase (pH 9.4, 4.6, 4.3)	Muscle fiber types
Oxidative enzymes (NADH, SDH, cytochrome oxidase)[a]	Mitochondrial disorders (ragged red fibers); T-tubular aggregates[b] target fibers, central cores
Oil red O	Lipid storage disease
PAS (periodic acid-Schiff)	Glycogen storage disease
Acid phosphatase	Lysosomes
Congo red, crystal violet	Amyloidosis
Myophosphorylase	McArdle's disease
Phosphofructokinase (PFK)	PFK deficiency
Myoadenylate deaminase (MADD)	MADD deficiency
Immunohistologic techniques	Most molecular defects of membrane, dystroskeletal, contractile apparatus

[a]NADH = nicotinamide adenine dehydrogenase; SDH = succinic dehydrogenase. [b]T-tubular aggregates are stained by NADH but not SDH.

with cytochrome oxidase, a respiratory chain enzyme. Oil red O demonstrates neutral fat and is especially useful in lipid-storage myopathies. Glycogen content can be assessed by the periodic acid-Schiff (PAS) reaction. In patients with muscle fatigue and rhabdomyolysis syndromes, specific enzymes that can be assessed by histochemistry include myophosphorylase, phosphofructokinase, and myoadenylate deaminase.

ELECTRON MICROSCOPY

Electron microscopy is only necessary under very specific conditions. One form of inflammatory myopathy, inclusion body myositis, can be confirmed by ultrastructural examination (see chapter 10); mitochondrial myopathies (chapter 8); myofibrillar myopathies, and certain congenital myopathies (chapter 6) such as nemaline (rod) myopathy can be better characterized by electron microscopy. Usually the presence of tubular aggregates, which may be strongly suspected on the basis of histochemical profile of NADH-TR-positive and SDH-negative material in type 2 fibers, requires ultrastructural confirmation. Ultrastructural examination is not necessary in biopsy analysis for muscular dystrophy.

IMMUNE STAINING

The demonstration of immune deposits is particularly relevant in dermatomyositis, where immunoglobulin (especially IgM and IgG) and complement (C5 through C9, and membrane attack complex) are distinctive (chapter 10). Localization of antibody to the sarcolemmal membrane is now available for assessment of many muscular dystrophies (Figure 2–24).[35] Lymphocyte subclasses can be identified using mononuclear antibody staining (chapter 10).

Differentiating Neuropathy From Myopathy

HISTOLOGIC FEATURES OF NEUROPATHY

When muscle weakness is neurogenic, histologic changes are usually easy to recognize (Table 2–7). The most characteristic change is atrophy, resulting in the appearance of small *angular* fibers not selective for fiber types. Early in the disease, scattered atrophic fibers are present, which stain darkly with oxidative enzymes. Later, groups of angular fibers can be seen. In H&E and trichrome stains, the loss of myofibrils leaves behind clumps of pyknotic nuclei. In some denervating disorders, *target fibers*, which may be a sign of reinnervation, are present. Target fibers generally have a clear central or eccentric zone surrounded by a dense intermediate zone and a relatively normal periphery, giving the appearance of three zones (Figure 2–25). Not all target fibers exhibit the densely stained intermediate region, however. Target fibers are usually type 1 fibers. *Type grouping*, unequivocal evidence of reinnervation, is a loss of the usual mosaic pattern of fiber types, which is replaced by large groups

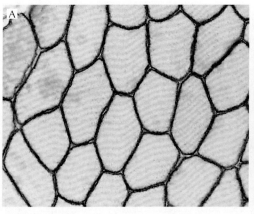
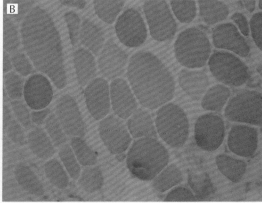

Figure 2–24. Immunofluorescent demonstration of dystrophin: control (A) and boy with Duchenne muscular dystrophy (B).

Table 2–7 **Muscle Biopsy Features Differentiating Myopathy from Neuropathy**

Features	Myopathy	Neuropathy
Muscle fiber size/shape	Variability in size (small to hypertrophied) or grouped round fibers	Small angular fibers; groups of small fibers
Nuclei	Increased internal nuclei	Atrophied fibers with nuclear clumps (pyknotic)
Necrosis/phagocytosis	Common	Rare
Inflammation	Variable	None
Connective tissue	Increased	Normal (unless end stage)
Fiber-type changes	Type predominance or preferential involvement in some diseases	Type grouping

(>40 in number) of homogeneous fiber types (Figure 2–26). Type grouping occurs because reinnervation converts the muscle-fiber types of a denervated motor unit to that of the adopting motor neuron.

In spinal muscular atrophy, where denervation occurs very early in life, the muscle biopsy appearance is distinctive: large groups of hypertrophied type 1 fibers are intermixed with fascicles of small type 1 and type 2 fibers. In these atrophic fascicles, the type 1 fibers are usually smaller than the type 2 fibers.

Type grouping must be distinguished from fiber *type predominance*. In most muscle biopsies, fiber types 1, 2A, and 2B are relatively equally represented, each comprising about one-third of the total. In type predominance, one type of fiber makes up more than 55%[18] (Figure 2–26). Although type predominance can be caused by reinnervation, some myopathies alter the ratio of fiber types: Type 1 fiber predominance appears in Duchenne and Becker muscular dystrophies and in congenital myopathies, including central core disease and nemaline (rod) myopathy.

HISTOLOGIC FEATURES OF MYOPATHY

Muscle has substantial regenerative capabilities. When the muscle fiber is injured, resting mononucleated muscle precursor cells, called satellite cells, are stimulated to proliferate and either fuse with the injured muscle fiber or fuse with one another to form *regenerating fibers*. These are typically basophilic in the H&E stain because of high RNA content. During regeneration, muscle fiber nuclei often assume a central or paracentral location. An increase to more than 3% internal nuclei is considered abnormal.

Fiber splitting (Figures 2–27 and 2–28) is prominent in chronic myopathies such as limb-girdle dystrophy. It is a normal occurrence at a myotendinous junction, since the muscle fiber splits as it inserts into the tendon; a section through this area must be interpreted with caution. Fiber splitting usually occurs in a previously injured area of the muscle fiber. *Ring fibers* are another change seen in chronic myopathy (Figures 2–29 and 2–30).

Connective tissue frequently proliferates when muscle fibers are lost. This endomysial connective tissue proliferation is especially prominent in disorders, such as Duchenne muscular dystrophy (Figure 2–30A). In chronic myopathies, irrespective of their cause, excess endomysial connective tissue typically is accompanied by increased variability in fiber size, internal nuclei, and fiber splitting (Figure 2–30B).

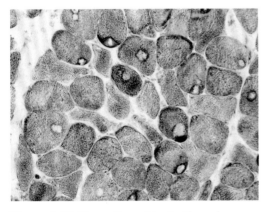

Figure 2–25. Target fibers. Muscle fibers show central light zone surrounded by a densely stained region (NADH-TR).

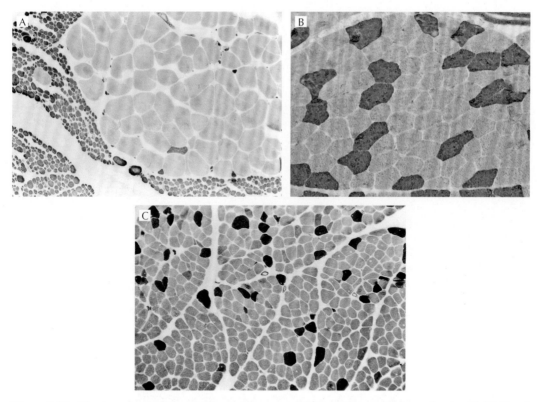

Figure 2–26. Fiber type abnormalities. (A) Fiber type-grouping. (B) Type 1 fiber predominance (moderate). (C) Type 1 fiber predominance (marked). ATPase reaction, pH 9.4 preincubation.

Cell infiltration or inflammation occurs in many conditions. When muscle fibers undergo necrosis, macrophages are recruited to the site of injury. In addition, mononuclear inflammatory cells participate in muscle fiber breakdown and can be seen invading muscle fibers prior to necrosis, especially in polymyositis (Figure 2–31). Using mononuclear antibodies, invading cells can be further subtyped. In the inflammatory myopathies, T cells, both helper (CD4) and cytotoxic/suppressor (CD8) participate in the process (chapter 10). Even

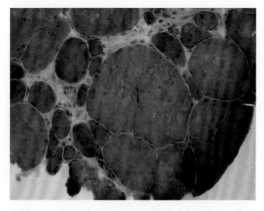

Figure 2–27. Chronic myopathy: Fiber splitting, Gomori trichrome.

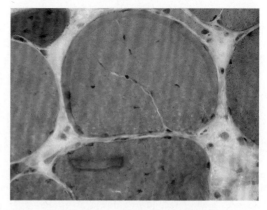

Figure 2–28. Chronic myopathpy: A split fiber, which is also a ring fiber. Gomori trichrome.

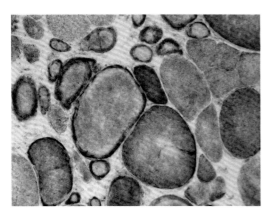

Figure 2–29. Chronic myopathy: Numerous ring fibers; marked variation in fiber size, increased endomysial connective tissue. Many fibers are "rounded" as opposed to polygonal.

in conditions that are not primarily immune mediated (e.g., Duchenne muscular dystrophy), CD8-positive cells invade muscle fibers. Cellular and perivascular infiltration are the hallmark of the three major types of inflammatory myopathies: dermatomyositis, polymyositis, and inclusion body myositis. Perifascicular atrophy (Figure 2–32) is virtually pathognomonic of dermatomyositis and often occurs in the absence of cellular infiltrates. The muscle biopsy can be a diagnostic source for vasculitis; mononuclear cells can be seen invading the walls of small- and medium-sized arteries.

Preferential Fiber Type Involvement

Preferential atrophy of muscle fiber types occurs in certain conditions (Table 2–7). Type 2 fibers, particularly type 2B, are selectively affected in hyperthyroidism, corticosteroid excess (endogenous or exogenous), disuse, cachexia, and upper motor neuron disease (Figure 2–33). Type 1 fiber atrophy is less common but is prominent in myotonic dystrophy and in infants and children with centronuclear myopathy and congenital fiber-type disproportion.

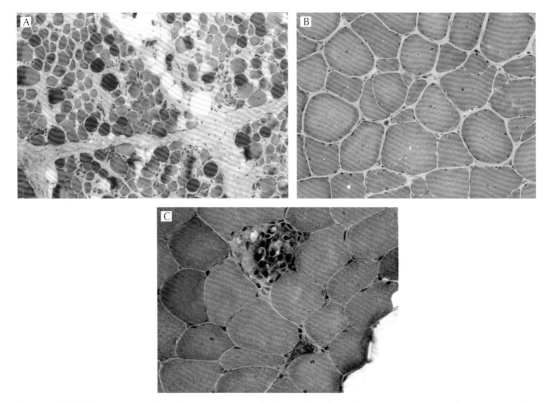

Figure 2–30. Chronic myopathy. (A) Duchenne muscular dystrophy. Marked variation in fiber size, abnormally rounded fibers, opaque fibers, increased endomysial connective tissue. Hematoxylin and eosin. (B) Chronic myopathy. Gomori trichrome. (C) Necrotic fiber, present in active myopathies, both acute and chronic. Gomori trichrome.

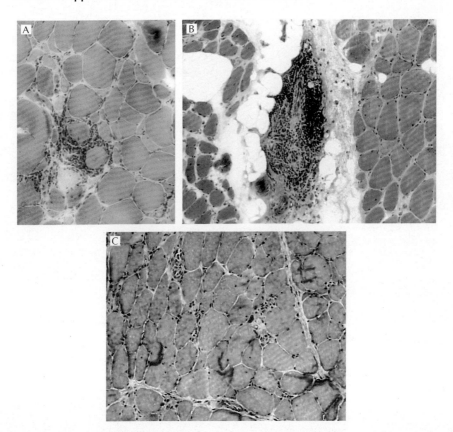

Figure 2–31. Inflammatory myopathy. (A) Endomysial inflammatory cells. Gomori trichrome. (B) Perivascular inflammatory cells. Gomori trichrome. (C) Necrotizing myopathy. Hematoxylin and eosin.

Certain cytoarchitectural abnormalities also have a fiber-type predilection, usually involving type 1 fibers. *Target fibers*, which affect mainly type 1 fibers, have already been discussed as a feature of neurogenic disorders (see Figure 2–25). *Central cores* resemble

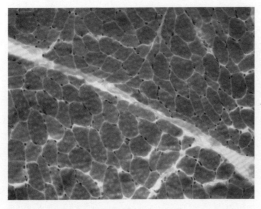

Figure 2–32. Inflammatory myopathy. Perifascicular atrophy. Gomori trichrome.

target fibers and are diagnostic of the congenital myopathy, central core disease (chapter 6). Central cores like target fibers affect mainly type 1 fibers and have a central zone unreactive with NADH-TR; they do not have the densely stained zone surrounding the central region. In nemaline myopathy, rod *bodies,* originating from the Z disc, accumulate predominantly in type 1 fibers. Rod bodies appear as dark red or purple structures in the modified trichrome stain. Ultrastructural examination demonstrates an osmiophilic, latticelike appearance of Z-disc origin, into which thin filaments insert (chapter 6). Centronuclear myopathy (Figure 2–34) and other congenital myopathies (see chapter 6) can be identified by light microscopy.

Mitochondrial abnormalities also preferentially affect type 1 fibers. Ragged red fibers are so named because of the clusters of red-staining material under the sarcolemma in the trichrome stain (see chapter 8). Electron microscopy of ragged red fibers

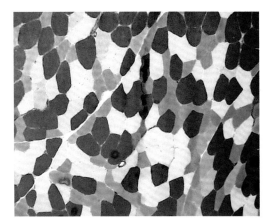

Figure 2–33. Type 2B fiber atrophy.

demonstrates clusters of enlarged, often bizarrely shaped mitochondria, many of which have closely packed cristae with intramitochondrial inclusions. This fiber abnormality is indicative of a mitochondrial disorder (see chapter 8).

Tubular aggregates are one of the few cytoarchitectural abnormalities preferentially affecting type 2 fibers. Tubular aggregates are clusters of tubular proliferation arising from the sarcoplasmic reticulum. They demonstrate positive staining with NADH-TR, a negative reaction for SDH, and a prominent red appearance in the trichrome stain. They may be seen in periodic paralysis, but are also present in other conditions and often confer little or no diagnostic specificity.

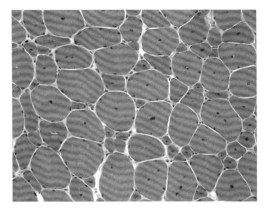

Figure 2–34. Centronuclear myopathy. Hematoxylin and eosin.

Sources of Diagnostic Error

In addition to the risk of overlooking multifocal disease because of sampling error, in many instances the results of the muscle biopsy may be misleading. Moreover, the range of normal for muscle fiber diameters varies widely within, and especially between, different muscles.

NERVE BIOPSY

Indications for Biopsy

Nerve biopsy may be indicated for patients with myopathies, because both proximal and distal muscle diseases often include neuropathic disorders in their differential diagnosis. Because the repertoire of pathologic changes of the nerve is limited, the indications for nerve biopsy are more restricted than for muscle biopsy. The nerve biopsy is most valuable to identifying changes in the blood vessels and in the supporting connective tissue elements of the nerve. The leading indication for nerve biopsy is a search for vasculitis. Other indications include suspected amyloidosis, or granulomatous diseases such as sarcoidosis as well as in various immune-mediated neuropathies. A diagnosis of leprosy can also be made from a nerve biopsy.

Nerve biopsies are of very limited use in hereditary disorders; molecular testing is available for most disorders. In hereditary conditions such as the lysosomal storage diseases, the biopsy can demonstrate the presence of certain storage products (for example, metachromatic granules), but a definitive diagnosis can only be established by biochemical assay of white blood cells or other appropriate tissue or by molecular genetic testing.

Selection of Biopsy Sites

SURAL NERVE

Biopsies are performed most commonly on the sural nerve. It may be reached through an incision over the calf or at the lateral malleolus. A convenient site for biopsy is in the lower leg, through an incision approximately 25 cm above the plantar surface of the heel, 1 cm lateral to the midline. The advantage of this site is that the nerve usually has not yet branched, and pressure-induced changes are unlikely. (At the level of the lateral malleolus, the nerve is chronically exposed to pressure from shoes.) In addition, the usual curvilinear incision at the ankle may heal slowly.

SUPERFICIAL PERONEAL NERVE

The next most accessible site for nerve biopsy is the anterior compartment of the lower leg, where the superficial peroneal nerve (a sensory branch of the common peroneal nerve) can be obtained. Biopsy of this nerve is done with the patient lying in a supine position, which is more comfortable than the prone position required for sural nerve biopsies. Positioning for sural nerve biopsy may be very difficult for some patients, such as those on a ventilator. When searching for vasculitis, the superficial peroneal nerve biopsy also offers the advantage of the close apposition of this nerve to the peroneus brevis muscle, facilitating a combined muscle/nerve biopsy and avoiding a second incision. Vasculitis is found in vessels in the peroneus brevis muscle at least as frequently as in the superficial peroneal nerve.

The disadvantages of a biopsy of the superficial peroneal nerve are that fewer fascicles are found than in the sural nerve, and the nerve takes a more variable course, making the biopsy procedure potentially more difficult. In addition, potential pressure-induced changes of the common peroneal nerve at the fibular head may be reflected downstream at the site of the superficial peroneal nerve biopsy.

SUPERFICIAL RADIAL NERVE

A third nerve available for biopsy is the superficial radial nerve. The incision is made at the wrist; identification of the nerve may be difficult because of confusion with the surrounding tendons. In addition, the removal of this nerve results in a sensory loss over the thumb, which is disconcerting to some patients. Although it is a pure sensory nerve, biopsy is performed only as a last resort, such as in a patient who has a suspected vasculitis but has findings confined to the upper extremities.

Tissue Removal and Preparation

An important consideration for patient comfort at the time of nerve biopsy is direct infiltration of local anesthetic into the sheath of the nerve. Cutting the nerve without appropriate nerve block is very painful and should be avoided. Removal of a specimen approximately 4 cm long is ideal. A 1-cm segment of this specimen is separated, mounted on a chuck with gum tragacanth, and frozen for 10 to 15 seconds in isopentane cooled to $-160°C$. This procedure is identical to the method used for freezing muscle. Frozen sections are valuable for identification of immune deposits (immunoglobulin and complement) and for mononuclear cell typing (T cells, B cells, macrophages). Another 1-cm segment of nerve is placed in buffered formalin and processed for paraffin sections, which are used to demonstrate vasculitis and connective tissue abnormalities such as inflammatory cells and granulomas. A portion of the remaining nerve is fixed at its in situ length (e.g., attached to a tongue blade) in 3% phosphate-buffered glutaraldehyde for 30 minutes before dissection into 1- to 2-mm blocks, which are returned to the same fixative for 1.5 hours. These blocks are placed in 1% phosphate-buffered osmium tetroxide for 2 hours, followed by dehydration in graded alcohols and propylene oxide; they are subsequently embedded in a resin plastic media. Plastic sections 1 μm thick and stained with toluidine blue or paraphenylenediamine provide a basis for study by high-resolution light microscopy. For nerve fiber teasing, individual nerve fascicles are separated and put in 2% osmium tetroxide for 24 hours, then into 60% glycerol. Single nerve fibers are teased and placed on slides for further study. The combination of high resolution light microscopy and nerve fiber teasing allows careful assessment of the type of nerve pathology: axonal versus demyelinating, and primary versus secondary demyelination. Electron microscopy is not necessary for most biopsies, but it is indicated in the rare cases in which a storage material is being sought.

For skin biopsy for cutaneous nerve assessment, punch biopsies obtained from skin under local anesthesia permit quantification of small intradermal nerves. A reduction in the number of these nerves (which requires careful quantification in experienced laboratories) can point to small fiber neuropathy as a diagnosis.

REFERENCES

1. Askanas V, Engel WK, DiMauro S, Brooks BR, and Mehler M: Adult-onset acid maltase efficiency: Morphologic and biochemical abnormalities reproduced in cultured muscle. N Engl J Med 294:573, 1976.

2. Koster JR, Slee RG, Van der Klei-Van Moorsel JM, Rietra PJGM, and Lucas CJ: Physico-chemical and immunological properties of acid α-glucosidase from various human tissues in relation to glycogenosis type II (Pompe's disease). Clin Chim Acta 68:49, 1976.

3. McComas AJ, Kereshi S, and Quinlan J: A method for detecting functional weakness. J Neurol Neurosurg Psychiatry 46:280, 1983.

4. Shahani BT: Electromyography in CNS Disorders: Central EMG. Butterworth, Stoneham, MA, 1984.

5. Weiner IH and Weiner HL: Nocturnal leg muscle cramps. JAMA 244:2332, 1980.

6. Pearson CM, Rimer DG, and Mommaerts WFHM: A metabolic myopathy due to absence of muscle phosphorylase. Am J Med 30:502, 1961.

7. Costill DL: Sweating: Its composition and effects on body fluids. Ann N Y Acad Sci 301:160, 1977.

8. Medical Research Council. Aids to the Investigation of Peripheral Nerve Injuries. Her Majesty's Stationery Office, London, 1976.

9. Osher RH and Griggs RC: Orbicularis fatigue: The "peek" sign of myasthenia gravis. Arch Ophthalmol 97:677, 1979.

10. Patel AN and Swami RK: Muscle percussion and neostigmine test in the clinical evaluation of neuromuscular disorders. N Engl J Med 281:523, 1969.

11. Mizusawa H, Takagi A, Sugita H, and Toyokura Y: Mounding phenomenon: An experimental study in vitro. Neurology 33:90, 1983.

12. Roth G: The origin of fasciculations. Ann Neurol 12:542, 1982.

13. Fleet WS and Watson RT: From benign fasciculations and cramps to motor neuron disease. Neurology 36:997, 1986.

14. Albers JW, Allen AA, Bastron JA, and Daube JR: Limb myokymia. Muscle Nerve 4:494, 1981.

15. Spiro AJ: Minipolymyoclonus A neglected sign in childhood spinal muscular atrophy. Neurology 20:1124, 1970.

16. Said G, Bathien N, and Cesaro P: Peripheral neuropathies and tremor. Neurology 32:480, 1982.

17. Adams RD, Shahani BT, and Young RR: Tremor in association with polyneuropathy. Transactions of the American Neurological Association 97:44, 1972.

18. Sladky JT, Brown MJ, and Berman PH: Chronic inflammatory demyelinating polyneuropathy of infancy: A corticosteroid-responsive disorder. Ann Neurol 20:76, 2986

19. Tsung SH: Several conditions causing elevation of serum CK-MB and CK-BB. Am J Clin Pathol 75:711, 1981.

20. Siegel AJ, Silverman LM, and Holman BL: Elevated creatine kinase MB isoenzyme levels in marathon runners: Normal myocardial scintigrams suggest noncardiac source. JAMA 246:2049, 1981.

21. Sunohara N, Takagi A, Nonaka I, Sugita H, and Satoyoshi E: Idiopathic hyperCKemia. Neurology 34:544, 1984.

22. Alevizos B, Spengos M, Vassilopoulos D, and Stefanis C: γ-glutamyl transpeptidase. Elevated activity in myotonic dystrophy. J Neurol Sci 28:225, 1976.

23. Griggs RC. Forbes G. Moxley RT, and Herr BE: The assessment of muscle mass in progressive neuromuscular disease. Neurology 33:158, 1983.

24. Orwoll ES, Oviatt SK, Biddle JA: Precision of dual-energy x-ray absorptiometry: development of quality control rules and their application in longitudinal studies. J Bone Miner Res 8:693, 1993.

25. Fischmann A, Morrow JM, Sinclari CD, Reilly MM, Hanna MG et al: Improved anatomical reproducibility in quantitataive lower-limb muscle MRI. J Magn Reson Imaging. 2013 Oct 7. Doi: 10.1002/jmri.24220. [Epub ahead of print].

26. Lamminen AE: Magnetic resonance imaging of primary skeletal muscle disease patterns of distribution and severity of involvement. Br. J. Radiol 63:946, 1990.

27. Griggs R, Vihola A, Hackman P, Talvinen K, Haravuori H, Faulkner G, Eymard B, Richard I, Selcen D, Engel A, Carpen O, Udd B: Zaspopathy in a large classic late onset distal myopathy family. Brain, 130(Pt 6, June):1477, 2007.

28. Mahjneh I, Lamminen AE, Udd B, et al: Muscle magnetic resonance imaging chows distinct diagnostic patterns in Welander and tibial muscular dystrophy. Acta Neurol Scan, 110:87, 2004.

29. Flanigan KM, Kerr I, Bromberg MB, et al: Congenital muscular dystrophy with rigid spine syndrome: a clinical pathological, radiological, and genetic study. Ann Neurol, 47:152, 2000.

30. Studýnková JT, Charvát F, Jarosová K, Vencovský J: MRI in the assessment of polymyositis and dermatomyositis. Rheumatology, 46:1174, 2007.

31. Phillips BA, Cala LA, Thickbroom GW, et al: Patterns of muscle involvement in inclusion body myositis: clinical and magnetic resonance imaging study. Muscle Nerve, 24:1526, 2001.

32. Forbes SC, Watler GA, Rooney WD, et al: Skeletal muscles of ambulant children with Duchenne muscular dystrophy: validation of multicenter study of evaluation with MR imaging and MR spectroscopy. Radiology, published online before print May 21, 2013, doi:10.1148/radiol.13121948

33. Buchthal F and Kamieniecka Z: The diagnostic yield of quantified electromyography and quantified muscle biopsy in neuromuscular disorders. Muscle Nerve 5:265, 1982.

34. Sanders DB and Howard JF: AAEE minimonograph #25: Single-fiber electromyography in myasthenia gravis. Muscle Nerve 9:809, 1986.

35. Sewry CA, Molnar MJ: Histopathology and immunoanalysis of muscle. In: Karpati G, et al (eds), Disorders of Voluntary Muscle, 8th ed. Cambridge University Press, 2010, p.5–6

36. Miller RG, Kuntz JL: Nerve conduction studies in infants and children. J Chil Neurol 1:19, 1986.

Chapter 3

Genetic Evaluation of the Patient and Family

Gerald Pfeffer
Patrick F. Chinnery

Many neuromuscular diseases are inherited as single gene disorders, and the last 20 years have seen an explosion of knowledge identifying novel gene defects in patients with well-recognized clinical phenotypes. The molecular dissection of the limb-girdle muscular dystrophies has been particularly fruitful in identifying novel phenotypes associated with mutations in specific genes.[1] Taking this still further, a single gene such as titin (*TTN*) has been associated with several remarkably different phenotypes, depending on which region of the gene is mutated.

Some *TTN* mutations cause cardiomyopathy,[2] others cause an early-onset myopathy with cardiomyopathy,[3] mutations of the 119th fibronectin type III domain of *TTN* present in late adult life with distal weakness and early respiratory muscle failure,[4,5] and mutations at the distal end of the protein cause a milder, late-onset distal myopathy, tibial muscular dystrophy.[6]

Given this important expansion in our understanding of the genetic basis of muscle disease, there has been a general trend to perform genetic testing earlier in the clinical evaluation.

For specific diagnoses such as facioscapulo-humeral dystrophy and myotonic dystrophy, the clinical picture often points directly to a specific genetic lesion that can be confirmed at the first clinic visit with a molecular genetic blood test. As a result, muscle biopsies and neurophysiological studies may not be required in both of these contexts. However, if the clinical picture is incomplete, or not characteristic for a particular disorder, then a systematic clinical evaluation involving clinical tests, aimed at defining the phenotype, is an essential step before proceeding to molecular genetic testing. This is particularly important in mitochondrial disorders, which can present in a variety of different ways, and it may not be apparent on first clinic visit where the underlying gene defect lies. In this situation it may be essential to carry out a muscle biopsy to enable immunocytochemical analysis, immunoblotting of specific muscle proteins, or biochemical studies, to provide guidance for targeted genetic testing. However, it should be noted that this approach has already begun to change as next-generation sequencing (NGS) approaches are validated in the clinical context. It is therefore likely that the need for invasive diagnostic tests will further decrease over the next few years.

This chapter considers the role of the contemporary clinical and molecular genetic approach, focusing on the core principles. The genetics and details of testing for specific disease are considered in other chapters. However, the reader would be well advised to consult the literature and online resources before considering which specific genetic tests to perform in many patients with neuromuscular disorders, and when to perform them, because the field is evolving so rapidly.

CLINICAL EVALUATION

Clinical History

A detailed family history is an essential component of the clinical assessment of a patient with muscle disease. Careful questioning can reveal family members who either clearly had the same underlying muscle disorder affecting the index case, or may have had a diagnosis that is consistent with the same disorder, but was not accurately diagnosed at the time. The history should not only involve neuromuscular symptoms, but also should encompass cardiac symptoms if appropriate, or the multisystem features seen in patients with mitochondrial disorders, myotonic dystrophy, or other disorders. Piecing together the inheritance pattern can be difficult, but it is a crucial step in informing subsequent molecular genetic investigations.

All forms of inheritance have been described in inherited muscle disease: autosomal dominant, such as titinopathy and certain forms of limb-girdle muscular dystrophy; autosomal recessive, including the limb-girdle muscular dystrophies and forms of congenital myasthenia; X linked, including Duchenne, Becker, and Emery-Dreifuss muscular dystrophy; and maternally inherited mitochondrial disorders due to mitochondrial DNA mutations.

Although the family history may be very revealing, the absence of a family history should not put the clinician off the diagnosis of an inherited muscle disease. Dominant disorders often have variable penetrance, and thus can appear to skip generations. Autosomal-recessive disorders often appear as sporadic cases in an outbred population, and de novo mutations are well recognized for many inherited muscle diseases (e.g., up to one-third of patients with Duchenne muscular dystrophy). Thus, the possibility of an inherited disorder should not be rejected in the absence of a family history, and the apparent inheritance patterns can be misleading at times. However, when present, a clear-cut pedigree with multiple affected individuals is enormously valuable in directing further investigation.

As well as the diagnostic considerations, the history also should focus on the functional effect of the patient's disability: whether the patient is able to be independent at home or the office, and is otherwise able to manage activities of daily living. Most patients with muscle disease will require some type of supportive care, and this can range from a referral for ankle orthoses for foot drop, to home occupational therapy assessment, to adapting the home and providing caregivers for more disabled patients. Physicians should regularly inquire whether the assistance available to the patient is sufficient for the maintenance of daily and dignified living, and should advocate for further support when indicated. The social impact of genetic disease on patients and their families is often substantial, and providing access to patient groups or other forms of emotional support can be invaluable.

Physical Examination

Owing to significant phenotypic overlap, the various disorders, when defined genetically, are impossible to define on strictly clinical grounds. Nonetheless, an attentive and detailed clinical examination is critical in establishing the diagnosis. Patients should always be examined in a hospital gown so that evaluation of proximal musculature and particularly the shoulder girdle are possible. On simple observation, several findings may already be apparent, such as lordosis, head drop, or other postural abnormalities. The pattern of muscle atrophy or hypertrophy should be sought, if present, as well as the presence of scapular winging. Joint deformities due to contractures, congenital myopathy, or longstanding neuropathy should be appreciated if present. Abnormalities of motor tone or tendon reflexes are important in providing evidence for the localization. On testing of muscle power, the pattern of weakness should be documented (particularly, predominantly proximal or distal, or specific damage patterns such as scapuloperoneal syndrome). Sensory examination typically focuses on the lower extremities and is important in providing evidence for neuropathy or for localization when it is caused by more proximal lesions. Findings such as hammer toes suggest long-standing neuropathy. The autonomic nervous system should also be interrogated when indicated, usually with orthostatic blood pressure measurements. The cerebellar system is usually unaffected in neuromuscular disorders but should still be carefully examined to exclude a multisystem disease or to differentiate sensory ataxia. Cranial nerve examination should not be forgotten, because the presence or absence of bulbar weakness or external ophthalmoplegia contributes significantly to establishing the differential diagnosis. The general medical examination is important, particularly of the cardiac system, which is affected in some muscle diseases (chapter 13). A low threshold should exist to order pulmonary and cardiac function testing in patients with supine respiratory symptoms or in patients suspected of having diseases known to affect ventilation (see chapter 12), since neuromuscular ventilatory failure in particular has signs that are difficult to recognize or are subclinical. Skeletal abnormalities such as rigid spine or scoliosis can be of diagnostic significance as well.

Clinical Investigations Guiding Genetic Testing

Other clinical testing provides guidance for the selection of accurate genetic testing; a broad review of this is beyond the scope of this chapter, and is considered in later chapters. However, it is worth mentioning that some investigations are generally useful in stratifying neuromuscular disorders, such as serum creatine kinase levels, or nerve conduction and electromyography studies. MRI is increasingly useful as a noninvasive test for muscle disease and can be used to help define the likely genetic cause[7] and assist with selection of muscle biopsy sites if needed. Muscle or nerve biopsy are invasive investigations that can help guide genetic testing when the appropriate differential diagnosis is not obvious.

MOLECULAR GENETIC TESTING IN A CLINICAL CONTEXT

Technological advances have dramatically changed the molecular genetic approach within the last decade. Early studies involving radioactive techniques, such as Southern blotting, have been largely superseded by fluorescence-based methods including the extensive use of targeted resequencing of candidate genes. The molecular approach now falls into major groups encompassing conventional and next-generation sequencing techniques, as detailed in the following sections.

Conventional Genetic Testing

ALLELE-SPECIFIC MUTATION ANALYSIS

Specific mutation analysis can involve assays directed at individual nucleotide changes that are a frequent cause of neuromuscular disease, particularly if a particular mutation is common within the same population (such as from a founder effect). Likewise, recurring rearrangements of a gene (deletions or duplications) or trinucleotide repeat expansions can also be tested rapidly using this approach. The key point here is that if the test is negative, the clinician should not necessarily be put off the diagnosis, because other specific mutations could be causing the phenotype in the patient. However, if the test is positive, then the diagnosis may be confirmed rapidly using DNA extracted from a blood sample, or sometimes from a buccal swab in children.

SANGER SEQUENCING

Chain-termination sequencing with a fluorescent Sanger-based approach is now widespread in diagnostic laboratories through the world. The approach is used to screen for mutations in areas of the genome known to be associated with disease where different mutations are clustered together. This could involve a segment of a gene known to cause a muscle disease (e.g., exon hot spots) or could involve the entire gene. Typically, mutations occur within the region that codes for amino acids, or alternatively may be in adjacent regulatory regions, where base substitutions can affect the splicing of the gene, or the degree of expression of the gene in a particular tissue. If this approach identifies a known mutation, then confirming the diagnosis can be relatively straightforward. However, if the variant has not been seen before, then the clinician and patient may be left with some uncertainty about its clinical significance.

Bioinformatic/computational approaches can help predict whether an individual nucleotide base change is likely to be causing the disease. A key step is to perform segregation analysis within a family, if this is possible. This involves looking for the mutation in affected individuals, and confirming that it is not present in unaffected individuals. Last, it may not be possible to work out whether the mutation is causing the disease without functional studies, which can be very time consuming and costly, and are rarely used in a routine diagnostic context. Functional studies require expressing the new mutation in a cell culture system and determining if the mutation results in abnormal function.

SCREENING FOR REARRANGEMENTS

Point mutations typically account for approximately 80% of known pathogenic mutations in inherited muscle diseases, and both deletions and duplications account for a large proportion of the remaining molecular lesions. Deletions and duplications can be missed by a targeted sequencing approach, and specific molecular assays are required to identify these rearrangements. As mentioned, Southern blot techniques were used in the past, but increasingly fluorescence-based methods have become more widespread in their application. Comparative genomic hybridization (CGH) is now widely used to detect large-scale gene rearrangements across the whole human genome. Different CGH arrays have different degrees of resolution, but typically resolves changes in copy number with probes approximately every 300 kilobases. Multiplex ligation-dependent probe amplification analysis is a PCR-based technique that can be employed to detect deletions and duplications (with resolution depending upon the spacing of the probes) within specific disease genes, and are enormously valuable in several different neuromuscular disorders.

Next-Generation Sequencing

The advent of next-generation sequencing (NGS, also called massively parallel sequencing) is having a dramatic impact on our capacity to make a molecular diagnosis in patients with inherited muscle disease. Several NGS platforms are commercially available, each having important technological differences. In general, however, all of the "second generation" NGS technologies have in common the requirement for amplification of DNA prior to sequencing, as well as repetitive "wash and detect" cycles to measure the addition of individual nucleotides during resequencing.[8] The major advantage of these technologies over Sanger sequencing is that the sequencing of all targets occurs simultaneously (in parallel). Thus when compared with Sanger sequencing, second-generation sequencing has much greater automation, much higher throughput, and much lower cost per base sequenced.

Using this technology, multigene panels have been devised to enable the cost- and time-efficient screening of all genes associated with particular phenotypes, which is important because of the massive number of genetic etiologies in muscle disease, and the phenotypic overlap between them (a summary of the available panels is available from reference 9). NGS also has utility in testing for single genes, for example in the case of the giant dystrophin protein, in which a single platform can identify rearrangements and single nucleotide variants.[10] Other giant genes, such as *TTN*, cannot feasibly be sequenced by conventional approaches and NGS would be the only option available.[11] However, the diagnostic gold standard remains Sanger sequencing and therefore genetic lesions found with NGS must also be confirmed with conventional methods.

Outside of diagnostic testing, the most common use for NGS is in exome sequencing. The *exome* is the sum of all exons in the human genome, accounts for approximately 1% of the human genome, and includes the DNA sequences known to code for proteins. Exome sequencing kits are designed to sequence the exome as well as flanking regions involved in splicing and gene regulation. It is estimated that approximately 85% of pathogenic mutations in human genetic diseases will be found within the exome sequence. However, there are numerous limitations that prevent this technique from being used in diagnostic testing, namely (a) coverage of the exome is usually 85% to 90%, which may miss important regions relevant to the patient's phenotype; (b) hundreds or thousands of potentially pathogenic genetic variants are detected in each individual, and determining which (if any) of these are relevant requires the coordinated effort of a research group; (c) data storage becomes a problematic and expensive consideration; and (d) privacy, disclosure, and other ethical issues relating to incidental findings. For these reasons it is likely that diagnostic testing using NGS will remain restricted to targeted testing for relevant genes or gene panels, at least in the short term, although the preceding limitations eventually may be resolved with technological improvements (for both sequencing technology and data storage), greater completeness of databases for known genetic variants (both disease causing and non–disease causing), improved bioinformatic methods, and greater experience with the possible ethical complications. It is also worth mentioning that for the time being, certain genetic lesions (such as lengthy polynucleotide repeats and large-scale rearrangements) are not detectable using most NGS technologies and still require conventional sequencing methods.

Many of the current technological limitations may become nonissues once "third generation" NGS technology becomes commercially available. Several different technologies are currently in development, and in general these have in common the ability to sequence DNA without the initial enrichment step (avoiding artifacts that can be introduced at this stage) as well as the ability to perform continuous sequencing without interruption of the reaction for repetitive "wash/detect" cycles. These technologies, once available, are expected to be more fully automated; have higher throughput; be capable of sequencing from even a single molecule; and involve less equipment, fewer reagents, and lower cost compared with current NGS technologies. A review of the technologies in development at the time of writing is recommended.[12]

IMPLICATIONS OF A POSITIVE GENETIC TEST RESULT

A positive genetic test result has the most direct impact for the patient by establishing a precise diagnosis. The physician is then able to provide expectations regarding treatment and prognosis, which provide closure for the patient and allow planning for the future. Some genetic diseases have specific treatments that would only be available to the patient with a confirmed diagnosis. For example, late-onset Pompe disease (acid maltase deficiency) is treated with alglucosidase alfa,[13] a recombinant protein to replace the deficient enzyme in the disease (see chapter 7). Equally important is that a precise diagnosis will avoid the use of inappropriate treatments for other speculative diagnoses. Last, having a diagnosis also allows patients to identify themselves within relevant patient groups, which can be a strong source of support for them and their families.

The genetic diagnosis is also instrumental to inform genetic counseling, in order to address the indirect implications of the test result, namely (a) diagnostic testing for other affected family members, (b) predictive testing for unaffected family members, and (c) preimplantation or prenatal diagnosis.

Diagnostic Testing for Affected Family Members

For the same reasons that diagnostic confirmation is important for the index patient, it is important to validate the diagnosis in other affected family members. When the mutation is discovered in the proband, testing for the other family members is technically straightforward, but still should always be done with the availability of proper genetic counseling.

Ethical complications can arise in situations where patients do not want their family members to know of the diagnosis. These situations require careful genetic counseling and must be managed on an individual basis depending on the disease in question (particularly whether a diagnosis will affect treatment or eligibility for benefits), and other factors in the context.

Predictive Testing for Unaffected Family Members

Knowing the underlying molecular basis of a muscle disease provides the opportunity for other family members to have genetic testing to determine whether they are carriers, or are likely to become affected by the muscle disease in future. However, testing should only proceed with great caution, after careful counseling of the patient and family members to ensure that individual patients are aware of the potential implications of a predictive genetic test. These can be significant, and include the physiological consequences of inheriting and not inheriting the disorder (so-called survivor guilt), in addition to the potential impact on insurance prospects and career aspirations. Note that this will vary by jurisdiction: in the United States such discrimination is not permitted under the 2008 Genetic Information Nondiscrimination Act. In the case of Huntington disease (although not a neuromuscular disease, it is the prototype disease for predictive testing), it would appear that such testing is seldom requested by asymptomatic at-risk family members.[14] Carrier testing for autosomal-recessive disorders is less contentious, and enables an individual to accurately determine the risk of them having an affected child of their own. This may involve carrier testing in their partner before they plan to start a family.

Prenatal Diagnosis

Knowing the molecular basis of a disorder enables reliable and accurate prenatal diagnosis, which is now routine in most major centers. Again, the key first step is defining the pathogenic mutation in affected family members. It is then possible to test pregnancy in the first trimester, either by chorionic villus biopsy or amniocentesis, to determine whether the fetus is at risk of developing the same disease. This is generally only undertaken if a couple has agreed to proceed with a termination of pregnancy, should the underlying genetic disorder be detected prenatally.

Knowing the precise molecular basis of a muscle disease also enables preimplantation genetic diagnosis, which is carried out on a blastocyst developed following in vitro fertilization. Unaffected blastocysts are reimplanted in the mother and allowed to develop normally. Although less widely available, preimplantation diagnosis is now routinely considered in several centers worldwide for muscle diseases.

It is worth noting that the prenatal diagnosis of mitochondrial disorders remains challenging, if the underlying disease is caused by a mutation in mitochondrial DNA (mtDNA). Although the mutation may be inherited down the maternal line, a mixed proportion of mutated in a wild-type DNA (mtDNA heteroplasmy) leads to unpredictable outcomes of pregnancy. Recent published guidelines support the use of prenatal diagnosis, but with certain caveats.[15] It is important that prospective parents realize that that risk prediction is less certain than for nuclear genetic disorders; in many instances it is not possible to give clear guidance on the recurrence risk. This is usually because the fetus may have an intermediate level of heteroplasmy which is of uncertain long-term significance. Preimplantation diagnosis in mitochondrial disorders has been carried out, enabling the successful reintroduction of blastocysts with a very low mutation load, thus drastically reducing the risk of recurrence.[15] Last, novel techniques are under development to enable the prevention of mitochondrial disorders by nuclear transfer or spindle transfer techniques, which enable mutated mtDNA to be separated from the nuclear genome, and transferred to a donor oocyte or embryo that lacks the mtDNA mutation, thus theoretically preventing the transmission of the disorder.[16] Following public consultation, the United Kingdom is moving to a position where this approach may become legal as a treatment to prevent the transmission of mitochondrial diseases.

Personalized or Precision Medicine

Identifying the specific molecular basis for a disease allows a highly precise form of patient categorization, enabling "personalized" or "precision" medicine. On one level, the precise diagnosis allows the clinician and patient to refer to other patients who have been described in the literature with a similar or identical molecular lesion, thus facilitating more appropriate prognostic guidance and disease surveillance. If genotype–phenotype correlations exist, then a personalized prognosis can be given based on the genetic lesion. For example, splice site or frameshift mutations are associated with better prognosis in *LAMA2* mutations (merosin-deficient congenital muscular dystrophy 1A; see chapter 6).[17]

On the next level, it is hoped that molecular stratification will enable highly personalized targeted therapies. In the absence of available therapies for most muscle diseases, significant scientific effort has been directed toward tailored therapies that address specific molecular defects or even individual genetic lesions. An example of this includes exome-skipping strategies for Duchenne muscular dystrophy(see chapter 4).[18]

In other branches of medicine, differences in treatment response can be predicted based on the presence of certain genetic variants, and once more treatments are available in neuromuscular disease, similar studies hopefully will allow for personalized care to occur.

REFERENCES

1. Bushby K. Diagnosis and management of the limb girdle muscular dystrophies. Pract Neurol 9(6):314–323, 2009.
2. Herman DS, Lam L, Taylor MR, Wang L, Teekakirikul P, Christodoulou D, et al. Truncations of titin causing dilated cardiomyopathy. N Engl J Med 366(7):619–628, 2012.
3. Carmignac V, Salih MA, Quijano-Roy S, Marchand S, Al Rayess MM, Mukhtar MM, et al. C-terminal titin deletions cause a novel early-onset myopathy with fatal cardiomyopathy. Ann Neurol 61(4):340–351, 2007.
4. Palmio J, Evila A, Chapon F, Tasca G, Xiang F, Bradvik B, et al. Hereditary myopathy with early respiratory failure: Occurrence in various populations. J Neurol Neurosurg Psychiatry. 2013 Apr 19. [epub ahead of print, DOI: 10.1136/jnnp-2013-304965]
5. Pfeffer G, Barresi R, Wilson IJ, Hardy SA, Griffin H, Hudson J, et al. Titin founder mutation is a common cause of myofibrillar myopathy with early respiratory failure. J Neurol Neurosurg Psychiatry. 2013 Mar 13. [epub ahead of print, DOI: 10.1136/jnnp-2012-304728]
6. Udd B, Vihola A, Sarparanta J, Richard I, Hackman P. Titinopathies and extension of the M-line mutation phenotype beyond distal myopathy and LGMD2J. Neurology 64(4):636–642, 2005.
7. Wattjes MP, Kley RA, Fischer D. Neuromuscular imaging in inherited muscle diseases. Eur Radiol 20(10):2447–2460, 2010.
8. Schadt EE, Turner S, Kasarskis A. A window into third-generation sequencing. Hum Mol Genet 19(R2):R227–R240, 2010.
9. Rehm HL. Disease-targeted sequencing: A cornerstone in the clinic. Nat Rev Genet 14(4):295–300, 2013.
10. Lim BC, Lee S, Shin JY, Kim JI, Hwang H, Kim KJ, et al. Genetic diagnosis of Duchenne and Becker muscular dystrophy using next-generation sequencing technology: Comprehensive mutational search in a single platform. J Med Genet 48(11):731–736, 2011.
11. Pfeffer G, Elliott HR, Griffin H, Barresi R, Miller J, Marsh J, et al. Titin mutation segregates with hereditary myopathy with early respiratory failure. Brain 135(Pt 6):1695–1713, 2012.
12. Morey M, Fernandez-Marmiesse A, Castineiras D, Fraga JM, Couce ML, Cocho JA. A glimpse into past, present, and future DNA sequencing. Mol Genet Metab. 2013 Sep–Oct;110(1–2):3–24.
13. van der Ploeg AT, Clemens PR, Corzo D, Escolar DM, Florence J, Groeneveld GJ, et al. A randomized study of alglucosidase alfa in late-onset Pompe's disease. N Engl J Med 15;362(15):1396–1406, 2010.
14. Creighton S, Almqvist EW, MacGregor D, Fernandez B, Hogg H, Beis J, et al. Predictive, pre-natal and diagnostic genetic testing for Huntington's disease: The experience in Canada from 1987 to 2000. Clin Genet 63(6):462–475, 2003.
15. Hellebrekers DM, Wolfe R, Hendrickx AT, de Coo IF, de Die CE, Geraedts JP, et al. PGD and heteroplasmic mitochondrial DNA point mutations: A systematic review estimating the chance of healthy offspring. Hum Reprod Update 18(4):341–349, 2012.
16. Craven L, Tuppen HA, Greggains GD, Harbottle SJ, Murphy JL, Cree LM, et al. Pronuclear transfer in human embryos to prevent transmission of mitochondrial DNA disease. Nature 6;465(7294):82–85, 2010.
17. Geranmayeh F, Clement E, Feng LH, Sewry C, Pagan J, Mein R, et al. Genotype-phenotype correlation in a large population of muscular dystrophy patients with LAMA2 mutations. Neuromuscul Disord 20(4):241–250, 2010.
18. van Deutekom JC, Janson AA, Ginjaar IB, Frankhuizen WS, Aartsma-Rus A, Bremmer-Bout M, et al. Local dystrophin restoration with antisense oligonucleotide PRO051. N Engl J Med 27;357(26):2677–2686, 2007.

Specific Myopathies

Chapter 4

The Muscular Dystrophies

Emma Ciafaloni
Robert C. Griggs

DUCHENNE AND BECKER MUSCULAR DYSTROPHIES

Duchenne and Becker muscular dystrophy (DBMD) are X-linked recessive muscular dystrophies caused by mutations in the dystrophin gene resulting in deficiency of dystrophin, a muscle membrane protein. Prior to the discovery of the dystrophin gene in 1987,[1] the distinction between Duchenne and Becker dystrophies was based on clinical features: onset of symptoms before age 5 and loss of ambulation prior to age 12 in Duchenne; onset of symptoms after age 5 (mean age of onset = 11 years) and ability to ambulate beyond age 15 and frequently into adulthood, in Becker. Intermediate cases, termed "outliers," fell in between these two phenotypes. Since the discovery of dystrophin deficiency as the cause of DBMD,[2] the term *dystrophinopathies* has described the spectrum of severe, intermediate, and mild phenotypes. Mutations that cause complete absence of dystrophin usually result in the more severe phenotype of Duchenne muscular dystrophy (DMD), while mutations causing a truncated but partially functioning dystrophin result in the milder "outlier" and Becker muscular dystrophy (BMD) phenotypes (see section on Genetics of Duchenne and Becker Muscular Dystrophies below).

Epidemiology

Duchenne muscular dystrophy is the most common form of muscular dystrophy in children. A population-based assessment of DMD prevalence in the United States in 2007 estimated its prevalence at four U.S. sites at 1.3–1.8 per 10,000 males age 5–24 years, and a majority of surveillance subjects were surviving into adulthood.[3] Data from newborn screening worldwide show a birth prevalence of DMD ranging from 1 in 7,730 (1.3 per 10,000) to 1 in 3,871 (2.6 per 10,000).[4,5]

Newborn screening is not yet routine in the United States, reflecting the lack of definitive evidence that treatment at an early presymptomatic age improves outcome. Due in part to the recent promising advancements in exon-skipping and gene replacement therapeutic trials, interest for newborn screening has been rekindled by the Centers for Disease Control and Prevention, the Muscular Dystrophy Association, and others. A two-tier system of analysis that uses predetermined levels of CK on dried blood spots to predict DMD gene mutations has been shown effective and practical.[6]

A proposal to add Duchenne muscular dystrophy to the panel of diseases for which newborns are routinely screened has been recently presented to the U.S. Department of Health and Human Services Secretary's Discretionary Advisory Committee on Heritable Disorders in Newborns and Children, and a decision is currently pending.[7-9]

Genetics of Duchenne and Becker Muscular Dystrophies

The dystrophinopathies are inherited recessive X-linked disorders caused by mutation in the dystrophin gene at locus Xp21.2. New spontaneous mutations account for about 30% of all cases. This is the largest known gene, spanning 2.5 million base pairs (bp) and encompassing about 1.5% of the X chromosome. The coding sequence consists of 79 exons and seven promoters. The full 14,000-bp messenger RNA (mRNA) transcribed from the dystrophin gene is expressed mostly in skeletal and cardiac muscle, with small amounts also expressed in the brain (Figure 4–1).[10] The 427-kilodalton (kDa), full-length dystrophin protein is localized to the inner muscle membrane and is part of a protein complex that links the muscle membrane to the cytoskeleton and the extracellular matrix (Figure 4–2). This dystrophin-glycoprotein complex stabilizes the sarcolemma and prevents contraction-induced damage and necrosis. Shorter isoforms of dystrophin are expressed in the retina, brain, kidney, liver, lung, heart, and peripheral nerves.

There is no correlation between the size of the mutation and the resulting phenotypic severity. For example, deletions of a single exon such as exon 44 frequently result in classic DMD, while mutations encompassing as much as 50% of the gene have been described in a mild Becker phenotype.[11-13] Generally, frame-shifting mutations that cause complete lack of dystrophin expression are responsible for the more severe phenotype (DMD) while in-frame mutations that result in an abnormal but partially functional dystrophin account for the milder phenotype (BMD).

Disease penetrance is complete in males. Carrier females have a 50% chance to transmit the pathogenic mutation in each pregnancy; their daughters will have a 50% chance of being carriers and their son will have a 50% chance of having DMD. Female carriers are usually asymptomatic, but can rarely manifest a moderate to severe DMD phenotype due to skewed X chromosome inactivation defined by >75% of nuclei harboring the mutant DMD gene on the active X chromosome (manifesting carriers). The DMD or BMD phenotype can also be rarely observed in females with an XO genotype (Turner's syndrome), with a structurally abnormal X chromosome or with an X–autosome translocation.

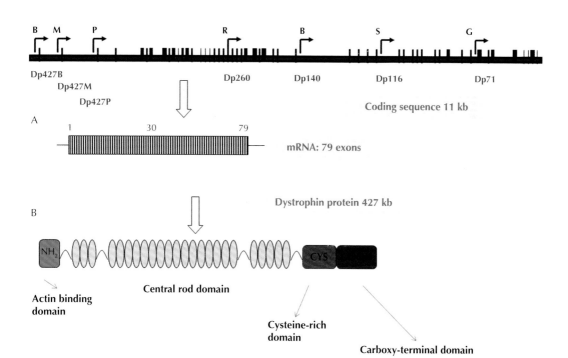

Figure 4–1. A: The dystrophin gene, located in Xp21.2. The white lines represent the 79 exons distributed over the 2.5-million-bp genomic sequence. The white arrows mark the promoters for the different isoforms: B = brain; M = muscle; P = Purkinje; R= retinal; S = Schwann cells; G= general. Isoforms size is in red. B: The full-size dystrophin protein and its domains. (Adapted from Levenson, 2012.)

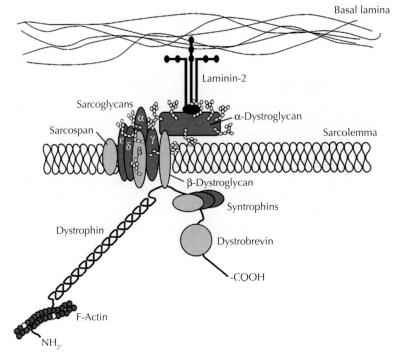

Figure 4–2. The dystrophin-associated protein complex. Bushby K M D Brain 1999;122:1403–1420.

Carrier Detection and Prenatal Testing

When the proband's disease-causing mutation is known, carrier testing can be performed in at-risk females in the family. Prenatal testing in pregnant carriers is possible if their specific mutation is known. Fetal sex is determined by chromosome analysis from cells obtained from chorionic villus sampling at 10 to 12 weeks gestation or by amniocentesis at approximately 15 to18 weeks gestation ; if the phenotype is XY, the known disease-causing mutation can be analyzed in DNA extracted from fetal cells to establish disease status.

Clinical Features: DMD

Although DMD can be diagnosed at birth based on family history and elevated CK, clinical abnormalities at birth are uncommon. First

signs and symptoms are usually recognized by the parents or schoolteachers between ages 2 and 5.[14] Delayed motor milestones (especially walking) are common, and some have advocated for CK screening in all boys with delayed walking.[15] Common presenting motor symptoms include difficulty with running, climbing, going upstairs and keeping up with peers; inability to jump; and frequent falling. Delayed speech is not uncommon and more rarely global developmental delay is present.[14] A wide-based waddling gait, exaggerated lumbar lordosis, and a Gowers' sign when getting up from the floor are typical (Figure 4–3). Neck flexion weakness and inability to lift the head against gravity is common in all stages of disease, but when detected prior to age 5, it indicates a more severe phenotype (DMD rather than BMD). The ankles' plantar flexor and invertor muscles remain remarkably strong until late in the illness. Proximal lower extremity weakness always precedes upper extremity weakness. Strength worsens over time in

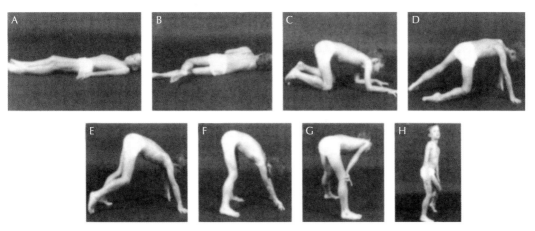

Figure 4–3. Gowers' sign. A patient with Duchenne motor dystrophy (DMD) is shown rising from the floor. The most common cause of weakness in young boys is DMD, but Gowers' sign is present in any disorder characterized by proximal weakness. To stand, the patient must roll from supine to prone (A and B), push off the floor (C–E), lock his knees (F), and then "climb up his legs" (G and H).

a stereotypical manner with progressive loss of functions such as running, getting up from the floor, climbing stairs, and eventually walking. Muscles that are innervated by the cranial nerves are unaffected except for the tongue, which often is enlarged. Pseudohypertrophy of the calves is common (Figure 4–4 and 4–5).

Joint contractures are an important clinical manifestation. By age 6 most patients have contractures at the iliotibial bands, hip joints, and heel cords. Heel-cord contractures produce "toe walking" (Figure 4–2). Knee, elbow, and wrist contractures develop later, usually after loss of ambulation, and progress once patients

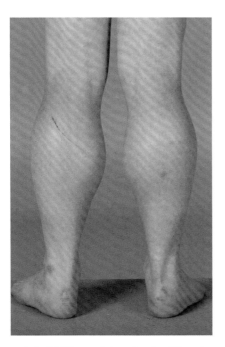

Figure 4–4. DMD: pseudohypertrophy of the calves.

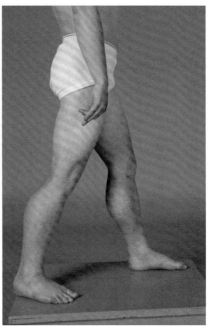

Figure 4–5. DMD patient demonstrating heel cord tightness and face-forward hands from shoulder girdle weakness.

are confined to a wheelchair. Without respiratory support, death is usually due to respiratory failure and pneumonia and occurs age 18 to 20. With use of corticosteroids DMD patients are now living longer and frequently into their third decade.[3]

Long bone and vertebral fractures are common in all patients with DMD[16] and full-time use of wheelchair and use of corticosteroids increases the risk for fractures. Low-impact fractures in ambulatory and nonambulatory patients may lead to the difficult-to-recognize fat emboli syndrome, with presentation of acute respiratory distress and altered mental status[17, 18] (Figure 4–6A–D). Fractures often go undiagnosed, causing a delay in the diagnosis of this potentially fatal syndrome. Recognition of this syndrome is important as prompt supportive treatment may change the outcome. This syndrome has been reported after falls from wheelchairs, which are not uncommon and frequently due to inconsistent use of seat belts.

Scoliosis is very common, occurring rarely before age 11, and most frequently after the ability to walk is lost. Curvatures increase over time with wheelchair use. Increasing scoliosis together with progressive diaphragmatic weakness compromises respiratory function over time.

As many as 90% of patients with DMD have abnormalities on electrocardiogram (ECG).[19-21] Tall right precordial R waves with an increased R/S amplitude ratio in V1 and deep narrow Q waves in left precordial leads are the most common and distinctive changes. Most patients demonstrate labile or persistent sinus tachycardia or other sinus arrhythmias. Ectopic rhythms, including atrial and ventricular premature beats, arise less frequently; ectopic tachyarrhythmias occur rarely. Intra-atrial

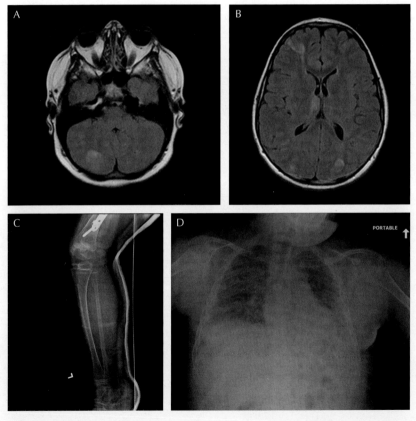

Figure 4–6. Fat emboli syndrome in a 15-year-old ambulatory boy with DMD on deflazacort after falling at home. A & B: Brain MRI axial FLAIR images showing several focal lesions in the cerebellum (largest in the right cerebellum), basal ganglia, and right frontal and left occipital cortex. C: Left tibia and fibula in lateral projection shows a comminuted undisplaced fracture of the diaphysis of the proximal tibia. D: Chest X-ray showing diffuse interstitial edema.

conduction-system defects are more common than atrioventricular and infranodal disturbances. Atrioventricular nodal block seldom occurs. Progressive cardiomyopathy is an important cause of morbidity and mortality in DMD, especially now that patients survive longer with the disease.[22,23]

A restrictive pattern of progressive weakness of respiratory muscles is a cardinal feature of DMD. Forced vital capacity (FVC) increases until age 10 and after a plateau phase, it progressively decreases.[24] When the FVC reaches the value of 1 L, 5-year survival is less than 10%.[25] The first sign of respiratory muscle weakness is a weak cough as measured by peak cough flow (PCF), followed by nocturnal hypoventilation and disturbed sleep, and finally diurnal hypoventilation. A weak cough contributes to prolonged upper respiratory infection due to inability to clear secretions.

Clinical and pathologic involvement of smooth muscle of the gastrointestinal tract, although frequently overlooked, can be an important manifestation. Constipation is common throughout the disease. A syndrome of acute gastric dilatation, also referred as pseudo-obstruction, consists of sudden episodes of vomiting, associated with abdominal pain and distention, and may lead to death.[26] The acute gastric dilatation probably results from gastric hypomotility, which can be demonstrated by delayed gastric emptying using a standard radiolabeled meal of oatmeal.[27] Patients who died from this syndrome showed degeneration of the outer, longitudinal smooth-muscle layer of the stomach, likely due to dystrophin deficiency.[28]

In his original description of the disorder in 1886, Duchenne described decreased intellectual abilities. While there is clear evidence of overall cognitive, psychosocial, and behavioral deficits in DMD,[29] there is great heterogeneity in nonmotor deficits; only about 30% of boys with DMD will display such deficits, with most boys demonstrating a pure "motor DMD" phenotype with normal intelligence.[30] Full-length dystrophin is normally expressed in the cerebral cortex, hippocampus, and cerebellum. The shorter isoforms of dystrophin, Dp 71, Dp 116, Dp 140, and Dp 260 are also located in the brain (Figure 4–1). A correlation between mutation affecting the Dp140 isoform and intellectual impairment has been reported.[31] Dystrophin is absent in the DMD brain, and gliosis and neuronal loss has been described.[32]

Reduced overall intellectual functioning compared to the general population and to unaffected siblings also has been described.[33,34] Verbal intelligence seems more affected than nonverbal performance-based skills in DMD and the intellectual deficit, unlike the progressive muscle weakness, does not worsen over time.[35,36] Consistent deficits in executive function and inhibition have also been shown versus children with rheumatoid arthritis and unaffected siblings.[37] An increased comorbidity between DMD and autism spectrum disorders (3.1%), attention-deficit/hyperactivity disorder (ADHD; 11.7%), and obsessive-compulsive disorder (4.8%) has been described.[38] No relationship between the use of corticosteroids and ADHD has been found. A study investigating psychosocial functioning in a large group of boys with DMD ages 5 to 17 years compared with a control group with other chronic conditions by using the Personal Adjustment and Role Skills Scale–III (PARS–III) found that patients with DMD have significantly more difficulty with peer relationships and suggested that social relations may worsen over time.[39] No difference was found between boys who did or did not take corticosteroids.

Clinical Features: Becker Muscular Dystrophy

BMD is characterized by onset of proximal lower extremity weakness after age 5 and by the ability to ambulate, always past age 15 and frequently well into adulthood. Proximal upper extremity weakness develops after the onset of leg weakness. Scoliosis, joint contractures, and cognitive abnormalities are less common than in DMD. The spectrum of weakness severity is much wider than in DMD. Some patients have subclinical muscle weakness, calf hypertrophy, myalgias, and muscle cramps; some patients maintain the ability to walk into their fifties. Heart failure from dilated cardiomyopathy is a common cause of morbidity and mortality in BMD.[40]

Differential Diagnosis

Emery-Dreifuss muscular dystrophy (EDMD) is characterized by early childhood contractures of the elbow flexors, neck extensor and Achilles tendons, followed by slowly progressive muscle weakness and wasting, and cardiomyopathy and arrhythmias (see section on Emery-Dreifuss Muscular Dystrophy). Unlike DMD, elbow contractures are prominent early in the course of the disease and precede loss of ambulation. Cardiac transplantation is frequently necessary well before patients lose the ability to walk. The disease is inherited in an X-linked manner due to mutations in the EMD gene (encoding emerin) or the *FHL1* gene, or in an autosomal dominant or recessive manner when mutations are in the *LMNA* gene encoding lamin A and C.

Limb-girdle muscular dystrophy (LGMD; discussed later in this chapter) is a group of disorders characterized by progressive muscle weakness with onset in childhood or adulthood and inherited in an autosomal-recessive or dominant manner. LGMD is caused by mutations in genes encoding proteins in the sarcoglycan complex or other membrane proteins. LGMD types with childhood onset, highly elevated CK, and calf hypertrophy such as LGMD2L caused by mutations in the *FKRP* gene encoding fukutin-related protein and the sarcoglyconopathies (LGMD2C, 2D, 2E, and 2F) most resemble DMD.

Juvenile spinal muscular atrophy (SMA) is characterized by hypotonia, symmetric limb muscle weakness sparing face and ocular muscles, absent tendon reflexes, and tongue fasciculations. SMA is a disease of anterior horn cells and is transmitted in an autosomal-recessive manner. CK is not as elevated as in DMD and EMG can easily distinguish SMA from a muscular dystrophy.

X-linked myopathy with excessive autophagy is a very rare childhood disorder characterized by very slowly progressive weakness predominantly in the legs. It is caused by mutations in the *VMA21* gene. The X-linked recessive inheritance with full expression in males only, together with the onset of weakness between 5 and 10 years of age and elevated CK, makes this disease clinically similar to DMD. Muscle biopsy distinguishes it from DMD due to the absence of necrotic fibers and the presence of prominent membrane-bound vacuoles, which are dystrophin- and lysosome-associated membrane protein-2 positive. Deposition of the C5b-9 complement attack complex, subsarcolemmal deposition of calcium, and expression of MHC1 complex is also typical.

Diagnosis and Tests

Serum CK is the most useful screening test for the diagnosis of DMD.

Whole-blood DNA analysis for dystrophin gene mutations has largely replaced the clinical need for muscle biopsy to confirm the diagnosis.

CREATINE KINASE

Serum CK measurement is the most important screening test when suspecting a diagnosis of dystrophinopathy. Creatine kinase is highly elevated (10–100 times normal) in all patients with DMD, even in the first years of life and before symptoms become apparent. Serum CK concentration decreases with advancing age and in the late stages of the disease due to the progressive loss of muscle fibers and replacement by connective tissue.[41] Creatine kinase testing can be used to screen boys with a known family history of DMD. A CK less than 10 times normal, except in the very advanced stage of the disease, is strong evidence against the diagnosis of DMD. Increased serum CK (2–10 times normal) can be found in 30% to 50% of DMD female carriers with higher mean concentration in carriers younger than 20 years of age.[42]

CK testing is inexpensive and easily available but is underutilized in screening for DMD. Delay in CK testing accounts for much of the persistent diagnostic delay in DMD[14] (Figures 4–4 and 4–5). Once CK is found to be elevated, DNA testing can confirm the diagnosis.

DNA ANALYSIS

In almost all cases the diagnosis can be confirmed by DNA analysis, which is now 95% sensitive in detecting mutations in the dystrophin gene.

Dystrophin gene analysis on DNA isolated from peripheral blood leucocytes is clinically available and able to identify a deletion in about 65% of DMD cases and up to 85% of BMD cases by Southern blot and PCR. Deletions are more common in two hot spots, one in the distal portion of the gene between exons 44 and 53 (70%) and one more proximal between exons 2 and 20.[43]

Smaller rearrangements such as point mutations, nonsense mutations, and microdeletions are detected in 25% to 35% and duplications in about 5% to 10% of cases. The size of the deletion does not correlate with the severity of the clinical manifestations. Mutations that disrupt the mRNA reading frame lead to complete lack of dystrophin and cause the severe DMD phenotype, while in-frame mutations that allow for translation of some shorter but partially functional dystrophin with intact N and C termini cause the milder BMD phenotype. This "reading frame" rule is accurate in about 92% of cases in predicting phenotype severity.[44] Exceptions to this rule exist[45] and are likely due to exon-skipping and differences in intronic deletion breakpoints.

Confirmation of the diagnosis by DNA testing and knowledge of the specific mutation in each patient is very important for genetic counseling in the family members and because some of the new treatments that are presently being developed are mutation specific (e.g., splicing correction, exon skipping).

MUSCLE BIOPSY AND HISTOLOGY

Distinctive features characterize the muscle biopsy in Duchenne and Becker dystrophy: increased variability in fiber size, with both small and hypertrophied fibers, and altered fiber-type distribution consisting of type 1 fiber predominance and type 2B fiber deficiency. Type 2C fibers frequently appear. Mononuclear cells, commonly seen in the endomysial connective tissue and occasionally in the invading necrotic fibers, consist of 80% cytotoxic T cells and 20% macrophages.[46] Small groups of basophilic regenerating and necrotic fibers are a distinctive, common feature. Large, opaque, darkly stained fibers are very frequent and most likely result from segmental hypercontraction. These fibers often show small tears in the plasma membrane.[47] Proliferation of endomysial connective tissue (fibrosis) is a consistent feature that progresses over time. Fat gradually replaces degenerating muscle fibers. Internal nuclei and split fibers occur less often than in the other muscular dystrophies.

DYSTROPHIN ANALYSIS

Dystrophin is a cytoskeletal protein localized in the inner surface of the sarcolemma and is demonstrable by immune staining of fresh frozen sections using dystrophin antibodies.

Immune staining by using dystrophin antibodies shows complete or almost complete absence of dystrophin in Duchenne cases and reduced or patchy dystrophin stain in Becker cases (Figure 4–6). A mosaic pattern is seen in female carriers. Approximately 1% of the muscle fibers in DMD biopsies will demonstrate sarcolemmal staining. These dystrophin-positive fibers are called revertants (Figure 4–6C). They arise from spontaneous mutations superimposed on the underlying disease-causing mutation. This new mutation restores the reading frame and allows for dystrophin expression in some muscle fibers.

Western blot analysis, a technique by which electrophoresis of muscle components measures proteins with specific molecular weights, is the best method to detect reduced amounts or variants of dystrophin with lower molecular weights.[48]

ELECTROMYOGRAPHY AND NERVE CONDUCTION STUDIES

Electromyography (EMG) can differentiate between a myopathic process and a neurogenic disorder, but in current practice it is no longer used as a diagnostic tool for DBMD due to its low specificity and the improved sensitivity and availability of DNA testing. If done, it shows fibrillation potentials and positive sharp waves and short-duration, low-amplitude, polyphasic, and rapidly recruited motor unit potentials consistent with a myopathy with muscle fiber irritability. Decreased insertional activity and reduced number of motor units are seen in the advance stages of the disease once muscle has been replaced by connective tissue. These findings occur late in many of the muscular dystrophies and do not differentiate DBMD from other forms of muscular dystrophies or inflammatory myopathies. Sensory and motor nerve conduction studies are usually normal.

Treatment

Treatment for DBMD is targeted at prolonging ambulation for as long as possible and preventing and managing the secondary complications, especially respiratory failure, cardiomyopathy, and scoliosis. Corticosteroids are the only treatment option currently available.[49,50] Corticosteroids and noninvasive ventilatory support have changed the natural history of and significantly improved life expectancy in DMD, and the majority of patients now survive into adulthood.[51–54]

Prospective, randomized, controlled clinical trials have demonstrated that prednisone increases muscle strength, improves motor performance and pulmonary function, and slows the progression of the disease in boys between 5 and 15 years.[49,50,55–60] Studies ranged between 6 and 18 months in duration and included patients between 5 and 15 years old. The Report of the Quality Standards Subcommittee of the American Academy of Neurology and the Practice Committee of the Child Neurology Society, as well as a Cochrane Review, concluded that prednisone at a dose of 0.75 mg/kg/day should be offered as treatment to all patients with DMD.[49,50] Use of a higher dose of 1.5 mg/kg/day does not add more benefit, and a lower dose of 0.3 mg/kg/day is less beneficial but still effective. Although best evidence supports a daily regimen as the most effective,[57] alternate day dosing and intermittent dosing of 10 days on/10 days off and a high dose (5 mg/kg) twice weekly are also currently used in practice.[57,61–65] Deflazacort at a dose of 0.9 mg/kg/day produces similar effects in muscle strength and function in DMD but is not currently FDA approved in the United States.[66–70] Limited data suggests that starting corticosteroids before age 5 is more effective. Corticosteroid therapy is currently recommended to be initiated between the age of 5 and 15, although many experts in the field in more recent years have started using steroids before age 5 when symptoms and signs first become evident.[63,64,71–74] There is insufficient evidence regarding the optimal duration of treatment and whether treatment should be continued after ambulation is lost; however, in recent years, many recommend continuing corticosteroid treatment in nonambulatory patients due to some evidence for beneficial effects on upper extremities and cardiopulmonary function, and for delay in scoliosis development.[68,75]

Despite class 1 evidence of the therapeutic effectiveness of corticosteroids treatment in DMD, many patients still do not receive this treatment as part of their standard of care,[76] and there is no agreed-upon optimum regimen.[77]

The most common side effects are weight gain, development of a Cushingoid facial appearance, and slowed growth. Side effects should be fully discussed with the patient and his or her family, and strategies to prevent weight gain and optimize bone health should be implemented prior to initiating corticosteroid treatment. If side effects develop from daily prednisone, the dose is often decreased to a minimum of 0.3 mg/kg/day; if the side effects are still unmanageable at this lower dose, consideration should be given to discontinuation or to switching to either deflazacort or an intermittent schedule of prednisone.[78]

Comprehensive care recommendations have been published to provide a framework of standardization for corticosteroids use and management of side effects among practitioners involved in the multidisciplinary care of patients with DMD.[78,79] Treatment with corticosteroids requires commitment from the patients, their family, and all the care providers involved in order to be most effective. There is a clinical trial in progress comparing the three most frequent regimens used in DMD; standard measures to prevent corticosteroid side effects and addresses complications of DMD are part of this study.[77]

Other Drugs and Supplements

Creatine supplementation in the mdx mouse model for DMD decreased muscle necrosis and stress-induced elevation of intracellular calcium, increased myogenesis, and improved mitochondrial respiration.[80] Based on the results of this study, a double-blind randomized trial of creatine 0.10 mg/kg/day in boys with DMD showed an increase in hand grip strength and free-fat mass.[81] However, a second randomized, placebo-controlled, double-blind, three-arm trial compared creatine 5 g/day or glutamine 0.6 g/kg/day to placebo in ambulatory boys with Duchenne aged 4 to 10 and found no difference in the primary outcome measures of manual and quantitative muscle strength. Creatine was well tolerated.[82] There is currently no consensus recommendation about use of creatine in DMD. If creatine is used, good hydration should be maintained and kidney function should be monitored. Creatine should be stopped in case of kidney dysfunction.

Coenzyme Q10 (CoQ10) is a potent antioxidant that has shown to preserve muscle strength in mdx mice.[83] An open label pilot trial in steroid-treated boys with DMD showed an 8.5% increase in total quantitative muscle test.[84] Larger controlled studies have not been done, and there is no consensus on the use of CoQ10 for the treatment of DMD. Losartan, an angiotensin II type 1 receptor blocker improved muscle regeneration, decreased fibrosis, and significantly slowed disease progression in the diaphragm, cardiac, and gastrocnemius muscles of mdx mice.[85-88] Clinical trials of losartan in boys with DMD have not been done.

Respiratory Care

Patients with DMD should be proactively monitored for the expected complications caused by the progressive weakness of respiratory muscles at the different stages of the disease: weak cough, nocturnal hypoventilation and disturbed sleep, diurnal hypoventilation, and respiratory failure. The use of nocturnal noninvasive nasal ventilation and assisted cough has changed the natural history and prolonged life expectancy in DMD.[52,54] Detailed guidelines for respiratory management in the different disease stages of DMD are available.[89-91] In the ambulatory phase of the disease, yearly monitoring of FVC is usually sufficient and should start at age 6. In the nonambulatory phase of FVC, PCF and maximum inspiratory and expiratory pressures should be monitored twice a year. Manual or mechanical assisted cough should be used when respiratory infection is present and PCF is < 270 L/min, when baseline PCF is < 160 L/min or maximum expiratory pressure is < 40 cm water, and when baseline FVC is < 40% or < 1.25 L in older teenagers/young adults. Nocturnal noninvasive ventilation is indicated whenever signs and symptoms of hypoventilation are present, when baseline SpO_2 is < 95% and/or end-tidal CO_2 is > 45 mm Hg while awake, when an apnea/hypopnea index is > 10 per hour on polysomnogram or four or more episodes of SpO_2 <92% or drops in SpO_2 of at least 4% per hour of sleep.[79] Tracheostomy should be discussed in the nonambulatory phase of disease so that the patient and his family have time to learn about this option and decide based on preference. Tracheostomy should be considered when noninvasive ventilation is not tolerated or feasible, whenever there is failure to achieve extubation during a critical illness or perioperatively, and when there is recurrent aspiration of secretions into the lungs with drops of SpO_2 < 95% despite cough assistance.[79,90,91] Long-term use of noninvasive ventilation up to 24 hours/day should be considered as an alternative option to tracheostomy in eligible patients.[92]

Immunization with 23-valent pneumococcal polysaccharide vaccine should be given to all patients 2 years and older. Yearly immunization with trivalent inactivated influenza vaccine is indicated in all patients 6 months and older. These vaccines are not live vaccines and therefore are safe in patients taking corticosteroids.

Treatment of respiratory infection should be prompt and include assisted cough and antibiotics whenever cultures are positive or oxygen saturation < 95%. Hypoxemia from atelectasis, hypoventilation, and difficulty mobilizing secretions is best treated with noninvasive ventilatory support and assisted cough. Supplemental oxygen therapy should be used with caution as it may exacerbate hypercapnea by reducing central respiratory drive.

Other considerations in respiratory management are discussed in chapter 13; particular note should be taken of the value of glossopharyngeal breathing and of the need to monitor FVC without its aid.[93]

Perioperative Management

Patients with DMD and a FVC < 50% undergoing surgery with anesthesia or sedation should be trained preoperatively in the use of manual or mechanically assisted cough and noninvasive ventilation to reduce the postoperative risk of failure of extubation, atelectasis, and pneumonia.[90,94] Depolarizing muscle relaxants such as succinylcholine and inhalation anesthetic agents should be avoided due to the risk for fatal reactions, malignant hyperthermialike reaction, hyperkalemia, and rhabdomyolysis.[95-97]

Cardiac Care

Guidelines for the cardiac care of patients with Duchenne dystrophy are available.[98,99] Baseline cardiac evaluation is currently recommended to be done at diagnosis or by age 6 years with electrocardiogram and an echocardiogram. Biannual follow-up screenings are recommended until age 10. Yearly cardiac assessment should be done starting at age 10 or as soon as cardiac signs and symptoms arise.[79] Ventricular abnormalities should prompt initiation of angiotensin-converting-enzyme inhibitors as first-line therapy; beta-blockers and diuretics are also used.[100-104] Established guidelines for the management of heart failure should be followed.[98,105,106] Some studies suggest that starting treatment before any signs of abnormal cardiac function are evident can delay the onset of cardiomyopathy.[107–109] The best time for inititation of cardiac medications is uncertain.[110]

Cardiac transplant is an option in milder BMD phenotypes with prominent and early symptomatic cardiomyopathy that develop before loss of ambulation and while the muscle weakness is still mild.[111–114]

Bone Health and Orthopedic Management

Vitamin D levels should be assessed annually and vitamin D replacement should be used for documented deficiency. Daily calcium intake in the diet should be review and supplementation considered.

Dual-energy X-ray absorptiometry (DEXA) should be obtained annually in patients with a history of fractures and in patients taking corticosteroids.

Long bone and vertebral fractures are common in DMD. Treatment strategies and consensus guidelines are available.[89,115-117] Back pain should prompt spine X-ray to rule out vertebral fractures. Vertebral fractures should be treated with intravenous bisphosphonate. There is currently no consensus on the use of oral bisphosphonates for the prevention or treatment of fractures in DMD.

Severe fractures of the lower extremities in ambulatory patients should be treated with internal fixation if necessary, and prompt and careful rehabilitation should follow the surgery to maximize the chance of resuming ambulation. In nonambulatory patients splinting and casting is appropriate if there is severe pain.

Scoliosis occurs in the majority of wheelchair-bound Duchenne patients.[118,119] Monitoring should be done by clinical exam during the ambulatory phase, and by radiography when the patient begins using a wheelchair full time. Surgery should be considered when the Cobb angle is between 20° and 40°, and before cardiac and respiratory functions have declined to a point that makes surgery too risky. Corticosteroid treatment significantly decreases the risk of scoliosis.[75] Surgical spinal instrumentation and fusion correct the scoliosis, help preventing further deformity and respiratory restriction, and improve sitting and comfort. Some of the function in the upper extremities can be lost after spinal fusion and this possibility needs to be discussed with the patient and family prior to surgery.

Heel-cord lengthening or tenotomy to correct severe equinus foot deformity should be considered in nonambulatory patients with the goal of improving pain and pressure and skin breakdown, or to allow the patient to wear shoes or to better position himself or herself in the wheelchair and during pivot transfers.[120,121]

Surgical interventions are not effective in improving or preserving independent ambulation in the late ambulatory phase of the disease.

Nutrition

Education of patients and their families about the importance of maintaining a healthy weight is important for the long-term management of DMD. Strategies to maintain a weight or BMI for age between the 10th and the 85th percentile of national percentile charts should be discussed and implemented throughout the disease. Enrolling the expertise of a nutritionist may be helpful at different stages of the disease and especially prior to initiation of corticosteroid treatment. Analysis of the patient's diet can reveal a need for specific vitamins or food supplements. Particular attention should be given to the daily calcium intake as patients with DMD are more prone to osteopenia and fractures. Daily fiber intake is an important tool for management of the constipation common in DMD.[89]

Physical Therapy

A physical therapy program should be introduced early in the course of the disease to gradually familiarize the patient and the family with the long-term need for exercises to prevent contractures, and with adaptive devices to maximize mobility and independence. Regular active, active-assisted, or passive stretching at the ankles, knees, and hip is important in both ambulatory and nonambulatory phases and should be done at school and/or at home, ideally every day but at least 4 to 6 days per week.[122-124] During the nonambulatory phase, stretching of the wrist, elbows, and fingers and the use of hand splints should be started to preserve and maximize upper extremity function.[89] Occupational therapy evaluation is very helpful to address tasks related to dressing, driving, and computer use, and to recommend an adaptive plan at home, school, and work, such as angled writing surfaces and adjustable tables, modified utensils, and other equipment for environmental control.

Aquatic therapy can maintain mobility, strength, and flexibility and provides aerobic exercise to promote cardiopulmonary fitness.

A physical therapist or other expert familiar with Duchenne dystrophy should be involved in ordering a wheelchair that is best designed to optimize mobility in the community, provides truncal support and best positioning of the lower extremities, and preferably allows for tilting.

The regular use of a standing frame should be introduced while the patient can still walk to facilitate standing after ambulation is lost and to help prevent contractures, scoliosis, osteopenia, and decubitus ulcers. Using the tilting capability of a wheelchair to get into a standing position is an alternative to standing frames. Ankle-foot orthotics (AFOs) during the day are not indicated in ambulatory patients as they can compromise the ability to walk by limiting toe-walking, which is a compensatory mechanism for weakness of the quadriceps. Some experts advocate for the use of AFOs at nighttime but there is no uniform agreement among providers at this point due to lack of definitive evidence. Use of AFOs in conjunction with stretching may be helpful in the ambulatory phase to prevent ankle contractures. Use of AFOs during the day may be helpful to prevent ankle contractures and foot deformities in full-time wheelchair users and to help with standing and limited walking in part-time wheelchair users. Knee-ankle-foot orthotics may prolong assisted walking and standing.[125,126]

In the late phase of the disease when transfers have become difficult, the use of a mobile or overhead tracking hoist should be introduced to transfer patients into the shower, wheelchair, and bed and to the toilet. Teaching the proper use of such devices to caregivers is important to prevent excessive abdominal pressure and incorrect body positioning during transfers that might lead to anxiety and respiratory compromise.

Speech, Cognitive, and Behavioral Management

Assessment of speech and language should be done at the time of diagnosis and thereafter at each clinic visit, and a referral to speech and language therapy should be initiated as soon as a delay in speech or language development is suspected. Neuropsychological assessment should be done prior to entering school to identify deficits and to create an individualized education plan. Pharmacological treatment with stimulants should be considered for concomitant ADHD. Selective serotonin reuptake inhibitors are used for anxiety, depression, and obsessive-compulsive disorder. In patients displaying aggression and anger outbursts, mood stabilizers are indicated.[78]

Palliative Care

Palliative care should be considered in the late stage of the disease to help with difficult treatment decisions about end-stage respiratory failure and cardiomyopathy and to clarify goals of care.[127-131] Palliative teams can provide emotional and spiritual support to patients and their families and help coping with grief and loss.[78]

Therapies Under Investigation

GENE REPLACEMENT THERAPY

Gene therapy in DMD has been challenging due to the large size of the dystrophin gene. Gene therapy for DMD may be possible with a mini-dystrophin gene less than 4 kilobases (kb) that fits into an adeno-associated virus (AAV) vector and translates a smaller but functional dystrophin protein.[132-135]

Delivery of a functional mini-dystrophin transgene in six boys with DMD by biceps intramuscular injection showed evidence of transient but not long-term transgene expression due to the unexpected T-cell immunity targeting self- and non-self dystrophin epitopes.[136] Revertant fibers, which were thought to induce tolerance, may in fact play an important role in priming and sustaining this immune response and further study of this possibility is needed.[137] Mendell's pivotal study identified cellular immunity as the next challenge that needs to be overcome in order for dystrophin gene replacement to be successful.

Gene therapy by vascular delivery is also being actively studied for possible human clinical trials.[138-143]

SUPPRESSION OF STOP CODONS

Gene manipulation using small molecules targeted at RNA modulation to restore the reading frame and produce full-length functional dystrophin is being actively pursued in parallel with gene replacement therapy. Suppression of stop codon mutations is one of these alternative molecular strategies. The possible therapeutic role of this novel therapeutic strategy is reserved to the 15% of patients in whom the disease is caused by a stop codon mutation.[144, 145]

The therapeutic potential of gentamicin has been demonstrated in preclinical studies in the mdx mouse and in a 6-month clinical trial in patients with DMD caused by stop codon mutations. This trial showed significant improvement in dystrophin expression levels, stabilization of muscle weakness, and mild improvement in FVC,[146,147] but the associated renal toxicity and the need for intravenous administration limited clinical effectiveness and further development of this treatment.

Ataluren is an oral agent that selectively induces ribosomal read-through of premature disease-causing stop codons while still respecting normal stop codons. Ataluren restores full-length dystrophin expression in skeletal and cardiac muscle, and improves muscle function in the mdx mice treated for 2 to 8 weeks.[148,149] Ataluren treatment in a phase 2a open-label trial in DMD increased dystrophin in the extensor digitorum brevis (EDB) muscle of 23 out of 38 patients (61%) after 28 days (mean increase = 11.1%).[150]

A double-blind placebo-controlled phase 2b trial in ambulatory patients aged 5 years or older showed improvement in 6 minutes' walk, the primary outcome measure for this 48-week trial.[151]

A phase 3 trial is currently ongoing, and FDA approval will depend on the results of this trial and further analysis of the results of the phase 2b open-label extension phase.

EXON SKIPPING

Exon skipping allows restoration of the mRNA reading frame and dystrophin expression by omitting one or more exons. Skipping of specific exons corrects a series of different deletions. For example, skipping of exon 51 is applicable to about 13% of all deletions (del. 45–50, 47–50, 48–50, 49–50, 50, 52, 52–63). Skipping 9 other exons will correct about 70% of all mutations.

Preclinical efficacy of exon skipping has been demonstrated in the mdx and dog animal models.[152,153] Skipping exon 51 with an antisense oligonucleotide (PRO051) and a morpholino oligomer (AVI-4658) delivered directly into muscle has been studied in two human clinical trials and has shown restoration of dystrophin expression.[154,155] Further studies using systemic delivery of PRO051 and AVI-4658 have also been carried out and showed both agents to be well tolerated. Weekly subcutaneous administration of PRO051 for 5 weeks showed dystrophin expression in the majority of muscle fibers in 10 out of 12 patients and a mild improvement in the 6-minute walk test.[156,157] Weekly intravenous delivery of AVI-4658 (eteplirsen) for 12 weeks in a phase 2 dose escalation study showed safety and biochemical efficacy, and a variable range of new dystrophin expression from 8.9% to 16.4% in 7 out of 19 patients.[157] These results are encouraging and have prompted the planning of currently ongoing multicenter phase 3 clinical trials.

EMERY-DREIFUSS MUSCULAR DYSTROPHY

Emery-Dreifuss muscular dystrophy (EDMD) was recognized as an entity distinct from Duchenne and Becker dystrophies in 1966.[158] Dreifuss and Hogan had identified many of the typical clinical features of EDMD in 1961,[159] and subsequent reports have further emphasized its distinctive phenotype.[160-164] Due to the frequent cardiac manifestations and risk for sudden cardiac death characteristic of EDMD, early diagnosis is important.

Genetics

EDMD is inherited most frequently in an X-linked or autosomal-dominant manner; genetically confirmed AR-EDMD due to homozygous *LMNA* mutation is rare.[165,166]

The overall prevalence of EDMD is not known but XL-EDMD prevalence is estimated at 1:100,000 and XL-EDMD is considered the third most common X-linked dystrophy (after Duchenne and Becker muscular dystrophy).[167]

Mutations in three genes cause the EDMD phenotype: the *EMD* gene (Xq28) encoding emerin and the *FHL1* gene (Xq26.3) encoding FHL1 for XL-EDMD, and the *LMNA* gene (1q22) encoding lamins A/C for AD-EDMD and AR-EDMD. These genes encode proteins that localize to the nuclear membrane or to the nucleoplasm and cytoplasm.

In normal individuals emerin is expressed in the inner nuclear membrane and can be detected in muscle biopsy, skin biopsy, lymphocytes, and buccal cells by western blot and immunofluorescence. Emerin is absent in 95% of patients with XL-EDMD.[168]

Three isoforms of FHL1 are expressed in the nucleus and cytoplasm where they can be detected by western blot and immunofluorescence in myoblasts, muscle biopsy, fibroblasts, and cardiomyocytes. In patient with XL-EDMD caused by mutation in the FHL1 gene, FHL1 protein is absent or decreased.[169]

Lamins A/C are expressed in the nuclear membrane and in the nucleoplasm. Mutations in the *LMNA* gene account for less than 50% of AD-EDMD cases, suggesting that other genes not yet identified are involved in EDMD.[170,171]

When trying to confirm a diagnosis of EDMD, if the family history points to a pattern of inheritance, defects for *EMD* and *FHL1* should be tested first in suspected XL-EDMD, and *LMNA* defects should be tested in AD or AR-EDMD. When family history is absent, emerin expression should be tested first in males to help distinguish XL from AD-EDMD

and guide DNA testing. Because it is rare for XL-EDMD female carriers to manifest symptoms, female patients should be tested for *LMNA* mutations first.

Defects in the *LMNA* gene account for many allelic disorders referred as laminopathies, including some affecting the skeletal muscle (*LGMD1B*, LMNA-related congenital muscular dystrophy), the peripheral nerve (*CMT2B1*), the heart (AD dilated cardiomyopathy with conduction system defects), and other tissues (progeria syndromes, mandibuloacral dysplasia, Dunningam partial lypodystrophy).[172]

Other emerinopathies include a form of rare X-linked LGMD[173] and an X-linked cardiac disease with sinus node disease and atrial fibrillation.[174]

Allelic disorders caused by a defect in the *FHL1* gene include X-linked scapuloperoneal myopathy,[175] some cases of rigid spine syndrome,[176] X-linked hypertrophic cardiomyopathy,[169,177] and reducing body myopathy.[178]

Clinical Features

EDMD is characterized by the clinical triad of early joint contractures, slowly progressive muscle weakness and wasting, and cardiac arrhythmias and/or cardiomyopathy. Contractures of elbow flexors, neck extensors, and Achilles tendons develop early in the course of the disease, usually in the first two decades in both XL-EDMD and AD-EDMD (Figure 4–7A & B). In XL-EDMD contractures are usually the first sign of the disease and precede the onset of muscle weakness. In AD-EDMD contractures may develop after the onset of muscle weakness. Contractures of neck extensors cause limitation of neck flexion and can progress to limit the movement of the entire spine, which can then contribute to the loss of ambulation when combined with the lower extremity contractures and weakness. Scoliosis is rare. Neck extension involvement from weakness and contracture is a consistent clinical sign in EDMD especially due to lamins A/C mutations. Limb muscle weakness and wasting are slowly progressive and start in a humero-peroneal distribution and progress into the scapular and hip girdle muscles (Figure 4–7A & B). Toe walking, frequent falls, poor balance, and difficulty running are common. Loss of ambulation seldom occurs and then only late in the course of

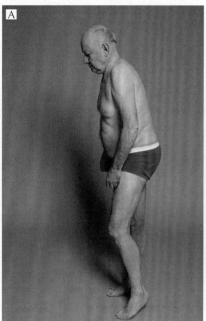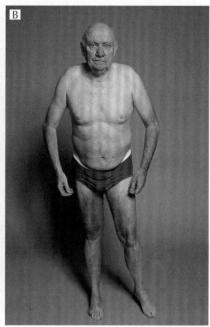

Figure 4–7. A and B: Man in his fifth decade with EDMD with typical elbow, neck, and knee contractures while still ambulatory.

AD-EDMD. Patients with XL-EDMD usually remain ambulatory.

Cardiac manifestations are potentially life-threatening and can affect even patients with minimal limb muscle weakness.[179] Patients may present with syncope, presyncope, or exercise intolerance. Arrhythmias include atrial fibrillation and atrial paralysis, as well as atrioventricular heart block varying from first degree to complete.[180,181] Dilated or hypertrophic cardiomyopathy is also common.[182,183] Patients with EDMD are at risk for embolic strokes, syncope, and sudden cardiac death.[184] Unpredictable cardiac death has been reported in patients without prior cardiac symptoms. Sudden death has also been reported in some cases despite pacemaker or defibrillator implant.[185-189] Carriers can occasionally have conduction defects.

Significant inter- and intrafamilial variation in the spectrum of clinical symptoms is common in EDMD, and it is more frequent in AD-EDMD than in XL-EDMD.[190] Some family members may present with only cardiac involvement, others with only muscle weakness and wasting, and some with only contractures. Cases with onset in the first few years of life and severe EDMD phenotype have been described. A floppy infant having a maternal uncle with onset of classic EDMD symptoms in his third decade has been described in a family with the same emerin mutation.[191]

Laboratory Features and Diagnostic Tests

Serum CK varies from normal to 20 times normal. Elevated CK concentration is more common in the early phase of the disease than in later stages. CK level may be normal in the autosomal-dominant EDMD due to mutations in the *LMNA* gene.

EMG usually shows nonspecific myopathic features and nerve conduction studies are normal. Motor unit potentials (MUPs) with longer duration, larger area, and increased amplitude and phases have been observed, suggesting a possible "neurogenic" variant of the disease.[160,192-194] Such neurogenic MUPs could result from reorganization of the motor unit and the increased variability of muscle fiber size and fiber density in this slowly progressive myopathy. EMG is seldom useful for diagnosis of EDMD due to lack of specificity.

Muscle CT and MRI in EDMD show fatty infiltration in the posterior thigh and posterior leg and can differentiate EDMD from other disorders with contractures such as collagen-VI-related myopathy.[195] In AD-EDMD due to lamin A/C mutations, muscle MRI shows a typical involvement of the posterior calf muscle with the medial head of the gastrocnemius predominantly involved and the lateral head relatively spared.[196-200] Muscle MRI can also show muscle abnormalities in cases with predominant cardiac symptoms and subclinical muscle involvement.[199]

Muscle histology shows nonspecific changes such as variation in fiber size, necrotic fibers, increased number and variation in size of myonuclei, and increase in endomysial and perimysial connective tissue.[201] Nuclear ultrastructural abnormalities including abnormal distribution of heterochromatin and loss of peripheral heterochromatin may be detected with electron microscopy.[202-204] Perivascular cuffing or endomysial and perimysial lymphocyte infiltration have been described in patients with *LMNA* mutations initially misdiagnosed as having childhood onset inflammatory myopathy.[205] Type 1 or 2 fiber disproportion can occur.[206]

In patients with XL-EDMD, muscle biopsy shows emerin absence in 95% of cases.[168,191] In female carriers of XL-EDMD, emerin nuclear immunostaining shows absence in a mosaic pattern. Emerin expression is normal in AD-EDMD.

In patients with AD-EDMD, lamins A/C are expressed normally at the nuclear membrane of skeletal and cardiac muscle due to the expression of the wild-type allele, and therefore this test is not useful to confirm the diagnosis of AD-EDMD.[207] Western blot analysis of lamins A/C may demonstrate normal level in many affected patients.[207]

In patients with XL-EDMD due to FHL1 mutations, FHL1 is absent or significantly decreased on immunofluorescence and western blot in fresh muscle biopsy, fibroblasts, and cardiomyocytes.[169]

Other muscle membrane proteins including dystrophin are normally detected in EDMD. Genetic testing is clinically available for mutation detection in the *EMD* gene (60% of XL-EDMD), *FHL1* gene (~10% of XL-EDMD), and *LMNA* gene (~45% of AD-EDMD).[172] Molecular confirmation of XL-EDMD or AD/AR-EDMD

diagnosis is important for accurate genetic counseling.

Dilated or hypertrophic cardiomyopathy is detected by echocardiography.

Various arrhythmias can be detected by EKG or 24-hour Holter monitor, including supraventricular and ventricular arrhythmias, atrial fibrillation, and atrioventricular and bundle-branch blocks.[188, 208]

Differential Diagnosis

While other muscular dystrophies can have similar scapulo-peroneal weakness, the development of joint contractures, cardiac arrhythmias, and cardiomyopathy occurs later. The concomitant triad of these clinical features is typical of EDMD. In the dystrophinopathies the contractures always follows the onset of muscle weakness and they never are the first sign of the disease; CK is always highly elevated, and cardiomyopathy is more frequent than conduction abnormalities and occurs usually in the advanced stage of the disease.

Bethlem myopathy caused by collagen VI gene mutations is characterized by proximal weakness and contractures but is not associated with cardiac abnormalities.

Rigid spine syndrome due to selenopathies usually presents with hypotonia and respiratory insufficiency. In X-linked vacuolar myopathy with cardiomyopathy (Danon disease), joint contractures and spine rigidity are not present.

Patients with EDMD with decreased spinal mobility and joint contractures as the main features may be misdiagnosed as having ankylosing spondylitis and be seen initially by a rheumatologist.[209]

Treatment

While there is no treatment for the underlying disease, early placement of pacemakers may be lifesaving. Early screening and detection of cardiac arrhythmias and cardiomyopathy is essential. Patients with EDMD should be screened with an EKG and an echocardiogram at the time of diagnosis and yearly thereafter. Holter monitor and electrophysiologic studies are indicated if there are cardiac symptoms. Antyarrhythmic drugs and pacemaker or cardioverter defibrillator implantation should be used as indicated for cardiac arrhythmias.[185] In patients with atrial fibrillation/flutter or atrial standstill, antithrombotic prophylaxis is recommended to prevent embolic strokes.[185] Pharmacological treatment of heart failure should follow standard guidelines. Cardiac transplant is a lifesaving option for end-stage heart failure indicated especially in those patients without severe skeletal or respiratory muscle weakness.[210,211]

Monitoring of pulmonary function annually and prior to any surgery is indicated.

Consultation with an orthopedic surgeon is appropriate for evaluation and consideration of surgical correction of joint contractures and scoliosis.

Physical therapy should focus on stretching exercises to help prevent contractures and strategies to improve mobility and maintain safe ambulation. Occupational therapy evaluation can improve function in the upper extremities when elbow and wrist contractures are a problem.

Potential difficulties and complications during anesthesia should be anticipated: difficult tracheal intubation (due to neck contractures), arrhythmias, and malignant hypertermia[212-216] as well as management of delivery by C-section in women with EDMD.[214,217]

THE MYOTONIC MUSCULAR DYSTROPHIES

The myotonic muscular dystrophies, unlike other common muscular dystrophies caused by abnormal expression of muscle membrane proteins, are caused by a toxic RNA–mediated gain-of-function. Abnormal expansion of a CTC repeat in myotonic dystrophy type 1 (DM1) and a CCTG in myotonic dystrophy Type 2 (DM2) leads to alteration of cellular function through alternative splicing of different genes due to the effect of the untranslated pathologic RNAs. This distinct and complex pathogenesis is associated with an equally complex phenotype that affects many tissues other than skeletal muscles, including brain, smooth muscle, eyes, heart, and the endocrine system.

DM1, originally described in 1909 and referred to as Steinert disease, is the most common muscular dystrophy in adults. In certain

regions such as Quebec, the disease reaches an incidence of almost 1 in 500. DM2 and proximal myotonic myopathy were originally thought to be clinically distinct entities but are now recognized as the same disease referred to as DM2.

Genetics

MYOTONIC DYSTROPHY TYPE 1

DM1 is caused by an unstable expansion of a CTG repeat on chromosome 19q13.3 in the untranslated region of the *DMPK* gene.[218,219] The accumulation of toxic RNA in the nucleus leads to disruption of alternative splicing with reversion to embryonic form of some proteins: the chloride channel, resulting in myotonia[220]; the insulin receptor, resulting in insulin resistance[221]; and the microtubule-associated protein tau, encoded by *MAPT*, a gene associated with cognitive function.[222] Misregulated splicing and altered gating of the Ca (V) 1.1. calcium channel is correlated with the severity of weakness in the tibialis anterior muscle of patients with DM1.[223] This misregulated splicing of many gene transcripts is mediated by sequestration of two muscleblind RNA-CUG binding proteins, CUG-BP and MBNL1, by the expanded repeats.[224,225] The disease is inherited in an autosomal-dominant manner. Normal alleles have 5 to 34 CTG repeats. Alleles with 50 or more CTG repeats are always associated with disease manifestations. Individuals with 35 to 49 CTG repeats in the premutation range do not have symptoms,[226] but their children have a greater risk of inheriting a larger repeat and being affected. Larger CTG expansions are associated with more severe disease and earlier onset of symptoms.[227] The *DMPK* CTG repeat is mitotically unstable and may expand during meiosis causing more severe and earlier onset disease in successive generations.[228,229] Anticipation is most common with maternal transmission, but possible with paternal transmission. Congenital DM1, a more severe form of the disease with manifestations starting in utero, is caused by very large expansions usually greater than 1,000 and is almost always inherited through maternal transmission.[230,231]

Prevalence worldwide is approximately 1:20,000 but much higher in certain regions such as Quebec due to a founder effect.[232]

Penetrance is almost 100% by age 50. *De novo* mutations due to expansion of a normal allele with < 34 repeats into the abnormal range are rare. *DMPK* is the only gene in which mutations are known to cause DM1.

MYOTONIC DYSTROPHY TYPE 2

DM2 is inherited in an autosomal-dominant manner and it is caused by an expansion of a CCTG repeat in exon 1 of the *CNBP* gene on chromosome 3q21.3 (previously known as *ZNF9*) encoding cellular nucleic acid–binding protein (zinc finger protein 9).[233] Pathogenic alleles contain between 75 and 11,000 CCTG repeats, with a usual mean of 5,000.[234] This is the only gene in which mutations are known to cause DM2, and DM2 is the only phenotype known to be associated with defects in *CNBP*. The exact prevalence of DM2 is not known as this disease is still underdiagnosed and misdiagnosed. Prevalence is higher in people of Northern European origin, in Germany and Poland, and in Finland, where DM2 is more common than DM1. Penetrance is almost 100%. There is no significant correlation between the number of the pathologic CCTG repeats and the disease severity or the age at onset of clinical manifestations.[235] There is no congenital form of DM2.[236] Current molecular testing techniques that include routine PCR and Southern blot have a detection sensitivity of 99%.

Clinical Features

DM1

The appearance of myotonic dystrophy patients can be so characteristic that a diagnosis becomes evident at first glance. Temporalis muscle wasting, hollow cheeks from masseter muscle atrophy, frontal baldness, ptosis, and facial weakness produce a typical "hatchet-faced" appearance (Figure 4–8). Distal limb muscles and neck flexors and sternocleidomastoids are involved early. Hand function is impaired by the myotonia and the weakness of the wrist and finger extensors, and the intrinsic hand muscles. Triceps are commonly weaker than biceps. Ankle dorsiflexion weakness may cause a foot drop, which can be mistaken for a peripheral neuropathy. The proximal muscles remain stronger than

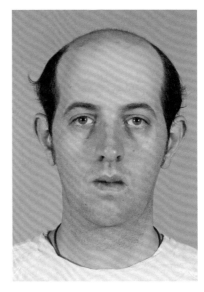

Figure 4–8. Typical facial features of DM1 with temporal wasting and frontal bolding.

the distal ones throughout the course, although the quadriceps muscles may undergo preferential atrophy and weakness at any time. The combination of weakness in knee extension and ankle dorsiflexion causes "back kneeing" (genu recurvatum). Palatal, pharyngeal, and tongue involvement produces a dysarthric speech, a nasal voice, and swallowing problems. Tongue atrophy can be severe.

Myotonia seldom causes complaints from patients with DM1 but has helpful, diagnostic importance. Myotonia can be easily detected by percussion of the thenar, wrist extensor, and tongue muscles (percussion myotonia) or by evaluation of grip release (grip myotonia). Tongue myotonia can be elicited by percussion of a tongue blade placed across the tongue (Figure 4–9A & B), producing sustained contraction ("napkin ring sign"). Handgrip myotonia improves with repeated contractures ("warm-up phenomenon"). Myotonia, clinical and electrical, does not develop until after age 5.

Cardiac

Cardiac involvement including heart failure, atrial or ventricular tachyarrhythmias, and atrioventricular conduction disease occur in 30% of DM1 patients.[237, 238] Both AV block and ventricular tachyarrhythmias are a common

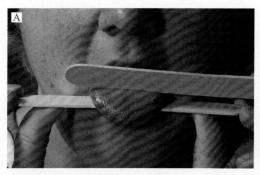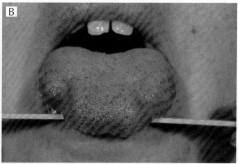

Figure 4–9. Myotonia demonstrated by percussion of the tongue (A) producing a sustained typical contracture or "napkin ring signs" (B).

cause of sudden death and early mortality. EKG with a rhythm other than sinus, PR interval of 240 ms or more, QRS duration of 120 ms or more, or second-degree or third-degree atrioventricular block, predict sudden death.[237] Cardiomyopathy and congestive heart failure occur far less frequently than conduction disturbances. Heart failure, if present, usually results from cor pulmonale secondary to respiratory failure and hypoxia (see chapter 13).

Sleep and Respiratory

Excessive daytime sleepiness (EDS) is the most common nonmuscular complaint in DM1and is frequently disabling.[239] Some DM1 patients have REM dysregulation on polysomnogram and multiple sleep latency test similar to narcolepsy without cataplexy.[240] However, the pathophysiology of this sleep disturbance is distinct from narcolepsy as patients with DM1 do not have a defect of hypocretin (Hcrt) release or Hcrt receptor splicing.[241] Patients with otherwise very mild disease and subclinical muscle weakness may experience daytime hypersomnolence and abnormal sleep patterns severe enough to cause inability to hold a job or participate in school. Obstructive and central sleep apneas, nocturnal hypoventilation, and diurnal ventilatory insufficiency and hypercapnea are common.[242,243]

Progressive restrictive lung disease is present in 34% of patients and correlates with the degree of skeletal muscle weakness, CTG repeat expansion size, and body mass index.[244] Neuromuscular respiratory failure is the most common cause of death.[237,238]

Perioperative pulmonary complications are common and include acute ventilatory failure,

apnea, atelectasis, pneumonia, and failure to extubate.[245,246] Sensitivity to anesthetic and sedating medications is common in DM1 as compared to DM2, especially with suxamethonium, thiopentone, neostigmine, and halothane.[245,247,248]

DM1 is associated with increased obstetric risks including preterm delivery (31%), abnormal fetal presentation (35%), and labor abnormalities in all three stages with increased number of operative deliveries (Cesarean section rate = 36%).[249-251] Severe urinary tract infections are also common (19%).[251]

CNS

Impaired visual-spatial processing, low IQ, abnormal executive function, depression, apathy, and avoidant personality are all common in DM1.[252,253] Frontal lobe function worsens overtime.[254] Single-photon emission computed tomography of the brain showed frontal and parieto-occipital hypoperfusion.[255] Brain MRI shows white-matter hyperintense lesions with a typical temporo-insular pattern.[256-259] Cognitive and radiographic changes are less frequent in DM2 patients.

Eyes

Iridescent multicolored posterior capsular lens opacities ("Christmas tree cataracts") are common in adult DM1 and they usually occur before age 50.[260] They can usually be seen by direct ophthalmoscopy, although some will be appreciated only by slit lamp evaluation. Cataracts may be the sole sign in very mildly affected family members with low numbers of CTG repeats. Over time cataracts becomes symptomatic and interfere with vision. Less common ocular abnormalities include retinal pigmentary degeneration (peripheral or involving the macula), low intraocular pressure, extraocular muscle myotonia, and extraocular muscle weakness. Meibomian cysts occur often and may require surgical resection.

Endocrine abnormalities are common in DM1, including hyperparathyroidism with increased PTH, type 2 diabetes, hyperinsulinism, thyroid dysfunction, androgen insufficiency, and abnormal growth hormone secretion.[261] Testicular atrophy with fibrosis of the seminiferous tubules is common. Male patients with impotence often have decreased plasma testosterone levels; androgen administration may restore potency. No evidence, however, suggests that androgen deficiency contributes to muscle weakness.[262] As the disease progresses, infertility occurs in both males and females. Women may have a high rate of fetal loss.[249,251] The frequent occurrence of cranial hyperostosis in DM1 may be mistaken, especially in men, for an underlying brain tumor such as meningioma.

Symptoms affecting many regions of the gastrointestinal tract occur in as many as 80% of patients with DM1. In the upper digestive tract, dyspepsia, heartburn, and dysphagia are most common. Oropharyngeal dysphagia and esophageal motility disorders are a common cause of aspiration pneumonia.[46] Impaired swallowing, posing a risk for aspiration, can result from delayed relaxation of pharyngeal muscles. Dysphagia may result from diminished esophageal motility associated with dilatation of the esophagus.[263] In the lower GI tract, abdominal pain, bloating, and constipation are common. Reduced colon motility leads to megacolon and fecal impaction, and the anal sphincter may undergo reflex myotonic contractions.[264]

Patients with DM1 have an increased risk of cancer overall, and especially in the endometrium, brain, ovary, and colon.[265,266]

The most common causes of death in DM1 are pneumonia, respiratory failure, sudden cardiac death, cardiovascular disease, and cancer.[238,267] Patients sometimes die from falling asleep while driving due to the pathologic EDS.

DM2

The distribution of muscle weakness in DM2 is more proximal than in DM1 and hip flexors, hip extensors, neck flexors, and finger flexors are often the most affected muscles.[268-270] The muscle wasting is not as pronounced as in DM1. Myotonia, clinically and electromyographically, is not as easily and consistently detected as in DM1. Widespread musculoskeletal pain is a typical symptom in DM2.[271] Facial weakness is not as prominent as in DM1. Cognitive impairment and radiologic abnormalities are not as pronounced as in DM1.[256] There is no congenital form of DM2.

CONGENITAL DM1

Congenital DM1 presents in utero with decreased fetal movement, uni- or bilateral talipes, and polyhydramnios.[272] It is caused by a large number of CTG repeats, almost always inherited from the mother. Mothers of newborns affected by congenital DM1 may be only mildly affected and still undiagnosed at the time of pregnancy. After delivery, affected infants have severe generalized weakness and hypotonia, club foot, weak cry, inability to feed, failure to thrive, and a typical "tented mouth" due to severe facial weakness[273] (Figure 4–10). Clinical and electromyographic myotonia is not present at this stage. Respiratory failure is common and may require prolonged ventilatory support and tracheostomy. Mortality rate from respiratory failure is 25% in the first year of life.[274] Infants surviving the first year will experience slow improvement in muscle strength and motor function during childhood and are eventually able to walk. This improvement is eventually followed by the typical progressive muscle weakness and wasting and multiorgan involvement as in the adult form of the disease. Cognitive impairment, frequently severe, is present in up to 60% of cases.

Laboratory Features and Diagnostic Tests

Serum CK level may be normal or mildly elevated in DM1 and DM2.

EMG evidence of typical waxing-waning myotonia is readily found in most muscles of patients affected with DM1 and is helpful in identifying family members with mild clinical symptoms. In patients with DM2, myotonia may be absent in some muscles, or have

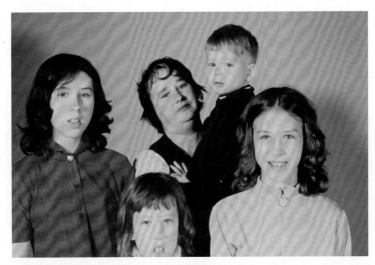

Figure 4–10. Mother with mild DM1 and her four children. The two girls on the left both have the congenital form of DM1, whereas the other two children have not inherited the disease.

a waning pattern only, and can be therefore often missed on EMG.[275] In some cases myotonia can be mistaken by waning p waves and interpreted as a sign of acute denervation, leading to the wrong diagnosis of motor neuron disease. In some patients with a mild, not yet diagnosed form of the disease, the myotonia may be discovered incidentally during an EMG ordered for other reasons, and this can lead to an unexpected diagnosis of DM1 or DM2. In evaluating a floppy infant for congenital DM1, however, it is important to note that myotonia will not be present at this stage and does not appear until after age 5 or older. In this situation the mother should be examined, and if a clinical diagnosis of DM1 cannot be made on the basis of clinical features, a maternal EMG may be helpful to look for myotonia.

Myopathic features with low-amplitude, short duration, polyphasic MUPs are usually present in weak muscles of affected patients with DM1 and DM2.

There is no single feature diagnostic of DM1 or DM2 on muscle biopsy. Muscle atrophy, selectively involving type 1 fibers, occurs in about 50% of DM1 cases, whereas preferential type 2 fiber atrophy has been reported in DM2. Increased numbers of central nuclei are typical. Fiber atrophy may be so severe that only nuclear clamps remain. Ring fibers and sarcoplasmic masses (homogeneous areas of disorganized myofibrillar material) occur with increased frequency. Necrosis of muscle fibers

and increased connective tissue, common in other muscular dystrophies, are uncommon in DM1 and DM2. Muscle biopsy is not necessary to make the diagnosis of DM1 or DM2 due to the high sensitivity and clinical availability of DNA testing.

Molecular genetic testing is the test of choice to confirm the diagnosis in DM1 and DM2. In DM1 patientsm expanded CTG repeats ≥ 50 on 19q13.3 can be detected in 100% of cases.

In DM2 molecular genetic testing from peripheral blood is able to detect the abnormal *CNBP* CCTG expansion and confirm the diagnosis in 99% of cases. CCTG repeat expansions ≥ 75 are considered disease-causing mutations.

Genetic testing is not necessary in patients with definite clinical features of DM1 or DM2 and a first-degree family relative with a positive genetic test. Best practice guidelines are available for clinical molecular genetic analysis and reporting in DM1 and DM2, including presymptomatic and prenatal testing.[276]

In DM1 and DM2, many laboratory abnormalities are common including elevated liver function test, abnormal cholesterol panels, and low albumin and red and white cell counts.[277,278]

Differential Diagnosis

DM2 has a more benign phenotype than DM1 with more proximal than distal weakness (hip flexion and extension, neck flexion, and finger flexion), less muscle wasting, less pronounced facial abnormalities, and less common cardiac conduction defects. Pain is a more common feature of DM2 and can sometimes lead to the misdiagnosis of fibromyalgia in cases with mild muscle weakness.[279] Some patients with DM1 with mild muscle weakness but prominent hypersomnia, cognitive delay, and abnormal facial features are sometimes misdiagnosed as narcolepsy, Parkinson syndrome, or mental retardation.

Some patients with DM2 are misdiagnosed as having motor neuron disease due to the atypical myotonia on EMG.

Clinical and electrical myotonia occurs in chloride and sodium channel nondystrophic myotonias, which are also frequently inherited in an autosomal manner. These can be distinguished clinically from DM1 and DM2 by the lack of muscle weakness and wasting, or other multisystem abnormalities.

Electrical but not clinical myotonia occurs in adult onset acid maltase deficiency (Pompe disease) in which elevated CK, a recessive pattern of inheritance, typical findings on muscle biopsy, and the lack of other organ involvement help distinguish it from DM1 and DM2.

Due to the predominant distal weakness, DM1 is sometimes misdiagnosed as hereditary inclusion body myopathy (HIBM), distal myopathy, or myofibrillar myopathy.

Desmin-related myopathies occur in children and adults, and due to the distal weakness pattern, lens opacity, and cardiomyopathy it can sometimes be misdiagnosed as DM1. Accumulation of desmin on muscle biopsy and the lack of clinical or electrical myotonia help differentiate this heterogeneous group of myopathies from DM1.

The mild, late-onset, autosomal-dominant or sporadic form of centronuclear myopathy has myotonic discharges on EMG and the typical central nuclei in the majority of muscle fibers on muscle biopsy and can be mistaken by DM1.[280] In floppy infants, it is important to differentiate congenital DM1 from X-linked myotubular myopathy. These two entities have clinical and pathological features in common including severe floppiness and weakness, difficulty with respiration and feeding, hip and knee contractures, and central nuclei on muscle biopsy. Additional features in myotubular myopathy, not typical in congenital DM1, are thin ribs, puffy eyelids, ophtalmoplegia, and normal cognitive development.[281]

Treatment

No specific treatment for the progressive muscle weakness and wasting is available in DM1 and DM2. Treatment is directed toward symptom prevention and management and requires a multidisciplinary approach. Physical therapy evaluation is useful in helping maintaining safe ambulation. Molded AFOs, which control foot drop and stabilize the ankle, help prevent falls. Patients frequently opt to use high-top shoes instead. Quadriceps weakness, common in many myotonic dystrophy patients, causes the knee to give way suddenly and can be difficult to treat. For severe quadriceps weakness, an extension above the knee may be added to the standard AFOs, but most patients will not tolerate these modified long leg braces. Use of a wheelchair may become necessary in severe cases.

No improvement in muscle strength or function has been demonstrated in an open-label trial of recombinant human insulin-like growth factor (IGF) 1 complexed with IGF binding protein 3 in DM.[282]

Mexiletine at a dose of 150 and 200 mg 3 times daily is effective, safe, and well tolerated as an antimyotonia treatment in DM1.[283] Mexilitine should not be used in patients with AV block greater than first degree. Other agents used empirically to treat the myotonia include procainamide, phenytoin, acetazolamide, taurine, imipramine, and clomipramine.

Polysomnogram to screen for obstructive sleep apnea, nocturnal hypoventilation, and central apnea should be used and CPAP should be ordered as indicated. Many patients with DM1are unable to tolerate CPAP and some continue to have significant EDS despite correct use of CPAP for sleep apnea. CNS stimulants such as modafinil (200–400 mg/day), methylphenidate, and dexamphetamine are used for severe EDS.[284-288] Their effect on improved activity level remains to be established.[289]

Patient with DM1 and DM2 should have yearly EKG to monitor for P–R interval lengthening, QRS prolongation, and conduction block. Identification of conduction disease and prompt use of prophylactic pacemakers is important to decrease the risk of sudden death. Patients with cardiac symptoms such as syncope, presyncope, chest pain, palpitations, and shortness of breath on exertion are referred to a cardiologist for evaluation. There are no specific guidelines on how to best reduce the risk of sudden cardiac death in DM1, and while wide practice variation exists, some have proposed aggressive use of prophylactic pacemakers and cardioverter defibrillators.[290-293]

Patients should be monitored yearly for cataracts and referred for surgery once these become symptomatic.

No specific medication is beneficial in treating the pain typical of DM2.

Future Directions

The use of antisense oligonucleotides as a therapeutic strategy to reverse the toxic RNA gain-of-function in DM1 has recently achieved great success in vitro and in animal models[294-297] and is likely to translate to human clinical trials in the near future. A morpholino antisense oligonucleotide reversed the defect of ClC-1 alternative splicing and eliminated myotonia in a DM1 mouse model.[297] These advances have proved that antisense-induced exon skipping is a powerful method to correct alternative splicing defects in DM1 and may become successful in human clinical use in the near future.

FACIOSCAPULOHUMERAL MUSCULAR DYSTROPHY

Facioscapulohumeral muscular dystrophy (FSHD) is the third most common muscular dystrophy after Duchenne muscular dystrophy and myotonic dystrophy. The characteristic features of facial weakness, dominant family history, and weakness that affects the shoulder girdle and the anterior compartment of the legs, frequently in an asymmetric pattern, make it a distinct disease easy to differentiate from limb-girdle and other muscular dystrophies. The molecular abnormality that causes FSHD has proven to be one of the most challenging to unravel among the muscular dystrophies, but sensitive and specific DNA testing is now available to confirm the diagnosis.

Genetics

The estimated incidence of FSHD is 1:20,000.[298] Higher rates have been reported since molecular diagnosis has become available.[299] An autosomal-dominant pattern of inheritance with almost complete penetrance has been established. Careful examination of family members is necessary because approximately 30% of those affected are unaware of involvement due to the mild degree of disease manifestations. *De novo* mutations account for 10% to 30% of cases. In 95% of patients with FSHD (FSHD1) there is a deletion in the number of *D4Z4* repeats in the subtelomeric region of chromosome 4q35. In normal individuals both chromosome 4 *D4Z4* alleles have between 11 and 100 repeats. Patients affected with FSHD have one chromosome 4 *D4Z4* allele contracted to between 1 and 10 repeats, and the other with a normal number of repeats.[300,301]

When the number of repeats falls below 11, the chromatin structure becomes more permissive, allowing the expression of the only gene sequence within the *D4Z4* repeats, the *DUX4* gene. Although necessary, the deletions alone are not sufficient to cause FSHD unless they occur on the permissive 4qA haplotype chromosomal background. The 4qA sequence allows the production of a stable *DUX4* message. It is the inappropriate expression of *DUX4* protein, a gene normally silenced in somatic tissues, that results in FSHD. *D4Z4* allele contractures occurring on 4B haplotypes are nonpathogenic. An almost identical *D4Z4* repeat sequence is present on chromosome 10q26 but deletions in this repeat do not cause FSHD.

About 5% of patients with FSHD (FSHD2) do not have a contraction of *D4Z4*. FSHD2 is, in a majority of cases, caused by mutations in *SMCHD1* (the encoding *structural maintenance of chromosomes flexible hinge domain containing 1* gene) on chromosome 18. Reduced levels of *SMCHD1* in muscle cause hypomethylation of the *D4Z4* locus on chromosome 4 and 10.[302]

Hypomethylation of the *D4Z4* locus results in a more permissive chromatin structure and, just as in FSHD1, when in the presence of a 4qA background it results in the inappropriate expression of *DUX4*. FSHD2 is clinically indistinguishable from FSHD1 and was discovered only recently.[302] No other allelic phenotypes are associated with the *D4Z4* contraction mutation. Although genetic anticipation has been suspected,[303] more recent observations suggest that apparent anticipation is in fact due to a gender difference in penetrance, with males being more severely and more frequently affected than females.[304]

An absence of anticipation in large kindreds has been noted.[305]

Clinical Features

The diagnosis of FSHD should be considered in patients with slowly progressive muscle weakness with distinct facial weakness and scapular winging in the setting of a positive family history. Onset of symptoms varies from infancy to late in life but it is most common in the second decade. Facial weakness is the initial manifestation in most cases but is mild and often unrecognized initially. Difficulty smiling, whistling, and drinking from a straw, as well as pouty lips, inability to bury the eyelashes, and partially open eyelids during sleep are common signs (Figure 4–11). Patients may appear mildly exophthalmic or depressed due to facial weakness. Extraocular and bulbar muscles are typically spared.

Facial weakness is followed by shoulder-girdle muscle weakness affecting scapular stabilizer muscles, including the lower portion of the trapezius, rhomboid, and serratus anterior. The sternocostal head of the pectoral muscle is also often atrophic and weak. This weakness makes arm elevation difficult or impossible. Scapular winging, frequently asymmetric, becomes apparent with abduction and forward movement of the arms (Figure 4–12). Deep axillary folds, horizontal clavicles, and sloping of the shoulders contribute also to the typical appearance of the shoulders, one of the most distinguishing features of FSHD (Figure 4–11). Biceps and triceps may be severely affected in the arms. The deltoid muscles usually remain strong, although they appear weak unless tested with the scapula mechanically fixed against the chest wall by the examiner holding it in place (Figure 4–13). Wrist extension weakness invariably exceeds that of wrist flexion.

Weakness in the anterior compartment of the legs is another early manifestation, and patients may present with foot drop. Abdominal wall and back muscle weakness is also common and cause a protruding abdomen and a severe lordotic posture. Abdominal muscle weakness often produces a Beevor's sign: when the patient is supine and relaxed, head flexion results in movement of the umbilicus, usually upward.

Prominent asymmetry in facial, limb, and even truncal muscle weakness is a frequent feature and a very useful clinical clue in supporting the diagnosis of FSHD.

About 20% of patients become wheelchair bound. Life expectancy is not usually decreased.

Common extramuscular manifestations include hearing loss and retinal vasculopathy, both of which are usually mild except when associated with large D4Z4 contractions resulting in fragments < 20 kb.[306] High-frequency sensorineural hearing loss (between 4000–6000 Hz) occurs in 75% of patients but remains asymptomatic in most cases. In childhood-onset FSHD hearing loss can be severe and may lead

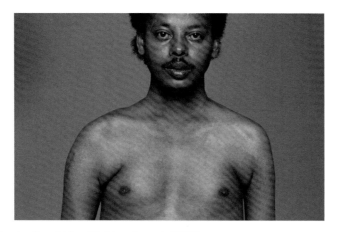

Figure 4–11. Prominent axillary fold and facial weakness in FSHD.

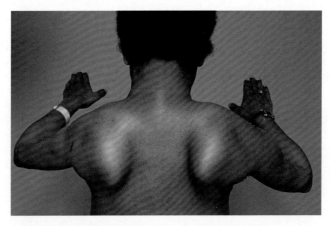

Figure 4–12. Typical scapular winging in FSHD.

to cognitive delay if not promptly recognized and treated.[307-309] The retinal vasculopathy is characterized by retinal microaneurysms and telengiectases, and failure of peripheral retina vascularization, but is usually largely asymptomatic.[308,310] In severe cases with large D4Z4 contractions the retinal vasculopathy can progress to Coats' syndrome, resulting in retinal detachment and vision loss.[306] ECG is usually

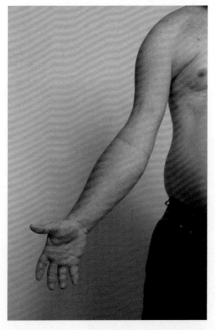

Figure 4–13. Biceps and triceps atrophy with relative sparing of the deltoid and forearm muscles resulting in the typical upper arm atrophy or "Popeye arms."

normal and cardiac manifestations are rare in FSHD; atrial tachyarrhythmias are observed in about 5% of patients.[311-315] Chronic musculoskeletal pain is common and unrecognized as typical in patients with FSHD.[316,317] Pain may disrupt sleep in some patients.[318] Pregnancy is usually uncomplicated in women with FSHD but increased rates of low birth weight and a need for operative deliveries have been reported. During gestation a quarter of women with FSHD experience disease worsening after delivery.[319] Respiratory dysfunction is not common in FSHD[315,320] and ventilatory support is needed only in rare patients with severe muscle disease, wheelchair dependency, and kyphoscoliosis.[321,322] Sleep-disordered breathing and impaired sleep quality can occur.[323,324] A severe, childhood-onset form of the disease affects about 4% of cases and is associated with greater disability, deafness, visual loss, severe progression of weakness, cognitive impairment, and sometimes seizures.[325-327] The severe facial diplegia affecting some children with congenital FSHD can be misdiagnosed as Möbius syndrome.[328] Early-onset FSHD is usually associated with larger contraction mutations of the D4Z4 fragment.

Laboratory Features and Diagnostic Tests

CK serum level is often normal and seldom greater than five times normal. A CK level greater than 10 times normal makes the diagnosis of FSHD unlikely.

EMG usually shows mild myopathic changes[302,329-332] but is rarely used for diagnosis of FSHD due to its lack of specificity compared to clinical DNA testing. Occasionally patients with undiagnosed FSHD are referred for EMG due to asymmetric scapular winging to rule out a long thoracic neuropathy or brachial plexopathy and a myopathy is found instead. EMG can aid in distinguishing Möbius syndrome from FSHD with facial diplegia.

Muscle biopsy shows isolated, angular, and necrotic fibers and moderate endomysial connective tissue proliferation with a multifocal distribution: one region of a biopsy may be severely affected, whereas an adjacent area shows minor abnormalities. The finding of a prominent inflammatory infiltrate in a biopsy can sometimes lead to a wrong diagnosis of inflammatory myopathy. Clinical genetic testing is the test of choice to confirm the diagnosis of FSHD and it is highly sensitive and specific. DNA from a blood sample is digested on Southern blot with EcoRI/BlnI restriction enzymes to assess the size of the chromosome 4q *D4Z4* repeats. FSHD patients have one allele in the normal size range of more than 50 kb and one allele of reduced size between 10 and 38 kb.[333] Approximately 5% of patients with a clinically typical presentation for FSHD have a negative DNA test. In these cases a muscle biopsy is an option to rule out other disorders that can mimic FSHD (see Differential Diagnosis, hereafter). If this additional testing is negative, FSHD2 should be considered. Guidelines for the genetic diagnosis of FSHD are available.[332,333] Quantitative MRI shows increased T2 signal and short tau-inversion recovery brightness consistent with edema and inflammation with a pattern of different degree in different muscles. The role of muscle edema and inflammation as a possible biomarker and the usefulness of MRI in clinical research are under investigation.[334,335]

Differential Diagnosis

The typical facial weakness and an autosomal-dominant family history, when present, help distinguishing FSHD from the LGMDs with scapuloperoneal weakness. Distinct muscle pathology is most useful in differentiating disorders that can sometimes clinically mimic FSHD such as nemaline and centronuclear myopathy, inclusion body myositis, polymyositis, mitochondrial myopathies, adult-onset acid maltase deficiency, and myofibrillary myopathy. Congenital FSHD is sometimes misdiagnosed as Möbius syndrome. When FSHD patients come to clinical attention because of a foot drop, they may be misdiagnosed as having CMT or other neurogenic disorders known to cause foot drop.

Treatment

Treatment of FSHD is centered on the symptomatic management of muscle weakness and the extramuscular manifestations of the disease. Therapeutic trials with albuterol have failed to demonstrate a definite effect on muscle strength.[336-338] Corticosteroids do not benefit patients.[339] Aerobic training and exercise with moderate weights have been shown to be beneficial in FSHD, unlike in other muscular dystrophies where muscle membrane fragility and muscle breakdown make exercise potentially injurious.[338,340,341] Foot drop may be helped by molded AFOs. When concomitant quadriceps weakness is present, a floor reaction AFO may be a better option because it prevents buckling of the knee ("back-kneeing") by providing extension support to the knee upon floor contact. Nonambulatory patients benefit from a motorized wheelchair with an adjustable height control. Some patients with severe weakness may find a hospital bed useful. In some patients with FSHD in whom the deltoid muscle has good strength, the range of motion of the shoulder can be improved by surgical fixation of the scapula to the thorax.[342] Several different surgical techniques are used to achieve scapular fixation.[343-346] Surgery should be reserved for patients with mild disease and should be done only on the side of dominant hand function. A shoulder brace may provide comfort to those patients experiencing musculoskeletal shoulder pain.

Screening audiometry is recommended in all patients and is particularly important in children affected by the early-onset form of the disease to prevent cognitive delay from unrecognized and untreated hearing loss. Standard therapy for hearing loss including amplification should be used when indicated.

Use of lubricants or taping of the eyes at night in those patients with incomplete eye closure is useful in preventing drying of the sclera and exposure keratitis. Surgical placement of small weights in the upper lids can restore lid closure.[347] Children with severe, early-onset disease should be screened with indirect ophthalmoscopy. Fluorescein angiography is indicated to screen for retinal vasculopathy and possible progression to Coats' syndrome. Early laser photocoagulation can prevent Coats' syndrome and visual loss.

Treatment of chronic musculoskeletal pain often improves quality of life and improves sleep. Use of nocturnal BiPAP should be considered when there is a restrictive pattern of respiratory weakness causing nocturnal hypoventilation.

LIMB-GIRDLE MUSCULAR DYSTROPHIES

The limb-girdle muscular dystrophies (LGMDs) consist of a group of inherited muscle diseases characterized by childhood or adult onset; symmetric, progressive, proximal muscle weakness; elevated CK; and muscle degeneration/regeneration on muscle biopsy. Clinical manifestations outside of skeletal muscle are rare, and inheritance is most commonly autosomal recessive and less frequently autosomal dominant. Phenotypic overlap exists between some LGMDs, distal myopathies, and congenital muscular dystrophies. The number of genes in which mutations cause LGMDs has rapidly increased in the past 20 years, and diagnosis by genetic subtype is challenging.

Genetics

LGMDs are caused by defects in genes encoding for muscle proteins associated with the sarcolemma (α, β, γ, δ-sarcoglycans, dysferlin, caveolin), proteins associated with the contractile apparatus, the sarcomere (telethonin, titin, myotilin), and various glycosyltranferases involved in the addition of carbohydrate residues to alpha-dystroglycan (*POMT1, POMT2, POMGNT1, FKTN, FKRP*).Whereas the primary defect in many LGMDs is known and the mechanism leading to the dystrophic

phenotype has been elucidated, in others the underlying pathophysiology has not yet been established.

Prevalence for all form of LGMD ranges from 1:14,500 to 1:123,000 and has been difficult to estimate due to disease heterogeneity and limited molecular confirmation.[348,349] Prevalence for specific subtypes varies greatly in different region of the world and founder mutations account for a high prevalence of some subtypes in some populations. Calpainopathy (LGMD2A) is the most frequent subtype, accounting for about 30% of all LGMD cases worldwide.[350] Dysferlinopathy (LGMD2B) is the second most prevalent in some populations (Italian, Brazilian, American, Australian, and Dutch), and in Libyan Jews the prevalence is 1:1,300 with a carrier risk of 10%.[351] LGMD2I (*FKRP*) is the second most common LGMD in North Europe.[352,353] α-sarcoglycanopathy is the most common of the sarcoglycanopathies (SGs) in Europe and North America, whereas γ-sarcoglycanopathy accounts for 100% of the SGs in North Africa. SGs are the cause of 68% of the severe, childhood-onset AR-LGMDs in Brazil.[354]

AD-LGMDs are very rare, accounting for less than 10% of all the LGMDs, and most AD subtypes (LGMD1s D–H) have been described only in single large pedigrees or in a few families in the world.[355-358]

Clinical Features

The clinical manifestations of LGMDs are characteristically limited to the skeletal muscle with proximal, symmetric progressive weakness. Clinical phenotypic overlap is prominent between the different subtypes but the different age at onset and variable pace of progression combined with some typical additional clinical features help direct the diagnosis for some specific subtypes (Tables 4–1 and 4–2). For example, respiratory insufficiency that occurs in patients who are still ambulatory is seen in SGs and LGMD2I but is otherwise seen only in the advanced stage of disease in other LGMDs. Calf hypertrophy is more common in SGs, LGMD2I, and LGMD1C. Muscle rippling is a special clue for the diagnosis of LGMD1C. In LGMD2B (dysferlinopathy) distinctive clinical clues include biceps atrophy with preservation of deltoid bulk resulting in a typical "deltoid

Table 4–1 Autosomal-Dominant Limb-Girdle Muscular Dystrophies

Disease Name	Gene	Ch Locus	Age at Onset (Years)	CK	Clinical Features	Other Features
LGMD1A Myotilinopathy	MYOT	5q31.2	18 and older	Normal to moderately high	Proximal weakness, distal weakness late, ankle contractures	Dysarthria, dysphagia, respiratory insufficiency
LGMD1B	LMNA	1q22	Birth to adulthood	Normal to moderately high	Lower extremity weakness, late upper extremity weakness	Atrioventricular conduction defects, DCM
LGMD1C caveolinopathy	CAV3	3p25.3	Any	Moderately to very high	Mild to moderate proximal weakness, cramps after exercise, myalgias	Calf hypertrophy, muscle rippling, HCM
LGMD1D	DES	2q35	Early adulthood	Normal to moderately high	Mostly lower extremity weakness, sparing quadriceps; ambulation preserved	Cardiac conduction defects, DCM
LGMD1E	DNAJB6	7q36.3	18–40; late onset in females	Normal to moderately high	Slowly progressive weakness in lower extremities, sparing quadriceps	Calf hypertrophy, loss of ambulation 20–30 years from onset
LGMD1F	?	7q32.1-q32.2	Any	Normal to high	Fast progression in early onset cases, facial weakness	Scoliosis, respiratory failure
LGMD1G	?	4q21	Adulthood	Normal to very high	Proximal lower extremity weakness	Finger and toe flexion limitation
LGMD1H	?	3p25-p23	2nd–5th decade	Normal to very high	Slowly progressive upper and lower extremity weakness	Calf hypertrophy, muscle atrophy, high serum lactate

Note. Ch locus = chromosome locus; DCM= dilated cardiomyopathy; HCM = hypertrophic cardiomyopathy.

Table 4–2 Autosomal-Recessive Limb-Girdle Muscular Dystrophies

Disease Name	Gene	Age at Onset (Years)	CK	Clinical Features	Other Features	Other Phenotypes
LGMD2A Calpainopathy	CAPN3	8–15; rarely late	High to very high	Mild to severe weakness, difficulty running, calf atrophy	Toe walking, early ankle contractures, scoliosis	NA
LGMD2B Dysferlinopathy	DYSF	15–25	High to very high	Weakness and atrophy of pelvic worse thanshoulder girdle muscles, difficulty running, late UEs involvement	Calf and biceps atrophy, deltoid "bulge", mean age at loss of ambulation = 45	Miyoshi myopathy; DMAT
LGMD2C, 2D, 2E, 2F/ Sarcoglycanopathies	γ-, α-, β-, & δ-SG	Childhood	High to very high	Severe, "Duchenne-like" progression; milder course also possible	Calf hypertrophy	Dilated cardiomyopathy (δ-SG)
LGMD2G	TCAP	2–15	Moderately high	Proximal and distal weakness, difficulty running	Calf hypertrophy, foot drop	Dilated cardiomyopathy 1N
LGMD2H	TRIM32	1st–2nd decade	Normal to very high	Waddling gait, facial weakness, flat smile	Muscle wasting	Sarcotubular myopathy
LGMD2I	FKRP	High to very high	Severe to mild; low FVC in 50% of cases		Calf and tongue hypertrophy, pectoralis atrophy	MDC1C
LGMD2J	TTN	2–25	High to very high	Severe, progressive proximal weakness	Distal weakness late in 50% of cases	Distal myopathy; dilated cardiomyopathy
LGMD2K LGMD2L	POMT1 ANO5	First decade Adulthood	Very high Very high	Mild proximal weakness Pelvic girdle weakness or calf hypertrophy, difficulty walking on tiptoe	Microcephaly, low IQ Asymmetric quadriceps and biceps atrophy	WWS NA
LGMD2M	FKTN	Infancy	Very high	Rigid spine, virally induced worsening weakness	Facial and axial weakness	Fukuyama CMD
LGMD2N	POMT2	First decade	Very high	Scapular winging, slow running, motor delay	Calf hypertrophy	WWS

Note. CMD: congenital muscular dystrophy, DMAT = distal myopathy with anterior tibial involvement, SG = sarcoglycanopathy; WWS= Walker-Warburg Syndrome bulge" and a commonly reported history of preserved ability to participate successfully in sports prior to the onset of symptoms.[359,360] Cardiac involvement is not seen in LGMD1C, 2A, 2B, 2G, 2H, or 2J, whereas dilated cardiomyopathy is seen in LGMD2I and the β, δ, and γ SGs.[361-363] Joint contractures are common in the advanced stage of LGMDs like in many muscular dystrophies, but are typically seen earlier in LGMD1B, LGMD2A, LGMD2I, and in the SGs. Scoliosis is seen earlier in the SGs but is common after patients become wheelchair dependent in most LGMDs. An increased risk for malignant hyperthermia and other general anesthesia reactions is seen in LGMD2I. Cognitive impairment or radiologic brain abnormalities are not common in LGMDs and should suggest a different diagnosis such as dystrophinopathy or congenital muscular dystrophy. Neonatal hypotonia is not a clinical feature of LGMD, except for LGMD1B.

Laboratory Features and Diagnostic Tests

CK level is high or very high in most AR-LGMDs and in caveolinopathy (LGMD1C) but can be normal in the AD-LGMDs (Tables 4–1 and 4–2). In LGMDs, CK level, as in other muscular dystrophies, decreases over time as muscle atrophy progresses. A normal CK level early in the disease excludes the diagnosis of an AR-LGMD.

Electrodiagnostic testing is not helpful in differentiating the subtypes of LGMD but has a role early in the diagnostic process to exclude spinal muscular atrophy, myotonic dystrophy, or myasthenic syndromes.

Muscle biopsy is crucial in the diagnostic process to differentiate the subtypes of LGMDs and in directing genetic testing. Histology is usually nonspecific and shows either a myopathic or a dystrophic pattern. Myopathic changes with variability in fiber size; necrotic fibers and endomysial fibrosis are typical of the AD-LGMDs. A more dystrophic pattern with prominent endomysial fibrosis, fiber degeneration and regeneration, and increased central nuclei is also common, more so in the AR-LGMDs. Type 1 fibers may be predominant. Some clues provided by histology may be useful. For example, prominent inflammatory infiltrates are common in dysferlinopathy (LGMD2B) and may lead to a misdiagnosis of acquired myositis[364-368]; amyloid deposits are also seen and this feature is unique to LGMD2B among the LGMDs[359]; rimmed vacuoles are seen in LGMD2G, 2J, and 2H[369]; and rimmed vacuoles and desmin accumulation may be seen in LGMD1A.[370]

Muscle immunoanalysis is crucial to demonstrate a primary deficit of a specific muscle protein associated to a particular subtype of LGMD, but some caution in interpretation needs to be used due to partial secondary deficiencies. In LGMD2A (calpainopathy), complete absence of calpain 3 by immunoblot or immunohistochemical analysis is seen in 58% of patients and confirms the diagnosis. A partial reduction on immunoblot is seen in 22% of patients with LGMD2A but can also be seen in LGMD2B and Udd myopathy,[371,372] and a normal amount of protein is seen in 20% of patients with confirmed molecular diagnosis of LGMD2A.[373,374] Antibodies to dysferlin show complete deficiency or patchy sarcolemmal and cytoplasmic staining on muscle biopsy of patients with LGMD2B.[375,376] Secondary deficiency of dysferlin can be seen in LGMD1C (caveolinopathy). Immunoblot to confirm a primary dysferlin deficiency has high predictive value and is therefore recommended.[377] The four sarcoglycans (α, β, γ, δ) are glycosylated transmembrane proteins that form a tetrameric complex associated to the DGC. A primary deficiency of one sarcoglycan causes a partial deficiency of all other sarcoglycans[378-380]; therefore immunoanalysis and immunoblot are highly predictive for a sarcoglycanopathy, but not for a specific one. In SGs dystrophin can also show a reduced expression pattern when β-dystroglycan is also reduced, and reduction of the N-terminal dystrophin domain is more pronounced than that of the C-terminal domain.[378] Secondary calpain 3 reduction is seen in dysferlinopathy (LGMD2B) and in LGMD2J.[371]

Muscle MRI can distinguish some LGMD subtypes from other muscular dystrophies or myopathies with overlapping clinical features.[381] For example, significant involvement of posterior thigh muscles, the soleus muscle, and the medial head of the gastrocnemius is typical of LGMD1A but not seen in other diseases with early contractures such as EDMD and Bethlem myopathy.[382] Although muscle

MRI is currently used mostly outside the United States and in specialized centers, it may become more routinely used in clinical practice in the near future.

Genetic testing to establish a specific subtype diagnosis in LGMDs is challenging due to the many genes involved, the ongoing discovery of new causative genes, the lack of common mutations in many of the known genes, and the clinical overlap between the different types. Even in specialized centers molecular diagnosis is not possible in up to half of cases. The cost and clinical availability of DNA testing for LGMDs varies in different countries, and even if multigene panels are available, they are usually very expensive. The development of a cheaper and more sensitive high-throughput DNA microarray ("gene chip") able to sequence multiple genes at low cost will improve the diagnostic process for LGMDs in the near future.

Differential Diagnosis

Any male with clinical features of a muscular dystrophy and high CK needs to be tested for dystrophinopathy before the diagnosis of LGMD is considered. Females with high CK and clinical evidence of muscle weakness but no family history should also be tested for a dystrophinopathy as their chance of being an isolated manifesting carrier for DMD is nearly as likely as having a subtype of AR-LGMD[383,384] and has obvious genetic counseling implication for the family.

Facial weakness is the most helpful feature in differentiating FSHD from LGMD, but FSHD patients with only mild facial weakness can resemble those with LGMD. The typical asymmetry in muscle weakness as well as the dominant family history helps differentiate FSHD from LGMD (see previous section on FSHD).

EDMD is differentiated from LGMD by the early onset joint contractures and the prominent cardiac manifestations (see previous section on EDMD).

Congential muscular dystrophies (CMDs) are inherited in an autosomal-recessive manner and there is phenotypic overlap between some CMD and LGMD subtypes. The presence of eye and brain abnormalities typical of the alpha-dystroglycanopathies and of prominent spine and limb contractures in COL6-related CMDs helps distinguish CMDs from LGMDs clinically. LGMD2A (calpainopathy) can manifest early contractures like EDMD and COL6-related CMD. Immunostaining and western blot from muscle biopsy help to more definitely establish a specific diagnosis based on the affected protein (see next section on CMD).

Inflammatory myopathies have symmetric proximal weakness and high CK but their acute or subacute onset of symptoms and response to immunosuppressive treatment help differentiate them from LGMD. Inflammatory infiltrates are common in dysferlinopathy (LGMD2B) and this diagnosis should be considered before a diagnosis of polymyositis and particularly if such "polymyositis" does not respond to prednisone therapy.[364,365]

Treatment

There is currently no specific treatment for any of the LGMDs. A double-blind placebo-controlled clinical trial of deflazacort in dysferlinopathy showed no improvement but instead a trend of worsening in muscle strength.[385,386]

Management is directed toward surveillance and treatment for cardiac arrhythmias and cardiomyopathy, nocturnal hypoventilation, respiratory insufficiency, and orthopedic complications (contractures and scoliosis; see chapter 13). Patients with LGMDs should be evaluated for cardiac and respiratory function prior to general anesthesia. Consultation with physical therapy at the different stages of disease is useful to maximize function and adaptation in the school and home environment. Weight and diet should be monitored to avoid obesity (see chapter 13).

Future Directions

Persistent α sarcoglycan gene expression has been demonstrated in two out of three patients with LGMD2D following gene transfer mediated by AVV.[387,388] Therapeutic approaches directed toward the LGMDs, including exon skipping with antisense technology and gene replacement, are undergoing further study.[389]

OCULOPHARYNGEAL MUSCULAR DYSTROPHY

Oculopharyngeal muscular dystrophy (OPMD), when first described by Taylor in 1915, was thought to represent a neuronal disorder. Kiloh and Nevin first recognized this disorder as a form of muscular dystrophy (ocular myopathy).[390] The term *oculopharyngeal muscular dystrophy* was introduced later by Victor et al.[391] OPMD is a dominantly inherited trinucleotide repeat disorder with distinctive clinical features of late onset, slowly progressive ptosis and ophthalmoparesis, dysphagia, and proximal muscle weakness.

Genetics

OPMD is autosomal-dominant and inherited with complete penetrance. *De novo* mutations are rare. French Canadians are the most commonly affected ethnic group, originating from a common ancestor who emigrated to Quebec in 1634. The disease also occurs with increased frequency in Spanish American families in southern Colorado, northern New Mexico, and Arizona,[392,393] and in large kindreds of Jewish families of Eastern European background. OPMD has been observed in more than 35 countries. The prevalence of OPMD varies from 1:600 among Bukhara Jews and 1:1,000 in French Canadians to 1:100,000 in France.[394-398]

OPMD is caused by an alanine GCG triplet expansion of variable size in the first exon of the PABPN1 gene on 14q11.2 coding for the polyadenylate binding protein nuclear 1.[398] Normal alleles have 10 GCG repeats, whereas autosomal-dominant alleles have 12 to 17. A much rarer autosomal-recessive form of OPMD has been described with alleles containing 11 GCG repeats.[399-402]

Some rare cases of OPMD caused by a point mutation or a microinsertion in exon 1 have been reported.[403-405] Polyalanine gain of function mechanisms such as abnormal aggregation, insufficient protein degradation, and intranuclear accumulation of misfolded protein have been proposed as possible pathogenic explanations.[406] PABPN1 is the only gene known to cause OPMD. The abnormal triplet repeat[407] in the PABPN1 gene is mitotically and meiotically stable and therefore, unlike other trinucleotide repeat disorders such as DM1, clinical anticipation is not observed. There is no clear correlation between the size of the triplet repeat and clinical severity or age of onset of the disease.[402] There are no other known disorders allelic to the PABPN1 gene.

Clinical Features

OPMD most frequently presents with the initial symptom of late onset ptosis, usually in the fourth to sixth decade (mean age at onset = 48 years), followed by the other cardinal symptom, dysphagia, after a few years. Ptosis is usually symmetric and associated with the typical compensatory mechanisms of frontalis muscle contraction and retroflexion of the head resulting, in the so called "astronomist's posture" (Figure 4–14). Rarely, dysphagia can precede ptosis. Dysphagia is progressive and over time becomes the most debilitating manifestation of this disease.

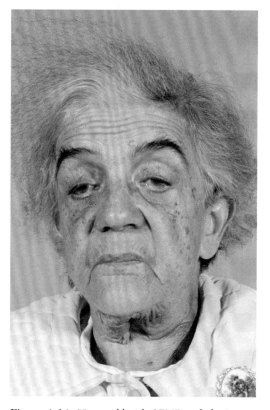

Figure 4–14. 80-year-old with OPMD and classic symmetric ptosis.

Extraocular muscle impairment varies in degree, but rarely progresses into complete ophthalmoplegia. Upward gaze is usually impaired first. Diplopia is seldom a symptom in OPMD, perhaps due to the symmetric and slow progression of the extraocular muscle weakness.

Laryngeal weakness may cause dysphonia. Tongue weakness and atrophy are common and facial weakness is sometimes present. Neck flexion and lower more than upper extremity weakness are also common. Limb weakness is usually mild and its progression is very slow, only rarely leading to severe functional disability or loss of independent ambulation. No other organs outside of skeletal muscle are affected in OPMD. The overall course of OPMD is very slow and life expectancy is not reduced if dysphagia is managed appropriately.

In rare patients with homozygous mutations, the onset of symptoms is much earlier, the severity and progression of disease manifestations are much worse, and life span is reduced.[408,409]

Laboratory Features and Diagnostic Tests

CK serum levels are usually normal, elevated from two to seven times the normal limit.

EMG of weak muscles is not specific and shows myopathic MUPs without spontaneous activity, consistent with a myopathy without muscle fiber irritability. Occasionally, neurogenic MUPs can be seen and are likely related to the typical old age of these patients.[410, 411] Currently EMG is used mostly as a screening tool to rule out a neurogenic process.

Muscle biopsy is characterized by intranuclear inclusions consisting of tubular filaments and small, often subsarcolemmal rimmed vacuoles lined with granular material (Figure 4–15). These unbranched tubular filaments are 8.5 nm in diameter, may reach 0.5 μm in length, often show striations with a periodicity of 7 to 7.5 nm, and differ from the larger, 15- to 18-nm intranuclear and extranuclear filaments seen in inclusion body myositis.[412-417] Small, atrophied, angulated fibers, as well as other nonspecific findings typically present in dystrophies—such as increased internal nuclei, type 1 fiber predominance, variation in fiber size,

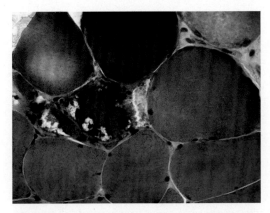

Figure 4–15. Muscle biopsy in OPMD: trichromic Gomori showing subsarcolemmal rimmed vacuoles.

and degenerating and regenerating fibers—are also common. Muscle biopsy is currently indicated only in those patients in whom the diagnosis is clinically suspected but the DNA testing is negative.

DNA testing determines the size of the GCG triplet expansion in the first exon of the *PABPN1* gene and is available in many commercial laboratories. It has 100% specificity and 99% sensitivity and is the test of choice to confirm the diagnosis of OPMD.[398]

MRI shows abnormal fat infiltration in the tongue and masseter, but also in posterior neck, shoulder girdle, lumbar paraspinal, and gluteus muscles.[418] Muscular involvement by MRI can detect subclinical disease and has been proposed as a possible outcome measure to detect disease progression in future clinical trials.[418-420]

Pharyngogram is used to evaluate the degree and progression of dysphagia and can show pooling in the pharyngeal vallecula, aspiration, and cricopharyngeal achalasia.

Differential Diagnosis

Chronic progressive external ophthalmoplegia results from many mitochondrial disorders (chapter 8) that predominantly affect the eye muscles, frequently in isolation, but may also cause an associated, slowly progressive, symmetric proximal myopathy. Ragged red fibers are frequently seen on muscle biopsy. Dysphagia is uncommon and ophthalmoplegia is more severe than in OPMD and manifests much earlier in life.

Myasthenia gravis (MG) can be differentiated from OPMD by the lack of autosomal-dominant family history and the fluctuating nature of the ptosis, limb weakness, and dysphagia. Ptosis is more frequently asymmetric in MG than in OPMD, and although diplopia is a very common and frequently disabling symptom in MG, it is infrequent in OPMD. Electrodiagnostic evaluation and serum antibody test help with the diagnosis.

In myotonic dystrophy, also a dominantly inherited trinucleotide repeat disorder, ptosis and dysphagia are common, but clinical and electromyographic myotonia easily distinguish it from OPMD. The involvement of multiple organs and the earlier onset of symptoms also help differentiate myotonic dystrophy from OPMD.

In distal hereditary motor neuropathy type VII (HMN7), spinal muscular atrophy is associated with pharyngeal and vocal cord weakness without ptosis.

Ophthalmoparesis is also a typical feature of some congenital myopathies such as centronuclear or myotubular myopathy.

Oculopharyngodistal myopathy (OPDM) is characterized by ptosis, external ophtalmoplegia, and dysphagia with weakness and wasting of distal muscles rather than proximal ones, and may have concomitant respiratory involvement, hearing loss, and cardiac conduction-system abnormalities.[421-424] OPDM is inherited in an autosomal-dominant or recessive manner and is considered genetically distinct from OPMD.

Treatment

Treatment for OPMD is symptomatic as there is no therapy targeted to the disease mechanism. Mild ptosis can be managed initially with eyelid crutches on glasses. When ptosis interferes with vision or causes neck pain from constant neck extension, blepharoplasty is indicated. Resection of the aponeurosis of the levator palpebrae is least invasive but usually needs to be repeated over time. Frontal suspension of the eyelids is more permanent but requires general anesthesia.[425-427] Mild exposure keratitis is a common complication of these procedures but usually resolves over a few weeks.

Mild to moderate dysphagia that does not cause choking or aspiration pneumonia is best managed by diet modifications such as thickening of liquids, pureeing of solid food, slow chewing, and increasing protein intake through pudding supplements to compensate for difficulty swallowing meat and other difficult-to-swallow foods. When dysphagia is more severe and causes aspiration pneumonia, weight loss, or frequent or severe choking, cricopharyngeal myotomy is helpful in many cases, although its benefit may lessen over time due to progression of the disease. Upper esophageal sphincter dilation by endoscopy is an alternative option that does not require general anesthesia, but it usually needs to be repeated over time.[428] In advanced cases gastrostomy tube placement is a more permanent option. Botulinum toxin injections in the upper esophageal muscle have been tried with some reported benefit but are not routinely used.[429]

Severe dysphonia is uncommon and can be managed with speech therapy or, in rare severe cases, the use of communication devices.

Patients with OPMD should receive the flu vaccine annually. Patients are at risk for aspiration pneumonia, especially after general anesthesia,[430,431] but can usually clear their airway because respiratory muscles and cough are normal.

Physical therapy evaluation is recommended, as progression of the lower extremity weakness may require a walker or wheelchair in the late stages.

THE CONGENITAL MUSCULAR DYSTROPHIES

The congenital muscular dystrophies (CMDs) are a clinically and genetically heterogeneous group of inherited muscle diseases with onset of muscle weakness at birth or early infancy and with muscle biopsy features consistent with a dystrophic process. Great advances in the past decade have resulted in the identification of mutations in 13 genes as causes of CMD. The classification of CMD remains challenging due to the overlap of phenotypes caused by mutations in different genes and because mutations in one gene can result in a spectrum of phenotypes. One important differentiating feature is the presence of clinical and radiographic brain abnormalities and eye abnormalities in some CMDs. They are caused by defects in structural proteins of the extracellular matrix, basement membrane, endoplasmic reticulum, and nuclear envelope, as well as by a defect in glycosylation of alpha-dystroglycan.

Genetics

The classification of CMDs has changed rapidly in the past 10 years as new causative genes have been discovered, and the nomenclature for the many CMDs subtypes is still evolving (Table 4–3). There is phenotypic overlap between CMDs and the congenital myopathies (see chapter 6) and the LGMDs (see Limb-Girdle Muscular Dystrophies section, earlier). CMDs are caused by mutations in at least 13 genes resulting in abnormalities in proteins localized in the sarcolemma, basal lamina, extracellular matrix, endoplasmic reticulum, and nuclear envelope and by abnormal glycosylation of alpha-dystroglycan.[432,433] Incidence and prevalence data for the CMD are limited. Prevalence ranges from 0.68 to 2.5 per 100,000 and is probably underestimated due to the different diagnostic classifications used and the limited availability of genetic confirmation until recent years.[434-436] The most common subtypes in populations of European descent are laminin alpha-2 and COL6-deficient CMDs. In Japan, COL6-related CMDs account for only 7% of cases,[437] while Fukuyama CMD with mutations in the *FKTN* gene is the most common form due to a founder effect.[438] *FKTN* mutations are very rare in the rest of the world.

The CMD are predominantly inherited in an autosomal-recessive manner except for the COL6-related CMDs, which can also be inherited in a dominant manner, and *LMNA*-related CMD, which is caused by dominant *de novo* mutations.[432,439] Currently, a diagnosis of CMD can be genetically confirmed in only 24% to 46% of cases.[440,441]

Clinical Features

The severity of muscle weakness in CMDs ranges from severe hypotonia at birth with failure to gain the ability to ambulate, to delayed motor milestones and ambulation preserved into adulthood. In laminin alpha-2 deficiency (MDC1A) hypotonia, difficulty feeding at birth and delayed motor milestones are typical. Patients are eventually able to sit but never walk.[442,443] In COL6-related CMD some patients may never achieve ambulation, whereas others can walk independently into adulthood.[444] The alpha-dystroglycanopathies encompass the greatest phenotypic spectrum, with Walker-Warburg syndrome (WWS) representing the most severe clinical phenotype with severe psychomotor delay and eye abnormalities; MDC1C with no eye or brain abnormality; and mild dystrophy (Table 4–3).[445] In LMNA-related CMD, hypotonia and weakness of the cervical and axial muscles are severe and rapidly progressive, causing either lack of head and trunk tone in the first 6 months of life, or progressive loss of head control after acquisition of sitting or walking ability ("dropped head syndrome").[446]

Progressive restrictive respiratory insufficiency can occur over time as muscle weakness progresses in patients with CMDs, especially after loss of ambulation. Early respiratory failure requiring ventilator support in the first or second decade of life, even in patients who are still able to walk, is typical of *COL6*-related and *SEPN1*-related CMD.[442]

Cardiac involvement varies considerably between the different subtypes of CMDs and includes dilated cardiomyopathy and systolic and diastolic dysfunction. Cardiac dysfunction occurs in CMD caused by mutation in *FKRP, FKTN, POMT1,* and *LMNA* but is not seen in COL6-related CMD.[447-450] Dilated cardiomyopathy is seen in patients with laminin alpha-2–related CMD.[451] Right heart failure can be seen in any CMD as a consequence of untreated respiratory failure.

Contractures are characteristic of some subtypes of CMD and are a useful clinical clue to reach a specific diagnosis. For example, the combination of hyperlaxity of distal joints, with contractures of proximal joint, kyphosis, and hip dislocation, is typical of COL6-related CMD. Diffuse joint contractures and spine rigidity develop over time in patients with laminin alpha-2 deficincy.

Follicular hyperkeratosis and poor wound healing with keloid formation are also typical in patients with COL6-related CMD (Figure 4–16A–B).

Seizures are common in Fukuyama-type CMD and average age of onset is 3 years. Initial seizures occur during a febrile illness in two-thirds of patients. Generalized tonic-clonic seizures are most common, followed by

Table 4–3 Congenital Muscular Dystrophies: Classification by Protein and Gene Defect

Defect Type	Subtype Disease Name	Genes Affected	Protein Affected	Alternate Disease Name	Other Phenotype
Defects of proteins in the basement membrane	Laminin alpha-2 deficiency (MDC1A)	LAMA2	Laminin alpha 2	Merosin-deficient CMD	—
Defects of proteins in the extracellular matrix	Collagen VI-deficient CMD	Col6A1	Collagen VI	Ullrich CMD	Bethlem myopathy, autosomal-recessive myosclerosis myopathy
		Col6A2	Collagen VI		
		Col6A3	Collagen VI		
Defects of glycosyltransferase enzymes that result in abnormal glycosylation of alpha-dystroglycan	Dystroglycanopathy	POMT1	Protein-O-mannosyltransferase 1	WWS	LGMD2K
		POMT2	Protein-O-mannosyltransferase 2	WWS	LGMD2N
		FKTN	Fukutin	WWS, MEB-like CMD,FCMD	LGMD2M no intellectual disability
		FKRP	Fukutin-related protein	WWS, MEB-like CMD, MDC1C	LGMD2I
		LARGE	Like-glycosyltransferase	WWS, MDC1D	LGMD
		POMGNT1	Protein-O-linked mannose beta 1,2-N-acetylglucosaminyltransferase	MEB	LGMD
		ISPD	Isoprenoid synthase domain–containing protein	WWS	LGMD
Defects of proteins of the endoplasmic reticulum	SEPN1-related CMD	SEPN1	Selenoprotein N, 1	Rigid spine syndrome (RSMD1)	Multi-minicore myopathy, fiber-type disproportion myopathy, desminopathy
Defects of nuclear envelope proteins	LMNA-related CMD CMD with adducted thumbs	LMNA	Lamin A/C	Dropped-head syndromeCMD with adducted thumbs	EDMD
		SYNE1	Nesprin-1 (enaptin)		

Note. WWS = Walker-Warburg syndrome, MEB = muscle-eye-brain disease, FCMD = Fukuyama congenital muscular dystrophy, EDMD = Emery-Dreifuss muscular dystrophy.

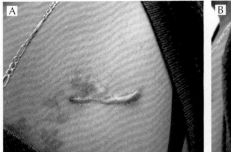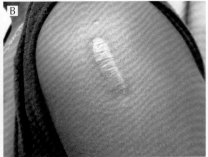

Figure 4–16. Patient with COL6-related CMD: Keloid is shown at the site of pacemaker insertion (A) and muscle biopsy (B).

complex partial and secondary generalized seizures.[452,453] Seizures occur in 20% to 30% of patients with laminin alpha-2 deficiency.

Intellectual disability varies from severe to mild in the dystroglycanopathies. No intellectual abnormalities are usually associated with laminin alpha-2 or COL6-related CMD.[454]

Brain MRI abnormalities are most common in the dystroglycanopathies and include hypoplastic cerebellum, hydrocephalus, cobblestone lissencephaly, frontoparietal polymicrogyria, cerebellar cysts, and brainstem hypoplasia (Figure 4–17A & B). In laminin alpha-2 CMD, MRI consistently shows white matter consistent with dysmyelination; rarely there are occipital lobe neuronal migration abnormalities. Cerebellar atrophy is seen in about one-third of patients.[433, 455]

Eye manifestations are common in the dystroglycanopathies and include hypoplastic or absent optic nerve, colobomas, cataracts, iris hypoplasia, retinal dysplasia or detachment, glaucoma, high myopia, and optic disc pallor.

Macrocephaly is seen in *POMGNT1* dystroglyconopathy and laminin alpha-2 deficiency.

Pseudohypertrophy of calves and tongue is seen in the dystroglyconopathies.

A peripheral neuropathy with slow conduction velocity may be present in laminin alpha-2 deficiency (MDC1A).

Laboratory Findings

Serum CK is normal or mildly elevated in CMD subtypes without abnormality in

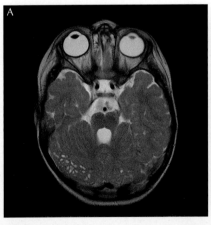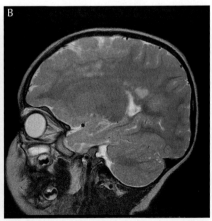

Figure 4–17. Brain MRI in a 2-year-old with dystroglycanopathy (muscle biopsy shown in Figure 4–18). A: Axial T2 image with dysmorphic brainstem with hypoplastic midbrain and pons and enlarged fourth ventricle; the upper part of the cerebellum including the vermis is dysplastic and the peripheral portions demonstrate clusters of tiny cysts. B: Sagittal T2 image with scattered ill-defined T2 hyperintense areas and some incomplete radial lines/bands in the pericallosal/periventricular region representing possible gliotic foci versus heterotopic gray matter.

merosin expression and in *SEPN1*-related and *COL6*-related CMD, whereas CK levels are greater than four times normal in CMD with primary merosin deficiency (laminin alpha-2 deficiency) or secondary merosin deficiency (dystroglyconopathies).

Eye examination by a pediatric ophthalmologist is important to evaluate for malformations of the anterior chamber (iris hypoplasia, cataracts, glaucoma), retinal dysplasia, or optic nerve hypoplasia typical of some dystroglycanopathies (WWS, muscle-eye-brain disease).

An MRI of the brain is useful in the diagnosis of the two CMDs with brain abnormalities, dystroglycanopathies, and LAMA2-related CMD. In the dystroglycanopathies the presence of cortical malformations, brainstem hypoplasia, and cerebellar cysts is common, whereas in LAMA2-related CMD white matter abnormalities on T2-weighted and fluid-attenuation inversion recovery images are typically found in all patients. No brain MRI abnormalities are found in CMD caused by defects in COL6, lamin A/C, and selenoprotein.

Electrodiagnostic studies are useful to exclude other causes of hypotonia and weakness, especially spinal muscular dystrophy, congenital peripheral neuropathies, and congenital myasthenic syndromes. EMG is either normal or shows myopathic changes in proximal muscles. Nerve conduction study can show a peripheral neuropathy associated with *LAMA2*-related CMD.[456]

Muscle MRI in COL6-related CMD shows a fatty infiltration in a peripheral rim pattern in the vasti muscles sparing the center of the muscle and relative sparing of the sartorius, gracilis, adductor longus and rectus femoris.[457] In SEPN1-related CMD, MRI shows selective involvement of adductor longus and sartorius muscles with sparing of the gracilis that correlates with the characteristic median thigh wasting seen on physical examination.[458,459]

Muscle biopsy is important in reaching a specific diagnosis as it provides useful clues to direct genetic testing. It is also important to rule out other disorders that may mimic a CMD such as mitochondrial myopathies, congenital myopathies, glycogen storage myopathies and spinal muscular atrophy. Histopathology usually shows a dystrophic pattern with fiber size variability, increased endomysial fibrosis, split fibers, hypercontracted fibers, and necrotic and regenerating fibers, or a nonspecific

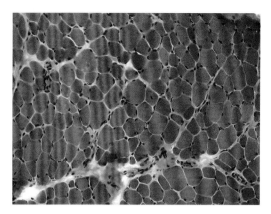

Figure 4–18. Skeletal muscle sample from patient with dystroglycanopathy, CK 2000, delayed walking, and brain abnormalities (Fig. 4–17): HE stain showing rounded fibers with increased variability in fiber size due to the presence of hypertrophy; one necrotic fiber undergoing phagocythosis; and increased interstitial fibrosis.

myopathic pattern without the specific features found in defined congenital myopathies (central cores and nemaline rods; Figure 4–18). Prominent necrosis is infrequent, and often absent. Immunohistochemical staining is critical in detecting deficiency of specific proteins and antibodies for laminin alpha-2 (merosin), COL6, and glycosylated alpha-dystroglycan (Figure 4–19A-B) should be used whenever a CMD is suspected. Reduction in labeling of laminin alpha-2 typical of mutations in *LAMA2* (MDC1A) is also common in the dystroglycanopathies (secondary merosin deficiency).

Genetic testing is now clinically available for many genes associated with specific subtypes of CMD (Table 4–3). The selection of a test for a specific gene should be guided by the clinical features and by brain MRI and muscle biopsy findings.

Differential Diagnosis

Among patients referred to neuromuscular centers for a possible diagnosis of CMD, congenital myasthenic syndromes, congenital myopathies, and LGMDs are the most common alternative diagnoses.[440]

In congenital myopathies joint contractures are rare, CK is normal or near normal, severe facial and ocular weakness is more common in the early stages, and the muscle weakness is frequently static or may improve over time.

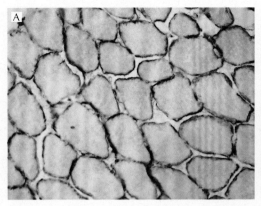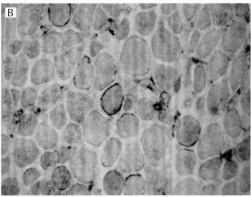

Figure 4–19. Immunohistochemical staining for alpha-dystroglycan using glycosylation-sensitive antibodies. Courtesy Dr. Rabi Tawil, University of Rochester, NY. A: Control with normal sarcolemmal staining pattern. B: Absent sarcolemmal staining in 2-year-old patient with CMD (brain MRI shown in CMD; Figure 4–17).

Muscle biopsy is most useful in differentiating specific congenital myopathies from CMD (see chapter 6).

Congenital myasthenic syndromes are characterized by normal CK, normal muscle biopsy histology, and abnormal neuromuscular transmission as documented by repetitive nerve stimulation and stimulated single-fiber EMG.

Limb-girdle muscular dystrophies and CMD have significant phenotype and genotype overlap: COL6 defects can cause Bethlem myopathy and Ullrich CMD, and defects in the genes associated with the dystroglycanopathies can also result in LGMD types (see Limb-Girdle Muscular Dystrophies section).

The infantile form of Pompe disease (acid maltase deficiency) presents with prominent hypotonia and respiratory insufficiency, but unlike CMD, it is frequently associated with hepatomegaly, cardiomyopathy, macroglossia, and typical PAS-positive vacuoles on muscle biopsy consistent with a glycogen storage disorder.

The congenital form of DM1 can be usually be differentiated from CMD based on family history and by examining the child's mother.

In the rare congenital form of FSHD, the prominent facial diplegia and the hearing loss help to distinguish it from CMD (see FHSD section earlier in this chapter).

SMA type 1 presents before age 6 months with hypotonia, muscle weakness, and respiratory difficulty and is differentiated from CMD by the presence of tongue atrophy and fasciculations, neurogenic motor units on EMG,

normal brain MRI, and fiber-type grouping on muscle biopsy. DNA testing for *SMN1* gene defects confirms the diagnosis.

Mitochondrial myopathies with infancy onset may have ocular and bulbar abnormalities in conjunction with brain abnormalities, and they are diagnosed based on specific histochemical and biochemical findings on muscle biopsy, as well as DNA mutations in mitochondrial DNA (see chapter 8).

Prader-Willi syndrome (PWS) presents in early infancy with severe hypotonia and feeding abnormality. It can be differentiated from CMD based on normal CK and normal muscle biopsy, presence of hypogonadism, and abnormal methylation of the PWS region on chromosome 15q11.

Marinesco-Sjögren syndrome can be misdiagnosed as CMD due to hypotonia, muscle weakness, mildly elevated CK, cataracts, cerebellar atrophy on MRI, and intellectual disability. Distinguishing features are the prominent cerebellar ataxia, positive gene testing for SIL1, and the autophagic vacuoles seen on muscle biopsy by electron microscopy.[460]

Treatment

No specific therapy currently exists for CMD, and management is directed at the prevention and treatment of the secondary complications (see chapter 13). A consensus statement on standard of care for CMD is available.[461] Optimal care is best achieved by a multidisciplinary team that includes neuromuscular, pulmonary, orthopedic, and physical and occupational therapy experts.

As in DMD, proactive and preventive pulmonary care is critical and should be guided by changes in FVC and peak cough flow. Management should include aggressive secretions clearance (cough assist), prompt treatment of respiratory infections (antibiotics, cough assist), and assisted ventilation (noninvasive positive-pressure ventilation, ventilation through tracheostomy; see chapter 13).

Patients with CMD should be screened for cardiac involvement at the time of diagnosis, and cardiac surveillance is indicated in those with CMD subtypes known to be associated with cardiac manifestations (see Clinical Features in this section).

Orthopedic evaluation should address the need for spinal bracing and scoliosis surgery as well as best prevention and correction of limb and spine contractures. Spinal bracing should aim at maximal abdomen, head, and spine support, and minimal restriction of chest excursion to avoid respiratory restriction.

Treatment of seizures should be chosen according to seizure type and guided by the MRI and EEG abnormalities. Seizures can sometimes be difficult to treat in the dystroglycanopathies due to the underlying brain malformations.[452,453,462] The role of nonpharmachological treatments such as surgery, ketogenic diet, and vagus nerve stimulation is unknown in CMD.

Referral to a child psychiatrist or psychologist should be considered in patient with behavioral or emotional symptoms or autistic features. Learning disability and mental retardation should be evaluated and addressed with early intervention programs and special services at school.

Eye exam should be performed at the time of initial diagnosis by a pediatric ophthalmologist to monitor for eye abnormalities. Visual impairment should be addressed promptly with referral to learning and adaptive services in order to maximize learning and quality of life.

DISTAL MUSCULAR DYSTROPHY

The term *distal myopathy* has persisted from the past when it was believed that myopathies were, by definition, proximal in distribution, but then rare cases of distal weakness were discovered to have convincing evidence for myopathy rather than neuropathy or anterior horn cell disease. Since the causes, courses, and pathologies of distal myopathies are similar to those of the muscular dystrophies, the term *distal muscular dystrophy* is now preferable. Moreover, as the causes of the distal dystrophies are defined, it is now clear that mutations of a single protein can cause either a proximal or distal phenotype. Nonetheless, it remains true that most patient presenting with distal weakness have either a peripheral neuropathy or anterior cell disease as the cause. In such patients it is important to be certain that both the clinical setting and the clinical neurophysiology are consistent with nerve cell disease; otherwise myopathy will be overlooked.

The distal muscular dystrophies, by definition, start either in the hands or the distal legs or feet. The specific mutations responsible for each of the diseases have now been identified (Table 4–4). In addition to the diseases characterized by their usually distal onset, many other hereditary and sporadic myopathies can have a distal presentation or prominent distal weakness (Box 4.1 lists the major diseases). The most frequently encountered and best characterized distal muscular dystrophies include Miyoshi myopathy, Nonaka myopathy (hereditary inclusion body myopathy), Udd myopathy (tibial muscular dystrophy), Welander myopathy, Liang myopathy (early onset distal dystrophy), and anoctominopathy.[463] These are summarized along with rarer conditions in Table 4–4. Some myofibrillar myopathies (discussed in chapter 5) were initially reported as distal myopathies (e.g., late-onset distal myopathy of Markesbery-Griggs and now known to be a zaspopoathy.[464,465] Here we consider the four most common distal myopathies/muscular dystrophies.

Miyoshi Myopathy

Miyoshi myopathy is caused by mutations in dysferlin (a dysferlinopathy). Dysferlinopathy was first discovered to have a distal phenotype but it subsequently has become clear that dysferlin mutations also present as a limb-girdle muscular dystrophy (LGMD2B)[466] and as an inflammatory myopathy resembling

Table 4–4 Classification of Distal Myopathies

Type	Initial Description	Locus/Gene	Onset Age (Years)	Initial Findings	CK Elevation	Muscle Biopsy
Miyoshi myopathy	Miyoshi, 1985	AR 2p13/DYSF	15–30	Posterior lower leg, calf	20–150×	Dystrophic
GNE myopathy	Nonaka, 1981	AR 9p1-q1/GNE	15–30	Anterior lower leg	3–4×	Dystrophic, rimmed vacuoles
Welander myopathy	Welander, 1951	AD 2p13/TIA1	>40	Hands, finger extensors	1–3×	Dystrophic, rimmed vacuoles
Tibial muscular dystrophy	Udd, 1993	AD 2q31/TTN	>35	Anterior lower leg	1–4×	Dystrophic, rimmed vacuoles
Laing myopathy (MPD1)	Laing, 1995	AD 14q/MYH7	35–60	Anterior lower leg	1–3×	Mild to moderately dystrophic
Vocal cord and pharyngeal weakness (MPD2)	Feit, 1998	AD 5q31/MATR3	35–60	Anterior lower leg, dysphonia	1–8×	Rimmed vacuoles
Anoctaminopathy	Bolduc, 2010	AD 11p14.3/ANO5	20–40	Posterior lower leg, calf	20–150×	Dystrophic
VCP-mutated distal myopathy	Palmio, 2011	AD 9p13.3/VCP	>35	Anterior leg (dementia during later years)	1–2×	Dystrophic, rimmed vacuoles
Distal ABD filaminopathy	Williams, 2005; Duff, 2011	AD 7q32-q35/FLNC	20–30	Thenar, anterior forearm, and posterior lower leg	1–2×	Dystrophic
KLH9-mutated distal myopathy	Cirak, 2010	AD 9p21.2-p22.3/KLH9	8–16	Anterior leg, glove and stocking sensory loss	1–8×	Dystrophic
Distal caveolinopathy	Tateyama, 2002	Sporadic 3p25/CAV3	>20	Hands and feet	20×	Dystrophic
Myofibrillar myopathies with distal phenotype						
Zaspopathy	Markesbery & Griggs, 1974	AD 10q22/ZASP (LDB3)	40–50	Clinically anterior, posterior on MRI	1–4×	Dystrophic, rimmed vacuoles, desmin bodies
Desminopathy	Milhorat & Wolf, 1943	AD 2q35/DES	Variable	Distal and proximal weakness, cardiomyopathy	1–4×	Dystrophic, rimmed vacuoles, desmin bodies
αB-crystallin-mutated distal myopathy	Reilich, 2010	AD 11q/CRYAB	50–60	Distal leg and hands	1.5–2.5×	Rimmed and nonrimmed vacuoles, Z-disk streaming, desmin and αB-crystallin aggregates
Myotilinopathy	Penisson-Besnier, 1998	AD 5q31/MYOT	50–60	Posterior more than anterior distal leg	1–3×	Dystrophic, rimmed and nonrimmed vacuoles, desmin-myotilin aggregates

---

Box 4.1 Other Myopathies That May Present With Distal Muscular Symptoms/Signs

Muscular dystrophies
Facioscapulohumeral muscular dystrophy
Myotonic dystrophy (DM1)
Congenital myopathies
Centronuclear
Myotubular
Nebulin
Metabolic
Glycogenoses
Mitochrondrial
Inflammatory myopathies
Inclusion body myositis

---

polymyositis.[467] Presymptomatic cases are often identified because of hyperCKemia (values 20-fold elevated or more).

GENETICS

Miyoshi myopathy was the first of the distal muscular dystrophies characterized by mutation and abnormal protein product. Mutations in the dysferlin gene must be identified on both chromosomes to provide strict genetic diagnosis, but demonstration of dysferlin absence by western blotting is sufficient for diagnosis. Dysferlin does not interact with dystrophin but appears to be important in cell signaling pathways.[468,469] Dysferlin also interacts with caveolin-3 and filamin C and may play a role in sarcolemmal repair.[470]

Mutations in dysferlin also cause a limb-girdle phenotype and, remarkably, the same mutation may cause either phenotype.[467]

EPIDEMIOLOGY

Miyoshi myopathy is the most frequent single cause of distal muscular dystrophy, but there are as yet no population-based studies of incidence or prevalence. As many as 30% of patients with the typical Miyoshi phenotype (onset of leg weakness in the posterior compartment and markedly elevated CK) do not have mutation in the dysferlin gene and have normal dysferlin on western blotting.[470]

CLINICAL

Many patients with dysferlinopathy present with isolated hyperCKemia in their teens. Onset of weakness is usually in the calf muscle and difficult to appreciate without testing function by having the patient walk on their toes or hop on one foot at a time. The calf muscles are often large even when weakness is demonstrable. The EDB muscle is frequently large (Figure 4–20) even when calf atrophy is marked (Figure 4–21). Anterior compartment

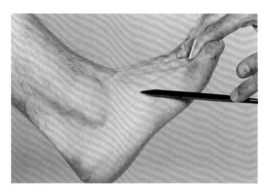

Figure 4–20. A patient with Miyoshi myopathy. The extensor digitorum brevis muscle (arrowhead) is spared.

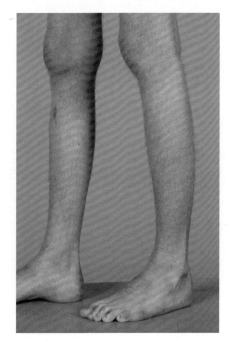

Figure 4–21. Gastrocnemious muscle wasting in Miyoshi myopathy.

muscles usually become weak and atrophied later but occasionally may be the first muscle affected. There is often preservation of the ability to "spread the toes" (Figure 4–22). Distal upper-limb strength is generally preserved, whereas biceps and triceps muscle involvement is developing. Knee extension becomes weak within 5 years and often progresses rapidly, resulting in loss of ambulation 10 to 20 years after disease onset. Respiratory, bulbar, and cardiac muscles are usually spared.

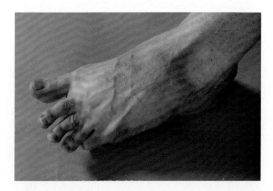

Figure 4–22. Preserved strength of the intrinsic foot muscles and ability to spread the toes in a patient with Miyoshi myopathy.

Approximately 10% of patients with dysferlinopathy present with evidence of inflammation on muscle biopsy and with proximal weakness leading to a diagnosis of polymyositis. Thus, the evaluation of "polymyositis" requires exclusion of dysferlinopathy (and many other muscular dystrophies; chapter 10).

LABORATORY STUDIES

The CK level is invariably elevated, usually 20-fold or more. Late in the disease, the CK level may fall as it does in other severely wasted patients. Other skeletal muscle enzymes are also elevated. The EMG shows small, brief MUPs with early recruitment. Muscle biopsy shows changes typical of a muscular dystrophy without vacuoles. Inflammation is present in some cases (see Clinical section above). There is no evidence for the involvement of cardiac muscles and respiratory function is usually normal. MRI of the legs can show fatty degeneration of the calf muscle before weakness is evident. Diagnostic testing for mutations in the dysferlin gene or western blotting for dysferlin are the specific diagnostic tests.

TREATMENT

There are no specific treatments yet for dysferlinopathies. Corticosteroids and immunosuppression with azathioprine have not slowed progression of weakness. Orthotics are often used for the posterior compartment leg weakness but are much less helpful than AFOs for anterior compartment weakness.

Welander Myopathy

Arguably the first well-established, true distal myopathy, Welander distal myopathy or dystrophy is of late onset and begins in the arms in most cases. The disorder was first identified in Sweden and a founder haplotype was identified before the mutated gene was discovered.[471,472]

GENETICS

Welander myopathy is autosomal dominant and results from a mutation in the C-terminal glutamine-rich prion-like domain of T-cell intracellular antigen-1 (TIA1).[472,473] TIA1 is an RNA-binding protein that regulates alternative splicing of certain pre-mRNAs. TIA1 appears to affect the assembly of "stress granules" that form in response to environmental stress.[474,475]

CLINICAL

Welander distal dystrophy is of late onset (20–40 years) and most often initially involves the hands with weakness of index finger extension and soon other finger muscles (Figure 4–23). The intrinsic hand muscles are also involved. Weakness is often asymmetrical. In 20% to 30% of patients foot dorsiflexor weakness is the initial sign, and the distal leg muscles become involved in almost all cases. Proximal leg and arm muscles are relatively spared so that ambulation is maintained. Rare instances of homozygous mutations have a more severe phenotype.[471]

LABORATORY STUDIES

Serum CK is usually 2- to 3-fold times normal but can be normal. The EMG shows small, brief MUP with pathological recruitment. Nerve conduction velocities are normal. Muscle biopsy shows changes of muscular dystrophy with the additional feature of rimmed vacuoles. There are no inflammatory cell infiltrates. MRI shows fatty replacement of calf and anterior compartment muscles, even before weakness has developed. Molecular testing demonstrating mutations in the *TIA1* gene is the definitive diagnostic test.[473]

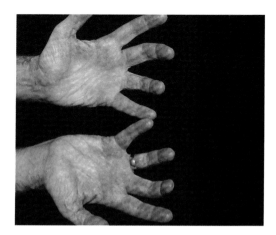

Figure 4–23. Prominent intrinsic atrophy of the hand muscles in a patient with Welander myopathy.

TREATMENT

Patients with foot drop obtain major benefit from AFOs. Various hand adaptive devices can improve hand function.

Tibial Muscular Dystrophy

This distal myopathy is relatively frequent in Finland (1:10,000) but occurs elsewhere both in subjects of Finnish descent and others. First recognized by Udd,[477] it presents with anterior compartment leg weakness in the fourth or fifth decade and progresses slowly to involve proximal leg muscles.

GENETICS

Udd myopathy is autosomal dominant and caused by mutations in the C-terminal domain of the large sarcolemmal protein, titin, which is located in the M-line of the sarcomere.[476,477] Homozygous mutations are rarely encountered and result in a more severe phenotype with limb-girdle distribution weakness.[478]

CLINICAL

The distribution of weakness closely resembles adult-onset Charcot-Marie-Tooth disease, with anterior compartment weakness starting in the fourth decade. As in Miyoshi myopathy, the EDB is preserved or enlarged, distinguishing these distal myopathies from peripheral neuropathic causes of distal weakness. Proximal weakness does not develop until late in the disease course and the upper extremities are generally spared.

LABORATORY STUDIES

The serum CK may be normal or slightly elevated. EMG is characteristic of myopathy with low-amplitude, brief MUP and early recruitment. Fibrillations are frequent. Biopsy shows changes typical of muscular dystrophy with the additional feature of rimmed vacuoles.

TREATMENT

AFOs are of major benefit in tibial muscular dystrophy (as they are in Charcot-Marie-Tooth disease). Respiratory, swallowing, and cardiac dysfunction do not occur.

GNE (Nonaka) Myopathy

This distal myopathy with rimmed vacuoles was initially described in Japan by Nonaka[479] and elsewhere decribed as a hereditary inclusion body myopathy (HIBM) with quadriceps muscle sparing.[480] Both Nonaka myopathy and HIBM have been found to result from mutations in the same gene: the (UDP-N-acetyl) 2-epimerase/N-acetylmannosamine kinase gene—usually termed the GNE gene.[481,482]

GENETICS

The disease is autosomal recessive. Many Japanese patients have a single founder mutation in GNE.[480] In other populations, patients have other mutations and are at times compound heterozygotes.

CLINICAL

GNE myopathy typical manifests in the third decade with distal leg weakness. Within a decade proximal weakness develops, generally paring the quadriceps (in contrast to the sporadic inflammatory myopathy, inclusion body myositis; see chapter 10). Neck flexors become involved but other cranial nerve–innervated muscles are spared. Respiratory and cardiac muscle involvement are not frequent.

LABORATORY STUDIES

The serum CK is usually elevated 3- to 5-fold. EMG is usually myopathic with prominent fibrillations. Biopsy shows rimmed vacuoles in addition to changes of chronic myopathy. Muscle MRI is distinctive: involvement of anterior leg muscles and thigh muscle sparing the quadriceps muscles. Diagnosis is most reliably made by sequencing the GNE gene.

TREATMENT

AFOs correct the foot drop and are of major benefit, but there is no treatment for the progressive weakness.

Distal Myofibrillar Myopathies

Most, if not all, of the lengthening list of myofibrillar myopathies have distal weakness and most can present as a distal myopathy with proximal weakness only appearing later in the course (see chapter 5). One of the myofibrillar myopathies, zaspopathy, was one of the earliest myopathies established to be a distal disorder.[464,465]

Other Distal Dystrophies/ Myopathies

There are many other very rare disorders; these are summarized in Table 4–4. Most have been reported in only single families or at most a handful of cases.

REFERENCES

1. Koenig M, Hoffman EP, Bertelson CJ, Monaco AP, Feener C, Kunkel LM. Complete cloning of the Duchenne muscular dystrophy (DMD) cDNA and preliminary genomic organization of the DMD gene in normal and affected individuals. *Cell*. 1987;50(3):509–517.
2. Koenig M, Monaco AP, Kunkel LM. The complete sequence of dystrophin predicts a rod-shaped cytoskeletal protein. *Cell*. 1988;53(2):219–228.
3. Centers for Disease Control and Prevention. Prevalence of Duchenne/Becker muscular dystrophy among males aged 5-24 years—four states, 2007. *MMWR Morb Mortal Wkly Rep*. 2009;58(40):1119–1122.
4. Parsons EP, Bradley DM, Clarke AJ. Newborn screening for Duchenne muscular dystrophy. *Arch Dis Child*. 2003;88(1):91–92.
5. Bradley DM, Parsons EP, Clarke AJ. Experience with screening newborns for Duchenne muscular dystrophy in wales. *BMJ*. 1993;306(6874):357–360.
6. Mendell JR, Shilling C, Leslie ND, et al. Evidence-based path to newborn screening for Duchenne muscular dystrophy. *Ann Neurol*. 2012;71(3):304–313. doi:10.1002/ana.23528.
7. Levenson D. Newborn screening for Duchenne muscular dystrophy gains support: Researchers to push for federal recommendation to have states add DMD test to newborn panel. *Am J Med Genet A*. 2012;158A(12):viii–ix. doi:10.1002/ajmg.a.35799.
8. Mendell JR, Lloyd-Puryear M. Report of MDA muscle disease symposium on newborn screening for Duchenne muscular dystrophy. *Muscle Nerve*. 2013;48(1):21–26. doi:10.1002/mus.23810.

9. Helderman-van den Enden AT, Madan K, Breuning MH, et al. An urgent need for a change in policy revealed by a study on prenatal testing for Duchenne muscular dystrophy. *Eur J Hum Genet*. 2013;21(1):21–26. doi:10.1038/ejhg.2012.101.

10. Muntoni F, Torelli S, Ferlini A. Dystrophin and mutations: One gene, several proteins, multiple phenotypes. *Lancet Neurol*. 2003;2(12):731–740.

11. Love DR, Flint TJ, Marsden RF, et al. Characterization of deletions in the dystrophin gene giving mild phenotypes. *Am J Med Genet*. 1990;37(1):136–142. doi:10.1002/ajmg.1320370132.

12. England SB, Nicholson LV, Johnson MA, et al. Very mild muscular dystrophy associated with the deletion of 46% of dystrophin. *Nature*. 1990;343(6254):180–182. doi:10.1038/343180a0.

13. Love DR, Flint TJ, Genet SA, Middleton-Price HR, Davies KE. Becker muscular dystrophy patient with a large intragenic dystrophin deletion: Implications for functional minigenes and gene therapy. *J Med Genet*. 1991;28(12):860–864.

14. Ciafaloni E, Fox DJ, Pandya S, et al. Delayed diagnosis in Duchenne muscular dystrophy: Data from the muscular dystrophy surveillance, tracking, and research network (MD STARnet). *J Pediatr*. 2009;155(3):380–385. doi:10.1016/j.jpeds.2009.02.007.

15. Mohamed K, Appleton R, Nicolaides P. Delayed diagnosis of Duchenne muscular dystrophy. *Eur J Paediatr Neurol*. 2000;4(5):219–223. doi:10.1053/ejpn.2000.0309.

16. McDonald DG, Kinali M, Gallagher AC, et al. Fracture prevalence in Duchenne muscular dystrophy. *Dev Med Child Neurol*. 2002;44(10):695–698.

17. Medeiros MO, Behrend C, King W, Sanders J, Kissel J, Ciafaloni E. Fat embolism syndrome in patients with Duchenne muscular dystrophy. *Neurology*. 2013;80(14):1350–1352. doi:10.1212/WNL.0b013e31828ab313.

18. McAdam LC, Rastogi A, Macleod K, Douglas Biggar W. Fat embolism syndrome following minor trauma in Duchenne muscular dystrophy. *Neuromuscul Disord*. 2012;22(12):1035–1039. doi:10.1016/j.nmd.2012.07.010.

19. Takami Y, Takeshima Y, Awano H, Okizuka Y, Yagi M, Matsuo M. High incidence of electrocardiogram abnormalities in young patients with Duchenne muscular dystrophy. *Pediatr Neurol*. 2008;39(6):399–403. doi:10.1016/j.pediatrneurol.2008.08.006.

20. James J, Kinnett K, Wang Y, Ittenbach RF, Benson DW, Cripe L. Electrocardiographic abnormalities in very young Duchenne muscular dystrophy patients precede the onset of cardiac dysfunction. *Neuromuscul Disord*. 2011;21(7):462–467. doi:10.1016/j.nmd.2011.04.005.

21. Ergul Y, Ekici B, Nisli K, et al. Evaluation of the North Star ambulatory assessment scale and cardiac abnormalities in ambulant boys with Duchenne muscular dystrophy. *J Paediatr Child Health*. 2012;48(7):610–616. doi:10.1111/j.1440-1754.2012.02428.x.

22. Politano L, Nigro G. Treatment of dystrophinopathic cardiomyopathy: Review of the literature and personal results. *Acta Myol*. 2012;31(1):24–30.

23. Wagner S, Knipp S, Weber C, et al. The heart in Duchenne muscular dystrophy: Early detection of contractile performance alteration. *J Cell Mol Med*. 2012;16(12):3028–3036. doi:10.1111/j.1582-4934.2012.01630.x.

24. Rideau Y, Jankowski LW, Grellet J. Respiratory function in the muscular dystrophies. *Muscle Nerve*. 1981;4(2):155–164. doi:10.1002/mus.880040213.

25. Phillips MF, Quinlivan RC, Edwards RH, Calverley PM. Changes in spirometry over time as a prognostic marker in patients with Duchenne muscular dystrophy. *Am J Respir Crit Care Med*. 2001;164(12):2191–2194. doi:10.1164/ajrccm.164.12.2103052.

26. Crowe GG. Acute dilatation of stomach as a complication of muscular dystrophy. *Br Med J*. 1961;1(5236):1371.

27. Barohn RJ, Levine EJ, Olson JO, Mendell JR. Gastric hypomotility in Duchenne's muscular dystrophy. *N Engl J Med*. 1988;319(1):15–18. doi:10.1056/NEJM198807073190103.

28. Leon SH, Schuffler MD, Kettler M, Rohrmann CA. Chronic intestinal pseudoobstruction as a complication of Duchenne's muscular dystrophy. *Gastroenterology*. 1986;90(2):455–459.

29. Snow WM, Anderson JE, Jakobson LS. Neuropsychological and neurobehavioral functioning in Duchenne muscular dystrophy: A review. *Neurosci Biobehav Rev*. 2013;37(5):743–752. doi:10.1016/j.neubiorev.2013.03.016.

30. Desguerre I, Christov C, Mayer M, et al. Clinical heterogeneity of Duchenne muscular dystrophy (DMD): Definition of sub-phenotypes and predictive criteria by long-term follow-up. *PLoS One*. 2009;4(2):e4347. doi:10.1371/journal.pone.0004347.

31. Felisari G, Martinelli Boneschi F, Bardoni A, et al. Loss of Dp140 dystrophin isoform and intellectual impairment in Duchenne dystrophy. *Neurology*. 2000;55(4):559–564.

32. Dubowitz V, Crome L. The central nervous system in Duchenne muscular dystrophy. *Brain*. 1969;92(4):805–808.

33. Hinton VJ, De Vivo DC, Nereo NE, Goldstein E, Stern Y. Poor verbal working memory across intellectual level in boys with Duchenne dystrophy. *Neurology*. 2000;54(11):2127–2132.

34. Hinton VJ, De Vivo DC, Fee R, Goldstein E, Stern Y. Investigation of poor academic achievement in children with Duchenne muscular dystrophy. *Learn Disabil Res Pract*. 2004;19(3):146–154. doi:10.1111/j.1540-5826.2004.00098.x.

35. Cotton SM, Voudouris NJ, Greenwood KM. Association between intellectual functioning and age in children and young adults with Duchenne muscular dystrophy: Further results from a meta-analysis. *Dev Med Child Neurol*. 2005;47(4):257–265.

36. Cotton S, Voudouris NJ, Greenwood KM. Intelligence and Duchenne muscular dystrophy: Full-scale, verbal, and performance intelligence quotients. *Dev Med Child Neurol*. 2001;43(7):497–501.

37. Mento G, Tarantino V, Bisiacchi PS. The neuropsychological profile of infantile Duchenne muscular dystrophy. *Clin Neuropsychol*. 2011;25(8):1359–1377. doi:10.1080/13854046.2011.617782.

38. Hendriksen JG, Vles JS. Neuropsychiatric disorders in males with Duchenne muscular dystrophy: Frequency rate of attention-deficit hyperactivity disorder (ADHD), autism spectrum disorder, and obsessive-compulsive disorder. *J Child Neurol*. 2008;23(5):477–481. doi:10.1177/0883073807309775.

39. Hendriksen JG, Poysky JT, Schrans DG, Schouten EG, Aldenkamp AP, Vles JS. Psychosocial adjustment in males with Duchenne muscular dystrophy: Psychometric properties and clinical utility of a parent-report questionnaire. *J Pediatr Psychol.* 2009;34(1):69–78. doi:10.1093/jpepsy/jsn067.

40. Cox GF, Kunkel LM. Dystrophies and heart disease. *Curr Opin Cardiol.* 1997;12(3):329–343.

41. Brooke MH, Fenichel GM, Griggs RC, et al. Clinical investigation in Duchenne dystrophy: 2. determination of the "power" of therapeutic trials based on the natural history. *Muscle Nerve.* 1983;6(2):91–103. doi:10.1002/mus.880060204.

42. Sumita DR, Vainzof M, Campiotto S, et al. Absence of correlation between skewed X inactivation in blood and serum creatine-kinase levels in Duchenne/Becker female carriers. *Am J Med Genet.* 1998;80(4):356–361.

43. Den Dunnen JT, Grootscholten PM, Bakker E, et al. Topography of the Duchenne muscular dystrophy (DMD) gene: FIGE and cDNA analysis of 194 cases reveals 115 deletions and 13 duplications. *Am J Hum Genet.* 1989;45(6):835–847.

44. Aartsma-Rus A, Van Deutekom JC, Fokkema IF, Van Ommen GJ, Den Dunnen JT. Entries in the Leiden Duchenne muscular dystrophy mutation database: An overview of mutation types and paradoxical cases that confirm the reading-frame rule. *Muscle Nerve.* 2006;34(2):135–144. doi:10.1002/mus.20586.

45. Chelly J, Gilgenkrantz H, Lambert M, et al. Effect of dystrophin gene deletions on mRNA levels and processing in Duchenne and Becker muscular dystrophies. *Cell.* 1990;63(6):1239–1248.

46. Arahata K, Engel AG. Monoclonal antibody analysis of mononuclear cells in myopathies. I: Quantitation of subsets according to diagnosis and sites of accumulation and demonstration and counts of muscle fibers invaded by T cells. *Ann Neurol.* 1984;16(2):193–208. doi:10.1002/ana.410160206.

47. Mokri B, Engel AG. Duchenne dystrophy: Electron microscopic findings pointing to a basic or early abnormality in the plasma membrane of the muscle fiber. *Neurology.* 1975;25(12):1111–1120.

48. Hoffman EP, Fischbeck KH, Brown RH, et al. Characterization of dystrophin in muscle-biopsy specimens from patients with Duchenne's or Becker's muscular dystrophy. *N Engl J Med.* 1988;318(21):1363–1368. doi:10.1056/NEJM198805263182104.

49. Moxley RT 3rd, Ashwal S, Pandya S, et al. Practice parameter: Corticosteroid treatment of Duchenne dystrophy: Report of the quality standards subcommittee of the American Academy of Neurology and the Practice Committee of the Child Neurology Society. *Neurology.* 2005;64(1):13–20. doi:10.1212/01.WNL.0000148485.00049.B7.

50. Manzur AY, Kuntzer T, Pike M, Swan A. Glucocorticoid corticosteroids for Duchenne muscular dystrophy. *Cochrane Database Syst Rev.* 2008;(1):CD003725. doi(1):CD003725. doi:10.1002/14651858.CD003725.pub3.

51. Centers for Disease Control and Prevention. Prevalence of Duchenne/Becker muscular dystrophy among males aged 5-24 years—four states, 2007. *MMWR Morb Mortal Wkly Rep.* 2009;58(40):1119–1122.

52. Eagle M, Baudouin SV, Chandler C, Giddings DR, Bullock R, Bushby K. Survival in Duchenne muscular dystrophy: Improvements in life expectancy since 1967 and the impact of home nocturnal ventilation. *Neuromuscul Disord.* 2002;12(10):926–929.

53. Moxley RT 3rd, Pandya S, Ciafaloni E, Fox DJ, Campbell K. Change in natural history of Duchenne muscular dystrophy with long-term corticosteroid treatment: Implications for management. *J Child Neurol.* 2010;25(9):1116–1129. doi:10.1177/0883073810371004.

54. Gomez-Merino E, Bach JR. Duchenne muscular dystrophy: Prolongation of life by noninvasive ventilation and mechanically assisted coughing. *Am J Phys Med Rehabil.* 2002;81(6):411–415.

55. Griggs RC, Moxley RT 3rd, Mendell JR, et al. Prednisone in Duchenne dystrophy. A randomized, controlled trial defining the time course and dose response. clinical investigation of Duchenne dystrophy group. *Arch Neurol.* 1991;48(4):383–388.

56. Mendell JR, Moxley RT, Griggs RC, et al. Randomized, double-blind six-month trial of prednisone in Duchenne's muscular dystrophy. *N Engl J Med.* 1989;320(24):1592–1597. doi:10.1056/NEJM198906153202405.

57. Fenichel GM, Mendell JR, Moxley RT 3rd, et al. A comparison of daily and alternate-day prednisone therapy in the treatment of Duchenne muscular dystrophy. *Arch Neurol.* 1991;48(6):575–579.

58. Griggs RC, Moxley RT 3rd, Mendell JR, et al. Duchenne dystrophy: Randomized, controlled trial of prednisone (18 months) and azathioprine (12 months). *Neurology.* 1993;43(3 Pt 1):520–527.

59. Backman E, Henriksson KG. Low-dose prednisolone treatment in Duchenne and Becker muscular dystrophy. *Neuromuscul Disord.* 1995;5(3):233–241.

60. Rahman MM, Hannan MA, Mondol BA, Bhoumick NB, Haque A. Prednisolone in Duchenne muscular dystrophy. *Bangladesh Med Res Counc Bull.* 2001;27(1):38–42.

61. Escolar DM, Hache LP, Clemens PR, et al. Randomized, blinded trial of weekend vs daily prednisone in Duchenne muscular dystrophy. *Neurology.* 2011;77(5):444–452. doi:10.1212/WNL.0b013e318227b164.

62. Connolly AM, Schierbecker J, Renna R, Florence J. High dose weekly oral prednisone improves strength in boys with Duchenne muscular dystrophy. *Neuromuscul Disord.* 2002;12(10):917–925.

63. Dubowitz V, Kinali M, Main M, Mercuri E, Muntoni F. Remission of clinical signs in early Duchenne muscular dystrophy on intermittent low-dosage prednisolone therapy. *Eur J Paediatr Neurol.* 2002;6(3):153–159.

64. Kinali M, Mercuri E, Main M, Muntoni F, Dubowitz V. An effective, low-dosage, intermittent schedule of prednisolone in the long-term treatment of early cases of Duchenne dystrophy. *Neuromuscul Disord.* 2002;12 Suppl 1:S169–74.

65. Sansome A, Royston P, Dubowitz V. Steroids in Duchenne muscular dystrophy; pilot study of a new low-dosage schedule. *Neuromuscul Disord.* 1993;3(5–6):567–569.

66. Mesa LE, Dubrovsky AL, Corderi J, Marco P, Flores D. Steroids in Duchenne muscular dystrophy—deflazacort trial. *Neuromuscul Disord.* 1991;1(4):261–266.

67. Biggar WD, Politano L, Harris VA, et al. Deflazacort in Duchenne muscular dystrophy: A comparison of two different protocols. *Neuromuscul Disord.* 2004;14(8–9):476–482. doi:10.1016/j.nmd.2004.05.001.

68. Biggar WD, Harris VA, Eliasoph L, Alman B. Long-term benefits of deflazacort treatment for boys with Duchenne muscular dystrophy in their second decade. *Neuromuscul Disord*. 2006;16(4):249–255. doi:10.1016/j.nmd.2006.01.010.

69. Angelini C, Pegoraro E, Turella E, Intino MT, Pini A, Costa C. Deflazacort in Duchenne dystrophy: Study of long-term effect. *Muscle Nerve*. 1994;17(4):386–391. doi:10.1002/mus.880170405.

70. Angelini C. The role of corticosteroids in muscular dystrophy: A critical appraisal. *Muscle Nerve*. 2007;36(4):424–435. doi:10.1002/mus.20812.

71. Merlini L, Gennari M, Malaspina E, et al. Early corticosteroid treatment in 4 Duchenne muscular dystrophy patients: 14-year follow-up. *Muscle Nerve*. 2012;45(6):796–802. doi:10.1002/mus.23272.

72. Merlini L, Cicognani A, Malaspina E, et al. Early prednisone treatment in Duchenne muscular dystrophy. *Muscle Nerve*. 2003;27(2):222–227. doi:10.1002/mus.10319.

73. Drachman DB, Toyka KV, Myer E. Prednisone in Duchenne muscular dystrophy. *Lancet*. 1974;2(7894):1409–1412.

74. DeSilva S, Drachman DB, Mellits D, Kuncl RW. Prednisone treatment in Duchenne muscular dystrophy. long-term benefit. *Arch Neurol*. 1987;44(8):818–822.

75. King WM, Ruttencutter R, Nagaraja HN, et al. Orthopedic outcomes of long-term daily corticosteroid treatment in Duchenne muscular dystrophy. *Neurology*. 2007;68(19):1607–1613. doi:10.1212/01.wnl.0000260974.41514.83.

76. Matthews DJ, James KA, Miller LA, et al. Use of corticosteroids in a population-based cohort of boys with Duchenne and Becker muscular dystrophy. *J Child Neurol*. 2010;25(11):1319–1324. doi:10.1177/0883073810362762.

77. Griggs RC, Herr BE, Reha A, et al. Corticosteroids in Duchenne muscular dystrophy: Major variations in practice. *Muscle Nerve*. 2013. doi:10.1002/mus.23831; 10.1002/mus.23831.

78. Bushby K, Finkel R, Birnkrant DJ, et al. Diagnosis and management of Duchenne muscular dystrophy, part 1: Diagnosis, and pharmacological and psychosocial management. *Lancet Neurol*. 2010;9(1):77–93. doi:10.1016/S1474-4422(09)70271-6.

79. Bushby K, Finkel R, Birnkrant DJ, et al. Diagnosis and management of Duchenne muscular dystrophy, part 2: Implementation of multidisciplinary care. *Lancet Neurol*. 2010;9(2):177–189. doi:10.1016/S1474-4422(09)70272-8.

80. Passaquin AC, Renard M, Kay L, et al. Creatine supplementation reduces skeletal muscle degeneration and enhances mitochondrial function in mdx mice. *Neuromuscul Disord*. 2002;12(2):174–182.

81. Tarnopolsky MA, Mahoney DJ, Vajsar J, et al. Creatine monohydrate enhances strength and body composition in Duchenne muscular dystrophy. *Neurology*. 2004;62(10):1771–1777.

82. Escolar DM, Buyse G, Henricson E, et al. CINRG randomized controlled trial of creatine and glutamine in Duchenne muscular dystrophy. *Ann Neurol*. 2005;58(1):151–155. doi:10.1002/ana.20523.

83. Granchelli JA, Pollina C, Hudecki MS. Pre-clinical screening of drugs using the mdx mouse. *Neuromuscul Disord*. 2000;10(4–5):235–239.

84. Spurney CF, Rocha CT, Henricson E, et al. CINRG pilot trial of coenzyme Q10 in steroid-treated Duchenne muscular dystrophy. *Muscle Nerve*. 2011;44(2):174–178. doi:10.1002/mus.22047.

85. Cohn RD, van Erp C, Habashi JP, et al. Angiotensin II type 1 receptor blockade attenuates TGF-beta-induced failure of muscle regeneration in multiple myopathic states. *Nat Med*. 2007;13(2):204–210. doi:10.1038/nm1536.

86. Nelson CA, Hunter RB, Quigley LA, et al. Inhibiting TGF-beta activity improves respiratory function in mdx mice. *Am J Pathol*. 2011;178(6):2611–2621. doi:10.1016/j.ajpath.2011.02.024.

87. Bish LT, Yarchoan M, Sleeper MM, et al. Chronic losartan administration reduces mortality and preserves cardiac but not skeletal muscle function in dystrophic mice. *PLoS One*. 2011;6(6):e20856. doi:10.1371/journal.pone.0020856.

88. Spurney CF, Sali A, Guerron AD, et al. Losartan decreases cardiac muscle fibrosis and improves cardiac function in dystrophin-deficient mdx mice. *J Cardiovasc Pharmacol Ther*. 2011;16(1):87–95. doi:10.1177/1074248410381757.

89. Bushby K, Finkel R, Birnkrant DJ, et al. Diagnosis and management of Duchenne muscular dystrophy, part 2: Implementation of multidisciplinary care. *Lancet Neurol*. 2010;9(2):177–189. doi:10.1016/S1474-4422(09)70272-8.

90. Birnkrant DJ, Bushby KM, Amin RS, et al. The respiratory management of patients with Duchenne muscular dystrophy: A DMD care considerations working group specialty article. *Pediatr Pulmonol*. 2010;45(8):739–748. doi:10.1002/ppul.21254.

91. Finder JD, Birnkrant D, Carl J, et al. Respiratory care of the patient with Duchenne muscular dystrophy: ATS consensus statement. *Am J Respir Crit Care Med*. 2004;170(4):456–465. doi:10.1164/rccm.200307-885ST.

92. Bach JR, Alba AS, Saporito LR. Intermittent positive pressure ventilation via the mouth as an alternative to tracheostomy for 257 ventilator users. *Chest*. 1993;103(1):174–182.

93. Bach JR, Bianchi C, Vidigal-Lopes M, Turi S, Felisari G. Lung inflation by glossopharyngeal breathing and "air stacking" in Duchenne muscular dystrophy. *Am J Phys Med Rehabil*. 2007;86(4):295–300. doi:10.1097/PHM.0b013e318038d1ce.

94. Birnkrant DJ. The American College of Chest Physicians consensus statement on the respiratory and related management of patients with Duchenne muscular dystrophy undergoing anesthesia or sedation. *Pediatrics*. 2009;123 Suppl 4:S242–4. doi:10.1542/peds.2008-2952J.

95. Yemen TA, McClain C. Muscular dystrophy, anesthesia and the safety of inhalational agents revisited; again. *Paediatr Anaesth*. 2006;16(2):105–108. doi:10.1111/j.1460-9592.2005.01801.x.

96. Hayes J, Veyckemans F, Bissonnette B. Duchenne muscular dystrophy: An old anesthesia problem revisited. *Paediatr Anaesth*. 2008;18(2):100–106. doi:10.1111/j.1460-9592.2007.02302.x.

97. Breucking E, Reimnitz P, Schara U, Mortier W. Anesthetic complications. the incidence of severe anesthetic complications in patients and families with progressive muscular dystrophy of the Duchenne and Becker types. *Anaesthesist*. 2000;49(3):187–195.

98. American Academy of Pediatrics Section on Cardiology and Cardiac Surgery. Cardiovascular health supervision for individuals affected by Duchenne or Becker muscular dystrophy. *Pediatrics*. 2005;116(6):1569–1573. doi:10.1542/peds.2005-2448.

99. Bushby K, Muntoni F, Bourke JP. 107th ENMC international workshop: The management of cardiac involvement in muscular dystrophy and myotonic dystrophy. 7th–9th June 2002, Naarden, The Netherlands. *Neuromuscul Disord*. 2003;13(2):166–172.

100. Saito T, Matsumura T, Miyai I, Nozaki S, Shinno S. Carvedilol effectiveness for left ventricular-insufficient patients with Duchenne muscular dystrophy. *Rinsho Shinkeigaku*. 2001;41(10):691–694.

101. Kajimoto H, Ishigaki K, Okumura K, et al. Beta-blocker therapy for cardiac dysfunction in patients with muscular dystrophy. *Circ J*. 2006;70(8):991–994.

102. Kwon HW, Kwon BS, Kim GB, et al. The effect of enalapril and carvedilol on left ventricular dysfunction in middle childhood and adolescent patients with muscular dystrophy. *Korean Circ J*. 2012;42(3):184–191. doi:10.4070/kcj.2012.42.3.184.

103. Doing AH, Renlund DG, Smith RA. Becker muscular dystrophy-related cardiomyopathy: A favorable response to medical therapy. *J Heart Lung Transplant* 2002;21(4):496–498.

104. Matsumura T, Tamura T, Kuru S, Kikuchi Y, Kawai M. Carvedilol can prevent cardiac events in Duchenne muscular dystrophy. *Intern Med*. 2010;49(14):1357–1363.

105. Hunt SA, American College of Cardiology, American Heart Association Task Force on Practice Guidelines: ACC/AHA 2005 guideline update for the diagnosis and management of chronic heart failure in the adult: A report of the American College of Cardiology/American Heart Association Task Force on Practice Guidelines. *J Am Coll Cardiol*. 2005;46(6):e1–e82. doi:10.1016/j.jacc.2005.08.022.

106. Radford MJ, Arnold JM, Bennett SJ, et al. ACC/AHA key data elements and definitions for measuring the clinical management and outcomes of patients with chronic heart failure: A report of the American College of Cardiology/American Heart Association Task Force on Clinical Data Standards. *Circulation*. 2005;112(12):1888–1916. doi:10.1161/CIRCULATIONAHA.105.170073.

107. McNally EM. New approaches in the therapy of cardiomyopathy in muscular dystrophy. *Annu Rev Med*. 2007;58:75–88. doi:10.1146/annurev.med.58.011706.144703.

108. Duboc D, Meune C, Pierre B, et al. Perindopril preventive treatment on mortality in Duchenne muscular dystrophy: 10 years' follow-up. *Am Heart J*. 2007;154(3):596–602. doi:10.1016/j.ahj.2007.05.014.

109. Duboc D, Meune C, Lerebours G, Devaux JY, Vaksmann G, Becane HM. Effect of perindopril on the onset and progression of left ventricular dysfunction in Duchenne muscular dystrophy. *J Am Coll Cardiol*. 2005;45(6):855–857. doi:10.1016/j.jacc.2004.09.078.

110. Meune C, Duboc D. How should physicians manage patients with Duchenne muscular dystrophy when experts' recommendations are not unanimous? *Dev Med Child Neurol*. 2006;48(10):863–864. doi:10.1017/S0012162206221856.

111. Wu RS, Gupta S, Brown RN, et al. Clinical outcomes after cardiac transplantation in muscular dystrophy patients. *J Heart Lung Transplant*. 2010;29(4):432–438. doi:10.1016/j.healun.2009.08.030.

112. Ruiz-Cano MJ, Delgado JF, Jimenez C, et al. Successful heart transplantation in patients with inherited myopathies associated with end-stage cardiomyopathy. *Transplant Proc*. 2003;35(4):1513–1515.

113. Orlov YS, Brodsky MA, Allen BJ, Ott RA, Orlov MV, Jay CA. Cardiac manifestations and their management in Becker's muscular dystrophy. *Am Heart J*. 1994;128(1):193–196.

114. Finsterer J, Bittner RE, Grimm M. Cardiac involvement in Becker's muscular dystrophy, necessitating heart transplantation, 6 years before apparent skeletal muscle involvement. *Neuromuscul Disord*. 1999;9(8):598–600.

115. Quinlivan R, Shaw N, Bushby K. 170th ENMC international workshop: Bone protection for corticosteroid treated Duchenne muscular dystrophy. 27–29 November 2009, Naarden, The Netherlands. *Neuromuscul Disord*. 2010;20(11):761–769. doi:10.1016/j.nmd.2010.07.272.

116. Quinlivan R, Roper H, Davie M, Shaw NJ, McDonagh J, Bushby K. Report of a muscular dystrophy campaign funded workshop Birmingham, UK, January 16th 2004. Osteoporosis in Duchenne muscular dystrophy; its prevalence, treatment and prevention. *Neuromuscul Disord*. 2005;15(1):72–79. doi:10.1016/j.nmd.2004.09.009.

117. Biggar WD, Bachrach LK, Henderson RC, Kalkwarf H, Plotkin H, Wong BL. Bone health in Duchenne muscular dystrophy: A workshop report from the meeting in Cincinnati, Ohio, July 8, 2004. *Neuromuscul Disord*. 2005;15(1):80–85. doi:10.1016/j.nmd.2004.09.010.

118. Kinali M, Main M, Eliahoo J, et al. Predictive factors for the development of scoliosis in Duchenne muscular dystrophy. *Eur J Paediatr Neurol*. 2007;11(3):160–166. doi:10.1016/j.ejpn.2006.12.002.

119. Kinali M, Messina S, Mercuri E, et al. Management of scoliosis in Duchenne muscular dystrophy: A large 10-year retrospective study. *Dev Med Child Neurol*. 2006;48(6):513–518. doi:10.1017/S0012162206001083.

120. Scher DM, Mubarak SJ. Surgical prevention of foot deformity in patients with Duchenne muscular dystrophy. *J Pediatr Orthop*. 2002;22(3):384–391.

121. Wright JG. Surgical prevention of foot deformity in patients with Duchenne muscular dystrophy. *J Pediatr Orthop*. 2003;23(3):419.

122. Hyde SA, FlŁytrup I, Glent S, et al. A randomized comparative study of two methods for controlling Tendo Achilles contracture in Duchenne muscular dystrophy. *Neuromuscul Disord*. 2000;10(4–5):257–263.

123. Scott OM, Hyde SA, Goddard C, Dubowitz V. Prevention of deformity in Duchenne muscular dystrophy. A prospective study of passive stretching and splintage. *Physiotherapy*. 1981;67(6):177–180.

124. McDonald CM. Limb contractures in progressive neuromuscular disease and the role of stretching, orthotics, and surgery. *Phys Med Rehabil Clin N Am*. 1998;9(1):187–211.

125. Hyde SA, Scott OM, Goddard CM, Dubowitz V. Prolongation of ambulation in Duchenne muscular dystrophy by appropriate orthoses. *Physiotherapy*. 1982;68(4):105–108.

126. Bakker JP, de Groot IJ, Beckerman H, de Jong BA, Lankhorst GJ. The effects of knee-ankle-foot orthoses in the treatment of Duchenne muscular dystrophy: Review of the literature. *Clin Rehabil*. 2000;14(4):343–359.

127. Arias R, Andrews J, Pandya S, et al. Palliative care services in families of males with Duchenne muscular dystrophy. *Muscle Nerve*. 2011;44(1):93–101. doi:10.1002/mus.22005.

128. Simonds AK. Living and dying with respiratory failure: Facilitating decision making. *Chron Respir Dis*. 2004;1(1):56–59.

129. Penner L, Cantor RM, Siegel L. Joseph's wishes: Ethical decision-making in Duchenne muscular dystrophy. *Mt Sinai J Med*. 2010;77(4):394–397. doi:10.1002/msj.20196.

130. Fraser LK, Childs AM, Miller M, et al. A cohort study of children and young people with progressive neuromuscular disorders: Clinical and demographic profiles and changing patterns of referral for palliative care. *Palliat Med*. 2012;26(7):924–929. doi:10.1177/0269216311419989.

131. Weidner NJ. Developing an interdisciplinary palliative care plan for the patient with muscular dystrophy. *Pediatr Ann*. 2005;34(7):546–552.

132. Gregorevic P, Allen JM, Minami E, et al. rAAV6-microdystrophin preserves muscle function and extends lifespan in severely dystrophic mice. *Nat Med*. 2006;12(7):787–789. doi:10.1038/nm1439.

133. Wang B, Li J, Qiao C, et al. A canine minidystrophin is functional and therapeutic in mdx mice. *Gene Ther*. 2008;15(15):1099–1106. doi:10.1038/gt.2008.70.

134. Wang Z, Kuhr CS, Allen JM, et al. Sustained AAV-mediated dystrophin expression in a canine model of Duchenne muscular dystrophy with a brief course of immunosuppression. *Mol Ther*. 2007;15(6):1160–1166. doi:10.1038/sj.mt.6300161.

135. Fabb SA, Wells DJ, Serpente P, Dickson G. Adeno-associated virus vector gene transfer and sarcolemmal expression of a 144 kDa micro-dystrophin effectively restores the dystrophin-associated protein complex and inhibits myofibre degeneration in nude/mdx mice. *Hum Mol Genet*. 2002;11(7):733–741.

136. Mendell JR, Campbell K, Rodino-Klapac L, et al. Dystrophin immunity in Duchenne's muscular dystrophy. *N Engl J Med*. 2010;363(15):1429–1437. doi:10.1056/NEJMoa1000228.

137. Gussoni E, Pavlath GK, Miller RG, et al. Specific T cell receptor gene rearrangements at the site of muscle degeneration in Duchenne muscular dystrophy. *J Immunol*. 1994;153(10):4798–4805.

138. Rodino-Klapac LR, Montgomery CL, Bremer WG, et al. Persistent expression of FLAG-tagged micro dystrophin in nonhuman primates following intramuscular and vascular delivery. *Mol Ther*. 2010;18(1):109–117. doi:10.1038/mt.2009.254.

139. Rodino-Klapac LR, Janssen PM, Montgomery CL, et al. A translational approach for limb vascular delivery of the micro-dystrophin gene without high volume or high pressure for treatment of Duchenne muscular dystrophy. *J Transl Med*. 2007;5:45. doi:10.1186/1479-5876-5-45.

140. Rodino-Klapac LR, Montgomery CL, Mendell JR, Chicoine LG. AAV-mediated gene therapy to the isolated limb in rhesus macaques. *Methods Mol Biol*. 2011;709:287–298. doi:10.1007/978-1-61737-982-6_19.

141. Liang KW, Nishikawa M, Liu F, Sun B, Ye Q, Huang L. Restoration of dystrophin expression in mdx mice by intravascular injection of naked DNA containing full-length dystrophin cDNA. *Gene Ther*. 2004;11(11):901–908. doi:10.1038/sj.gt.3302239.

142. Zhang G, Wooddell CI, Hegge JO, et al. Functional efficacy of dystrophin expression from plasmids delivered to mdx mice by hydrodynamic limb vein injection. *Hum Gene Ther*. 2010;21(2):221–237. doi:10.1089/hum.2009.133.

143. Gregorevic P, Blankinship MJ, Allen JM, et al. Systemic delivery of genes to striated muscles using adeno-associated viral vectors. *Nat Med*. 2004;10(8):828–834. doi:10.1038/nm1085.

144. Flanigan KM, Dunn DM, von Niederhausern A, et al. Mutational spectrum of DMD mutations in dystrophinopathy patients: Application of modern diagnostic techniques to a large cohort. *Hum Mutat*. 2009;30(12):1657–1666. doi:10.1002/humu.21114.

145. Flanigan KM, von Niederhausern A, Dunn DM, Alder J, Mendell JR, Weiss RB. Rapid direct sequence analysis of the dystrophin gene. *Am J Hum Genet*. 2003;72(4):931–939.

146. Malik V, Rodino-Klapac LR, Viollet L, et al. Gentamicin-induced readthrough of stop codons in Duchenne muscular dystrophy. *Ann Neurol*. 2010;67(6):771–780. doi:10.1002/ana.22024.

147. Barton-Davis ER, Cordier L, Shoturma DI, Leland SE, Sweeney HL. Aminoglycoside antibiotics restore dystrophin function to skeletal muscles of mdx mice. *J Clin Invest*. 1999;104(4):375–381. doi:10.1172/JCI7866.

148. Hirawat S, Welch EM, Elfring GL, et al. Safety, tolerability, and pharmacokinetics of PTC124, a nonaminoglycoside nonsense mutation suppressor, following single- and multiple-dose administration to healthy male and female adult volunteers. *J Clin Pharmacol*. 2007;47(4):430–444. doi:10.1177/0091270006297140.

149. Welch EM, Barton ER, Zhuo J, et al. PTC124 targets genetic disorders caused by nonsense mutations. *Nature*. 2007;447(7140):87–91. doi:10.1038/nature05756.

150. Bönnemann C, Finkel R, Wong B, Flanigan K, Sampson J, Sweeney L, Reha A, Elfring G, Miller L, Hirawat S. Phase 2 study of PTC124 for nonsense mutation suppression therapy of Duchenne muscular dystrophy (DMD) *Neuromuscular Disorders*, 2007;17(9):783.

151. McDonald CM, Henricson EK, Abresch RT, et al. The 6-minute walk test and other endpoints in Duchenne muscular dystrophy: Longitudinal natural history observations over 48 weeks from a multicenter study. *Muscle Nerve*. 2013. doi:10.1002/mus.23902.

152. Goyenvalle A, Babbs A, Powell D, et al. Prevention of dystrophic pathology in severely affected dystrophin/utrophin-deficient mice by morpholino-oligomer-mediated exon-skipping. *Mol Ther*. 2010;18(1):198–205. doi:10.1038/mt.2009.248.

153. Yokota T, Lu QL, Partridge T, et al. Efficacy of systemic morpholino exon-skipping in Duchenne dystrophy dogs. *Ann Neurol.* 2009;65(6):667–676. doi:10.1002/ana.21627.

154. Kinali M, Arechavala-Gomeza V, Feng L, et al. Local restoration of dystrophin expression with the morpholino oligomer AVI-4658 in Duchenne muscular dystrophy: A single-blind, placebo-controlled, dose-escalation, proof-of-concept study. *Lancet Neurol.* 2009;8(10):918–928. doi:10.1016/S1474-4422(09)70211-X.

155. van Deutekom JC, Janson AA, Ginjaar IB, et al. Local dystrophin restoration with antisense oligonucleotide PRO051. *N Engl J Med.* 2007;357(26):2677–2686. doi:10.1056/NEJMoa073108.

156. Goemans NM, Tulinius M, van den Akker JT, et al. Systemic administration of PRO051 in Duchenne's muscular dystrophy. *N Engl J Med.* 2011;364(16):1513–1522. doi:10.1056/NEJMoa1011367.

157. Cirak S, Arechavala-Gomeza V, Guglieri M, et al. Exon skipping and dystrophin restoration in patients with Duchenne muscular dystrophy after systemic phosphorodiamidate morpholino oligomer treatment: An open-label, phase 2, dose-escalation study. *Lancet.* 2011;378(9791):595–605. doi:10.1016/S0140-6736(11)60756-3.

158. Emery AE, Dreifuss FE. Unusual type of benign x-linked muscular dystrophy. *J Neurol Neurosurg Psychiatry.* 1966;29(4):338–342.

159. Dickey RP, Ziter FA, Smith RA. Emery-Dreifuss muscular dystrophy. *J Pediatr.* 1984;104(4):555–559.

160. Hopkins LC, Jackson JA, Elsas LJ. Emery-Dreifuss humeroperoneal muscular dystrophy: An x-linked myopathy with unusual contractures and bradycardia. *Ann Neurol.* 1981;10(3):230–237. doi:10.1002/ana.410100306.

161. Rotthauwe HW, Mortier W, Beyer H. New type of recessive X-linked muscular dystrophy: Scapulo-humeral-distal muscular dystrophy with early contractures and cardiac arrhythmias. *Humangenetik.* 1972;16(3): 181–200.

162. Rowland LP, Fetell M, Olarte M, Hays A, Singh N, Wanat FE. Emery-Dreifuss muscular dystrophy. *Ann Neurol.* 1979;5(2):111–117. doi:10.1002/ana.410050203.

163. Thomas PK, Calne DB, Elliott CF. X-linked scapuloperoneal syndrome. *J Neurol Neurosurg Psychiatry.* 1972;35(2):208–215.

164. Waters DD, Nutter DO, Hopkins LC, Dorney ER. Cardiac features of an unusual X-linked humeroperoneal neuromuscular disease. *N Engl J Med.* 1975;293(20):1017–1022. doi:10.1056/NEJM197511132932004.

165. Raffaele Di Barletta M, Ricci E, Galluzzi G, et al. Different mutations in the LMNA gene cause autosomal dominant and autosomal recessive Emery-Dreifuss muscular dystrophy. *Am J Hum Genet.* 2000;66(4):1407–1412. doi:10.1086/302869.

166. Jimenez-Escrig A, Gobernado I, Garcia-Villanueva M, Sanchez-Herranz A. Autosomal recessive Emery-Dreifuss muscular dystrophy caused by a novel mutation (R225Q) in the lamin A/C gene identified by exome sequencing. *Muscle Nerve.* 2012;45(4):605–610. doi:10.1002/mus.22324.

167. Zacharias AS, Wagener ME, Warren ST, Hopkins LC. Emery-Dreifuss muscular dystrophy. *Semin Neurol.* 1999;19(1):67–79. doi:10.1055/s-2008-1040827.

168. Yates JR, Wehnert M. The Emery-Dreifuss muscular dystrophy mutation database. *Neuromuscul Disord.* 1999;9(3):199.

169. Gueneau L, Bertrand AT, Jais JP, et al. Mutations of the FHL1 gene cause Emery-Dreifuss muscular dystrophy. *Am J Hum Genet.* 2009;85(3):338–353. doi:10.1016/j.ajhg.2009.07.015.

170. Bonne G, Mercuri E, Muchir A, et al. Clinical and molecular genetic spectrum of autosomal dominant Emery-Dreifuss muscular dystrophy due to mutations of the lamin A/C gene. *Ann Neurol.* 2000;48(2):170–180.

171. Ellis JA. 81st Enmc international workshop: 4th meeting on Emery-Dreifuss muscular dystrophy 7th and 8th July 2000, Naarden, The Netherlands. *Neuromuscul Disord.* 2001;11(4):417–420.

172. Bonne G, Leturcq F, Ben Yaou R. Emery-Dreifuss muscular dystrophy. In: Pagon RA, Adam MP, Bird TD, Dolan CR, Fong CT, Stephens K, eds. *GeneReviews.* Seattle (WA): University of Washington, Seattle; 1993.

173. Fanin M, Nascimbeni AC, Aurino S, et al. Frequency of LGMD gene mutations in Italian patients with distinct clinical phenotypes. *Neurology.* 2009;72(16):1432–1435. doi:10.1212/WNL.0b013e3181a1885e.

174. Karst ML, Herron KJ, Olson TM. X-linked nonsyndromic sinus node dysfunction and atrial fibrillation caused by emerin mutation. *J Cardiovasc Electrophysiol.* 2008;19(5):510–515. doi:10.1111/j.1540-8167.2007.01081.x.

175. Quinzii CM, Vu TH, Min KC, et al. X-linked dominant scapuloperoneal myopathy is due to a mutation in the gene encoding four-and-a-half-LIM protein 1. *Am J Hum Genet.* 2008;82(1):208–213. doi:10.1016/j.ajhg.2007.09.013.

176. Shalaby S, Hayashi YK, Goto K, et al. Rigid spine syndrome caused by a novel mutation in four-and-a-half LIM domain 1 gene (FHL1). *Neuromuscul Disord.* 2008;18(12):959–961. doi:10.1016/j.nmd.2008.09.012.

177. Friedrich FW, Wilding BR, Reischmann S, et al. Evidence for FHL1 as a novel disease gene for isolated hypertrophic cardiomyopathy. *Hum Mol Genet.* 2012;21(14):3237–3254. doi:10.1093/hmg/dds157.

178. Shalaby S, Hayashi YK, Nonaka I, Noguchi S, Nishino I. Novel FHL1 mutations in fatal and benign reducing body myopathy. *Neurology.* 2009;72(4):375–376. doi:10.1212/01.wnl.0000341311.84347.a0.

179. van Tintelen JP, Hofstra RM, Katerberg H, et al. High yield of LMNA mutations in patients with dilated cardiomyopathy and/or conduction disease referred to cardiogenetics outpatient clinics. *Am Heart J.* 2007;154(6):1130–1139. doi:10.1016/j.ahj.2007.07.038.

180. Parmar MS, Parmar KS. Emery-Dreifuss humeroperoneal muscular dystrophy: Cardiac manifestations. *Can J Cardiol.* 2012;28(4):516.e1–516.e3. doi:10.1016/j.cjca.2012.01.012.

181. Wozakowska-Kaplon B, Bakowski D. Atrial paralysis due to progression of cardiac disease in a patient with Emery-Dreifuss muscular dystrophy. *Cardiol J.* 2011;18(2):189–193.

182. Pasotti M, Klersy C, Pilotto A, et al. Long-term outcome and risk stratification in dilated cardiolaminopathies. *J Am Coll Cardiol*. 2008;52(15):1250–1260. doi:10.1016/j.jacc.2008.06.044.

183. Nigro G, Russo V, Ventriglia VM, et al. Early onset of cardiomyopathy and primary prevention of sudden death in X-linked Emery-Dreifuss muscular dystrophy. *Neuromuscul Disord*. 2010;20(3):174–177. doi:10.1016/j.nmd.2009.12.004.

184. Becane HM, Bonne G, Varnous S, et al. High incidence of sudden death with conduction system and myocardial disease due to lamins A and C gene mutation. *Pacing Clin Electrophysiol*. 2000;23(11 Pt 1):1661–1666.

185. Boriani G, Gallina M, Merlini L, et al. Clinical relevance of atrial fibrillation/flutter, stroke, pacemaker implant, and heart failure in Emery-Dreifuss muscular dystrophy: A long-term longitudinal study. *Stroke*. 2003;34(4):901–908. doi:10.1161/01. STR.0000064322.47667.49.

186. Redondo-Verge L, Yaou RB, Fernandez-Recio M, Dinca L, Richard P, Bonne G. Cardioembolic stroke prompting diagnosis of LMNA-associated Emery-Dreifuss muscular dystrophy. *Muscle Nerve*. 2011;44(4):587–589. doi:10.1002/mus.22179.

187. Tanaka K, Uehara T, Sato K, Amano T, Minematsu K, Toyoda K. Successful intravenous rt-PA thrombolysis for a childhood cardioembolic stroke with Emery-Dreifuss muscular dystrophy. *Cerebrovasc Dis*. 2012;33(1):92–93. doi:10.1159/000331930.

188. Sanna T, Dello Russo A, Toniolo D, et al. Cardiac features of Emery-Dreifuss muscular dystrophy caused by lamin A/C gene mutations. *Eur Heart J*. 2003;24(24):2227–2236.

189. Zaim S, Bach J, Michaels J. Sudden death in an Emery-Dreifuss muscular dystrophy patient with an implantable defibrillator. *Am J Phys Med Rehabil*. 2008;87(4):325–329. doi:10.1097/PHM.0b013e318168b9d4.

190. Mercuri E, Poppe M, Quinlivan R, et al. Extreme variability of phenotype in patients with an identical missense mutation in the lamin A/C gene: From congenital onset with severe phenotype to milder classic Emery-Dreifuss variant. *Arch Neurol*. 2004;61(5):690–694. doi:10.1001/archneur.61.5.690.

191. Wehnert M, Muntoni F. 60th ENMC international workshop: Non X-linked Emery-Dreifuss muscular dystrophy 5-7 June 1998, Naarden, The Netherlands. *Neuromuscul Disord*. 1999;9(2):115–121.

192. Cruz Martinez A, Du Theil LA. Electrophysiologic evaluation of Emery-Dreifuss muscular dystrophy. A single fiber and quantitative EMG study. *Electromyogr Clin Neurophysiol*. 1989;29(2):99–103.

193. Rowinska-Marcinska K, Szmidt-Salkowska E, Fidzianska A, et al. Atypical motor unit potentials in Emery-Dreifuss muscular dystrophy (EDMD). *Clin Neurophysiol*. 2005;116(11):2520–2527. doi:10.1016/j.clinph.2005.01.017.

194. Witt TN, Garner CG, Pongratz D, Baur X. Autosomal dominant Emery-Dreifuss syndrome: Evidence of a neurogenic variant of the disease. *Eur Arch Psychiatry Neurol Sci*. 1988;237(4):230–236.

195. Deconinck N, Dion E, Ben Yaou R, et al. Differentiating Emery-Dreifuss muscular dystrophy and collagen VI-related myopathies using a specific CT scanner pattern. *Neuromuscul Disord*. 2010;20(8):517–523. doi:10.1016/j.nmd.2010.04.009.

196. Mercuri E, Counsell S, Allsop J, et al. Selective muscle involvement on magnetic resonance imaging in autosomal dominant Emery-Dreifuss muscular dystrophy. *Neuropediatrics*. 2002;33(1):10–14. doi:10.1055/s-2002-23593.

197. Mercuri E, Clements E, Offiah A, et al. Muscle magnetic resonance imaging involvement in muscular dystrophies with rigidity of the spine. *Ann Neurol*. 2010;67(2):201–208. doi:10.1002/ana.21846.

198. Carboni N, Mura M, Marrosu G, et al. Muscle imaging analogies in a cohort of patients with different clinical phenotypes caused by LMNA gene mutations. *Muscle Nerve*. 2010;41(4):458–463. doi:10.1002/mus.21514.

199. Carboni N, Mura M, Marrosu G, et al. Muscle MRI findings in patients with an apparently exclusive cardiac phenotype due to a novel LMNA gene mutation. *Neuromuscul Disord*. 2008;18(4):291–298. doi:10.1016/j.nmd.2008.01.009.

200. Semnic R, Vucurevic G, Kozic D, Koprivsek K, Ostojic J, Sener RN. Emery-Dreifuss muscular dystrophy: MR imaging and spectroscopy in the brain and skeletal muscle. *AJNR Am J Neuroradiol*. 2004;25(10):1840–1842.

201. Mittelbronn M, Hanisch F, Gleichmann M, et al. Myofiber degeneration in autosomal dominant Emery-Dreifuss muscular dystrophy (AD-EDMD) (LGMD1B). *Brain Pathol*. 2006;16(4):266–272. doi:10.1111/j.1750-3639.2006.00028.x.

202. Sabatelli P, Lattanzi G, Ognibene A, et al. Nuclear alterations in autosomal-dominant Emery-Dreifuss muscular dystrophy. *Muscle Nerve*. 2001;24(6): 826–829.

203. Sewry CA, Brown SC, Mercuri E, et al. Skeletal muscle pathology in autosomal dominant Emery-Dreifuss muscular dystrophy with lamin A/C mutations. *Neuropathol Appl Neurobiol*. 2001;27(4):281–290.

204. Mittelbronn M, Sullivan T, Stewart CL, Bornemann A. Myonuclear degeneration in LMNA null mice. *Brain Pathol*. 2008;18(3):338–343. doi:10.1111/j.1750-3639.2008.00123.x.

205. Komaki H, Hayashi YK, Tsuburaya R, et al. Inflammatory changes in infantile-onset LMNA-associated myopathy. *Neuromuscul Disord*. 2011;21(8):563–568. doi:10.1016/j.nmd.2011.04.010; 10.1016/j.nmd.2011.04.010.

206. Merlini L, Granata C, Dominici P, Bonfiglioli S. Emery-Dreifuss muscular dystrophy: Report of five cases in a family and review of the literature. *Muscle Nerve*. 1986;9(6):481–485. doi:10.1002/mus.880090602.

207. Menezes MP, Waddell LB, Evesson FJ, et al. Importance and challenge of making an early diagnosis in LMNA-related muscular dystrophy. *Neurology*. 2012;78(16):1258–1263. doi:10.1212/WNL.0b013e318250d839.

208. Russo V, Rago A, Palladino A, et al. P-wave duration and dispersion in patients with Emery-Dreifuss muscular dystrophy. *J Investig Med*. 2011;59(7):1151–1154. doi:10.231/JIM.0b013e31822cf97a.

209. Goncu K, Guzel R, Guler-Uysal F. Emery-Dreifuss muscular dystrophy in the evaluation of decreased spinal mobility and joint contractures. *Clin*

Rheumatol. 2003;22(6):456–460. doi:10.1007/s10067-003-0771-9.

210. Dell'Amore A, Botta L, Martin Suarez S, et al. Heart transplantation in patients with Emery-Dreifuss muscular dystrophy: Case reports. *Transplant Proc.* 2007;39(10):3538–3540. doi:10.1016/j.transproceed.2007.06.076.

211. Kichuk Chrisant MR, Drummond-Webb J, Hallowell S, Friedman NR. Cardiac transplantation in twins with autosomal dominant Emery-Dreifuss muscular dystrophy. *J Heart Lung Transplant.* 2004;23(4):496–498. doi:10.1016/S1053-2498(03)00204-3.

212. Funnell A, Morgan J, McFadzean W. Anaesthesia and orphan disease: Management of cardiac and perioperative risks in a patient with Emery-Dreifuss muscular dystrophy. *Eur J Anaesthesiol.* 2012;29(12):596–598. doi:10.1097/EJA.0b013e3283585457.

213. Shende D, Agarwal R. Anaesthetic management of a patient with Emery-Dreifuss muscular dystrophy. *Anaesth Intensive Care.* 2002;30(3):372–375.

214. Sariego M, Bustos A, Guerola A, Romero I, Garcia-Baquero A. Anesthesia for cesarean section in a case of Emery-Dreifuss muscular dystrophy. *Rev Esp Anestesiol Reanim.* 1996;43(8):288–290.

215. Jensen V. The anaesthetic management of a patient with Emery-Dreifuss muscular dystrophy. *Can J Anaesth.* 1996;43(9):968–971. doi:10.1007/BF03011813.

216. Aldwinckle RJ, Carr AS. The anesthetic management of a patient with Emery-Dreifuss muscular dystrophy for orthopedic surgery. *Can J Anaesth.* 2002;49(5):467–470. doi:10.1007/BF03017922.

217. Kim OM, Elliott D. Elective caesarean section for a woman with Emery-Dreifuss muscular dystrophy. *Anaesth Intensive Care.* 2010;38(4):744–747.

218. Brook JD, McCurrach ME, Harley HG, et al. Molecular basis of myotonic dystrophy: Expansion of a trinucleotide (CTG) repeat at the 3' end of a transcript encoding a protein kinase family member. *Cell.* 1992;69(2):385.

219. Fu YH, Pizzuti A, Fenwick RG Jr, et al. An unstable triplet repeat in a gene related to myotonic muscular dystrophy. *Science.* 1992;255(5049):1256–1258.

220. Mankodi A, Takahashi MP, Jiang H, et al. Expanded CUG repeats trigger aberrant splicing of ClC-1 chloride channel pre-mRNA and hyperexcitability of skeletal muscle in myotonic dystrophy. *Mol Cell.* 2002;10(1):35–44.

221. Savkur RS, Philips AV, Cooper TA. Aberrant regulation of insulin receptor alternative splicing is associated with insulin resistance in myotonic dystrophy. *Nat Genet.* 2001;29(1):40–47. doi:10.1038/ng704.

222. Leroy O, Wang J, Maurage CA, et al. Brain-specific change in alternative splicing of tau exon 6 in myotonic dystrophy type 1. *Biochim Biophys Acta.* 2006;1762(4):460–467. doi:10.1016/j.bbadis.2005.12.003.

223. Tang ZZ, Yarotskyy V, Wei L, et al. Muscle weakness in myotonic dystrophy associated with misregulated splicing and altered gating of ca(V)1.1 calcium channel. *Hum Mol Genet.* 2012;21(6):1312–1324. doi:10.1093/hmg/ddr568.

224. Miller JW, Urbinati CR, Teng-Umnuay P, et al. Recruitment of human muscleblind proteins to (CUG)(n) expansions associated with myotonic dystrophy. *EMBO J.* 2000;19(17):4439–4448. doi:10.1093/emboj/19.17.4439.

225. Jiang H, Mankodi A, Swanson MS, Moxley RT, Thornton CA. Myotonic dystrophy type 1 is associated with nuclear foci of mutant RNA, sequestration of muscleblind proteins and deregulated alternative splicing in neurons. *Hum Mol Genet.* 2004;13(24):3079–3088. doi:10.1093/hmg/ddh327.

226. Martorell L, Monckton DG, Sanchez A, Lopez De Munain A, Baiget M. Frequency and stability of the myotonic dystrophy type 1 premutation. *Neurology.* 2001;56(3):328–335.

227. Harley HG, Rundle SA, MacMillan JC, et al. Size of the unstable CTG repeat sequence in relation to phenotype and parental transmission in myotonic dystrophy. *Am J Hum Genet.* 1993;52(6):1164–1174.

228. De Temmerman N, Sermon K, Seneca S, et al. Intergenerational instability of the expanded CTG repeat in the DMPK gene: Studies in human gametes and preimplantation embryos. *Am J Hum Genet.* 2004;75(2):325–329. doi:10.1086/422762.

229. Ashizawa T, Dubel JR, Dunne PW, et al. Anticipation in myotonic dystrophy. II. complex relationships between clinical findings and structure of the GCT repeat. *Neurology.* 1992;42(10):1877–1883.

230. Rakocevic-Stojanovic V, Savic D, Pavlovic S, et al. Intergenerational changes of CTG repeat depending on the sex of the transmitting parent in myotonic dystrophy type 1. *Eur J Neurol.* 2005;12(3):236–237. doi:10.1111/j.1468-1331.2004.01075.x.

231. Zeesman S, Carson N, Whelan DT. Paternal transmission of the congenital form of myotonic dystrophy type 1: A new case and review of the literature. *Am J Med Genet.* 2002;107(3):222–226.

232. Yotova V, Labuda D, Zietkiewicz E, et al. Anatomy of a founder effect: Myotonic dystrophy in northeastern Quebec. *Hum Genet.* 2005;117(2–3):177–187. doi:10.1007/s00439-005-1298-8.

233. Liquori CL, Ricker K, Moseley ML, et al. Myotonic dystrophy type 2 caused by a CCTG expansion in intron 1 of ZNF9. *Science.* 2001;293(5531):864–867. doi:10.1126/science.1062125.

234. Liquori CL, Ikeda Y, Weatherspoon M, et al. Myotonic dystrophy type 2: Human founder haplotype and evolutionary conservation of the repeat tract. *Am J Hum Genet.* 2003;73(4):849–862. doi:10.1086/378720.

235. Schoser BG, Kress W, Walter MC, Halliger-Keller B, Lochmuller H, Ricker K. Homozygosity for CCTG mutation in myotonic dystrophy type 2. *Brain.* 2004;127(Pt 8):1868–1877. doi:10.1093/brain/awh210.

236. Udd B, Meola G, Krahe R, et al. Myotonic dystrophy type 2 (DM2) and related disorders report of the 180th ENMC workshop including guidelines on diagnostics and management, 3–5 December 2010, Naarden, The Netherlands. *Neuromuscul Disord.* 2011;21(6):443–450. doi:10.1016/j.nmd.2011.03.013.

237. Groh WJ, Groh MR, Saha C, et al. Electrocardiographic abnormalities and sudden death in myotonic dystrophy type 1. *N Engl J Med.* 2008;358(25):2688–2697. doi:10.1056/NEJMoa062800.

238. Mathieu J, Allard P, Potvin L, Prevost C, Begin P. A 10-year study of mortality in a cohort of patients with myotonic dystrophy. *Neurology.* 1999;52(8):1658–1662.

239. Dauvilliers YA, Laberge L. Myotonic dystrophy type 1, daytime sleepiness and REM sleep dysregulation. *Sleep Med Rev.* 2012;16(6):539–545. doi:10.1016/j.smrv.2012.01.001.

240. Gibbs JW 3rd, Ciafaloni E, Radtke RA. Excessive daytime somnolence and increased rapid eye movement pressure in myotonic dystrophy. *Sleep.* 2002;25(6):662–665.

241. Ciafaloni E, Mignot E, Sansone V, et al. The hypocretin neurotransmission system in myotonic dystrophy type 1. *Neurology.* 2008;70(3):226–230. doi:10.1212/01.wnl.0000296827.20167.98.

242. Pincherle A, Patruno V, Raimondi P, et al. Sleep breathing disorders in 40 Italian patients with myotonic dystrophy type 1. *Neuromuscul Disord.* 2012;22(3):219–224. doi:10.1016/j.nmd.2011.08.010.

243. Monteiro R, Bento J, Goncalves MR, Pinto T, Winck JC. Genetics correlates with lung function and nocturnal ventilation in myotonic dystrophy. *Sleep Breath.* 2013. doi:10.1007/s11325-013-0807-6.

244. Kaminsky P, Poussel M, Pruna L, Deibener J, Chenuel B, Brembilla-Perrot B. Organ dysfunction and muscular disability in myotonic dystrophy type 1. *Medicine (Baltimore).* 2011;90(4):262–268. doi:10.1097/MD.0b013e318226046b.

245. Mathieu J, Allard P, Gobeil G, Girard M, De Braekeleer M, Begin P. Anesthetic and surgical complications in 219 cases of myotonic dystrophy. *Neurology.* 1997;49(6):1646–1650.

246. Owen PM, Chu C. Emergency caesarean section in a patient with myotonic dystrophy: A case of failed postoperative extubation in a patient with mild disease. *Anaesth Intensive Care.* 2011;39(2):293–298.

247. Kirzinger L, Schmidt A, Kornblum C, Schneider-Gold C, Kress W, Schoser B. Side effects of anesthesia in DM2 as compared to DM1: A comparative retrospective study. *Eur J Neurol.* 2010;17(6):842–845. doi:10.1111/j.1468-1331.2009.02942.x.

248. Weingarten TN, Hofer RE, Milone M, Sprung J. Anesthesia and myotonic dystrophy type 2: A case series. *Can J Anaesth.* 2010;57(3):248–255. doi:10.1007/s12630-009-9244-1.

249. Awater C, Zerres K, Rudnik-Schoneborn S. Pregnancy course and outcome in women with hereditary neuromuscular disorders: Comparison of obstetric risks in 178 patients. *Eur J Obstet Gynecol Reprod Biol.* 2012;162(2):153–159. doi:10.1016/j.ejogrb.2012.02.020.

250. Rudnik-Schoneborn S, Schneider-Gold C, Raabe U, Kress W, Zerres K, Schoser BG. Outcome and effect of pregnancy in myotonic dystrophy type 2. *Neurology.* 2006;66(4):579–580. doi:10.1212/01.wnl.0000198227.91131.1e.

251. Rudnik-Schoneborn S, Zerres K. Outcome in pregnancies complicated by myotonic dystrophy: A study of 31 patients and review of the literature. *Eur J Obstet Gynecol Reprod Biol.* 2004;114(1):44–53. doi:10.1016/j.ejogrb.2003.11.025.

252. Meola G, Sansone V. Cerebral involvement in myotonic dystrophies. *Muscle Nerve.* 2007;36(3):294–306. doi:10.1002/mus.20800.

253. Winblad S, Jensen C, Mansson JE, Samuelsson L, Lindberg C. Depression in myotonic dystrophy type 1: Clinical and neuronal correlates. *Behav Brain Funct.* 2010;6:25-9081-6-25. doi:10.1186/1744-9081-6-25.

254. Sansone V, Gandossini S, Cotelli M, Calabria M, Zanetti O, Meola G. Cognitive impairment in adult myotonic dystrophies: A longitudinal study. *Neurol Sci.* 2007;28(1):9–15. doi:10.1007/s10072-007-0742-z.

255. Meola G, Sansone V, Perani D, et al. Executive dysfunction and avoidant personality trait in myotonic dystrophy type 1 (DM-1) and in proximal myotonic myopathy (PROMM/DM-2). *Neuromuscul Disord.* 2003;13(10):813–821.

256. Weber YG, Roebling R, Kassubek J, et al. Comparative analysis of brain structure, metabolism, and cognition in myotonic dystrophy 1 and 2. *Neurology.* 2010;74(14):1108–1117. doi:10.1212/WNL.0b013e3181d8c35f.

257. Minnerop M, Weber B, Schoene-Bake JC, et al. The brain in myotonic dystrophy 1 and 2: Evidence for a predominant white matter disease. *Brain.* 2011;134(Pt 12):3530–3546. doi:10.1093/brain/awr299.

258. Franc DT, Muetzel RL, Robinson PR, et al. Cerebral and muscle MRI abnormalities in myotonic dystrophy. *Neuromuscul Disord.* 2012;22(6):483–491. doi:10.1016/j.nmd.2012.01.003.

259. Romeo V, Pegoraro E, Ferrati C, et al. Brain involvement in myotonic dystrophies: Neuroimaging and neuropsychological comparative study in DM1 and DM2. *J Neurol.* 2010;257(8):1246–1255. doi:10.1007/s00415-010-5498-3.

260. Reiter C, Gramer E. Anticipation in patients with iridescent multicoloured posterior capsular lens opacities ("Christmas tree cataract"): The role in the diagnosis of myotonic dystrophy. *Ophthalmologe.* 2009;106(12):1116–1120. doi:10.1007/s00347-009-1924-2.

261. Orngreen MC, Arlien-Soborg P, Duno M, Hertz JM, Vissing J. Endocrine function in 97 patients with myotonic dystrophy type 1. *J Neurol.* 2012;259(5):912–920. doi:10.1007/s00415-011-6277-5.

262. Griggs RC, Kingston W, Herr BE, Forbes G, Moxley RT 3rd. Myotonic dystrophy: Effect of testosterone on total body potassium and on creatinine excretion. *Neurology.* 1985;35(7):1035–1040.

263. Ercolin B, Sassi FC, Mangilli LD, Mendonca LI, Limongi SC, de Andrade CR. Oral motor movements and swallowing in patients with myotonic dystrophy type 1. *Dysphagia.* 2013. doi:10.1007/s00455-013-9458-9.

264. Bellini M, Biagi S, Stasi C, et al. Gastrointestinal manifestations in myotonic muscular dystrophy. *World J Gastroenterol.* 2006;12(12):1821–1828.

265. Win AK, Perattur PG, Pulido JS, Pulido CM, Lindor NM. Increased cancer risks in myotonic dystrophy. *Mayo Clin Proc.* 2012;87(2):130–135. doi:10.1016/j.mayocp.2011.09.005.

266. Gadalla SM, Lund M, Pfeiffer RM, et al. Cancer risk among patients with myotonic muscular dystrophy. *JAMA.* 2011;306(22):2480–2486. doi:10.1001/jama.2011.1796.

267. Mathieu J, Prevost C. Epidemiological surveillance of myotonic dystrophy type 1: A 25-year population-based study. *Neuromuscul Disord.* 2012;22(11):974–979. doi:10.1016/j.nmd.2012.05.017.

268. Ricker K. Myotonic dystrophy and proximal myotonic myopathy. *J Neurol.* 1999;246(5):334–338.

269. Moxley RT 3rd. Proximal myotonic myopathy: Mini-review of a recently delineated clinical disorder. *Neuromuscul Disord.* 1996;6(2):87–93.

270. Day JW, Ricker K, Jacobsen JF, et al. Myotonic dystrophy type 2: Molecular, diagnostic and clinical spectrum. *Neurology.* 2003;60(4):657–664.

271. Suokas KI, Haanpaa M, Kautiainen H, Udd B, Hietaharju AJ. Pain in patients with myotonic dystrophy type 2: A postal survey in Finland. *Muscle Nerve.* 2012;45(1):70–74. doi:10.1002/mus.22249.

272. Zaki M, Boyd PA, Impey L, Roberts A, Chamberlain P. Congenital myotonic dystrophy: Prenatal ultrasound findings and pregnancy outcome. *Ultrasound Obstet Gynecol.* 2007;29(3):284–288. doi:10.1002/uog.3859.

273. Mashiach R, Rimon E, Achiron R. Tent-shaped mouth as a presenting symptom of congenital myotonic dystrophy. *Ultrasound Obstet Gynecol.* 2002;20(3):312–313. doi:10.1046/j.1469-0705.2002.00785.x.

274. Campbell C, Sherlock R, Jacob P, Blayney M. Congenital myotonic dystrophy: Assisted ventilation duration and outcome. *Pediatrics.* 2004;113(4):811–816.

275. Logigian EL, Ciafaloni E, Quinn LC, et al. Severity, type, and distribution of myotonic discharges are different in type 1 and type 2 myotonic dystrophy. *Muscle Nerve.* 2007;35(4):479–485. doi:10.1002/mus.20792.

276. Kamsteeg EJ, Kress W, Catalli C, et al. Best practice guidelines and recommendations on the molecular diagnosis of myotonic dystrophy types 1 and 2. *Eur J Hum Genet.* 2012;20(12):1203–1208. doi:10.1038/ejhg.2012.108.

277. Heatwole C, Johnson N, Goldberg B, Martens W, Moxley R,3rd. Laboratory abnormalities in patients with myotonic dystrophy type 2. *Arch Neurol.* 2011;68(9):1180–1184. doi:10.1001/archneurol.2011.191.

278. Heatwole CR, Miller J, Martens B, Moxley RT 3rd. Laboratory abnormalities in ambulatory patients with myotonic dystrophy type 1. *Arch Neurol.* 2006;63(8):1149–1153. doi:10.1001/archneur.63.8.1149.

279. Auvinen S, Suominen T, Hannonen P, Bachinski LL, Krahe R, Udd B. Myotonic dystrophy type 2 found in two of sixty-three persons diagnosed as having fibromyalgia. *Arthritis Rheum.* 2008;58(11):3627–3631. doi:10.1002/art.24037.

280. Hawkes CH, Absolon MJ. Myotubular myopathy associated with cataract and electrical myotonia. *J Neurol Neurosurg Psychiatry.* 1975;38(8):761–764.

281. Jungbluth H, Wallgren-Pettersson C, Laporte JF, Centronuclear (Myotubular) Myopathy Consortium. 164th ENMC international workshop: 6th workshop on centronuclear (myotubular) myopathies, 16–18th January 2009, Naarden, The Netherlands. *Neuromuscul Disord.* 2009;19(10):721–729. doi:10.1016/j.nmd.2009.06.373.

282. Heatwole CR, Eichinger KJ, Friedman DI, et al. Open-label trial of recombinant human insulin-like growth factor 1/recombinant human insulin-like growth factor binding protein 3 in myotonic dystrophy type 1. *Arch Neurol.* 2011;68(1):37–44. doi:10.1001/archneurol.2010.227.

283. Logigian EL, Martens WB, Moxley RT 4th, et al. Mexiletine is an effective antimyotonia treatment in myotonic dystrophy type 1. *Neurology.* 2010;74(18):1441–1448. doi:10.1212/WNL.0b013e3181dc1a3a.

284. Hilton-Jones D, Bowler M, Lochmueller H, et al. Modafinil for excessive daytime sleepiness in myotonic dystrophy type 1—the patients' perspective. *Neuromuscul Disord.* 2012;22(7):597–603. doi:10.1016/j.nmd.2012.02.005.

285. Damian MS, Gerlach A, Schmidt F, Lehmann E, Reichmann H. Modafinil for excessive daytime sleepiness in myotonic dystrophy. *Neurology.* 2001;56(6):794–796.

286. Talbot K, Stradling J, Crosby J, Hilton-Jones D. Reduction in excess daytime sleepiness by modafinil in patients with myotonic dystrophy. *Neuromuscul Disord.* 2003;13(5):357–364.

287. Annane D, Moore DH, Barnes PR, Miller RG. Psychostimulants for hypersomnia (excessive daytime sleepiness) in myotonic dystrophy. *Cochrane Database Syst Rev.* 2006;(3)(3):CD003218. doi:10.1002/14651858.CD003218.pub2.

288. Orlikowski D, Chevret S, Quera-Salva MA, et al. Modafinil for the treatment of hypersomnia associated with myotonic muscular dystrophy in adults: A multicenter, prospective, randomized, double-blind, placebo-controlled, 4-week trial. *Clin Ther.* 2009;31(8):1765–1773. doi:10.1016/j.clinthera.2009.08.007.

289. Wintzen AR, Lammers GJ, van Dijk JG. Does modafinil enhance activity of patients with myotonic dystrophy?: A double-blind placebo-controlled crossover study. *J Neurol.* 2007;254(1):26–28. doi:10.1007/s00415-006-0186-z.

290. Ha AH, Tarnopolsky MA, Bergstra TG, Nair GM, Al-Qubbany A, Healey JS. Predictors of atrio-ventricular conduction disease, long-term outcomes in patients with myotonic dystrophy types I and II. *Pacing Clin Electrophysiol.* 2012;35(10):1262–1269. doi:10.1111/j.1540-8159.2012.03351.x.

291. Wahbi K, Meune C, Porcher R, et al. Electrophysiological study with prophylactic pacing and survival in adults with myotonic dystrophy and conduction system disease. *JAMA.* 2012;307(12):1292–1301. doi:10.1001/jama.2012.346.

292. Bhakta D, Shen C, Kron J, Epstein AE, Pascuzzi RM, Groh WJ. Pacemaker and implantable cardioverter-defibrillator use in a US myotonic dystrophy type 1 population. *J Cardiovasc Electrophysiol.* 2011;22(12):1369–1375. doi:10.1111/j.1540-8167.2011.02200.x.

293. Groh WJ, Bhakta D. Arrhythmia management in myotonic dystrophy type 1. *JAMA.* 2012;308(4):337–338; author reply 338. doi:10.1001/jama.2012.6807.

294. Mulders SA, van den Broek WJ, Wheeler TM, et al. Triplet-repeat oligonucleotide-mediated reversal of RNA toxicity in myotonic dystrophy. *Proc Natl Acad Sci U S A.* 2009;106(33):13915–13920. doi:10.1073/pnas.0905780106.

295. Leger AJ, Mosquea LM, Clayton NP, et al. Systemic delivery of a peptide-linked morpholino oligonucleotide neutralizes mutant RNA toxicity in a mouse model of myotonic dystrophy. *Nucleic Acid Ther.* 2013;23(2):109–117. doi:10.1089/nat.2012.0404.

296. Wheeler TM, Sobczak K, Lueck JD, et al. Reversal of RNA dominance by displacement of protein sequestered on triplet repeat RNA. *Science*. 2009;325(5938):336–339. doi:10.1126/science.1173110.

297. Wheeler TM, Lueck JD, Swanson MS, Dirksen RT, Thornton CA. Correction of ClC-1 splicing eliminates chloride channelopathy and myotonia in mouse models of myotonic dystrophy. *J Clin Invest*. 2007;117(12):3952–3957. doi:10.1172/JCI33355.

298. Emery AE. Population frequencies of inherited neuromuscular diseases—a world survey. *Neuromuscul Disord*. 1991;1(1):19–29.

299. Sposito R, Pasquali L, Galluzzi F, et al. Facioscapulohumeral muscular dystrophy type 1A in northwestern Tuscany: A molecular genetics-based epidemiological and genotype-phenotype study. *Genet Test*. 2005;9(1):30–36. doi:10.1089/gte.2005.9.30.

300. Lemmers RJ, van der Vliet PJ, Klooster R, et al. A unifying genetic model for facioscapulohumeral muscular dystrophy. *Science*. 2010;329(5999):1650–1653. doi:10.1126/science.1189044.

301. Lemmers RJ, Wohlgemuth M, van der Gaag KJ, et al. Specific sequence variations within the 4q35 region are associated with facioscapulohumeral muscular dystrophy. *Am J Hum Genet*. 2007;81(5):884–894. doi:10.1086/521986.

302. Lemmers RJ, Tawil R, Petek LM, et al. Digenic inheritance of an SMCHD1 mutation and an FSHD-permissive D4Z4 allele causes facioscapulohumeral muscular dystrophy type 2. *Nat Genet*. 2012;44(12):1370–1374. doi:10.1038/ng.2454.

303. Zatz M, Marie SK, Passos-Bueno MR, et al. High proportion of new mutations and possible anticipation in Brazilian facioscapulohumeral muscular dystrophy families. *Am J Hum Genet*. 1995;56(1):99–105.

304. Zatz M, Marie SK, Cerqueira A, Vainzof M, Pavanello RC, Passos-Bueno MR. The facioscapulohumeral muscular dystrophy (FSHD1) gene affects males more severely and more frequently than females. *Am J Med Genet*. 1998;77(2):155–161.

305. Flanigan KM, Coffeen CM, Sexton L, Stauffer D, Brunner S, Leppert MF. Genetic characterization of a large, historically significant Utah kindred with facioscapulohumeral dystrophy. *Neuromuscul Disord*. 2001;11(6–7):525–529.

306. Statland JM, Sacconi S, Farmakidis C, Donlin-Smith CM, Chung M, Tawil R. Coats syndrome in facioscapulohumeral dystrophy type 1: Frequency and D4Z4 contraction size. *Neurology*. 2013;80(13):1247–1250. doi:10.1212/WNL.0b013e3182897116.

307. Trevisan CP, Pastorello E, Tomelleri G, et al. Facioscapulohumeral muscular dystrophy: Hearing loss and other atypical features of patients with large 4q35 deletions. *Eur J Neurol*. 2008;15(12):1353–1358. doi:10.1111/j.1468-1331.2008.02314.x.

308. Padberg GW, Brouwer OF, de Keizer RJ, et al. On the significance of retinal vascular disease and hearing loss in facioscapulohumeral muscular dystrophy. *Muscle Nerve Suppl*. 1995;(2)(2):S73–80.

309. Brouwer OF, Padberg GW, Ruys CJ, Brand R, de Laat JA, Grote JJ. Hearing loss in facioscapulohumeral muscular dystrophy. *Neurology*. 1991;41(12):1878–1881.

310. Tekin NF, Saatci AO, Kavukcu S. Vascular tortuosity and coats'-like retinal changes in facioscapulohumeral muscular dystrophy. *Ophthalmic Surg Lasers*. 2000;31(1):82–83.

311. Finsterer J, Stollberger C. Clinical or subclinical cardiac involvement in facioscapulohumeral muscular dystrophy. *Neuromuscul Disord*. 2006;16(1):61–62; author reply 62–63. doi:10.1016/j.nmd.2005.10.002.

312. Laforet P, de Toma C, Eymard B, et al. Cardiac involvement in genetically confirmed facioscapulohumeral muscular dystrophy. *Neurology*. 1998;51(5):1454–1456.

313. Trevisan CP, Pastorello E, Armani M, et al. Facioscapulohumeral muscular dystrophy and occurrence of heart arrhythmia. *Eur Neurol*. 2006;56(1):1–5. doi:10.1159/000094248.

314. Galetta F, Franzoni F, Sposito R, et al. Subclinical cardiac involvement in patients with facioscapulohumeral muscular dystrophy. *Neuromuscul Disord*. 2005;15(6):403–408. doi:10.1016/j.nmd.2005.02.006.

315. Kilmer DD, Abresch RT, McCrory MA, et al. Profiles of neuromuscular diseases. facioscapulohumeral muscular dystrophy. *Am J Phys Med Rehabil*. 1995;74(5 Suppl):S131–9.

316. Jensen MP, Hoffman AJ, Stoelb BL, Abresch RT, Carter GT, McDonald CM. Chronic pain in persons with myotonic dystrophy and facioscapulohumeral dystrophy. *Arch Phys Med Rehabil*. 2008;89(2):320–328. doi:10.1016/j.apmr.2007.08.153; 10.1016/j.apmr.2007.08.153.

317. Bushby KM, Pollitt C, Johnson MA, Rogers MT, Chinnery PF. Muscle pain as a prominent feature of facioscapulohumeral muscular dystrophy (FSHD): Four illustrative case reports. *Neuromuscul Disord*. 1998;8(8):574–579.

318. Della Marca G, Frusciante R, Vollono C, et al. Pain and the alpha-sleep anomaly: A mechanism of sleep disruption in facioscapulohumeral muscular dystrophy. *Pain Med*. 2013;14(4):487–497. doi:10.1111/pme.12054.

319. Ciafaloni E, Pressman EK, Loi AM, et al. Pregnancy and birth outcomes in women with facioscapulohumeral muscular dystrophy. *Neurology*. 2006;67(10):1887–1889. doi:10.1212/01.wnl.0000244471.05316.19.

320. Stubgen JP, Schultz C. Lung and respiratory muscle function in facioscapulohumeral muscular dystrophy. *Muscle Nerve*. 2009;39(6):729–734. doi:10.1002/mus.21261; 10.1002/mus.21261.

321. Wohlgemuth M, van der Kooi EL, van Kesteren RG, van der Maarel SM, Padberg GW. Ventilatory support in facioscapulohumeral muscular dystrophy. *Neurology*. 2004;63(1):176–178.

322. Carter GT, Bird TD. Ventilatory support in facioscapulohumeral muscular dystrophy. *Neurology*. 2005;64(2):401; author reply 401.

323. Della Marca G, Frusciante R, Vollono C, et al. Sleep quality in facioscapulohumeral muscular dystrophy. *J Neurol Sci*. 2007;263(1–2):49–53. doi:10.1016/j.jns.2007.05.028.

324. Della Marca G, Frusciante R, Dittoni S, et al. Sleep disordered breathing in facioscapulohumeral muscular dystrophy. *J Neurol Sci*. 2009;285(1–2):54–58. doi:10.1016/j.jns.2009.05.014.

325. Klinge L, Eagle M, Haggerty ID, Roberts CE, Straub V, Bushby KM. Severe phenotype in

infantile facioscapulohumeral muscular dystrophy. *Neuromuscul Disord*. 2006;16(9–10):553–558. doi:10.1016/j.nmd.2006.06.008.

326. Bindoff LA, Mjellem N, Sommerfelt K, et al. Severe fascioscapulohumeral muscular dystrophy presenting with coats' disease and mental retardation. *Neuromuscul Disord*. 2006;16(9–10):559–563. doi:10.1016/j.nmd.2006.06.012.

327. Hobson-Webb LD, Caress JB. Facioscapulohumeral muscular dystrophy can be a cause of isolated childhood cognitive dysfunction. *J Child Neurol*. 2006;21(3):252–253.

328. Felice KJ, Jones JM, Conway SR. Facioscapulohumeral dystrophy presenting as infantile facial diplegia and late-onset limb-girdle myopathy in members of the same family. *Muscle Nerve*. 2005;32(3):368–372. doi:10.1002/mus.20344.

329. Pino LJ, Stashuk DW, Podnar S. Probabilistic muscle characterization using quantitative electromyography: Application to facioscapulohumeral muscular dystrophy. *Muscle Nerve*. 2010;42(4):563–569. doi:10.1002/mus.21742.

330. Podnar S, Zidar J. Sensitivity of motor unit potential analysis in facioscapulohumeral muscular dystrophy. *Muscle Nerve*. 2006;34(4):451–456. doi:10.1002/mus.20613.

331. Dorobek M, Szmidt-Salkowska E, Rowinska-Marcinska K, Gawel M, Hausmanowa-Petrusewicz I. Relationships between clinical data and quantitative EMG findings in facioscapulohumeral muscular dystrophy. *Neurol Neurochir Pol*. 2013;47(1):8–17.

332. Stubgen JP. Facioscapulohumeral muscular dystrophy. A quantitative electromyographic study. *Electromyogr Clin Neurophysiol*. 2007;47(3): 175–182.

333. Lemmers RJ, O'Shea S, Padberg GW, Lunt PW, van der Maarel SM. Best practice guidelines on genetic diagnostics of facioscapulohumeral muscular dystrophy: Workshop 9th June 2010, LUMC, Leiden, The Netherlands. *Neuromuscul Disord*. 2012;22(5): 463–470. doi:10.1016/j.nmd.2011.09.004.

334. Friedman SD, Poliachik SL, Otto RK, et al. Longitudinal features of stir bright signal in FSHD. *Muscle Nerve*. 2013. doi:10.1002/mus.23911; 10.1002/mus.23911.

335. Friedman SD, Poliachik SL, Carter GT, Budech CB, Bird TD, Shaw DW. The magnetic resonance imaging spectrum of facioscapulohumeral muscular dystrophy. *Muscle Nerve*. 2012;45(4):500–506. doi:10.1002/mus.22342.

336. Kissel JT, McDermott MP, Mendell JR, et al. Randomized, double-blind, placebo-controlled trial of albuterol in facioscapulohumeral dystrophy. *Neurology*. 2001;57(8):1434–1440.

337. Kissel JT, McDermott MP, Natarajan R, et al. Pilot trial of albuterol in facioscapulohumeral muscular dystrophy. FSH-DY group. *Neurology*. 1998;50(5): 1402–1406.

338. van der Kooi EL, Vogels OJ, van Asseldonk RJ, et al. Strength training and albuterol in facioscapulohumeral muscular dystrophy. *Neurology*. 2004;63(4): 702–708.

339. Tawil R, McDermott MP, Pandya S, et al. A pilot trial of prednisone in facioscapulohumeral muscular dystrophy. FSH-DY group. *Neurology*. 1997;48(1):46–49.

340. Olsen DB, Orngreen MC, Vissing J. Aerobic training improves exercise performance in facioscapulohumeral muscular dystrophy. *Neurology*. 2005;64(6):1064–1066. doi:10.1212/01. WNL.0000150584.45055.27.

341. Milner-Brown HS, Miller RG. Muscle strengthening through high-resistance weight training in patients with neuromuscular disorders. *Arch Phys Med Rehabil*. 1988;69(1):14–19.

342. Orrell RW, Copeland S, Rose MR. Scapular fixation in muscular dystrophy. *Cochrane Database Syst Rev*. 2010;(1):CD003278. doi(1):CD003278. doi:10.1002/14651858.CD003278.pub2.

343. Giannini S, Faldini C, Pagkrati S, et al. Fixation of winged scapula in facioscapulohumeral muscular dystrophy. *Clin Med Res*. 2007;5(3):155–162. doi:10.3121/cmr.2007.736.

344. Giannini S, Ceccarelli F, Faldini C, Pagkrati S, Merlini L. Scapulopexy of winged scapula secondary to facioscapulohumeral muscular dystrophy. *Clin Orthop Relat Res*. 2006;449:288–294. doi:10.1097/01. blo.0000218735.46376.c0.

345. Demirhan M, Uysal O, Atalar AC, Kilicoglu O, Serdaroglu P. Scapulothoracic arthrodesis in facioscapulohumeral dystrophy with multifilament cable. *Clin Orthop Relat Res*. 2009;467(8):2090– 2097. doi:10.1007/s11999-009-0815-9.

346. Ketenjian AY. Scapulocostal stabilization for scapular winging in facioscapulohumeral muscular dystrophy. *J Bone Joint Surg Am*. 1978;60(4):476–480.

347. Sansone V, Boynton J, Palenski C. Use of gold weights to correct lagophthalmos in neuromuscular disease. *Neurology*. 1997; 48(6):1500–1503.

348. van der Kooi AJ, Barth PG, Busch HF, et al. The clinical spectrum of limb girdle muscular dystrophy. A survey in the netherlands. *Brain*. 1996;119(Pt 5):1471–1480.

349. Urtasun M, Saenz A, Roudaut C, et al. Limb-girdle muscular dystrophy in Guipuzcoa (Basque country, Spain). *Brain*. 1998;121(Pt 9):1735–1747.

350. Guglieri M, Magri F, D'Angelo MG, et al. Clinical, molecular, and protein correlations in a large sample of genetically diagnosed Italian limb girdle muscular dystrophy patients. *Hum Mutat*. 2008;29(2):258–266. doi:10.1002/humu.20642.

351. Argov Z, Sadeh M, Mazor K, et al. Muscular dystrophy due to dysferlin deficiency in Libyan Jews. Clinical and genetic features. *Brain*. 2000;123(Pt 6):1229–1237.

352. Kang PB, Feener CA, Estrella E, et al. LGMD2I in a North American population. *BMC Musculoskelet Disord*. 2007;8:115. doi:10.1186/1471-2474-8-115.

353. Stensland E, Lindal S, Jonsrud C, et al. Prevalence, mutation spectrum and phenotypic variability in Norwegian patients with limb girdle muscular dystrophy 2I. *Neuromuscul Disord*. 2011;21(1):41–46. doi:10.1016/j.nmd.2010.08.008.

354. Vainzof M, Passos-Bueno MR, Pavanello RC, Marie SK, Oliveira AS, Zatz M. Sarcoglycanopathies are responsible for 68% of severe autosomal recessive limb-girdle muscular dystrophy in the Brazilian population. *J Neurol Sci*. 1999;164(1):44–49.

355. Bisceglia L, Zoccolella S, Torraco A, et al. A new locus on 3p23-p25 for an autosomal-dominant limb-girdle muscular dystrophy, LGMD1H. *Eur J Hum Genet*. 2010;18(6):636–641. doi:10.1038/ejhg.2009.235.

356. Greenberg SA, Salajegheh M, Judge DP, et al. Etiology of limb girdle muscular dystrophy 1D/1E determined by laser capture microdissection proteomics. *Ann Neurol*. 2012;71(1):141–145. doi:10.1002/ ana.22649.

357. Harms MB, Sommerville RB, Allred P, et al. Exome sequencing reveals DNAJB6 mutations in dominantly-inherited myopathy. *Ann Neurol*. 2012;71(3):407–416. doi:10.1002/ana.22683.

358. Palenzuela L, Andreu AL, Gamez J, et al. A novel autosomal dominant limb-girdle muscular dystrophy (LGMD 1F) maps to 7q32.1-32.2. *Neurology*. 2003;61(3):404–406.

359. Rosales XQ, Gastier-Foster JM, Lewis S, et al. Novel diagnostic features of dysferlinopathies. *Muscle Nerve*. 2010;42(1):14–21. doi:10.1002/mus.21650.

360. Klinge L, Aboumousa A, Eagle M, et al. New aspects on patients affected by dysferlin deficient muscular dystrophy. *J Neurol Neurosurg Psychiatry*. 2010;81(9):946–953. doi:10.1136/jnnp.2009.178038.

361. Melacini P, Fanin M, Duggan DJ, et al. Heart involvement in muscular dystrophies due to sarcoglycan gene mutations. *Muscle Nerve*. 1999;22(4):473–479.

362. Fanin M, Melacini P, Boito C, Pegoraro E, Angelini C. LGMD2E patients risk developing dilated cardiomyopathy. *Neuromuscul Disord*. 2003;13(4):303–309.

363. Kirschner J, Lochmuller H. Sarcoglycanopathies. *Handb Clin Neurol*. 2011;101:41–46. doi:10.1016/ B978-0-08-045031-5.00003-7.

364. Confalonieri P, Oliva L, Andreetta F, et al. Muscle inflammation and MHC class I up-regulation in muscular dystrophy with lack of dysferlin: An immunopathological study. *J Neuroimmunol*. 2003;142(1–2): 130–136.

365. Cenacchi G, Fanin M, De Giorgi LB, Angelini C. Ultrastructural changes in dysferlinopathy support defective membrane repair mechanism. *J Clin Pathol*. 2005;58(2):190–195. doi:10.1136/jcp.2004.018978.

366. Prelle A, Sciacco M, Tancredi L, et al. Clinical, morphological and immunological evaluation of six patients with dysferlin deficiency. *Acta Neuropathol*. 2003;105(6):537–542. doi:10.1007/ s00401-002-0654-1.

367. Fanin M, Angelini C. Muscle pathology in dysferlin deficiency. *Neuropathol Appl Neurobiol*. 2002;28(6):461–470.

368. Gallardo E, Rojas-Garcia R, de Luna N, Pou A, Brown RH, Jr, Illa I. Inflammation in dysferlin myopathy: Immunohistochemical characterization of 13 patients. *Neurology*. 2001;57(11):2136–2138.

369. Reilich P, Petersen JA, Vielhaber S, et al. LGMD 2I due to the common mutation 826C>A in the FKRP gene presenting as myopathy with vacuoles and paired-helical filaments. *Acta Myol*. 2006;25(2):73–76.

370. Selcen D, Engel AG. Mutations in myotilin cause myofibrillar myopathy. *Neurology*. 2004;62(8):1363–1371.

371. Anderson LV, Harrison RM, Pogue R, et al. Secondary reduction in calpain 3 expression in patients with limb girdle muscular dystrophy type 2B and Miyoshi myopathy (primary dysferlinopathies). *Neuromuscul Disord*. 2000;10(8):553–559.

372. Fanin M, Pegoraro E, Matsuda-Asada C, Brown RH, Jr, Angelini C. Calpain-3 and dysferlin protein screening in patients with limb-girdle dystrophy and myopathy. *Neurology*. 2001;56(5):660–665.

373. Fanin M, Nascimbeni AC, Tasca E, Angelini C. How to tackle the diagnosis of limb-girdle muscular dystrophy 2A. *Eur J Hum Genet*. 2009;17(5):598–603. doi:10.1038/ejhg.2008.193.

374. Groen EJ, Charlton R, Barresi R, et al. Analysis of the UK diagnostic strategy for limb girdle muscular dystrophy 2A. *Brain*. 2007;130(Pt 12):3237–3249. doi:10.1093/brain/awm259.

375. Piccolo F, Moore SA, Ford GC, Campbell KP. Intracellular accumulation and reduced sarcolemmal expression of dysferlin in limb-girdle muscular dystrophies. *Ann Neurol*. 2000;48(6):902–912.

376. Matsuda C, Hayashi YK, Ogawa M, et al. The sarcolemmal proteins dysferlin and caveolin-3 interact in skeletal muscle. *Hum Mol Genet*. 2001;10(17): 1761–1766.

377. Tagawa K, Ogawa M, Kawabe K, et al. Protein and gene analyses of dysferlinopathy in a large group of Japanese muscular dystrophy patients. *J Neurol Sci*. 2003;211(1–2):23–28.

378. Klinge L, Dekomien G, Aboumousa A, et al. Sarcoglycanopathies: Can muscle immunoanalysis predict the genotype? *Neuromuscul Disord*. 2008;18(12): 934–941. doi:10.1016/j.nmd.2008.08.003.

379. Kirschner J, Lochmuller H. Sarcoglycanopathies. *Handb Clin Neurol*. 2011;101:41–46. doi:10.1016/ B978-0-08-045031-5.00003-7.

380. Bonnemann CG, Modi R, Noguchi S, et al. Beta-sarcoglycan (A3b) mutations cause autosomal recessive muscular dystrophy with loss of the sarcoglycan complex. *Nat Genet*. 1995;11(3):266–273. doi:10.1038/ng1195-266.

381. Stramare R, Beltrame V, Dal Borgo R, et al. MRI in the assessment of muscular pathology: A comparison between limb-girdle muscular dystrophies, hyaline body myopathies and myotonic dystrophies. *Radiol Med*. 2010;115(4):585–599. doi:10.1007/ s11547-010-0531-2.

382. Mercuri E, Bushby K, Ricci E, et al. Muscle MRI findings in patients with limb girdle muscular dystrophy with calpain 3 deficiency (LGMD2A) and early contractures. *Neuromuscul Disord*. 2005;15(2):164–171. doi:10.1016/j.nmd.2004.10.008.

383. Hoffman EP, Pegoraro E, Scacheri P, et al. Genetic counseling of isolated carriers of Duchenne muscular dystrophy. *Am J Med Genet*. 1996;63(4):573–580. doi:2-F.

384. Hoffman EP, Arahata K, Minetti C, Bonilla E, Rowland LP. Dystrophinopathy in isolated cases of myopathy in females. *Neurology*. 1992;42(5):967–975.

385. Walter MC, Reilich P, Thiele S, et al. Treatment of dysferlinopathy with deflazacort: A double-blind, placebo-controlled clinical trial. *Orphanet J Rare Dis*. 2013;8:26-1172-8-26. doi:10.1186/1750-1172-8-26.

386. Wagner KR, Fleckenstein JL, Amato AA, et al. A phase I/II trial of MYO-029 in adult subjects with muscular dystrophy. *Ann Neurol*. 2008;63(5):561–571. doi:10.1002/ana.21338; 10.1002/ana.21338.

387. Mendell JR, Rodino-Klapac LR, Rosales XQ, et al. Sustained alpha-sarcoglycan gene expression after gene transfer in limb-girdle muscular dystrophy, type 2D. *Ann Neurol*. 2010;68(5):629–638. doi:10.1002/ ana.22251.

388. Mendell JR, Rodino-Klapac LR, Rosales-Quintero X, et al. Limb-girdle muscular dystrophy type 2D gene therapy restores alpha-sarcoglycan and associated proteins. *Ann Neurol*. 2009;66(3):290–297. doi:10.1002/ana.21732.

389. Barthelemy F, Wein N, Krahn M, Levy N, Bartoli M. Translational research and therapeutic perspectives in dysferlinopathies. *Mol Med*. 2011;17(9–10):875–882. doi:10.2119/molmed.2011.00084.

390. Kiloh LG, Nevin S. Progressive dystrophy of the external ocular muscles (ocular myopathy). *Brain*. 1951;74(2):115–143.

391. Victor M, Hayes R, Adams RD. Oculopharyngeal muscular dystrophy. A familial disease of late life characterized by dysphagia and progressive ptosis of the eyelids. *N Engl J Med*. 1962;267:1267–1272. doi:10.1056/NEJM196212202672501.

392. Becher MW, Morrison L, Davis LE, et al. Oculopharyngeal muscular dystrophy in Hispanic New Mexicans. *JAMA*. 2001;286(19):2437–2440.

393. Grewal RP, Karkera JD, Grewal RK, Detera-Wadleigh SD. Mutation analysis of oculopharyngeal muscular dystrophy in Hispanic American families. *Arch Neurol*. 1999;56(11):1378–1381.

394. Brunet G, Tome FM, Eymard B, Robert JM, Fardeau M. Genealogical study of oculopharyngeal muscular dystrophy in France. *Neuromuscul Disord*. 1997;7 Suppl 1:S34–7.

395. Brunet G, Tome FM, Samson F, Robert JM, Fardeau M. Oculopharyngeal muscular dystrophy. A census of French families and genealogic study. *Rev Neurol (Paris)*. 1990;146(6–7):425–429.

396. Blumen SC, Nisipeanu P, Sadeh M, et al. Epidemiology and inheritance of oculopharyngeal muscular dystrophy in Israel. *Neuromuscul Disord*. 1997;7 Suppl 1:S38–40.

397. Brais B, Xie YG, Sanson M, et al. The oculopharyngeal muscular dystrophy locus maps to the region of the cardiac alpha and beta myosin heavy chain genes on chromosome 14q11.2-q13. *Hum Mol Genet*. 1995;4(3):429–434.

398. Brais B, Bouchard JP, Xie YG, et al. Short GCG expansions in the PABP2 gene cause oculopharyngeal muscular dystrophy. *Nat Genet*. 1998;18(2):164–167. doi:10.1038/ng0298-164.

399. Hebbar S, Webberley MJ, Lunt P, Robinson DO. Siblings with recessive oculopharyngeal muscular dystrophy. *Neuromuscul Disord*. 2007;17(3):254–257. doi:10.1016/j.nmd.2006.11.009.

400. Semmler A, Kress W, Vielhaber S, Schroder R, Kornblum C. Variability of the recessive oculopharyngeal muscular dystrophy phenotype. *Muscle Nerve*. 2007;35(5):681–684. doi:10.1002/mus.20726.

401. Fried K, Arlozorov A, Spira R. Autosomal recessive oculopharyngeal muscular dystrophy. *J Med Genet*. 1975;12(4):416–418.

402. Brais B, Bouchard JP, Xie YG, et al. Short GCG expansions in the PABP2 gene cause oculopharyngeal muscular dystrophy. *Nat Genet*. 1998;18(2):164–167. doi:10.1038/ng0298-164.

403. Robinson DO, Hilton-Jones D, Mansfield D, et al. Two cases of oculopharyngeal muscular dystrophy (OPMD) with the rare PABPN1 c.35G>C; p.Gly12Ala point mutation. *Neuromuscul Disord*. 2011;21(11):809–811. doi:10.1016/j.nmd.2011.06.003.

404. Robinson DO, Wills AJ, Hammans SR, Read SP, Sillibourne J. Oculopharyngeal muscular dystrophy: A point mutation which mimics the effect of the PABPN1 gene triplet repeat expansion

mutation. *J Med Genet*. 2006;43(5):e23. doi:10.1136/jmg.2005.037598.

405. Maksimova NR, Nikolaeva IA, Korotkov MN, et al. The clinical-genealogic and molecular-genetic characteristics of oculopharyngeal muscular dystrophy in the republic of Sakha (Yakutia). *Zh Nevrol Psikhiatr Im S S Korsakova*. 2008;108(6):52–60.

406. Banerjee A, Apponi LH, Pavlath GK, Corbett AH. PABPN1: Molecular function and muscle disease. *FEBS J*. 2013. doi:10.1111/febs.12294.

407. Fan X, Rouleau GA. Progress in understanding the pathogenesis of oculopharyngeal muscular dystrophy. *Can J Neurol Sci*. 2003;30(1):8–14.

408. Blumen SC, Brais B, Korczyn AD, et al. Homozygotes for oculopharyngeal muscular dystrophy have a severe form of the disease. *Ann Neurol*. 1999;46(1):115–118.

409. Blumen SC, Bouchard JP, Brais B, et al. Cognitive impairment and reduced life span of oculopharyngeal muscular dystrophy homozygotes. *Neurology*. 2009;73(8):596–601. doi:10.1212/WNL.0b013e3181b388a3.

410. Jones LK, Jr, Harper CM. Clinical and electrophysiologic features of oculopharyngeal muscular dystrophy: Lack of evidence for an associated peripheral neuropathy. *Clin Neurophysiol*. 2010;121(6):870–873. doi:10.1016/j.clinph.2010.01.022; 10.1016/j.clinph.2010.01.022.

411. Bouchard JP, Brais B, Brunet D, Gould PV, Rouleau GA. Recent studies on oculopharyngeal muscular dystrophy in Quebec. *Neuromuscul Disord*. 1997;7 Suppl 1:S22–9.

412. Tome FM, Fardeau M. Nuclear inclusions in oculopharyngeal dystrophy. *Acta Neuropathol*. 1980;49(1):85–87.

413. Tome FM, Askanas V, Engel WK, Alvarez RB, Lee CS. Nuclear inclusions in innervated cultured muscle fibers from patients with oculopharyngeal muscular dystrophy. *Neurology*. 1989;39(7):926–932.

414. Tome FM, Chateau D, Helbling-Leclerc A, Fardeau M. Morphological changes in muscle fibers in oculopharyngeal muscular dystrophy. *Neuromuscul Disord*. 1997;7 Suppl 1:S63–9.

415. Blumen SC, Sadeh M, Korczyn AD, et al. Intranuclear inclusions in oculopharyngeal muscular dystrophy among Bukhara Jews. *Neurology*. 1996;46(5):1324–1328.

416. Coquet M, Vital C, Julien J. Presence of inclusion body myositis-like filaments in oculopharyngeal muscular dystrophy. Ultrastructural study of 10 cases. *Neuropathol Appl Neurobiol*. 1990;16(5):393–400.

417. Bouchard JP, Gagne F, Tome FM, Brunet D. Nuclear inclusions in oculopharyngeal muscular dystrophy in Quebec. *Can J Neurol Sci*. 1989;16(4):446–450.

418. King MK, Lee RR, Davis LE. Magnetic resonance imaging and computed tomography of skeletal muscles in oculopharyngeal muscular dystrophy. *J Clin Neuromuscul Dis*. 2005;6(3):103–108. doi:10.1097/01.cnd.0000152060.57673.25.

419. Fischmann A, Hafner P, Fasler S, et al. Quantitative MRI can detect subclinical disease progression in muscular dystrophy. *J Neurol*. 2012;259(8):1648–1654. doi:10.1007/s00415-011-6393-2.

420. Fischmann A, Gloor M, Fasler S, et al. Muscular involvement assessed by MRI correlates to motor function measurement values in oculopharyngeal

muscular dystrophy. *J Neurol.* 2011;258(7): 1333–1340. doi:10.1007/s00415-011-5937-9.

421. Uyama E, Uchino M, Chateau D, Tome FM. Autosomal recessive oculopharyngodistal myopathy in light of distal myopathy with rimmed vacuoles and oculopharyngeal muscular dystrophy. *Neuromuscul Disord.* 1998;8(2):119–125.

422. Satoyoshi E, Kinoshita M. Oculopharyngodistal myopathy. *Arch Neurol.* 1977;34(2):89–92.

423. van der Sluijs BM, ter Laak HJ, Scheffer H, van der Maarel SM, van Engelen BG. Autosomal recessive oculopharyngodistal myopathy: A distinct phenotypical, histological, and genetic entity. *J Neurol Neurosurg Psychiatry.* 2004;75(10):1499–1501. doi:10.1136/jnnp.2003.025072.

424. Durmus H, Laval SH, Deymeer F, et al. Oculopharyngodistal myopathy is a distinct entity: Clinical and genetic features of 47 patients. *Neurology.* 2011;76(3):227–235. doi:10.1212/WNL. 0b013e318207b043.

425. Codere F. Oculopharyngeal muscular dystrophy. *Can J Ophthalmol.* 1993;28(1):1–2.

426. Molgat YM, Rodrigue D. Correction of blepharoptosis in oculopharyngeal muscular dystrophy: Review of 91 cases. *Can J Ophthalmol.* 1993;28(1):11–14.

427. Rodrigue D, Molgat YM. Surgical correction of blepharoptosis in oculopharyngeal muscular dystrophy. *Neuromuscul Disord.* 1997;7 Suppl 1:S82–4.

428. Mathieu J, Lapointe G, Brassard A, et al. A pilot study on upper esophageal sphincter dilatation for the treatment of dysphagia in patients with oculopharyngeal muscular dystrophy. *Neuromuscul Disord.* 1997;7 Suppl 1:S100–4.

429. Restivo DA, Marchese Ragona R, Staffieri A, de Grandis D. Successful botulinum toxin treatment of dysphagia in oculopharyngeal muscular dystrophy. *Gastroenterology.* 2000;119(5):1416.

430. Pellerin HG, Nicole PC, Trepanier CA, Lessard MR. Postoperative complications in patients with oculopharyngeal muscular dystrophy: A retrospective study. *Can J Anaesth.* 2007;54(5):361–365. doi:10.1007/BF03022658.

431. Christopher K, Horkan C, Patterson RB, Yodice PC. Oculopharyngeal muscular dystrophy complicating airway management. *Chest.* 2001;120(6):2101–2103.

432. Sparks S, Quijano-Roy S, Harper A, et al. Congenital Muscular Dystrophy Overview. 2001 Jan 22 [Updated 2012 Aug 23]. In: Pagon RA, Adam MP, Bird TD, et al., editors. GeneReviews™ [Internet]. Seattle (WA): University of Washington, Seattle; 1993–2013. Available from: http://www.ncbi.nlm.nih.gov/books/ NBK1291/

433. Jimenez-Mallebrera C, Brown SC, Sewry CA, Muntoni F. Congenital muscular dystrophy: Molecular and cellular aspects. *Cell Mol Life Sci.* 2005;62(7–8): 809–823. doi:10.1007/s00018-004-4510-4.

434. Darin N, Tulinius M. Neuromuscular disorders in childhood: A descriptive epidemiological study from western Sweden. *Neuromuscul Disord.* 2000;10(1):1–9.

435. Norwood FL, Harling C, Chinnery PF, Eagle M, Bushby K, Straub V. Prevalence of genetic muscle disease in northern England: In-depth analysis of a muscle clinic population. *Brain.* 2009;132(Pt 11):3175–3186. doi:10.1093/brain/awp236.

436. Mostacciuolo ML, Miorin M, Martinello F, Angelini C, Perini P, Trevisan CP. Genetic epidemiology of congenital muscular dystrophy in a sample from north-east Italy. *Hum Genet.* 1996;97(3):277–279.

437. Okada M, Kawahara G, Noguchi S, et al. Primary collagen VI deficiency is the second most common congenital muscular dystrophy in Japan. *Neurology.* 2007;69(10):1035–1042. doi:10.1212/01. wnl.0000271387.10404.4e.

438. Matsumoto H, Hayashi YK, Kim DS, et al. Congenital muscular dystrophy with glycosylation defects of alpha-dystroglycan in Japan. *Neuromuscul Disord.* 2005;15(5):342–348. doi:10.1016/j.nmd.2005.01.009.

439. Quijano-Roy S, Mbieleu B, Bonnemann CG, et al. De novo LMNA mutations cause a new form of congenital muscular dystrophy. *Ann Neurol.* 2008;64(2):177–186. doi:10.1002/ana.21417.

440. Clement EM, Feng L, Mein R, et al. Relative frequency of congenital muscular dystrophy subtypes: Analysis of the UK diagnostic service 2001-2008. *Neuromuscul Disord.* 2012;22(6):522–527. doi:10.1016/j.nmd.2012.01.010.

441. Peat RA, Smith JM, Compton AG, et al. Diagnosis and etiology of congenital muscular dystrophy. *Neurology.* 2008;71(5):312–321. doi:10.1212/01. wnl.0000284605.27654.5a.

442. Bonnemann CG, Rutkowski A, Mercuri E, Muntoni F. CMD Outcomes Consortium. 173rd ENMC international workshop: Congenital muscular dystrophy outcome measures 5–7 March 2010, Naarden, The Netherlands. *Neuromuscul Disord.* 2011;21(7):513–522. doi:10.1016/j.nmd.2011.04.004.

443. Rajakulendran S, Parton M, Holton JL, Hanna MG. Clinical and pathological heterogeneity in late-onset partial merosin deficiency. *Muscle Nerve.* 2011;44(4):590–593. doi:10.1002/mus.22196.

444. Brinas L, Richard P, Quijano-Roy S, et al. Early onset collagen VI myopathies: Genetic and clinical correlations. *Ann Neurol.* 2010;68(4):511–520. doi:10.1002/ ana.22087.

445. Willer T, Lee H, Lommel M, et al. ISPD loss-of-function mutations disrupt dystroglycan O-mannosylation and cause Walker-Warburg syndrome. *Nat Genet.* 2012;44(5):575–580. doi:10.1038/ ng.2252.

446. Chemla JC, Kanter RJ, Carboni MP, Smith EC. Two children with "dropped head" syndrome due to lamin A/C mutations. *Muscle Nerve.* 2010;42(5):839–841. doi:10.1002/mus.21820.

447. Pane M, Messina S, Vasco G, et al. Respiratory and cardiac function in congenital muscular dystrophies with alpha dystroglycan deficiency. *Neuromuscul Disord.* 2012;22(8):685–689. doi:10.1016/j. nmd.2012.05.006.

448. Bello L, Melacini P, Pezzani R, et al. Cardiomyopathy in patients with POMT1-related congenital and limb-girdle muscular dystrophy. *Eur J Hum Genet.* 2012;20(12):1234–1239. doi:10.1038/ ejhg.2012.71.

449. Arimura T, Hayashi YK, Murakami T, et al. Mutational analysis of fukutin gene in dilated cardiomyopathy and hypertrophic cardiomyopathy. *Circ J.* 2009;73(1):158–161.

450. Finsterer J, Ramaciotti C, Wang CH, et al. Cardiac findings in congenital muscular dystrophies.

Pediatrics. 2010;126(3):538–545. doi:10.1542/peds. 2010-0208; 10.1542/peds.2010-0208.

451. Spyrou N, Philpot J, Foale R, Camici PG, Muntoni F. Evidence of left ventricular dysfunction in children with merosin-deficient congenital muscular dystrophy. *Am Heart J*. 1998;136(3):474–476.

452. Yoshioka M, Higuchi Y, Fujii T, Aiba H, Toda T. Seizure-genotype relationship in Fukuyama-type congenital muscular dystrophy. *Brain Dev*. 2008;30(1):59–67. doi:10.1016/j.braindev.2007.05.012.

453. Yoshioka M, Higuchi Y. Long-term prognosis of epilepsies and related seizure disorders in Fukuyama-type congenital muscular dystrophy. *J Child Neurol*. 2005;20(4):385–391.

454. Messina S, Bruno C, Moroni I, et al. Congenital muscular dystrophies with cognitive impairment. A population study. *Neurology*. 2010;75(10):898–903. doi:10.1212/WNL.0b013e3181f11dd5.

455. Muntoni F, Voit T. The congenital muscular dystrophies in 2004: A century of exciting progress. *Neuromuscul Disord*. 2004;14(10):635–649. doi:10.1016/j.nmd.2004.06.009.

456. Quijano-Roy S, Renault F, Romero N, Guicheney P, Fardeau M, Estournet B. EMG and nerve conduction studies in children with congenital muscular dystrophy. *Muscle Nerve*. 2004;29(2):292–299. doi:10.1002/mus.10544.

457. Mercuri E, Cini C, Pichiecchio A, et al. Muscle magnetic resonance imaging in patients with congenital muscular dystrophy and Ullrich phenotype. *Neuromuscul Disord*. 2003;13(7–8):554–558.

458. Mercuri E, Lampe A, Allsop J, et al. Muscle MRI in Ullrich congenital muscular dystrophy and Bethlem myopathy. *Neuromuscul Disord*. 2005;15(4):303–310. doi:10.1016/j.nmd.2005.01.004.

459. Flanigan KM, Kerr L, Bromberg MB, et al. Congenital muscular dystrophy with rigid spine syndrome: A clinical, pathological, radiological, and genetic study. *Ann Neurol*. 2000;47(2):152–161.

460. Senderek J, Krieger M, Stendel C, et al. Mutations in SIL1 cause Marinesco-Sjogren syndrome, a cerebellar ataxia with cataract and myopathy. *Nat Genet*. 2005;37(12):1312–1314. doi:10.1038/ng1678.

461. Wang CH, Bonnemann CG, Rutkowski A, et al. Consensus statement on standard of care for congenital muscular dystrophies. *J Child Neurol*. 2010;25(12):1559–1581. doi:10.1177/0883073810381924.

462. Di Rosa G, Messina S, D'Amico A, et al. A new form of alpha-dystroglycanopathy associated with severe drug-resistant epilepsy and unusual EEG features. *Epileptic Disord*. 2011;13(3):259–262. doi:10.1684/epd.2011.0461.

463. Mankodi A, Udd, B, Griggs RC: In Rosenberg RM and Pascual JM (eds): *Rosenberg's Molecular and Genetic Basis of Neurological and Psychiatric Disease*, 5th Edition, Elsevier, in press 2014.

464. Markesbery WR, Griggs RC, Leach RP, Lapham LW: Late onset hereditary distal myopathy. *Neurology*. 1974;24:127.

465. Griggs R, Vihola A, Hackman P, et al. Zaspopathy in a large classic late-onset distal myopathy family. *Brain*. 2007;130:1477–1484.

466. Liu J, Aoki M, Illa I, et al. Dysferlin, a novel skeletal muscle gene, is mutated in Miyoshi myopathy and limb girdle muscular dystrophy. *Nat Genet*. 1998;20:31–36.

467. Linssen WH, de Visser M, Notermans NC, et al. Genetic heterogeneity in Miyoshi-type distal muscular dystrophy. *Neuromuscul Disord*. 1998;8:317–320.

468. Anderson LV, Davison K, Moss JA, et al. Dysferlin is a plasma membrane protein and is expressed early in human development. *Hum Mol Genet*. 1999;8:855–861.

469. Bittner RE, Anderson LV, Burkhardt E, et al. Dysferlin deletion in SJL mice (SJL-Dysf) defines a natural model for limb girdle muscular dystrophy 2B. *Nat Genet*. 1999;23:141–142.

470. Jaiswal JK, Marlow G, Summerill G, et al. Patients with a non-dysferlin Miyoshi myopathy have a novel membrane repair defect. *Traffic*. 2007;8:77–88.

471. Welander L. Homozygous appearance of distal myopathy. *Acta Genet*. 1957;7:32.

472. Klar J, Sobol M, Melberg A, et al. Welander distal myopathy caused by an ancient founder mutation in TIA1 associated with perturbed splicing. *Hum Mutat*. 2013;34:572–577.

473. Hackman P, Sarparanta J, Lehtinen S, et al. Welander distal myopathy is caused by a mutation in the RNA-binding protein TIA1. *Ann Neurol*. 2012: 73 (4): 500–509.

474. Forch P, Puig O, Martinez C, Seraphin B, Valcarcel J. The splicing regulator TIA-1 interacts with U1-C to promote U1 snRNP recruitment to 5' splice sites. *EMBO J*. 2002;21:6882–6892.

475. Gilks N, Kedersha N, Ayodele M, et al. Stress granule assembly is mediated by prion-like aggregation of TIA-1. *Mol Biol Cell*. 2004;15:5383–5398.

476. Haravuori H, Vihola A, Straub V, et al. Secondary calpain3 deficiency in 2q-linked muscular dystrophy: titin is the candidate gene. *Neurology*. 2001;56:869–877.

477. Hackman P, Vihola A, Haravuori H, et al. Tibial muscular dystrophy is a titinopathy caused by mutations in TTN, the gene encoding the giant skeletal-muscle protein titin. *Am J Hum Genet*. 2002;71:492–500.

478. Udd B, Vihola A, Sarparanta J, Richard I, Hackman P. Titinopathies and extension of the M-line mutation phenotype beyond distal myopathy and LGMD2J. *Neurology*. 2005;64:636–642.

479. Nishino I, Malicdan MC, Murayama K, Nonaka I, Hayashi YK, Noguchi S. Molecular pathomechanism of distal myopathy with rimmed vacuoles. *Acta Myol*. 2005;24:80–83.

480. Nishino I, Noguchi S, Murayama K, et al. Distal myopathy with rimmed vacuoles is allelic to hereditary inclusion body myopathy. *Neurology*. 2002;59:1689–1693.

481. Eisenberg I, Avidan N, Potikha T, et al. The UDP-N-acetylglucosamine 2-epimerase/N-acetylmannosamine kinase gene is mutated in recessive hereditary inclusion body myopathy. *Nat Genet*. 2001;29:83–87.

482. Kayashima T, Matsuo H, Satoh A, et al. Nonaka myopathy is caused by mutations in the UDP-N-acetylglucosamine-2-epimerase/N-acetylmannosamine kinase gene (GNE). *J Hum Genet*. 2002;47:77–79.

Chapter 5

Myofibrillar Myopathies

Duygu Selcen

PATHOLOGICAL FEATURES

CLINICAL FEATURES
Desminopathy
αB-Crystallinopathy
Myotilinopathy
Zaspopathy
Filaminopathy

Bag3opathy
FHL1opathy
DNAJB6-Related MFM
Titin-Related MFM

TREATMENT

REFERENCES

The term *myofibrillar myopathies* (MFMs) was proposed in 1996 as a descriptive term for a group of chronic neuromuscular diseases associated with common morphologic features[1,2]: myofibrillar disorganization beginning at the Z-disk followed by accumulation of myofibrillar degradation products and ectopic expression of multiple proteins in the abnormal fiber regions (Figures 5–1 & 5–2). The clinical features of MFMs are more variable. Distal muscles are often involved but some patients present with limb-girdle or scapuloperoneal distribution of weakness. Cardiomyopathy and peripheral neuropathy can be associated features.[3]

EMG studies of affected muscles reveal mostly myopathic MUPs and abnormal electrical irritability including myotonic discharges. Rarely, neurogenic MUPs or slowing of nerve conduction velocities are seen.

The myofibrillar myopathies can be viewed as muscular dystrophies. They conform to Erb's definition of diseases caused by the primary degeneration of the muscle fibers.[4] Also, different forms of MFM have the clinical features of muscular dystrophies and some were first reported as such. For example, myotilinopathy was first classified as LGMD1A by the clinical criteria[5,6] and zaspopathy[7,8] was first reported as a distal muscular dystrophy. The

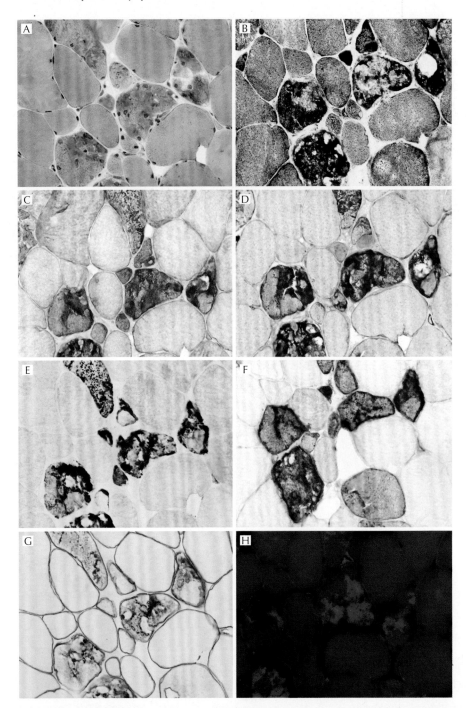

Figure 5–1. A, B, and H: Characteristic histologic findings of a patient with zaspopathy in trichrome (A), NADH dehydrogenase (B), and Congo red (H) stained sections. C–G: Nonconsecutive sections in the same series stained trichromatically (A), and immunoreacted for desmin (C), αB-crystallin (D), myotilin (E), NCAM (F), and dystrophin (G). Note abnormal accumulation of each protein in the structurally abnormal fibers.

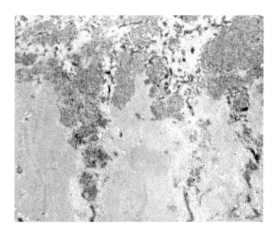

Figure 5–2. Early ultrastructural findings in αB-crystallinopathy. Normal Z-disks give rise to abnormal expanses of material of Z-disk density intermingled with pleomorphic dappled dense bodies. (Reproduced from Selcen et al., 2003)

kinship classified as LGMD1E was found to carry a splice site mutation in desmin.[9]

PATHOLOGICAL FEATURES

The muscle fibers vary abnormally in size. Some abnormal fibers contain large vesicular nuclei. Groups of small fibers, with three or more small fibers per group, are a common finding. In most cases, however, the atrophic fibers account for only a small proportion of the total. Some atrophic fibers arise by fiber splitting. Necrotic and regenerating fibers and increased fibrosis can be present. Sparse perivascular or endomysial mononuclear inflammatory cells were present in about 10% of the biopsy specimens in the Mayo Clinic cohort. The pathologic changes are best observed in trichrome-stained sections that reveal fibers displaying an admixture of amorphous, granular, or hyaline deposits that vary in shape and size, and are dark blue, blue-red, or dark green in color (Figure 5–1A). In a given fiber, the abnormal areas are single or multiple, and encompass from a small fraction to nearly the entire extent of the cross-sectional fiber area. Typical cytoplasmic bodies are conspicuous in less than 10% of the patients. Occasional abnormal fibers also contain nemaline rods. Pathologic alterations occur in both atrophic and nonatrophic fibers. The abnormal fibers can be distributed focally, so if only a small muscle specimen is obtained, if a clinically unaffected muscle is sampled, or if only paraffin-embedded tissue is examined, the characteristic changes could be overlooked. Many abnormal fiber regions, and especially the hyaline structures, lack or have little oxidative enzyme activity, but oxidative enzyme activity can be accentuated around the larger inclusions (Figure 5–1B). Some muscle fibers harbor small to large vacuoles containing membranous material, and some patients have enlarged, giant fibers. Many hyaline structures are intensely congophilic and the congophilia is best observed in Congo red–stained sections viewed under rhodamine optics (Figure 5–1H). The intensity of the fluorescent signal can vary from mild to intense. The congophilic inclusions are not metachromatic with the crystal violet stain and do not display apple-green birefringence in polarized light. Therefore, they are unlike the small amyloid deposits of inclusion body myositis. The large congophilic deposits are an important diagnostic feature of MFM biopsies. Increases of acid phosphatase appear in some vacuoles and in small foci of many abnormal fibers.

Signs of denervation, consisting of groups of atrophic fibers composed of fibers of either histochemical type, and increased reactivity of atrophic fibers for nonspecific esterase, are observed in some patients. A few patients show fiber type grouping. Many abnormal fibers contain small lakes of PAS-positive material. The muscle fiber lipid content is normal.

The pathologic findings in MFM patients are generally similar with the following exceptions. With mutations in desmin or αB-crystallin, the pathologic changes are often less severe and more monotonous, and the congophilic deposits are fewer and less intensely fluorescent than in other types of MFM. Preapoptotic and apoptotic nuclei occur at an increased frequency in α B-crystallinopathy and Bag3opathy. Reducing bodies, detected by the menadione-nitroblue tetrazolium transferase reaction, appear in some patients with FHL1opathy.

Immunohistochemical studies indicate ectopic accumulation of multiple proteins in the abnormal fiber regions that include desmin (Figure 5–1C), myotilin (Figure 5–1E), neural cell adhesion molecule (NCAM; Figure 5–1F), dystrophin (Figure 5–1G), sarcoglycans, actin, plectin, gelsolin, ubiquitin, filamin C, syncoilin, Bag3, synemin, Xin, TAR

DNA-binding protein 43, and co-chaperones including αB-crystallin (Figure 5–1D), heat shock protein (Hsp) 27, and DNAJB23.[3,10-17] Additional abnormal accumulation of several other proteins was documented in myotilinopathy and desminopathy. These include phospho-tau; β-amyloid; clusterin; a mutant nonfunctional ubiquitin; the multimeric signal protein p62; glycoxidation and lipoxidation markers; neuronal, inducible, and endothelial nitric oxide synthases; superoxide dismutase; neuron-related proteins such as ubiquitin carboxy-terminal hydrolase L1; synaptosomal-associated protein 25; synaptophysin; and α-internexin.[12,18,19, 20]

Electron microscopy (EM) demonstrates disintegration of myofibrils that begins at or in immediate proximity of the Z-disk. The earliest changes consist of Z-disk streaming or accumulation of material of Z-disk density intermingled with pleomorphic, dappled dense bodies in close proximity to the Z-disk (Figures 5–4). In FHL1opathy, tubulofilamentous material is arising from a proportion of Z disks. In patients with desminopathy, α B-crystallinopathy, and Bag3opathy, small pleomorphic dense structures or granulofilamentous material accumulate between the myofibrils (Figure 5–3). In more advanced stages, when the Z-disks have disintegrated, the sarcomeres fall apart and the myofibrils are no longer recognizable (Figure 5–4). Dislocated membranous organelles and glycogen accumulate in spaces vacated by disintegrating myofibrils

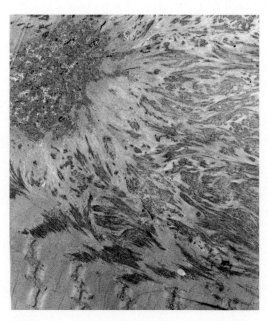

Figure 5–4. Ultrastructural findings in zaspopathy. Normal Z-disks are replaced by stripes of dense material, the myofibrils move out of register, and mitochondria accumulate in clusters.

(Figure 5–4). Other fiber regions harbor fragmented filaments or Z-disk remnants that aggregate into globoid inclusions (Figure 5–5A & C). On higher resolution, the globoid structures are composed of degraded filaments and some amorphous material (Figure 5–5D). Some fiber regions display bundles of filaments coated with dense material (Figure 5–5B). Some dislocated organelles are trapped and degraded in autophagic vacuoles (Figure 5–6) and some vacuoles undergo exocytosis.

Claeys et al.[21] report distinct EM patterns in different subtypes of MFMs and recommend EM to be included in the diagnostic workup of MFMs. They noted the following specific features: electron-dense granulofilamentous material under the sarcolemma in desminopathy and α B-crystallinopathy; filamentous bundles and floccular thin filamentous accumulations in zaspopathy; and filamentous bundles and tubulofilamentous inclusions in myotilinopathy. However, in our experience these morphologic features are not uniquely specific for the mutated protein, and the ultrastructural features in desminopathy and αB-crystallinopathy are more diverse than stated.

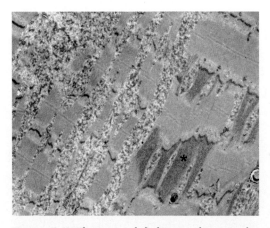

Figure 5–3. Ultrastructural findings in desminopathy. Note widened intermyofibrillar spaces are filled with dappled dense bodies and Z-disk streaming (asterisk). (Reproduced from Selcen & Engel, 2004).

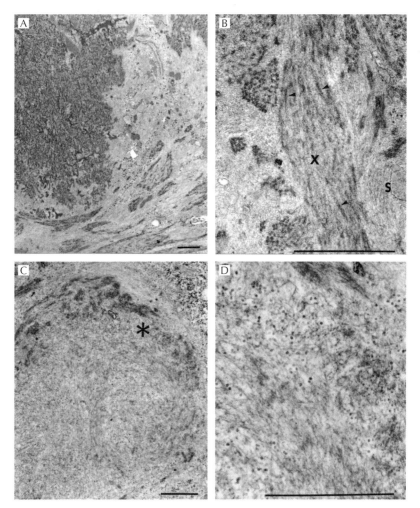

Figure 5–5. Large hyaline structures observed by light microcopy consist of compacted and fragmented filaments of variable electron density (A & C). Panel D shows a higher magnification of region marked by asterisk in panel C and resolves filamentous profiles. In panel B, an abnormal fiber region harbors longitudinally oriented bundles of filaments (X) coated by dense material (arrowheads). Note sarcomere remnant (S) containing thick and thin filaments. Bars = 1 μm. (Reproduced from Selcen & Engel, 2004).

CLINICAL FEATURES

Most patients with MFM present with progressive muscle weakness, but in some patients the cardiomyopathy may precede the muscle weakness. Most MFMs are transmitted by autosomal-dominant inheritance, but FHL1opathy is transmitted by X-linked inheritance, and some forms of α-crystallinopathy can be transmitted by autosomal-recessive inheritance. Sporadic cases are frequent either because a mutation arises in the germ line, or because the disease in the parents was unrecognized.

Desminopathy

In skeletal muscle, desmin is detected at the periphery of Z-disks, under the sarcolemma, and at the myotendinous and neuromuscular junctions. In cardiac muscle, it is abundant at intercalated disks and Purkinje fibers. Desmin is a type III intermediate filament (IF) protein primarily expressed in skeletal, cardiac, and smooth muscle cells. IFs are 10 nm in diameter, intermediate in size between thick (15 nm) and thin (5–6 nm) filaments. They serve to maintain structural integrity and resist externally applied mechanical stress.[22] Desmin

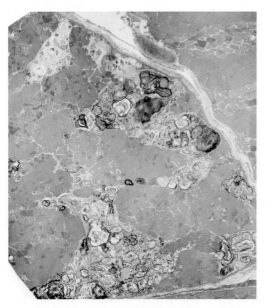

Figure 5–6. Multiple autophagic vacuoles harboring degraded membranous organelles and debris.

with other associated IFs forms a heteropolymeric lattice that organizes the myofibrils and links them to nuclei, mitochondria, and the sarcolemma.[22,23,24]

Since the first reports of mutations in desmin causing MFM by Goldfarb et al.[25] and Munoz-Marmol et al.,[26] more than 40 mutations have been reported. The distribution of weakness can be distal, limb-girdle, and scapuloperoneal. Muscle atrophy, mild facial weakness, dysphagia, dysarthria, and respiratory insufficiency can occur. Cardiomyopathy, especially arrhythmogenic type, is a common manifestation. The majority of patients present between 10 to 61 years of age, but a patient carrying a homozygous in-frame deletion of 7 amino acids (p.Arg173_Glu179del) in *DES* exon 6 presented with syncopal episodes in infancy.[27] An unusual presentation was observed in two brothers with childhood-onset progressive axial and proximal muscle weakness, calf hypertrophy, and severe joint contractures and dilated cardiomyopathy resembling the Emery-Dreifuss muscular dystrophy phenotype, but the disease was caused by a homozygous deletion of 22 bp in *DES* exon 6. Interestingly, the muscle biopsy did not show the typical MFM changes, but the pathologic changes were not detailed.[28]

αB-Crystallinopathy

The α-crystallins are small heat-shock proteins that associate into 15- to 20-nm high-molecular-weight soluble aggregates to become functional. The primary role of α-crystallins is to bind to unfolded and denatured proteins to suppress their nonspecific aggregation. Like other members of the small heat-shock protein family, αB-crystallin monomers contain an N-terminal domain (residues 1–63), an α-crystallin domain (residues 64–105), and a C-terminal extension (residues 106–175).[29] The A and B forms of α-crystallin are encoded by different genes but have highly homologous amino acid sequences.[29] Both forms are abundant in the lens where they prevent cataract formation. αB-crystallin is also found in nonlenticular tissues, with highest levels in cardiac and skeletal muscle. In these tissues, αB-crystallin is immunolocalized to the Z-disk and its expression is enhanced after stress[30] and exercise.[31] αB-crystallin chaperones actin and desmin filaments[32], tubulin subunits of microtubules,[33] and a variety of soluble enzymes,[34,35] protecting them from stress-induced damage.

In 1998, Vicart et al.[36] identified a heterozygous missense mutation in *CRYAB* in a large kinship. Subsequently, two heterozygous truncating mutations were observed in two patients in the Mayo MFM cohort.[37] The affected patients present in adult life, have symmetric proximal and distal muscle weakness and atrophy, and show respiratory involvement. Some patients also have hypertrophic cardiomyopathy, palato-pharyngeal weakness, and cataracts. Since then, two other patients were reported with muscle weakness and cardiomyopathy, and one of them also had a posterior polar cataracts.[38,39] The muscle biopsy was typical of MFM in both kinships.

Recently, a homozygous c.60delC (p.Ser21AlafsX24) in *CRYAB* was identified as the disease gene of the fatal infantile hypertonic muscular dystrophy of Canadian Aboriginals.[40] The affected infants present with progressive limb and axial muscle stiffness, and develop severe respiratory insufficiency; most die in the first year of life. MFMs are typically transmitted by dominant inheritance but in this disease the parental phenotype is rescued by limited expression of the highly truncated nonfunctional mutant gene product. Another similarly affected infant was reported carrying homozygous c.343delT (p.Ser115ProfsX14) mutation.[41]

Myotilinopathy

Myotilin is a 57 kDa Z-disk-associated protein expressed strongly in skeletal and weakly in cardiac muscle.[42] It contains a serine-rich amino-terminal region that also comprises a hydrophobic stretch, two immunoglobulin (Ig)-like domains and a carboxy terminal tail. The Ig-like repeats are required for the formation of antiparallel myotilin dimers.[42,43] Myotilin binds to α-actinin, the main component of Z-disk that cross link actin filaments at the Z-disk, and to filamin C, a peripheral Z-disk protein. The α-actinin binding site resides between myotilin residues 79 and 150[6]; and the filamin C binding site is located in the second Ig-like domain.[44] In addition, myotilin cross-links actin filaments and plays a role in the alignment of myofibrils during the later stages of myofibrillogenesis.[43]

In 2000, Hauser et al.[6] detected a missense mutation in *MYOT* in a large kinship that had previously been linked to the myotilin locus at 5q31. The disease was identified as LGMD1A. Two years later, a second kinship with a similar phenotype was found to have a missense mutation in myotilin.[45] One of the reports,[45] however, did not assess the pathology of the disease, and the other report[6] showed only Z-disk alteration in some muscle fibers. That myotilin is a Z-disk component prompted a search for myotilin mutations in the Mayo cohort of MFM patients and resulted in discovery of six mutations in eight unrelated patients.[14] In the identified patients, the mean age of onset was 60 years. In three patients the weakness was more prominent distally than proximally. Cardiac involvement without signs of coronary artery disease was evident in three patients. Peripheral neuropathy, reflected by clinical, EMG, and histologic criteria, or by a combination of these, was apparent in all patients. Subsequent studies by other investigators identified additional patients with mutations in *MYOT*,[12,46,47,48] including the kinship originally described under the rubric of "spheroid body myopathy."[47] Some kinships show intrafamily phenotypic variability. All myotilin mutations reported to date are heterozygous missense amino acid changes, and all but one mutation fall in *MYOT* exon 2, a sequence of unknown structure and function.[6,12,14,45,47-49]

Zaspopathy

ZASP (Z-band alternatively spliced PDZ motif-containing protein) is expressed predominantly in cardiac and skeletal muscle.[50] It binds to α-actinin,[51] the structural component of the Z-filaments that cross-link thin filaments of adjacent sarcomeres. Sixteen *ZASP*-associated exons have been detected in genomic DNA, and splice variants of these exist in cardiac and skeletal muscle. Skeletal muscle harbors three isoforms. The longest isoform lacks exons 4 and 9; another long isoform lacks exons 4, 9, and 10; and a short isoform lacks exon 4 and carries a stop codon in exon 9. In the mouse and human, three cardiac isoforms resemble those in skeletal muscle but contain exon 4 instead of exon 6.[52] Recently, however, exon 6 was also detected in the human heart.[53] All ZASP isoforms have an N-terminal PDZ domain important for protein-protein interactions[54] and a 26 residue ZM motif in exons 4 and 6 needed specifically for interaction with α-actinin.[55] The long isoforms have three C-terminal LIM domains that interact with protein kinase-C subtypes.[56] Targeted deletion of *ZASP* in the mouse (referred to as Cypher[51] or Oracle[57] in the mouse) causes skeletal and cardiac myopathy with fragmented Z-disks.[58]

Zaspopathy-causing MFM was first described in 2005 by Selcen and Engel[15] in 11 MFM patients who carried heterozygous missense mutations in *ZASP*. The mean age of onset was in sixth decade. Most patients presented with muscle weakness but one patient presented with palpitations and mild hyperCKemia. Seven of 11 patients had family histories consistent with autosomal-dominant inheritance. The patients had proximal and/or distal muscle weakness. Three patients had cardiac involvement without signs of coronary artery disease, and in one of these the cardiac symptoms antedated the muscle weakness by 10 years. Peripheral nerve involvement by clinical, EMG, or histologic criteria was detected in five patients. The mutations detected in these patients were Ala147Thr and Ala165Val in exon 6, and Arg268Cys in exon 9. The Ala165Val mutation is within, and the Ala147Thr mutation is immediately before, the ZM motif needed for interaction with α-actinin.[55] Subsequently, the large kinship, described by Markesbery et al. in 1974, and five other kinships with distal myopathy and MFM pathology, were shown to carry the Ala165Val mutation. These six kinships and the three of the zaspopathy kinships observed at the Mayo Clinic harboring this mutation may have a common founder.[7]

Recently, another family with onset of distal weakness in the first decade of life with c.349G>A (p.Asp117Asn) mutation was identified.[59] The same mutation was previously detected in patients with isolated cardiomyopathy without skeletal muscle involvement.[53] Interestingly, the patients did not have cardiomyopathy and the muscle specimen of one patient did not show classical MFM features.

Filaminopathy

The filamins are a family of high-molecular-weight cytoskeletal homodimeric proteins containing an N-terminal actin-binding domain followed by 24 Ig like repeats.[60] Whereas the expression of filamins A and B is ubiquitous, filamin C is largely restricted to skeletal and cardiac muscle. The filamins are involved in multiple processes, such as the organization of actin filaments, membrane stabilization, and they serve as a scaffold for signaling proteins. Filamin C also interacts with several Z-disc proteins and with γ- and δ-sarcoglycan at the sarcolemma.[61,60,62]

In 2005, Vorgerd et al.[17] identified a dominant Trp2710X mutation in the last exon of filamin C in 17 affected individuals of a large German kinship. Subsequently, the same nonsense mutation was observed in two other German families[63] and three MFM kinships in the Mayo MFM cohort. The age of onset is between 24 and 60 years. All patients have progressive muscle weakness. The serum CK level is normal to 10-fold elevated above the upper limit of normal. Cardiomyopathy, respiratory insufficiency, and peripheral neuropathy are associated features. Further MFM-related *FLNC* mutations were detected: an in-frame deletion (Val903_Thr933del)[64] and a complex deletion-insertion mutation (Lys899_Val904del and Val899_Cys900ins),[65] both in the seventh Ig-like repeat in exon 18. Interestingly, three patients in a large Chinese family had chronic diarrhea before the onset of muscle weakness.[65]

Recently, Duff et al.[66] identified two families with distal myopathy with heterozygous c.577G>A (p.Ala193Thr) and c.752T>C

(p.Met251Thr) mutations in the N-terminal actin-binding domain of *FLNC*. The patients have distinct involvement of hand muscles and lack MFM features in the muscle specimens. In other related families with adult-onset and predominantly upper limb weakness, a frameshift c.5160delC (p.Phe1720LeufsX63) mutation was identified. This mutation results nonsense-mediated mRNA decay and therefore haploinsufficiency of filamin C. Although the light microscopic features of MFM were lacking in the muscle, EM revealed some features of MFM.[67]

Bag3opathy

Bag3 (Bcl-2 associated athanogene 3), also referred to as CAIR-1 or Bis, is a multidomain co-chaperone protein interacting with many other polypeptides. Bag3 is strongly expressed in skeletal and cardiac muscle and at a lower level in other tissues. Like other members of the Bag family, it harbors a C-terminal BAG domain that mediates interaction with Hsp 70 and the antiapoptotic protein Bcl-2. It also has a proline-rich region that interacts with WW-domain proteins implicated in signal transduction, and with Src-3 homology (SH3)–domain proteins implicated in antiapoptotic pathways. Bag3 also has a unique N-terminal WW domain that binds proline-rich sequences. Bag3 forms a stable complex with the small Hsp 8 and thereby participates in the degradation of misfolded or aggregated proteins.[60,68,69] Its targeted deletion in mice results in a fulminant myopathy with early lethality.[71]

In 2009, Selcen et al.[16] described Bag3opathy in 3 MFM patients who were heterozygous for Pro209Leu in exon 3. All three presented in childhood with severe muscle weakness. All had cardiomyopathy and developed respiratory insufficiency with diaphragm paralysis by the second decade, and two had a rigid spine. The muscle weakness was proximal in one patient, proximal and distal in the second patient, and distal more than proximal in the third patient. The serum CK ranged from 3 to 15 times above the upper limit of normal. The EMG of one patient showed both axonal and demyelinating polyneuropathy. The light microscopy findings were typical of MFM (Figure 5–1). The affected patients differed from most other MFM patients in early age of onset, rapid evolution of the illness, and presence of the rigid spine. Apoptosis was found in 8% of the nuclei. The enhanced nuclear apoptosis in Bag3opathy is consistent with known antiapoptotic effect of Bag3[72,70,73] and indicates that Pro209 contributes to this effect. Three other kinships were reported to have the same Pro209Leu mutation in *BAG3*. All patients show the same severe phenotype. One asymptomatic parent was a somatic mosaic for the mutation. Nerve biopsies showed axonal neuropathy with loss of myelinated axons and scattered giant axons.[74] Recently, four patients with sensorimotor neuropathy as a dominant feature of the disease were reported with the same mutation in *BAG3*. EMG revealed axonal neuropathy and examination of the sural biopsy of two patients revealed giant axonal neuropathy[75] (Figure 5–7).

FHL1opathy

The four-and-a-half LIM domain protein 1 (FHL1) is highly expressed in skeletal and cardiac muscle and less abundantly in brain, placenta, lung, liver, kidney, pancreas, and testis. It has three recognized alternatively spiced isoforms with different tissue localizations and protein interactions. Mutations in *FHL1* have been associated with diverse chronic myopathies.[76] These include late-onset X-linked scapulo-axio-peroneal myopathy with bent spine syndrome (XMPMA),[77] reducing body myopathy (RBM),[78,79] X-linked dominant scapuloperoneal muscular dystrophy,[80] rigid spine syndrome,[81] and contractures and cardiomyopathy mimicking Emery-Dreifuss muscular dystrophy.[82,83] Most *FHL1* mutations appear in the second or fourth LIM domains with a single mutation in the third LIM domain and another between the first and second LIM domain. Some of the patients carrying missense *FHL1* mutation have MFM features in the muscle biopsy as well as reducing bodies identified by the menadione-NBT reaction without substrate[84] at the light microscopy level and closely packed tubulofilamentous inclusions in the electron microscope (Figure 5–8).

DNAJB6-Related MFM

DNAJB6 is a ubiquitously expressed member of DNAJ (Hsp40) family of proteins important in regulation of Hsp70 activity via their J-domain.[85]

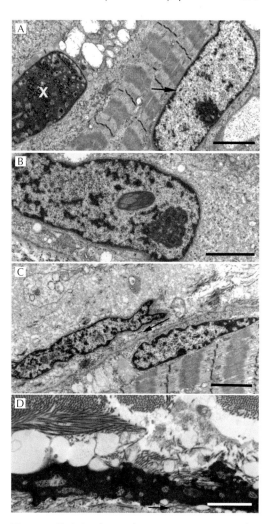

Figure 5–7. Nuclear alterations in Bag3opathy. (A) Ovoid nucleus with prominent nucleolus suggesting increased transcription (arrow) and apoptotic nucleus (X). (B) Large nucleus harboring clumps of heterochromatin. (C) A superficially positioned shrunken (pyknotic) nucleus in a muscle fiber is positioned under an exocytosed pyknotic nucleus. Arrow points to collagen fibrils in the extracellular space. (D) An exocytosed apoptotic nucleus. Arrow at bottom points to collagen in the extracellular space. Bars = 2 μm in (A) and (C) and 1 μm in (B) and (D). (Reproduced from Selcen et al., 2008)

Recently dominant missense mutations have been identified in families with LGMD, including one family who was originally assigned to LGMD1D.[86,87] The age of onset is between 14 and 60 years. The distribution of the weakness is proximal or distal predominant. None of the patients had cardiac or respiratory involvement. The muscle specimens reveal the features of myofibrillar myopathy including accumulation of multiple proteins.

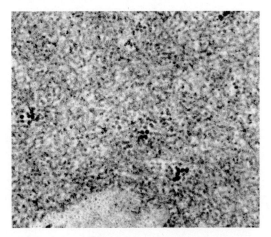

Figure 5–8. Tubulofilamentous profile in FHL1opathy.

Titin-Related MFM

Titin is a giant muscle protein that aligns with thick filaments and inserts into the Z-disk. It is important in regulating assembly of the contractile filaments, providing elasticity by its multiple spring elements, and may play a role in myofibrillar cell signaling.[88,89,90] Autosomal-dominant mutations in *TTN* have been associated with cardiomyopathy, distal muscular dystrophy, and recessive mutations with LGMD2J. A group of patients with progressive muscle weakness harboring a dominant missense mutation in *TTN* had early respiratory failure. The muscle biopsy features were characteristic of MFM.[91]

TREATMENT

No known measures mitigate the slow but relentless progression of MFM. Corticosteroids have not been shown to be of benefit. Physical therapy, consisting of passive exercises, orthoses, and other supporting devices, is helpful in the more advanced cases. Respiratory support consisting of continuous (CPAP) or BiPAP ventilation, initially at night and later in the daytime, are indicated in patients with respiratory failure and signs of hypercapnea.

Periodic monitoring of patients for appearance of cardiomyopathy should be done in all patients, and pacemaker and implantable cardioverter defibrillator should be considered in individuals with arrhythmia and/or cardiac conduction defects. Patients with progressive or life-threatening cardiomyopathy are candidates for cardiac transplantation.

REFERENCES

1. De Bleecker JL, Engel AG, Ertl BB. Myofibrillar myopathy with abnormal foci of desmin positivity. II. Immunocytochemical analysis reveals accumulation of multiple other proteins. J Neuropathol Exp Neurol. 1996;55:563–577.
2. Nakano S, Engel AG, Waclawik AJ, Emslie-Smith AM, Busis NA. Myofibrillar myopathy with abnormal foci of desmin positivity. I. Light and electron microscopy analysis of 10 cases. J Neuropathol Exp Neurol. 1996;55:549–562.
3. Selcen D, Ohno K, Engel AG. Myofibrillar myopathy: clinical, morphological and genetic studies in 63 patients. Brain. 2004;127:439–451.
4. Erb W. Dystrophia muscularis progressiva. Klinische und pathologisch-anatomische studien. Dtsch Z Nervenheilkd. 1891;1:173–261.
5. Gilchrist JM, Pericak-Vance M, Silverman L, Roses AD. Clinical and genetic investigation in autosomal dominant limb-girdle muscular dystrophy. Neurology. 1988 Jan;38(1):5–9.
6. Hauser MA, Horrigan SK, Salmikangas P, Torian UM, Viles KD, Dancel R, et al. Myotilin is mutated in limb girdle muscular dystrophy 1A. Hum Mol Genet. 2000;9:2141–2147.
7. Griggs R, Vihola A, Hackman P, Talvinen K, Haravuori H, Faulkner G, et al. Zaspopathy in a large classic late-onset distal myopathy family. Brain. 2007;130:1477–1484.
8. Markesbery WR, Griggs RC, Leach RP, Lapham LW. Late onset hereditary distal myopathy. Neurology. 1974;24:127–134.
9. Greenberg SA, Salajegheh M, Judge DP, Feldman MW, Kuncl RW, Waldon Z, et al. Etiology of limb girdle muscular dystrophy 1D/1E determined by laser capture microdissection proteomics. Ann Neurol. 2012 Jan;71(1):141–145.
10. Claeys KG, Sozanska M, Martin JJ, Lacene E, Vignaud L, Stockholm D, et al. DNAJB2 Expression in normal and diseased human and mouse skeletal muscle. Am J Pathol. 2010 Apr 15;176:2901–2910.
11. Ferrer I, Carmona M, Blanco R, Moreno D, Torrejon-Escribano B, Olive M. Involvement of clusterin and the aggresome in abnormal protein deposits in myofibrillar myopathies and inclusion body myositis. Brain Pathol. 2005 Apr;15(2):101–108.
12. Olive M, Goldfarb LG, Shatunov A, Fischer D, Ferrer I. Myotilinopathy: refining the clinical and myopathological phenotype. Brain. 2005;128:2315–2326.
13. Olive M, Janue A, Moreno D, Gamez J, Torrejon-Escribano B, Ferrer I. TAR DNA-Binding protein 43 accumulation in protein aggregate myopathies. J Neuropathol Exp Neurol. 2009 Mar;68(3):262–273.
14. Selcen D, Engel AG. Mutations in myotilin cause myofibrillar myopathy. Neurology. 2004;62:1363–1371

15. Selcen D, Engel AG. Mutations in ZASP define a novel form of muscular dystrophy in humans. Ann Neurol. 2005;57:269–276.

16. Selcen D, Muntoni F, Burton BK, Pegoraro E, Sewry C, Bite AV, et al. Mutation in *BAG3* causes severe dominant childhood muscular dystrophy. Ann Neurol. 2009;65:83–89.

17. Vorgerd M, van der Ven PF, Bruchertseifer V, Lowe T, Kley RA, Schroder R, et al. A mutation in the dimerization domain of filamin c causes a novel type of autosomal dominant myofibrillar myopathy. Am J Hum Genet. 2005;77:297–304.

18. Barrachina M, Moreno J, Juves S, Moreno D, Olive M, Ferrer I. Target genes of neuron-restrictive silencer factor are abnormally up-regulated in human myotilinopathy. Am J Pathol. 2007;171:1312–1323.

19. Janue A, Olive M, Ferrer I. oxidative stress in desminopathies and myotilinopathies: a link between oxidative damage and abnormal protein aggregation. Brain Pathol. 2007;17:377–388.

20. Olive M, van Leeuwen FW, Janue A, Moreno D, Torrejon-Escribano B, Ferrer I. Expression of mutant ubiquitin (UBB+1) and p62 in myotilinopathies and desminopathies. Neuropathol Appl Neurobiol. 2008;34:76–87.

21. Claeys KG, Fardeau M, Schroder R, Suominen T, Tolksdorf K, Behin A, et al. Electron microscopy in myofibrillar myopathies reveals clues to the mutated gene. Neuromuscul Disord. 2008 Aug;18(8):656–666.

22. Fuchs E, Weber K. Intermediate filaments: structure, dynamics, function, and disease. Annu Rev Biochem. 1994;63:345–382.

23. Herrmann H, Aebi U. Intermediate filaments and their associates: multi-talented structural elements specifying cytoarchitecture and cytodynamics. Curr Opin Cell Biol. 2000 Feb;12(1):79–90.

24. Schroder R, Furst DO, Klasen C, Reimann J, Herrmann H, van der Ven PF. Association of plectin with Z-discs is a prerequisite for the formation of the intermyofibrillar desmin cytoskeleton. Lab Invest. 2000 Apr;80(4):455–464.

25. Goldfarb LG, Park KY, Cervenakova L, Gorokhova S, Lee HS, Vasconcelos O, et al. Missense mutations in desmin associated with familial cardiac and skeletal myopathy. Nat Genet. 1998;19:402–403.

26. Munoz-Marmol AM, Strasser G, Isamat M, Coulombe PA, Yang Y, Roca X, et al. A dysfunctional desmin mutation in a patient with severe generalized myopathy. Proc Natl Acad Sci U S A. 1998;95:11312–11317.

27. Pinol-Ripoll G, Shatunov A, Cabello A, Larrode P, de la Puerta I, Pelegrin J, et al. Severe infantile-onset cardiomyopathy associated with a homozygous deletion in desmin. Neuromuscul Disord. 2009 Jun;19(6):418–422.

28. Carmignac V, Sharma S, Arbogast S, Fischer D, Serreri C, Serria M, et al. A homozygous desmin deletion causes an Emery-Dreifuss like recessive myopathy with desmin depletion. Neuromuscular Disorders. 2009 Sep;19(8–9):600.

29. Derham BK, Harding JJ. Alpha-crystallin as a molecular chaperone. Prog Retin Eye Res. 1999 Jul;18(4):463–509.

30. Djabali K, de Nechaud B, Landon F, Portier MM. AlphaB-crystallin interacts with intermediate filaments in response to stress. J Cell Sci. 1997 Nov;110 (Pt 21):2759–2769.

31. Neufer PD, Ordway GA, Williams RS. Transient regulation of c-fos, alpha B-crystallin, and hsp70 in muscle during recovery from contractile activity. Am J Physiol Cell Physiol. 1998 Feb 1;274(2):C341–C346.

32. Bennardini F, Wrzosek A, Chiesi M. Alpha B-crystallin in cardiac tissue. Association with actin and desmin filaments. Circ Res. 1992 Aug;71(2):288–294.

33. Arai H, Atomi Y. Chaperone activity of alpha B-crystallin suppresses tubulin aggregation through complex formation. Cell Struct Funct. 1997 Oct;22(5):539–544.

34. Bova MP, Yaron O, Huang Q, Ding L, Haley DA, Stewart PL, et al. Mutation R120G in alphaB-crystallin, which is linked to a desmin-related myopathy, results in an irregular structure and defective chaperone-like function. Proc Natl Acad Sci U S A. 1999 May 25;96(11):6137–6142.

35. Muchowski PJ, Clark JI. ATP-enhanced molecular chaperone functions of the small heat shock protein human alphaB crystallin. Proc Natl Acad Sci U S A. 1998 Feb 3;95(3):1004–1009.

36. Vicart P, Caron A, Guicheney P, Li Z, Prevost MC, Faure A, et al. A missense mutation in the alphaB-crystallin chaperone gene causes a desmin-related myopathy. Nat Genet. 1998;20:92–95.

37. Selcen D, Engel AG. Myofibrillar myopathy caused by novel dominant negative alpha B-crystallin mutations. Ann Neurol. 2003;54:804–810.

38. Casarin A, Giorgi G, Pertegato V, Siviero R, Cerqua C, Doimo M, et al. Copper and bezafibrate cooperate to rescue cytochrome c oxidase deficiency in cells of patients with SCO2 mutations. Orphanet Journal of Rare Diseases. 2012 Apr 19;7(1):21.

39. Reilich P, Schoser B, Schramm N, Krause S, Schessl J, Kress W, et al. The p.G154S mutation of the alpha-B crystallin gene (CRYAB) causes late-onset distal myopathy. Neuromuscul Disord. 2010 Apr;20(4):255–259.

40. Del Bigio MR, Chudley AE, Sarnat HB, Campbell C, Goobie S, Chodirker BN, et al. Infantile muscular dystrophy in Canadian Aboriginals is an αB-crystallinopathy. Ann Neurol. 2011; 69:866–871.

41. Forrest KM, Al-Sarraj S, Sewry C, Buk S, Tan SV, Pitt M, et al. Infantile onset myofibrillar myopathy due to recessive CRYAB mutations. Neuromuscular disorders: NMD. 2011 Jan;21(1):37–40.

42. Salmikangas P, Mykkanen OM, Gronholm M, Heiska L, Kere J, Carpen O. Myotilin, a novel sarcomeric protein with two Ig-like domains, is encoded by a candidate gene for limb-girdle muscular dystrophy. Hum Mol Genet. 1999 Jul;8(7):1329–1336.

43. Salmikangas P, van der Ven PF, Lalowski M, Taivainen A, Zhao F, Suila H, et al. Myotilin, the limb-girdle muscular dystrophy 1A (LGMD1A) protein, cross-links actin filaments and controls sarcomere assembly. Hum Mol Genet. 2003 Jan 15;12(2):189–203.

44. van der Ven PF, Obermann WM, Lemke B, Gautel M, Weber K, Furst DO. Characterization of muscle filamin isoforms suggests a possible role of gamma-filamin/ABP-L in sarcomeric Z-disc formation. Cell Motil Cytoskeleton. 2000 Feb;45(2):149–162.

45. Hauser MA, Conde CB, Kowaljow V, Zeppa G, Taratuto AL, Torian UM, et al. Myotilin mutation found in second pedigree with LGMD1A. Am J Hum Genet. 2002;71:1428–1432.

46. Berciano J, Gallardo E, Dominguez-Perles R, Garcia A, Garcia-Barredo R, Combarros O, et al. Autosomal

dominant distal myopathy with a myotilin S55F mutation: sorting out the phenotype. J Neurol Neurosurg Psychiatry. 2007;79:205–208.

47. Foroud T, Pankratz N, Batchman AP, Pauciulo MW, Vidal R, Miravalle L, et al. A mutation in myotilin causes spheroid body myopathy. Neurology. 2005;65:1936–1940.

48. Penisson-Besnier I, Talvinen K, Dumez C, Vihola A, Dubas F, Fardeau M, et al. Myotilinopathy in a family with late onset myopathy. Neuromuscul Disord. 2006;16:427–431.

49. Reilich P, Krause S, Schramm N, Klutzny U, Bulst S, Zehetmayer B, et al. A novel mutation in the myotilin gene (MYOT) causes a severe form of limb girdle muscular dystrophy 1A (LGMD1A). Journal of Neurology. 2011 Aug;258(8):1437–1444.

50. Faulkner G, Pallavicini A, Formentin E, Comelli A, Ievolella C, Trevisan S, et al. ZASP: a new Z-band alternatively spliced PDZ-motif protein. J Cell Biol. 1999 Jul 26;146(2):465–475.

51. Zhou Q, Ruiz-Lozano P, Martone ME, Chen J. Cypher, a striated muscle-restricted PDZ and LIM domain-containing protein, binds to alpha-actinin-2 and protein kinase C. J Biol Chem. 1999 Jul 9;274(28):19807–19813.

52. Huang C, Zhou Q, Liang P, Hollander MS, Sheikh F, Li X, et al. Characterization and in vivo functional analysis of splice variants of cypher. J Biol Chem. 2003 Feb 28;278(9):7360–7365.

53. Vatta M, Mohapatra B, Jimenez S, Sanchez X, Faulkner G, Perles Z, et al. Mutations in Cypher/ ZASP in patients with dilated cardiomyopathy and left ventricular non-compaction. J Am Coll Cardiol. 2003 Dec 3;42(11):2014–2027.

54. Harris BZ, Lim WA. Mechanism and role of PDZ domains in signaling complex assembly. J Cell Sci. 2001 Sep;114(Pt 18):3219–3231.

55. Klaavuniemi T, Kelloniemi A, Ylanne J. The ZASP-like motif in actinin-associated LIM protein is required for interaction with the alpha-actinin rod and for targeting to the muscle Z-line. J Biol Chem. 2004;279:26402–26410.

56. Arimura T, Hayashi T, Terada H, Lee SY, Zhou Q, Takahashi M, et al. A Cypher/ZASP mutation associated with dilated cardiomyopathy alters the binding affinity to protein kinase C. J Biol Chem. 2004 Feb 20;279(8):6746–6752.

57. Passier R, Richardson JA, Olson EN. Oracle, a novel PDZ-LIM domain protein expressed in heart and skeletal muscle. Mech Dev. 2000 Apr;92(2):277–284.

58. Zhou Q, Chu PH, Huang C, Cheng CF, Martone ME, Knoll G, et al. Ablation of Cypher, a PDZ-LIM domain Z-line protein, causes a severe form of congenital myopathy. J Cell Biol. 2001 Nov 12;155(4):605–612.

59. Strach K, Reimann J, Thomas D, Naehle CP, Kress W, Kornblum C. ZASPopathy with childhood-onset distal myopathy. Journal of Neurology. 2012 Jul; 259(7):1494–1496.

60. Takayama S, Reed JC. Molecular chaperone targeting and regulation by BAG family proteins. Nat Cell Biol. 2001 Oct;3(10):E237–E241.

61. van der Flier A, Sonnenberg A. Structural and functional aspects of filamins. Biochim Biophys Acta. 2001 Apr 23;1538(2–3):99–117.

62. Thompson TG, Chan YM, Hack AA, Brosius M, Rajala M, Lidov HG, et al. Filamin 2 (FLN2): A muscle-specific sarcoglycan interacting protein. J Cell Biol. 2000 Jan 10;148(1):115–126.

63. van der Ven PF, Wiesner S, Salmikangas P, Auerbach D, Himmel M, Kempa S, et al. Indications for a novel muscular dystrophy pathway. Gamma-filamin, the muscle-specific filamin isoform, interacts with myotilin. J Cell Biol. 2000 Oct 16;151(2):235–248.

64. Kley RA, Hellenbroich Y, van der Ven PFM, Furst DO, Huebner A, Bruchertseifer V, et al. Clinical and morphological phenotype of the filamin myopathy: a study of 31 German patients. Brain. 2007;130:3250–3264.

65. Shatunov A, Olive M, Odgerel Z, Stadelmann-Nessler C, Irlbacher K, van Landeghem F, et al. In-frame deletion in the seventh immunoglobulin-like repeat of filamin C in a family with myofibrillar myopathy. Eur J Hum Genet. 2009 May;17(5):656–663.

66. Luan X, Hong D, Zhang W, Wang Z, Yuan Y. A novel heterozygous deletion-insertion mutation (2695–2712 del/GTTTGT ins) in exon 18 of the filamin C gene causes filaminopathy in a large Chinese family. Neuromuscul Disord. 2010 Apr 21;20:390–396.

67. Duff RM, Tay V, Hackman P, Ravenscroft G, McLean C, Kennedy P, et al. Mutations in the N-terminal actin-binding domain of filamin C cause a distal myopathy. American Journal of Human Genetics. 2011 Jun 10;88(6):729–740.

68. Guergueltcheva V, Peeters K, Baets J, Ceuterick-de Groote C, Martin JJ, Suls A, et al. Distal myopathy with upper limb predominance caused by filamin C haploinsufficiency. Neurology. 2011 Dec 13;77(24):2105–2114.

69. Carra S, Seguin SJ, Lambert H, Landry J. HspB8 chaperone activity toward poly(Q)-containing proteins depends on its association with Bag3, a stimulator of macroautophagy. J Biol Chem. 2008 Jan 18;283(3):1437–1444.

70. Doong H, Vrailas A, Kohn EC. What's in the "BAG"?—A functional domain analysis of the BAG-family proteins. Cancer Lett. 2002 Dec 15;188(1–2):25–32.

71. Homma S, Iwasaki M, Shelton GD, Engvall E, Reed JC, Takayama S. BAG3 deficiency results in fulminant myopathy and early lethality. Am J Pathol. 2006 Sep;169(3):761–773.

72. Bonelli P, Petrella A, Rosati A, Romano MF, Lerose R, Pagliuca MG, et al. BAG3 protein regulates stress-induced apoptosis in normal and neoplastic leukocytes. Leukemia. 2004 Feb;18(2):358–360.

73. Liao Q, Ozawa F, Friess H, Zimmermann A, Takayama S, Reed JC, et al. The anti-apoptotic protein BAG-3 is overexpressed in pancreatic cancer and induced by heat stress in pancreatic cancer cell lines. FEBS Lett. 2001 Aug 17;503(2–3):151–157.

74. Odgerel Z, Sarkozy A, Lee HS, McKenna C, Rankin J, Straub V, et al. Inheritance patterns and phenotypic features of myofibrillar myopathy associated with a BAG3 mutation. Neuromuscul Disord. 2010 Jul;20(7):438–442.

75. Jaffer F, Murphy SM, Scoto M, Healy E, Rossor AM, Brandner S, et al. BAG3 mutations: another cause of giant axonal neuropathy. Journal of the Peripheral Nervous System: JPNS. 2012 Jun;17(2):210–216.

76. Cowling BS, Cottle DL, Wilding BR, D'Arcy CE, Mitchell CA, McGrath MJ. Four and a half LIM protein 1 gene mutations cause four distinct human myopathies: a comprehensive review of the clinical, histological and pathological features. Neuromuscul Disord. 2011 Apr;21(4):237–251.

77. Windpassinger C, Schoser B, Straub V, Hochmeister S, Noor A, Lohberger B, et al. An X-linked myopathy with postural muscle atrophy and generalized hypertrophy, termed XMPMA, is caused by mutations in FHL1. Am J Hum Genet. 2008 Jan;82(1):88–99.

78. Schessl J, Taratuto AL, Sewry C, Battini R, Chin SS, Maiti B, et al. Clinical, histological and genetic characterization of reducing body myopathy caused by mutations in FHL1. Brain. 2009 Feb;132(Pt 2): 452–464.

79. Schessl J, Zou Y, McGrath MJ, Cowling BS, Maiti B, Chin SS, et al. Proteomic identification of FHL1 as the protein mutated in human reducing body myopathy. J Clin Invest. 2008 Mar;118(3):904–912.

80. Quinzii CM, Vu TH, Min KC, Tanji K, Barral S, Grewal RP, et al. X-linked dominant scapuloperoneal myopathy is due to a mutation in the gene encoding four-and-a-half-LIM protein 1. Am J Hum Genet. 2008 Jan;82(1):208–213.

81. Shalaby S, Hayashi YK, Goto K, Ogawa M, Nonaka I, Noguchi S, et al. Rigid spine syndrome caused by a novel mutation in four-and-a-half LIM domain 1 gene (FHL1). Neuromuscul Disord. 2008 Dec;18(12): 959–961.

82. Gueneau L, Bertrand AT, Jais JP, Salih MA, Stojkovic T, Wehnert M, et al. Mutations of the FHL1 gene cause Emery-Dreifuss muscular dystrophy. Am J Hum Genet. 2009 Sep;85(3):338–353.

83. Knoblauch H, Geier C, Adams S, Budde B, Rudolph A, Zacharias U, et al. Contractures and hypertrophic cardiomyopathy in a novel FHL1 mutation. Ann Neurol. 2010 Jan;67(1):136–140.

84. Selcen D, Bromberg MB, Chin SS, Engel AG. Reducing bodies and myofibrillar myopathy features in FHL1 muscular dystrophy. Neurology. 2011 Nov 29;77(22):1951–1959.

85. Vos MJ, Hageman J, Carra S, Kampinga HH. Structural and functional diversities between members of the human HSPB, HSPH, HSPA, and DNAJ chaperone families. Biochemistry. 2008 Jul 8;47(27):7001–7011.

86. Harms MB, Sommerville RB, Allred P, Bell S, Ma D, Cooper P, et al. Exome sequencing reveals DNAJB6 mutations in dominantly-inherited myopathy. Ann Neurol. 2012 Mar;71(3):407–416.

87. Sarparanta J, Jonson PH, Golzio C, Sandell S, Luque H, Screen M, et al. Mutations affecting the cytoplasmic functions of the co-chaperone DNAJB6 cause limb-girdle muscular dystrophy. Nature Genetics. 2012 Apr;44(4):450–455, S1–S2.

88. Bang ML, Centner T, Fornoff F, Geach AJ, Gotthardt M, McNabb M, et al. The complete gene sequence of titin, expression of an unusual approximately 700-kDa titin isoform, and its interaction with obscurin identify a novel Z-line to I-band linking system. Circ Res. 2001 Nov 23;89(11):1065–1072.

89. Centner T, Yano J, Kimura E, McElhinny AS, Pelin K, Witt CC, et al. Identification of muscle specific ring finger proteins as potential regulators of the titin kinase domain. J Mol Biol. 2001 Mar 2;306(4):717–726.

90. Labeit S, Kolmerer B. Titins: giant proteins in charge of muscle ultrastructure and elasticity. Science. 1995 Oct 13;270(5234):293–296.

91. Ohlsson M, Hedberg C, Bradvik B, Lindberg C, Tajsharghi H, Danielsson O, et al. Hereditary myopathy with early respiratory failure associated with a mutation in A-band titin. Brain. 2012 Jun;135(Pt 6): 1682–1694.

Chapter 6

Congenital Myopathies

Francesco Muntoni
Caroline Sewry
Heinz Jungbluth

DEFINITION OF A CONGENITAL MYOPATHY

The congenital myopathies are a clinically and genetically heterogeneous group of neuro-muscular conditions characterized by variable degrees of muscle weakness and the presence of characteristic structural abnormalities on muscle biopsy. Based on these abnormalities—central cores, multi-minicores, nemaline rods, and central nuclei—specific conditions such

as central core disease (CCD),[1] multi-minicore disease (MmD),[2] nemaline myopathy (NM),[3] and centronuclear myopathy (CNM)[4] were defined in the second half of last century (Figure 6–1). Congenital fiber-type dispropor-tion (CFTD) is another congenital myopathy[5] whose status as a clear histopathological entity has, however, been disputed. Additional, much rarer structural congenital myopathies have been reported, often affecting only few fami-lies or even isolated cases.[6] Different congenital

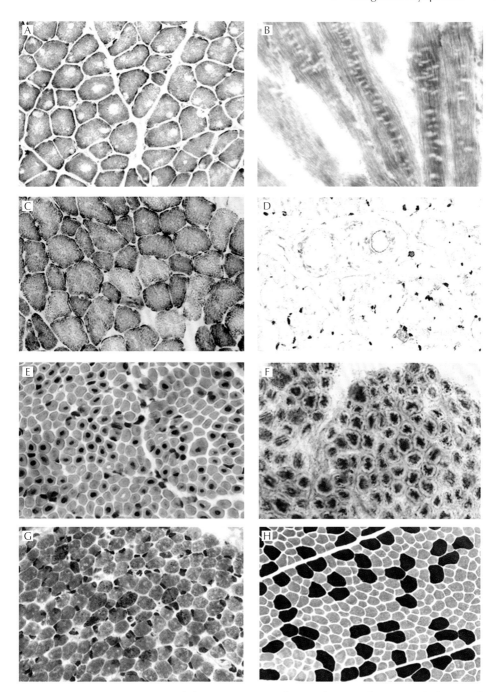

Figure 6–1. Main pathological features of the various congenital myopathies. Quadriceps muscle biopsies showing in (A) fiber type uniformity and prominent central and peripheral cores in a child with a C-terminal *RYR1* mutation (NADH-TR); (B) uniform fiber typing and multi-minicores in longitudinally sectioned fibers in a child with uncertain genetic background (NADH-TR); (C) unevenness of oxidative enzyme staining in both fiber types and small core-like areas in a child with *SEPN1* mutations; (D) a population of very small fibers positively immunolabeled for fetal myosin in a child with a variant of uncertain significance in the *RYR1* gene; (E) several central nuclei, a few central holes devoid of organelles, and central granular central basophilia (H & E); (F) dark staining centers with pale peripheral halos (NADH-TR) in a male neonate with a mutation in *MTM1*; (G) clusters of red-stained nemaline rods in many fibers in a neonate with an *ACTA1* mutation (Gomori trichrome); (H) type 1 fiber predominance and fiber type disproportion (with pale stained type 1 fibers signifantly smaller than the darkly stained type 2 fibers) in a child with an *ACTA1* mutation showing (ATPase pH 9.4).

Table 6–1 **Genes Implicated in the Major Structural Congenital Myopathies**

Myopathy	Gene Symbol	Protein	Locus	Inheritance
Central core disease (CCD)	*RYR1*	Skeletal muscle ryanodine receptor	19q13.1	**AD**, AR
Multi-minicore disease (MmD)	*SEPN1*	Selenoprotein N	1p35	AR
	RYR1	Skeletal muscle ryanodine receptor	19q13.1	AD, **AR**
Nemaline myopathy (NM)	*NEB*	Nebulin	2q21	AR
	ACTA1	Skeletal muscle α-actin	1q42	**AD**, AR[a]
	TPM3	Slow α-tropomyosin β-tropomyosin	1q22	**AD**, AR
	TPM2	Troponin T Cofilin-2	9p13.2	AR
	TNNT1	BTB/Kelch protein	19q13.4	AR
	CFL2		14q12	AR
	KBTBD13		15q22	AD
Centronuclear myopathy (CNM)	*MTM1*	Myotubularin	Xq28	XL
	DNM2	Dynamin 2	19p13.2	AD
	RYR1	Skeletal muscle ryanodine receptor	19q13.1	**AR**, (AD)[b]
	BIN1	Amphiphysin 2	2q14	AR
Congenital fiber type disproportion (CFTD)	*ACTA1*	Skeletal muscle α-actin	1q42	AD
	TPM3	Slow α-tropomyosin	1q22	AD
	SEPN1	Selenoprotein N	1p35	AR
	RYR1	Skeletal muscle ryanodine receptor	19q13.1	AR

Note. AD = autosomal dominant, AR = autosomal recessive, XL = X linked. The most common mode is indicated in bold where more than one mode of inheritance is implicated.
[a]Autosomal-dominant *ACTA1* mutations implicated in NM often occur *de novo*. [b]Autosomal-dominant inheritance of *RYR1*-related CNM has only been reported in one isolated case with a de novo dominant *RYR1* mutation, but no multigenerational families have been reported to date.

myopathies can rarely be distinguished on clinical grounds alone and a muscle biopsy is paramount, reflecting the essentially histopathological nature of the diagnosis. The definition of a congenital myopathy does not include other neuromuscular disorders with early onset such as congenital muscular dystrophies (CMDs) or mitochondrial and other metabolic myopathies. Many of the genes identified to date (Table 6–1) encode proteins involved in sarcomeric assembly or calcium homeostasis and excitation–contraction coupling. There is considerable overlap, with different mutations in the same gene giving rise to different histopathological features, and the same histopathological features caused by mutations in different genes, due to functional association of the respective gene products.

EPIDEMIOLOGY

The relative frequencies of individual congenital myopathies is unknown. Although some earlier studies have suggested NM as the most frequent form, more recent studies indicate CCD[7] and other congenital myopathies related to mutations in the skeletal muscle ryanodine receptor (*RYR1*) gene as the most common subgroup.[8] The true prevalence is likely to be underestimated, due to a substantial proportion of patients with mild clinical and/or nonspecific histopathological features, and the challenges of systematically studying all known genes, which include some of the largest genes known. In our own UK series, core myopathies, CCD and MmD, represented 56% of all cases.[9]

PRESENTATIONS OF A PATIENT WITH A CONGENITAL MYOPATHY

Presentation is usually at birth or in early infancy with hypotonia, variable weakness, and motor developmental delay. Associated respiratory and bulbar involvement is common, particularly in forms associated with *MTM1*, *NEB*, and *ACTA1* mutations, and may necessitate ventilatory support and nasogastric feeds. Severe joint contractures (arthrogryposis) within the fetal akinesia spectrum may be present in the most profoundly affected cases.[10] Weakness may be slight or unrecognized so that patients present later in childhood or, rarely, adulthood, with a history of motor developmental delay signs and symptoms of proximal weakness.

In most cases, distribution of weakness is predominantly axial and proximal, with some notable exceptions such as NM due to mutations in the *NEB* gene where distal involvement affecting foot dorsiflexion is common.[11] Facial involvement is highly variable. Extraocular muscle involvement is more common in the CNMs and recessive *RYR1*-related core myopathies. Corresponding to prominent axial weakness, there is often an associated scoliosis with or without spinal rigidity. Joint hypermobility is common[12] and contractures, particularly of the Achilles tendon, may evolve over time. With rare exceptions, an associated neuropathy is not a feature and CNS involvement is typically absent; however, secondary hypoxic insults may confound the clinical picture. The most profoundly affected neonates may show neurophysiological features mimicking an anterior horn cell disorder, leading to diagnostic confusion. Neurophysiological evidence of an associated neuromuscular transmission defect has been documented in core myopathies and CNM.[13] Often disproportionate respiratory impairment is common, particularly in patients with *SEPN1* or *NEB* mutations, emphasizing the need for regular monitoring of respiratory function and timely institution of ventilatory support. Cardiac involvement, namely right ventricular hypertrophy, is usually secondary to respiratory impairment. A primary cardiomyopathy is not a feature with the more common genetic backgrounds but may be prominent in much rarer genetic conditions that enter the differential diagnosis.

Apart from those who die from respiratory complications in infancy, in most patients the course is only slowly progressive, with the large majority achieving and maintaining independent ambulation. However, some deterioration may occur during intercurrent growth spurts. The degree of respiratory involvement is the most important prognostic factor.

Although different genetic forms can rarely be distinguished on clinical grounds alone, some clinical features are more common with certain genetic backgrounds than others (Table 6–2).

Table 6–2 Key Clinical and Histopathological Features Associated With Common Genetic Defects Implicated in the Congenital Myopathies

Gene	RYR1 AD	RYR1 AR	SEPN1	MTM1	DNM2	NEB	ACTA1
Frequency	+++	+++	++	++	+	++	++
Onset							
Infancy	++	+++	+	+++	+	+++	++
Childhood	+++	++	+++	+	+	+	++
Adulthood	++	+	−	−	+++	−	−
Clinical features							
External ophthalmoplegia	+	+++	−	+++	+++		−
Bulbar involvement	+	+++	++	+++	++	++	++
Respiratory Involvement	+	++	+++	+++	+	++	++
Cardiac Involvement	-	+	+[a]	−	−	−	+
Myalgia	+++	+	−	−	++	−	−
Malignant hyperthermia	+++	(++)[b]	−	−	−	−	−
Histopathology							
Cores	+++	+++	+++	−	+	+	+
FTD	+	+++	+	−	−	−	+
Connective issue/Fat	++	++	++	−	+	−	−
Central nuclei	++	++	−	+++	+++	−	−
Nemaline rods	++++	+++	−++	−+	−+++	++++++	++++
Muscle MRI (specify)							

Note. MTM1 = myotubularin gene, *DNM2* = dynamin gene, *NEB* = nebulin gene, *ACTA1* = skeletal muscle α-actin gene. − = not reported, + = infrequent, ++ = common, +++ = very common.
[a]Right ventricular impairment secondary to respiratory involvement. [b]Exact risk of MHS associated with recessive *RYR1* mutations currently unknown (modified from (ungbluth, Sewry, et al. (2011).[140]

DIAGNOSIS AND DIFFERENTIAL DIAGNOSIS

Floppiness in an infant is a common presentation of highly diverse disorders (summarized in Table 6–3), not all of them neuromuscular in origin. The clinician confronted with a floppy infant has to identify if the underlying cause is a systemic illness or a primary neurological, metabolic, or neuromuscular disorder; in the case of the latter, he or she has to decide which of the neuromuscular disorders with congenital onset is the most likely. Among the general causes, sepsis commonly causes floppiness in infants and may lead to the erroneous suspicion of a neuromuscular disorder, particularly if there is associated transient hyperCK-emia, not uncommon in the neonatal period. A number of chromosomal abnormalities, in particular Down syndrome and Prader-Willi syndrome, may give rise to profound floppiness, but affected infants, like those with other nonneuromuscular causes, are not typically weak. Amongst the primary neurological causes, severe hypoxia may result in initial hypotonia; epileptic and metabolic encephalopathies are other causes to be considered. Within the group of primary neuromuscular conditions, congenital myotonic dystrophy and SMA are amongst the most common and have

to be excluded in the first instance. There is substantial overlap with the genetic congenital myasthenic syndromes (CMS; as well as auto-immune transient neonatal MG), in particular in cases with prominent ptosis and extraocular/bulbar involvement. Although most CMDs are distinguished by variable degrees of CK elevation and dystrophic features on muscle biopsy, there is clearly a clinico-pathological continuum with the congenital myopathy spectrum, for example those due to mutations in the *COL6A1, 2* and *3*, the *SEPN1*, and the *RYR1* genes.

The key investigations in the assessment of the floppy infant (Table 6–3) have to be selected based on the history and specific clinical findings in individual patients. CK levels are usually normal, although mild to moderate elevations have been reported in some patients with *RYR1*-related myopathies. In case maternal MG is suspected, acetylcholine receptor antibody levels ought to be checked, bearing in mind that in a few instances infants with transient neonatal MG have been born to asymptomatic mothers. Other laboratory investigations mainly include those to exclude sepsis or an underlying metabolic disorder. Karyotype analysis (or increasingly, CGH array testing) is indicated to exclude underlying chromosomal abnormalities. Obtaining DNA

Table 6–3 Differential Diagnosis and Investigation of the Floppy Infant

	Examples	Key Investigations
Systemic illness	Sepsis	FBC, CRP, Blood cultures
Chromosomal abnormalities	Down syndrome Prader-Willi syndrome	Karyotype, CGH array
Neurological disorders	Hypoxic-ischemic encephalopathy (HIE) Epileptic encephalopathy	Brain MR imaging, EEG
Metabolic disorders	Urea cycle defect Non-ketotic hyperglycinemia Peroxisomal disorders Mitochondrial disorders Pompe disease Dyskinetic disorders	LFT, plasma lactate, ammonia, amino acids, bile acids, phytanic acid, pipecolic acid, VLCFA, acylcarnitines; urine amino and organic acids; CSF analysis
Neuromuscular disorders	Congenital myotonic dystrophy Spinal muscular atrophy (SMA) Congenital hypomyelinating neuropathy Congenital myasthenic syndromes Transient neonatal myasthenia gravis Congenital muscular dystrophies	CK, AChR antibodies, specific genetic testing; neurophysiology; muscle biopsy; muscle imaging

Note. The differential diagnosis of the floppy infant includes a wide range of primary general, neurological, metabolic, and neuromuscular conditions. Investigations have to be tailored based on the history and clinical findings in individual patients. LFT = liver function tests, VLCFA = very long chain fatty acids samples is paramount for specific genetic testing. A detailed neurophysiological assessment (including stimulated single-fiber EMG) may be required to exclude a CMS, or a severe congenital hypomyelinating neuropathy. A muscle biopsy is essential for the diagnosis and should include analysis of muscle histology, histochemistry, and in selected cases, ultrastructure by EM. Immunohistochemical studies are useful but not as informative as in the assessment of the muscular dystrophies. Muscle ultrasound and muscle magnetic resonance (MR) imaging may show selective involvement and have become an important diagnostic tool.[14] However, there are few data on muscle MR imaging in neonates and infants and interpretation of muscle ultrasound is largely user dependent.

SPECIFIC TYPES OF CONGENITAL MYOPATHIES

Congenital Myopathies With Cores

The core myopathies, CCD and MmD, are a heterogeneous group of conditions with the common defining histopathological feature of focally reduced oxidative activity of variable appearance ("central cores, multi-minicores").[15] Core myopathies are the most frequent form of congenital myopathy. Cores are, however, nonspecific and can occur in conditions other than congenital myopathies..

Following the original description by Magee and Shy in 1956,[1] numerous families with dominantly inherited CCD,[16] mostly associated with mutations in the *RYR1* gene, have been reported associated with fairly consistent *clinical features*. Onset is typically in infancy with proximal weakness pronounced in the hip girdle, but much milder as well as much more severe presentations have been documented. Clinical variability may be marked, even within the same family. Exertional myalgia is common and may be a presenting feature. Facial involvement is typically mild and extraocular muscles are usually spared, in contrast to recessively inherited *RYR1*-related core myopathies, often characterized by multi-minicores on muscle biopsy. Bulbar and respiratory involvement are often absent but have been observed in the most severe neonatal cases and occasionally in adults. An associated cardiomyopathy has not been reported in *RYR1*-related conditions. Orthopedic complications, in particular congenital dislocation of the hips, are common, as is marked distal ligamentous laxity. Most patients achieve independent ambulation, except the most severe neonatal cases, often due to *de novo* dominant *RYR1* mutations, and those with complex orthopedic problems. Many patients have a slowly progressive course, and intermittent deterioration, for example during or after pregnancy, has been reported. Serum CK levels are usually normal, but may rarely be elevated. Clinical features of MmD,[17] typically inherited in an autosomal-recessive fashion, are more variable depending on the genetic background. The most distinct, "classic" phenotype of MmD is due to recessive *SEPN1* mutations[18] and is characterized by early spinal rigidity, scoliosis, and respiratory impairment. Onset is often early in life and feeding difficulties with failure to thrive may be a presenting feature. Myopathic facial features are common, but extraocular muscle involvement is not typical. Axial muscle weakness is prominent and failure to acquire head control may be an early sign. Proximal muscle groups, particularly those of the shoulder girdle, are more affected than distal muscles. Muscle wasting mainly affects axial groups, the shoulder girdle and the inner thigh (so-called "bracket-like appearance"). The muscle MRIs of two patients with confirmed SEPN1 related myopathy are shown in Figure 6–2; the selective pattern of muscle involvement can help one suspect this condition. A progressive scoliosis and respiratory impairment typically characterize the second decade but may manifest earlier. In contrast, recessively inherited *RYR1*-related core myopathies with multi-minicores show a similar distribution of weakness and wasting but additional extraocular muscle involvement, pronounced on abduction and upward gaze.[19] Respiratory impairment is usually milder than in the classic form, although bulbar involvement may be pronounced. Other patients with recessively inherited *RYR1*-related core myopathy may show a distribution of weakness and wasting similar to the dominantly inherited variant, whereas others rarely have additional marked distal involvement.[20] A few severely affected neonates have been reported with generalized arthrogryposis, dysmorphic features, and mild

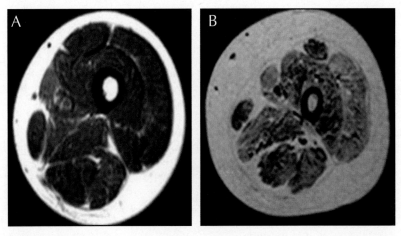

Figure 6–2. Axial T1-weighted images at thigh level in two patients with SEPN1 myopathy. Patient A had a selective sartorius muscle involvement with relative sparing of the other muscles, whereas Patient B had a more diffuse muscle involvement, but the sartorius was still relatively more severely involved when compared to the remaining muscles.

to moderate reduction of respiratory function.[10] Periodic paralysis has been reported in one isolated patient with a recessively inherited core myopathy and ophthalmoplegia.[21]

Respiratory impairment is common in recessively inherited core myopathies with congenital onset but mild or absent in forms with onset after infancy. Cardiac impairment may occur due to marked respiratory involvement but is not a primary feature of *SEPN1*- or *RYR1*-related forms of MmD. MHS has not been reported in *SEPN1*-related myopathies but is a potential risk in *RYR1*-related core myopathies, although the association is less certain for recessive than for dominant *RYR1* mutations. King-Denborough syndrome, a dysmorphic syndrome with marked musculoskeletal involvement,[22] as well as a distinct late-onset axial myopathy,[23] appear to be specific myopathic manifestations of certain MHS-related *RYR1* mutations. Precautions during general anesthesia such as avoidance of MH-triggering anesthetics or muscle relaxants should therefore be taken in patients with core myopathies, particularly in genetically unresolved cases or those with definite *RYR1* involvement.

RYR1–related core myopathies show a distinctive pattern of selective involvement on muscle MR imaging.[24] Muscle MR imaging is also a powerful tool to distinguish *SEPN1*-related MmD from other causes of rigid spine syndrome.[25]

Histopathological features in the core myopathies[26] are highly variable, ranging from extensive areas with reduced oxidative activity running along an appreciable proportion of the longitudinal axis of the muscle fiber (central cores) to multiple focal areas with reduced oxidative activity affecting only a few sarcomeres (multi-minicores). In *RYR1*–related, dominantly inherited CCD the cores are large and may be central or peripheral, whereas in *SEPN1*-related, recessively inherited MmD, cores are smaller, less well-defined, and on transverse sections they may only appear as unevenness of stain; there is, however, a continuum, particularly in cases due to recessive *RYR1* mutations. Cores are often more easily appreciated in longitudinal sections, where *SEPN1*-related MmD is typically associated with numerous small lesions scattered throughout the muscle fiber (minicores), whereas multiple larger lesions (multicores), often extending throughout the entire fiber diameter, are more commonly seen in forms of *RYR1*–related, recessively inherited MmD. In the latter group, there may be a continuum with the histopathologic appearance of *RYR1*–related, dominantly inherited CCD, evolving over time.[20] The cores in CCD show absence of both oxidative and phosphorylase enzymatic activity. They may be "structured" or, less commonly, "unstructured," with variable degrees of ATPase activity and sarcomeric disorganization. Like target fibers, some cores may have enhanced oxidative enzyme activity at their periphery. Central cores are usually found in type 1 fibers whereas minicores may affect both type 1 and type 2 fibers. In *RYR1*–related core myopathies there is often marked predominance or uniformity of type 1 fibers, which may precede the appearance of the cores. In *SEPN1*-related core myopathies, type 1 predominance may occur but is less pronounced. Both *RYR1*- and *SEPN1*-related myopathies can be associated with a disproportion in the size of type 1 versus type 2 fibers, with or without other pathologic features.[27] Increases in internal nucleation are also common in all *RYR1*-related core myopathies and in some cases they are central, resembling CNM.[28,29] Additionally nemaline rods staining red with the Gomori trichrome technique may be prominent in some *RYR1*-related myopathies (core-rod myopathy),[30] or may occur in occasional fibers. Substantial increases in fat and connective tissue have been described in both *SEPN1*- and *RYR1*-related core myopathies, although more overtly dystrophic features such as necrotic and regenerating fibers are usually absent. Isolated patients with *RYR1*-related core myopathies and respiratory chain enzyme abnormalities have been reported.[31]

On EM, both central and multi-minicores show reduction or absence of mitochondria. Cores may be structured or unstructured, with variable degrees of myofibrillar disorganization and accumulation of abnormal material within the usually sharply demarcated core area, although the area devoid of mitochondria may be more extensive than the area of disorganized myofibrils. The same biopsy may show different stages of core formation.

Abnormal expression of various sarcomeric and intermediate filament proteins, particularly desmin, has been demonstrated within or around the core area but is not specific. Abnormalities of proteins involved in calcium handling and homeostasis have been suggested to differentiate between distinct specific genetic backgrounds,[32] but variability of expression even within the same biopsy has to be considered. Immunoblotting of RyR1 can show a decreased amount.[33]

Understanding of the *genetics and pathogenesis* of the core myopathies has rapidly advanced in recent years: The majority of cases have been associated with mutations in *RYR1* and the *SEPN1* gene, but there is likely to be further heterogeneity.[15]

The largest proportion of cases with clinico-pathological features of CCD is due to dominant missense mutations in the skeletal muscle ryanodine receptor *(RYR1)* gene on chromosome 19q13.1.[34] MmD is genetically more heterogeneous, corresponding to more pronounced clinico-pathological variability, and has been associated with recessive mutations in the selenoprotein N *(SEPN1)* on chromosome 1p36[18] and recessive *RYR1* gene mutations,[19,35] respectively. There is also substantial overlap between *RYR1*-related core myopathies, particularly those with dominant inheritance, and the MHS trait.

RYR1 is arranged in 106 exons and encodes RyR1, a large protein of 5,037 amino acids that assembles as an oligotetramer.[36] The RyR1 receptor plays a crucial role in excitation–contraction (E–C) coupling by releasing Ca^{2+} from the sarcoplasmic reticulum, prompted by direct interaction with the voltage-sensing dihydropyridine receptor, its principal ligand. The C-terminal part of the RyR1 protein constitutes the actual Ca^{2+} channel, whereas the large hydrophobic N-terminal portion faces the myoplasm and forms the "foot structures" visible on electron microscopy. RyR1 receptors are expressed in a wide range of tissues other than skeletal muscle, including the immune system and neurons.

More than 200 *RYR1* mutations have been reported to date associated mainly with MHS, CCD,[37] and MmD[19,35] but also subgroups of CNM[29] and CFTD.[27] The majority of *RYR1* mutations associated with CCD and MHS identified to date are dominant missense mutations with only a few small deletions reported. In contrast, recessive inheritance of *RYR1* mutations is the most common mode of inheritance in MmD or other less common pathological phenotype.[19,27,29,33,38] Dominant *RYR1* mutations affecting the cytoplasmic N-terminal (MHS/CCD region 1, amino acids 35–614) and central (MHS/CCD region 2, amino acids 2163–2458) domains of the protein predominantly give rise to the MHS phenotype,[39] whereas the CCD phenotype is closely associated with dominant *RYR1* C-terminal (MHS/CCD region 3, amino acids 4550–4940) mutations.[33] Recessively inherited mutations are more widespread throughout the *RYR1* gene[29,33,34,38] and are often associated with severe reduction of the functional RyR1 protein.[33] It is important to realize that current diagnostic techniques involving genomic sequencing are not able to identify large genomic rearrangements such as deletions and duplications, which have been recently demonstrated.[40] This is relevant when assessing severe cases in whom an apparently single heterozygous mutation is also present in one of the asymptomatic parents.

The molecular mechanisms underlying *RYR1*-related disorders have been more extensively investigated for CCD and MHS compared to the more recently described recessively inherited *RYR1*-related myopathies.[36] MHS is generally thought to be associated with a "hyperactive" RyR1 channel, whereas two distinct models for RyR1 receptor malfunction in CCD have been proposed: depletion of sarcoplasmic reticulum calcium stores with resulting increase in cytosolic calcium levels ("leaky channel" hypothesis),[41] and disturbance of E–C coupling (E–C uncoupling hypothesis).[42] Based on a limited number of studies available to date, pathogenetic mechanisms underlying recessive *RYR1*-related myopathies appear to be more variable with loss of calcium conductance, probably mediated by marked RyR1 protein reduction, a relatively common observation.[15]

A number of animal models carrying knocked-in *RYR1* mutations related to MHS and CCD have emerged over recent years, providing valuable insights into the pathophysiology and the evolution of associated histopathological changes.[43] There is currently no murine model for recessive *RYR1*-related myopathies; however, the sporadic zebrafish *relatively relaxed* mutant[44] mimics one of the probable molecular mechanism underlying recessive core myopathies closely.

In addition to the *RYR1*-related form, another subgroup of MmD has been associated with recessive mutations in the selenoprotein N (*SEPN1*) gene on chromosome 1p36,[18] initially associated with CMD with rigidity of the spine (RSMD1). *SEPN1* mutations are predominantly truncating, with few reported missense mutations typically affecting functionally important domains of the protein such as the SECIS[45] or the selenocysteine redefinition element (SRE).[46] A multisystem disorder with associated myopathy resembling RSMD1 has been reported associated with mutations in the selenocysteine insertion sequence-binding protein 2 (SECISBP2).[47] Homozygous mutations are unexpectedly common due to the presence of founder mutations in different European populations. Selenoprotein N, a glycoprotein localized in the endoplasmic reticulum, belongs to a family of proteins mediating the effect of selenium and is involved in antioxidant defense systems and metabolic pathways. Selenoprotein N has a putative role in embryogenesis[48] and is more specifically involved in myogenesis, as suggested by abundant expression in fetal muscle precursor cells and the observation of a specific disturbance of satellite cell function in the sepn1 -/- knock-out mouse.[49] A role in calcium homeostasis is suggested by a structural motif similar to those found in calcium-binding proteins and the close functional and spatial relationship between selenoprotein N and RyR1 reported in normal zebrafish and the sepn1 -/- morphant.[50,51] The latter observation in conjunction with a proposed role of Selenoprotein N in redox-regulated calcium homeostasis may explain the clinico-pathological similarities between *RYR1*- and *SEPN1*-related core myopathies.

The *differential diagnosis* of the core myopathies[15] is wide: Core-formation is a nonspecific finding that may be observed in other contexts such as tenotomy, denervation ("target-fibers"), metabolic conditions, or even in healthy individuals following eccentric exercise. Focal areas of myofibrillar disruption are also common finding in other neuromuscular disorders, and may be extensive in myofibrillar myopathies ("wiped-out areas"). The presence of cores on muscle biopsy without associated weakness, as has been reported in some MHS individuals, is not sufficient to constitute a diagnosis of a core myopathy.

Once *RYR1* or *SEPN1* mutations have been excluded, other genetic defects associated with cores on muscle biopsy may be suggested by the presence of additional clinical or pathological features unusual in the context of *SEPN1*- or *RYR1*-related forms. Primary cardiomyopathies, for example, are not typically seen in the latter, but are a feature in those due to missense mutations in the ß-myosin heavy-chain gene, *MYH7*,[52] or other genetic backgrounds. Although many of the originally reported patients with this phenotype did not have any skeletal muscle weakness, a distinct associated myopathy phenotype has been recently reported that may mimic core myopathies and may not always have cardiac involvement.[53] A cardiomyopathy associated with cores on muscle biopsy has also been documented in one mildly affected family with dominant *ACTA1* mutations[54] and severely affected siblings with homozygous truncating titin mutations.[55] Also, mutations in the lamin A/C (*LMNA*) gene, a common cause of various muscular dystrophy phenotypes with prominent cardiac involvement, may also be associated with corelike structures on muscle biopsy. In cases without cardiac involvement, dominant and recessive mutations in *COL6A1*, 2 and 3, responsible for Bethlem myopathy and Ullrich CMD, respectively, are also often associated with corelike lesions.[26] Lastly, it is also of note that the congenital myasthenic syndromes (CMS) may mimic some of the histopathological appearance of core and other congenital myopathies.[56]

Congenital Myopathies With Central Nuclei

The congenital myopathies with central nuclei,[57] X-linked myotubular myopathy (XLMTM) and centronuclear myopathy (CNM), have been associated with all forms of Mendelian inheritance and are clinically heterogeneous, with some correlation between clinical severity and the mode of inheritance.

In addition to *clinical features* shared with other congenital myopathies, extraocular muscle involvement is the most consistent finding in all different genetic forms of MTM/CNM. XLMTM due to myotubularin (*MTM1*) mutations is the most severe form and often associated with reduced fetal movements and polyhydramnios. A history of miscarriages and male neonatal deaths in the maternal line is commonly obtained. Affected males may be macrosomic and show profound hypotonia and weakness, with associated bulbar and respiratory involvement almost always necessitating ventilation. Knee and hip contractures are common. With few exceptions, the condition is usually fatal over weeks or months unless constant respiratory support is provided.[58] Some long-term survivors show associated medical problems such as pyloric stenosis, gallstones, and hepatic peliosis. Neuromuscular junction abnormalities and/or an associated neuromuscular transmission defect have been reported in XLMTM and other forms of CNM and are due to involvement and simplification of the synaptic cleft.[59,60] Some XLMTM carriers may develop mild weakness, sometimes late in life,[61]

but more severe manifestations in females are usually due to skewed X-inactivation[62] or abnormalities of the X chromosome.[63]

Dominantly inherited CNM associated with *DNM2* mutations is frequently associated with a relatively mild condition, with onset from birth to the fifth decade.[64,65] Provided respiratory complications are managed proactively, even the most severe cases with neonatal onset may improve over time.[64,66,67] Facial weakness, ptosis, and ophthalmoplegia are common. Muscle weakness is mainly proximal, with additional truncal and distal involvement in many patients.[68,69] Marked muscle hypertrophy, particularly affecting the calves, has been occasionally reported.[70] Dominant intermediate Charcot-Marie-Tooth disease (CMTDIB) is an allelic condition[71] and subtle signs of peripheral or central nervous system involvement may also rarely be observed in *DNM2*-related CNM.[65,72,73] As in CMTDIB patients, nonmuscular features such as neutropenia[70] or cataracts[67] have been rarely reported in *DNM2*-related CNM. Muscle MR imaging shows a pattern of selective muscle involvement distinct from other genetically defined congenital myopathies.[74]

Recessively inherited CNM due to *RYR1* mutations[29] is typically of early-onset and moderate severity with improvement over time. Ptosis is common and extraocular muscle involvement is almost invariable. Bulbar involvement requiring nasogastric tube feeds and respiratory impairment needing ventilatory support are often transient, but a permanent ventilatory requirement has been reported in the most severe cases.

BIN1-related CNM has only been reported in few families,[75,76,77,78] mainly associated with early-onset and a severe phenotype. Marked intrafamilial variability and associated mental retardation has been reported in one consanguineous family.[76]

Different forms of MTM/CNM share similar *histopathological features*.[57] In addition to small fibers showing central nuclei, central areas with enhanced oxidative enzyme activity and a pale peripheral halo that has few mitochondria but myofibrils are present. The number of central nuclei may be low at birth, but increases with age and is variable between muscles. Features in common with other congenital myopathies are type 1 fiber predominance and small type 1 fibers. Central nuclei can be present in both fiber types and immuno-histochemistry shows they are present in fibers without developmental myosin isoforms, indicating that the fibers mature, at least in terms of myosin expression. Strictly centralized nuclei are more common than multiple internalized nuclei in the *MTM1*- and *DNM2*-related forms;[72] the opposite applies to *RYR1*-related cases.[29] *DNM2*- and *BIN1*-related forms can show peripheral as well as central nuclei, but this may be age-related. A radial distribution of sarcoplasmic strands with staining for NADH and with PAS staining is seen in some (particularly older) *DNM2*-related cases[79]; the latter may also exhibit features resembling a dystrophic pathology with excess endomysial connective tissue.[69] Cores in addition to the fibers with central nuclei may evolve over time in *RYR1*-related CNM,[80] but have also been reported in *DNM2*-related cases[68] and mildly affected patients harboring *MTM1* mutations.[70,81] "Necklace" fibers may be an additional feature in *MTM1* cases, in particular female carriers.[70,81] *MTM1*-, *DNM2*-, and *BIN1*–related cases show ultrastructural triad abnormalities, suggesting a pathogenic link.[82] Myotonic dystrophy is a histopathological phenocopy and should be considered early in the diagnostic process.[83]

Genetics and pathogenesis of CNM/MTM are complex.[57] Mutations in the myotubularin (*MTM1*) gene on chromosome Xq28 were the first to be identified,[84] and no other gene has to date been implicated in XLMTM. Most mothers of affected boys are carriers; mosaicism has been repeatedly documented. Although there are no clear mutational hotspots, seven *MTM1* mutations account for about 25% of cases and exons 12, 8, and 14 are most commonly involved. The majority are truncating mutations consistently associated with the more severe phenotype, whereas approximately 30% are missense mutations affecting conserved residues.[85,86,87,88,89] Some deep intronic mutations or genomic rearrangements involving the *MTM1* locus may not be detectable on routine sequencing.[90,91] A combination of XLMTM and intersexual genitalia has been reported in boys with a deletion extending beyond the *MTM1* locus.[92]

The dynamin 2 protein encoded by *DNM2* has 5 functional domains, two of them preferentially mutated in neuromuscular disorders: Mutations affecting the dynamin 2 middle domain are usually associated with milder presentations of dominantly inherited CNM,[79] whereas those concerning the pleckstrin homology domain give rise to more severe forms with earlier onset.[64,67,69] *RYR1*-related CNM is often due to compound heterozygosity for *RYR1* missense mutations and mutations inducing loss of open reading frame and a reduced amount of functional RyR1 protein.[28,29] *RYR1*-related CNM is common in South Africa due to the presence of founder mutations.[29] There is likely to be further heterogeneity: Tosch and colleagues reported two CNM patients with missense variations in the novel phosphoinositide phosphatase (hJUMPY), in one patient associated with a *de novo DNM2* mutation. The inheritance in these families is uncertain but could be either recessive with an undetected second allele, or digenic.[90] The possiblity that hJUMPY mutations have a modifying role has been proposed.

Most of the genes implicated in various forms of CNM to date encode proteins involved in membrane trafficking[93] and endocytosis. A number of animal models are now available.[94] *Myotubularin* belongs to the large family of dual-specificity phosphatases that play a role in the epigenetic regulation of signaling pathways involved in growth and differentiation,[95] particularly in membrane trafficking. The deleterious effect of specific *MTM1* mutations may be due to destabilization of its three-dimensional structure, loss of enzymatic activity, or disturbed protein–protein interactions,[96] with important secondary effects on T-tubule assembly,[97] endosomes,[98] desmin intermediate filament architecture, and mitochondrial dynamics.[99,100] Findings in a myotubularin knock-out mouse model[101] suggest that myotubularin is necessary for the maintenance of muscle fibers but not for myogenesis. In the animal model, the myotubularin-deficient phenotype may be correctable by delivery of the functional protein through viral vectors[102] or other therapeutic interventions.[103] Mutations in the dynamin 2 (*DNM2*) gene disturb specific enzymatic functions, dimerization of the mutant protein, and endocytosis pathways.[104] A knock-in mouse model of the common *DNM2* R465W mutation[105] exhibits impaired skeletal muscle structure and function, disturbed reticular assembly, and secondary mitochondrial alterations corresponding to findings in humans. Mutations in the *BIN1* gene encoding amphiphysin 2 have been demonstrated to abolish interactions with dynamin 2 and to disrupt the membrane tubulation properties of the mutant protein.[75]

Congenital Myopathies With Nemaline Rods

Congenital myopathies with nemaline rods, or NM, has been associated with mutations in seven genes to date, most commonly in nebulin (*NEB*)[106] and in slow skeletal muscle actin (*ACTA1*),[107] and less frequently in alpha-tropomyosin (*TPM3*),[108] beta-tropomyosin (*TPM2*),[109] slow troponin T (*TNNT1*),[110] cofilin-2 (*CFL2*),[111] and Kelch-repeat and BTB (POZ) domain containing 13 (*KBTBD 13*).[112] Most genes identified in NM to date encode thin filament proteins, but the function of the protein encoded by *KBTBD 13* is currently still unknown.

Clinical features of NM are variable depending on the genetic background[113] and have been studied in large series.[114] The most common form of NM due to recessive *NEB* mutations is characterized by onset in infancy with marked hypotonia, axial and proximal weakness, and pronounced bulbar involvement, the latter often the most prominent feature at presentation. Distal involvement in the lower limb becomes prominent later in life and may be presenting feature in some patients.[11] Respiratory involvement is almost universal in congenital NM and may present throughout life, with frequent respiratory infections, overt respiratory failure, or both. There is often marked discrepancy between respiratory and limb muscle involvement and some patients may develop insidious respiratory insufficiency while still ambulant, emphasizing the importance of regular monitoring of respiratory function and timely institution of ventilatory support. An associated cardiomyopathy is not a feature of *NEB*-related NM but has been reported rarely in patients with *ACTA1* mutations.[54] More specific clinical features include the tremor and progressive contractures in *TNNT1*-related NM prevalent in the Old Order Amish,[110] and the distinct slowness of movement seen in association with *KBTBD13* mutations.[112] In contrast to the typical congenital form, the few patients with *CFL2*-related NM

reported to date did not have facial weakness or foot drop.[111] There have been no reports of MHS associated with mutations in any of the seven known NM genes.

Different clinical categories of NM have been distinguished, (a) a severe congenital form, with severe contractures with or without bone fractures, and absence of spontaneous (respiratory) movements; (b) an intermediate congenital form, with some (respiratory) muscle movements but failure to achieve ambulation or to establish respiratory independence; (c) the typical congenital form as just outlined; (d) mild nemaline myopathy with childhood onset; (e) adult-onset nemaline myopathy; and (f) other forms of nemaline myopathy with unusual associated features. Sporadic late-onset NM[115] is mainly of autoimmune origin and not genetically determined.

The defining *histopathological feature* of NM is the presence of numerous nemaline rod bodies, most prominent on the Gomori trichrome sections or on semi-thin sections stained with Toluodine Blue and confirmed on EM.[26]

Nemaline rods derive from the Z-disk and contain mainly α-actinin, but also other proteins including myotilin, telethonin, actin, and tropomyosin; desmin is present at their periphery. Despite some differences that may direct genetic testing—for example, absence of specific nebulin epitopes in *NEB*-related myopathy,[116] or presence of intranuclear rods and/or accumulation of actin filaments in *ACTA1*-related NM[106]—the different genetic forms of NM cannot be distinguished on histopathological grounds alone. Nemaline rods are not specific for NM and have been reported as a secondary feature in other neuromuscular conditions, as a physiological finding in extraocular muscle, at myotendinous junctions, and as part of the normal aging process. Nemaline rods may also occur in HIV infection, occasionally associated with a clinical myopathy.[117] As in other congenital myopathies, fiber typing may be indistinct or type 1 fibers may be predominant and smaller in diameter. Rare cases with homozygous *ACTA1* null mutations show consistent presence of cardiac actin in skeletal muscle, in contrast to normal neonates in whom most of the cardiac actin isoform is replaced by the skeletal muscle isoform before birth.[118]

Recent advances in the *genetics* of NM have established common pattern of inheritance[113]:

In NM, autosomal-recessive inheritance is more common than autosomal-dominant inheritance, with many sporadic cases on record. Autosomal-recessive NM is most commonly due to mutations in the *NEB* gene,[106,119,120] whereas mutations in *ACTA1*,[107] *TPM2*, *TPM3*, *TNNT1*, and *CFL2* are much less frequently associated with recessive inheritance. In contrast to dominant *ACTA1* mutations, recessive *ACTA1* mutations are genetic or functional null mutations causing a severe myopathy.[121] A deletion in *NEB* exon 55 is a common founder mutation in the Ashkenazi Jewish[122] but possibly also other populations. Founder effects have also been demonstrated for *TNNT1* in the Amish[110] and *TPM3* in the Turkish population.[123] Autosomal-dominant nemaline myopathy is often due to *ACTA1* mutations[107] but may also be caused by mutations in *TPM2* or *TPM3*. In *ACTA1*-related but also in other dominantly inherited forms of NM, phenotypical variability may be significant, even within the same family. Sporadic cases of NM are most commonly caused by *de novo* dominant *ACTA1*,[124] and, probably less frequently, recessive *NEB* mutations.[125] The substantial difficulties of *NEB* screening related to the large size of this gene are likely to be overcome once novel approaches to genetic analysis become more widely available in a diagnostic setting.

With regard to genotype–phenotype correlations,[113,121,126] the typical form of congenital NM is most commonly caused by *NEB* mutations[106] and less frequently by mutations in the *ACTA1* and *TPM2* genes, whereas the most severe early-onset cases can often be attributed to *ACTA1* mutations[124] but less frequently to *NEB* mutations.[127] Both *ACTA1*- and *NEB*-related NM share generalized symmetrical weakness pronounced in the neck flexors, whereas ankle dorsiflexor weakness and knee flexor weakness is more marked in the *NEB*-related form. The intermediate form of NM may be caused by mutations in *TPM3*, *ACTA1*, or *NEB*, whereas the mild form has been associated with mutations in *ACTA1*, *NEB*, *TPM2*, *TPM3*, or *KBTBD13*. Of note, somatic and gonadal mosaicism has been observed in *ACTA1*-related NM.[128] Patients with NM have different patterns of selective involvement on muscle MRI, depending on the specific genetic background.[129]

The *pathogenetic mechanisms* underlying various forms of NM have been extensively studied.[112] Dominant mutations in the *ACTA1* gene exert a dominant negative effect on muscle function, possibly mediated by lower calcium sensitivity.[129] Recessively inherited *ACTA1* mutations do not express any functional protein, and severity of the phenotype is possibly dependent on compensatory expression of the cardiac isoform, developmentally expressed also in skeletal muscle. Therapeutic approaches in animal models of *ACTA1*-related NM are thus aimed at increasing the amount of the normal protein or the cardiac isoform.[130]

All known *NEB* mutations have been recessive, but despite their truncating nature there is usually residual protein expression,[116] probably due to differential isoform expression. Based on the limited number of studies published to date, *NEB* mutations are likely to affect the specifc role of nebulin in thin filament regulation and force generation.[131,132] A recently created *NEB* knock-out mouse[133] may advance understanding of the role of nebulin in the sarcomere, but it is an imperfect model as nemaline rod formation is inconsistent and a human null phenotype has not been reported to date.

Congenital Fiber Type Disproportion

CFTD is defined by type 1 fibers being 25% smaller than type 2 fibers in the absence of other pathological features on muscle biopsy.[134] The concept of CFTD as a distinct myopathy, however, is controversial, as type 1 fibers are often smaller than type 2 in all congenital myopathies and more specific histopathological features may evolve over time.

In the original series proposing CFTD as a distinct entity,[5] *clinical features* included marked hypotonia with variable weakness, myopathic facial appearance, frequent extraocular muscle involvement, ptosis and associated orthopedic complications; these cases, however, were assessed before the molecular era and are likely to have been genetically highly heterogeneous. The clinical course in genetically unresolved cases with CFTD is highly variable, ranging from slow improvement to continuous deterioration, the latter often due to progressive respiratory failure.

Recent advances in *genetics* have implicated genes also involved in other congenital myopathies. Heterozygous *ACTA1* missense mutations were the first mutations to be implicated in CFTD, in three Japanese patients with severe weakness and respiratory impairment but no extraocular muscle involvement.[135] A homozygous G943A mutation in the *SEPN1* gene[136] was identified in two sisters with CFTD and a complex clinical phenotype, featuring insulin resistance, severe scoliosis, and respiratory muscle weakness. Heterozygous missense mutations in the *TPM3* gene were identified in five CFTD families, associated with proximal and distal weakness, respiratory impairment, and ptosis but no extraocular muscle involvement.[137] In a sixth family, the recurrent p.Arg168His mutation was associated with both CFTD and NM in different family members, emphasizing the continuum between CFTD and other structural congenital myopathy phenotypes. Corresponding to the expanding spectrum of recessively inherited *RYR1*-related myopathies, CFTD in isolation has also been linked to compound heterozygous *RYR1* mutations recently in patients from seven families.[27] Extraocular muscle involvement was common in these patients and, as in other recessively inherited *RYR1*-related myopathies, appears to be a positive predictor of *RYR1* involvement. Features of CFTD and a myosin storage myopathy were found in a large family harboring a heterozygous mutation in the *MYH7* gene.[138] Last, Clarke and colleagues reported a presumably X-linked form of CFTD with facial, bulbar, and cardiorespiratory involvement and possible linkage to Xq.[139]

RARE CONGENITAL MYOPATHIES AND OTHER EARLY-ONSET MUSCLE DISORDERS

Rare congenital myopathies comprise those with definite dual pathology and those with unusual but distinct structural features, often reported only in few families or even isolated cases. There are also a number of early-onset muscle disorders with overlapping clinico-pathological features, in particular myosin storage (hyaline body) myopathy and reducing body myopathy, which are not consistently included with the structural congenital myopathies but which often enter the differential diagnosis.

Congenital myopathies with dual pathology have been reported before the molecular resolution of the structural congenital myopathies and have now been attributed to mutations in genes implicated in other, more clearly defined forms. The co-occurrence of cores and rods in the same muscle biopsy ("core-rod myopathy") is particularly common and has been associated with mutations in the *RYR1*[30] but also the *ACTA1*,[140] *DNM2*,[68] *CFL2*,[111] *KBTBD13*,[112] and *NEB*[141] genes.

Rare structural congenital myopathies comprise a wide range of highly diverse entities defined by the presence of a particular structural defect such as cap myopathy, zebra body myopathy, sarcotubular myopathy, spheroid body myopathy, fingerprint body myopathy, trilaminar myopathy, cylindrical spiral myopathy, and myopathy with tubular aggregates.[6] Some may not be genetic entities, whereas the underlying molecular defect is now known in others, suggesting a continuum with other myopathies. Identification of *ACTA1*, *TPM2*, and *TPM3* mutations in Cap myopathy and *ACTA1* mutations in zebra body myopathy suggest that these conditions are extensions of the NM spectrum rather than representing genetically distinct entities. Sarcotubular myopathy is caused by mutations in the *TRIM32* gene, responsible for a form of LGMD,[142] and spheroid body myopathy by mutations in the gene encoding myotilin, implicated in a form of myofibrillar myopathy.[143]

Reducing body myopathy (RBM) due to mutations in *FHL1* encoding the four-and-a-half LIM domain 1 protein[144] is characterized by intracytoplasmic inclusions staining strongly with the menadione-NBT stain. Despite some clinical overlap, the condition is usually more severe and more rapidly progressive than the typical structural congenital myopathies. Myosin storage (or hyaline body) myopathy due to mutations in the *MYH7* gene encoding the slow/β myosin heavy chain[145] is characterized by subsarcolemmal accumulation of slow myosin with a glassy (hyaline) appearance in type 1 muscle fibers that are unstained with NADH-TR, in contrast to caps. These "hyaline" areas are not visible in all cases but minicores, small type 1 fibers and ring fibers may be present.[53,138] Clinical features include proximal or scapuloperoneal weakness with variable cardiorespiratory involvement. Laing distal myopathy is an allelic condition.[146]

MANAGEMENT OF THE CONGENITAL MYOPATHIES

Management of the congenital myopathies is mainly supportive but rational therapies informed by ongoing research are on the horizon. Detailed guidelines for the management of patients with CMs have been recently published by a consortium of international experts.[147]

General management principles include a multidisciplinary team approach involving a neuromuscular neurologist, respiratory physicians, orthopedic surgeons, physiotherapists, occupational therapists, and speech language therapists. Regular monitoring of respiratory function (including overnight oximetry) and timely institution of ventilatory support are of particular importance and should be tailored according to clinical findings and the underlying genetic defect. In most patients respiratory insufficiency can be managed noninvasively. Although not invariable, the potential for respiratory deterioration during pregnancy ought to be anticipated. Cardiac follow-up is particularly important in patients with respiratory impairment because of the risk of cor pulmonale, but also in individuals where the genetic defect is uncertain, considering the potential risk of an associated primary cardiomyopathy. Swallowing difficulties and poor weight gain need to be managed proactively and may require at least temporary gastrostomy insertion. Dysarthria is common and often requires dedicated speech therapy input. Scoliosis surgery and other orthopedic interventions should be undertaken at a center with experience in the management of neuromuscular disorders and periods of immobilization should be kept as short as possible. Possible MHS has to be anticipated in the anesthetic management of patients with congenital myopathies, in particular those with known *RYR1* involvement or uncertain genetic background.

Trial pharmacological therapies in few small pilot studies include tyrosine supplementation in NM[148] and oral salbutamol treatment in *RYR1*-related myopathies.[149] Administration of antioxidants such as acetylcysteine has been proposed as a therapeutic approach for *SEPN1*-related myopathies.[150] Recently emerged evidence of an associated neuromuscular transmission defect in various forms of CNM[59] suggests that these conditions may at least be partly amenable to pharmacological agents enhancing neuromuscular transmission.

Upregulation of proteins with compensatory potential, for example cardiac actin in *ACTA1* null mutants,[151] has been promoted with some success in animal models of NM. Direct correction of the primary genetic defect via viral delivery has been demonstrated in a murine model of XLMTM[102] and carries promise for future therapeutic application in humans.

REFERENCES

1. Magee KR, Shy GM. A new congenital non-progressive myopathy. Brain 1956; 79: 610–621.
2. Engel AG, Gomez MR, Groover RV. Multicore disease. A recently recognized congenital myopathy associated with multifocal degeneration of muscle fibers. Mayo Clin Proc 1971; 46: 666–681.
3. Shy GM, Engel WK, Somers JE, Wanko T. Nemaline myopathy. A new congenital myopathy. Brain 1963; 86: 793–810.
4. Spiro AJ, Shy GM, Gonatas NK. Myotubular myopathy. Persistence of fetal muscle in an adolescent boy. Arch Neurol 1966; 14: 1–14.
5. Brooke MH. Congenital fiber type disproportion. Second International Congress on Muscle Diseases. Vol 2. Perth, Australia: Elsevier, Amsterdam, 1973.
6. Goebel HH, Bonnemann CG. 169th ENMC International Workshop Rare Structural Congenital Myopathies 6–8 November 2009, Naarden, The Netherlands. Neuromuscular Disorders: NMD 2011; 21: 363–374.
7. Norwood FL, Harling C, Chinnery PF, Eagle M, Bushby K, Straub V. Prevalence of genetic muscle disease in Northern England: in-depth analysis of a muscle clinic population. Brain. 2009; 132: 3175–3186.
8. Amburgey K, McNamara N, Bennett LR, McCormick ME, Acsadi G, Dowling JJ. Prevalence of congenital myopathies in a representative pediatric United States population. Ann Neurol. 2011; 70: 662–665.
9. Maggi L, Scoto M, et al. (2013). Congenital myopathies--clinical features and frequency of individual subtypes diagnosed over a 5-year period in the United Kingdom. Neuromus Dis. 2013; 23(3): 195–205.
10. Romero NB, Monnier N, Viollet L, Cortey A, Chevallay M, Leroy JP, et al. Dominant and recessive central core disease associated with RYR1 mutations and fetal akinesia. Brain 2003; 126: 2341–2349.
11. Lehtokari VL, Pelin K, Herczegfalvi A, Karcagi V, Pouget J, Franques J, et al. Nemaline myopathy

caused by mutations in the nebulin gene may present as a distal myopathy. Neuromuscular Disorders: NMD 2011; 21: 556–562.

12. Voermans NC, Bonnemann CG, Hamel BC, Jungbluth H, van Engelen BG. Joint hypermobility as a distinctive feature in the differential diagnosis of myopathies. J Neurol 2009; 256: 13–27.

13. Munot P, Lashley D, Jungbluth H, Feng L, Pitt M, Robb SA, et al. Congenital fibre type disproportion associated with mutations in the tropomyosin 3 (TPM3) gene mimicking congenital myasthenia. Neuromuscular Disorders: NMD 2010; 20: 796–800.

14. Wattjes MP, Kley RA, Fischer D. Neuromuscular imaging in inherited muscle diseases. European Radiology 2010; 20: 2447–2460.

15. Jungbluth H, Sewry CA, Muntoni F. Core myopathies. Seminars in pediatric neurology 2011; 18: 239–249.

16. Jungbluth H. Central core disease. Orphanet J Rare Dis 2007a; 2: 25.

17. Jungbluth H. Multi-minicore disease. Orphanet J Rare Dis 2007b; 2: 31.

18. Ferreiro A, Quijano-Roy S, Pichereau C, Moghadaszadeh B, Goemans N, Bonnemann C, et al. Mutations of the selenoprotein N gene, which is implicated in rigid spine muscular dystrophy, cause the classical phenotype of multiminicore disease: reassessing the nosology of early-onset myopathies. Am J Hum Genet 2002b; 71: 739–749.

19. Jungbluth H, Zhou H, Hartley L, Halliger-Keller B, Messina S, Longman C, et al. Minicore myopathy with ophthalmoplegia caused by mutations in the ryanodine receptor type 1 gene. Neurology 2005; 65: 1930–1935.

20. Ferreiro A, Monnier N, Romero NB, Leroy JP, Bonnemann C, Haenggeli CA, et al. A recessive form of central core disease, transiently presenting as multi-minicore disease, is associated with a homozygous mutation in the ryanodine receptor type 1 gene. Ann Neurol 2002a; 51: 750–759.

21. Zhou H, Lillis S, Loy RE, Ghassemi F, Rose MR, Norwood F, et al. Multi-minicore disease and atypical periodic paralysis associated with novel mutations in the skeletal muscle ryanodine receptor (RYR1) gene. Neuromuscul Disord 2010; 20: 166–173.

22. Dowling JJ, Lillis S, Amburgey K, Zhou H, Al-Sarraj S, Buk SJ, et al. King-Denborough syndrome with and without mutations in the skeletal muscle ryanodine receptor (RYR1) gene. Neuromuscular disorders: NMD 2011.

23. Jungbluth H, Lillis S, Zhou H, Abbs S, Sewry C, Swash M, et al. Late-onset axial myopathy with cores due to a novel heterozygous dominant mutation in the skeletal muscle ryanodine receptor (RYR1) gene. Neuromuscul Disord 2009; 19: 344–347.

24. Klein A, Jungbluth H, Clement E, Lillis S, Abbs S, Munot P, et al. Muscle magnetic resonance imaging in congenital myopathies due to ryanodine receptor type 1 gene mutations. Archives of Neurology 2011; 68: 1171–1179.

25. Mercuri E, Clements E, Offiah A, Pichiecchio A, Vasco G, Bianco F, et al. Muscle magnetic resonance imaging involvement in muscular dystrophies with rigidity of the spine. Annals of Neurology 2010; 67: 201–208.

26. Dubowitz V, Sewry CA. Muscle biopsy: A practical approach. London: WB Saunders, 2007.

27. Clarke NF, Waddell LB, Cooper ST, Perry M, Smith RL, Kornberg AJ, et al. Recessive mutations in RYR1 are a common cause of congenital fiber type disproportion. Hum Mutat 2010; 31: E1544–E1550.

28. Bevilacqua JA, Monnier N, Bitoun M, Eymard B, Ferreiro A, Monges S, et al. Recessive RYR1 mutations cause unusual congenital myopathy with prominent nuclear internalization and large areas of myofibrillar disorganization. Neuropathology and applied neurobiology 2011; 37: 271–284.

29. Wilmshurst JM, Lillis S, Zhou H, Pillay K, Henderson H, Kress W, et al. RYR1 mutations are a common cause of congenital myopathies with central nuclei. Ann Neurol 2010; 68: 717–726.

30. Monnier N, Romero NB, Lerale J, Nivoche Y, Qi D, MacLennan DH, et al. An autosomal dominant congenital myopathy with cores and rods is associated with a neomutation in the RYR1 gene encoding the skeletal muscle ryanodine receptor. Hum Mol Genet 2000; 9: 2599–2608.

31. Wortmann SB, Rodenburg RJ, Jonckheere A, de Vries MC, Huizing M, Heldt K, et al. Biochemical and genetic analysis of 3-methylglutaconic aciduria type IV: a diagnostic strategy. Brain 2009; 132: 136–146.

32. Herasse M, Parain K, Marty I, Monnier N, Kaindl AM, Leroy JP, et al. Abnormal distribution of calcium-handling proteins: a novel distinctive marker in core myopathies. J Neuropathol Exp Neurol 2007; 66: 57–65.

33. Zhou H, Jungbluth H, Sewry CA, Feng L, Bertini E, Bushby K, et al. Molecular mechanisms and phenotypic variation in RYR1-related congenital myopathies. Brain 2007; 130: 2024–2036.

34. Klein A, Lillis S, Munteanu I, Scoto M, Zhou H, Quinlivan R, et al. Clinical and genetic findings in a large cohort of patients with ryanodine receptor 1 gene-associated myopathies. Human Mutation 2012.;33(6):981–988.

35. Monnier N, Ferreiro A, Marty I, Labarre-Vila A, Mezin P, Lunardi J. A homozygous splicing mutation causing a depletion of skeletal muscle RYR1 is associated with multi-minicore disease congenital myopathy with ophthalmoplegia. Hum Mol Genet 2003; 12: 1171–1178.

36. Treves S, Anderson AA, Ducreux S, Divet A, Bleunven C, Grasso C, et al. Ryanodine receptor 1 mutations, dysregulation of calcium homeostasis and neuromuscular disorders. Neuromuscul Disord 2005; 15: 577–587.

37. Zhang Y, Chen HS, Khanna VK, De Leon S, Phillips MS, Schappert K, et al. A mutation in the human ryanodine receptor gene associated with central core disease. Nat Genet 1993; 5: 46–50.

38. Monnier N, Marty I, Faure J, Castiglioni C, Desnuelle C, Sacconi S, et al. Null mutations causing depletion of the type 1 ryanodine receptor (RYR1) are commonly associated with recessive structural congenital myopathies with cores. Hum Mutat 2008; 29: 670–678.

39. Ibarra MC, Wu S, Murayama K, Minami N, Ichihara Y, Kikuchi H, et al. Malignant hyperthermia in Japan: mutation screening of the entire ryanodine receptor type 1 gene coding region by direct sequencing. Anesthesiology 2006; 104: 1146–1154.

40. Monnier N, Laquerriere A, Marret S, Goldenberg A, Marty I, Nivoche Y, et al. First genomic rearrangement of the RYR1 gene associated with an atypical presentation of lethal neonatal hypotonia. Neuromuscul Disord 2009; 19: 680–684.

41. Tong J, McCarthy TV, MacLennan DH. Measurement of resting cytosolic Ca2+ concentrations and Ca2+ store size in HEK-293 cells transfected with malignant hyperthermia or central core disease mutant Ca2+ release channels. J Biol Chem 1999; 274: 693–702.

42. Dirksen RT, Avila G. Altered ryanodine receptor function in central core disease: leaky or uncoupled Ca(2+) release channels? Trends Cardiovasc Med 2002; 12: 189–197.

43. Maclennan DH, Zvaritch E. Mechanistic models for muscle diseases and disorders originating in the sarcoplasmic reticulum. Biochim Biophys Acta 2010. Biochim Biophys Acta. 2011; 1813(5):948–964.

44. Hirata H, Watanabe T, Hatakeyama J, Sprague SM, Saint-Amant L, Nagashima A, et al. Zebrafish relatively relaxed mutants have a ryanodine receptor defect, show slow swimming and provide a model of multi-minicore disease. Development 2007; 134: 2771–2781.

45. Allamand V, Richard P, Lescure A, Ledeuil C, Desjardin D, Petit N, et al. A single homozygous point mutation in a 3'untranslated region motif of selenoprotein N mRNA causes SEPN1-related myopathy. EMBO Rep 2006; 7: 450–454.

46. Maiti B, Arbogast S, Allamand V, Moyle MW, Anderson CB, Richard P, et al. A mutation in the SEPN1 selenocysteine redefinition element (SRE) reduces selenocysteine incorporation and leads to SEPN1-related myopathy. Hum Mutat 2009; 30: 411–416.

47. Schoenmakers E, Agostini M, Mitchell C, Schoenmakers N, Papp L, Rajanayagam O, et al. Mutations in the selenocysteine insertion sequence-binding protein 2 gene lead to a multisystem selenoprotein deficiency disorder in humans. J Clin Invest 2010; 120: 4220–4235.

48. Castets P, Maugenre S, Gartioux C, Rederstorff M, Krol A, Lescure A, et al. Selenoprotein N is dynamically expressed during mouse development and detected early in muscle precursors. BMC Dev Biol 2009; 9: 46.

49 Castets P, Bertrand AT, Beuvin M, Ferry A, Le Grand F, Castets M, et al. Satellite cell loss and impaired muscle regeneration in selenoprotein N deficiency. Hum Mol Genet 2011; 20: 694–704.

50. Deniziak M, Thisse C, Rederstorff M, Hindelang C, Thisse B, Lescure A. Loss of selenoprotein N function causes disruption of muscle architecture in the zebrafish embryo. Exp Cell Res 2007; 313: 156–167.

51. Jurynec MJ, Xia R, Mackrill JJ, Gunther D, Crawford T, Flanigan KM, et al. Selenoprotein N is required for ryanodine receptor calcium release channel activity in human and zebrafish muscle. Proc Natl Acad Sci U S A 2008; 105: 12485–12490.

52. Fananapazir L, Dalakas MC, Cyran F, Cohn G, Epstein ND. Missense mutations in the beta-myosin heavy-chain gene cause central core disease in hypertrophic cardiomyopathy. Proc Natl Acad Sci U S A 1993; 90: 3993–3997.

53. Muelas N, Hackman P, Luque H, Garces-Sanchez M, Azorin I, Suominen T, et al. MYH7 gene tail mutation causing myopathic profiles beyond Laing distal myopathy. Neurology 2010; 75: 732–741.

54. Kaindl AM, Ruschendorf F, Krause S, Goebel HH, Koehler K, Becker C, et al. Missense mutations of ACTA1 cause dominant congenital myopathy with cores. J Med Genet 2004; 41: 842–848.

55. Carmignac V, Salih MA, Quijano-Roy S, Marchand S, Al Rayess MM, Mukhtar MM, et al. C-terminal titin deletions cause a novel early-onset myopathy with fatal cardiomyopathy. Ann Neurol 2007; 61: 340–351.

56. Kinali M, Beeson D, Pitt MC, Jungbluth H, Simonds AK, Aloysius A, et al. Congenital myasthenic syndromes in childhood: diagnostic and management challenges. J Neuroimmunol 2008; 201–202: 6–12.

57. Romero NB, Bitoun M. Centronuclear myopathies. Seminars in Pediatric Neurology 2011; 18: 250–256.

58. Herman GE, Finegold M, Zhao W, de Gouyon B, Metzenberg A. Medical complications in long-term survivors with X-linked myotubular myopathy. J Pediatr 1999; 134: 206–214.

59. Robb SA, Sewry CA, Dowling JJ, Feng L, Cullup T, Lillis S, et al. Impaired neuromuscular transmission and response to acetylcholinesterase inhibitors in centronuclear myopathies. Neuromuscular Disorders: NMD 2011; 21(6):379–386.

60. Liewluck T, Shen XM, Milone M, Engel AG. Endplate structure and parameters of neuromuscular transmission in sporadic centronuclear myopathy associated with myasthenia. Neuromuscular Disorders: NMD 2011. 21(6):387–395.

61. Penisson-Besnier I, Biancalana V, Reynier P, Cossee M, Dubas F. Diagnosis of myotubular myopathy in the oldest known manifesting female carrier: a clinical and genetic study. Neuromuscul Disord 2007; 17: 180–185.

62. Jungbluth H, Sewry CA, Buj-Bello A, Kristiansen M, Orstavik KH, Kelsey A, et al. Early and severe presentation of X-linked myotubular myopathy in a girl with skewed X-inactivation. Neuromuscul Disord 2003; 13: 55–59.

63. Dahl N, Hu LJ, Chery M, Fardeau M, Gilgenkrantz S, Nivelon-Chevallier A, et al. Myotubular myopathy in a girl with a deletion at Xq27-q28 and unbalanced X inactivation assigns the MTM1 gene to a 600-kb region. Am J Hum Genet 1995; 56: 1108–1115.

64. Bitoun M, Bevilacqua JA, Prudhon B, Maugenre S, Taratuto AL, Monges S, et al. Dynamin 2 mutations cause sporadic centronuclear myopathy with neonatal onset. Annals of Neurology 2007; 62: 666–670.

65. Jeub M, Bitoun M, Guicheney P, Kappes-Horn K, Strach K, Druschky KF, et al. Dynamin 2-related centronuclear myopathy: clinical, histological and genetic aspects of further patients and review of the literature. Clinical Neuropathology 2008; 27: 430–438.

66. Melberg A, Kretz C, Kalimo H, Wallgren-Pettersson C, Toussaint A, Bohm J, et al. Adult course in dynamin 2 dominant centronuclear myopathy with neonatal onset. Neuromuscul Disord 2010; 20: 53–56.

67. Jungbluth H, Cullup T, Lillis S, Zhou H, Abbs S, Sewry C, et al. Centronuclear myopathy with cataracts due to a novel dynamin 2 (DNM2) mutation. Neuromuscul Disord 2010; 20: 49–52.

68. Schessl J, Medne L, Hu Y, Zou Y, Brown MJ, Huse JT, et al. MRI in DNM2-related centronuclear myopathy: evidence for highly selective muscle involvement. Neuromuscul Disord 2007; 17: 28–32.

69. Susman RD, Quijano-Roy S, Yang N, Webster R, Clarke NF, Dowling J, et al. Expanding the clinical, pathological and MRI phenotype of DNM2-related centronuclear myopathy. Neuromuscul Disord 2010; 20: 229–237.

70. Liewluck T, Lovell TL, Bite AV, Engel AG. Sporadic centronuclear myopathy with muscle pseudohypertrophy,

neutropenia, and necklace fibers due to a DNM2 mutation. Neuromuscular Disorders: NMD 2010; 20: 801–804.

71. Zuchner S, Noureddine M, Kennerson M, Verhoeven K, Claeys K, De Jonghe P, et al. Mutations in the pleckstrin homology domain of dynamin 2 cause dominant intermediate Charcot-Marie-Tooth disease. Nature Genetics 2005; 37: 289–294.

72. Hanisch F, Muller T, Dietz A, Bitoun M, Kress W, Weis J, et al. Phenotype variability and histopathological findings in centronuclear myopathy due to DNM2 mutations. Journal of Neurology 2011. 258(6):1085–1090.

73. Echaniz-Laguna A, Nicot AS, Carre S, Franques J, Tranchant C, Dondaine N, et al. Subtle central and peripheral nervous system abnormalities in a family with centronuclear myopathy and a novel dynamin 2 gene mutation. Neuromuscul Disord 2007; 17: 955–959.

74. Fischer D, Herasse M, Bitoun M, Barragan-Campos HM, Chiras J, Laforet P, et al. Characterization of the muscle involvement in dynamin 2-related centronuclear myopathy. Brain: A Journal of Neurology 2006; 129: 1463–1469.

75. Nicot AS, Toussaint A, Tosch V, Kretz C, Wallgren-Pettersson C, Iwarsson E, et al. Mutations in amphiphysin 2 (BIN1) disrupt interaction with dynamin 2 and cause autosomal recessive centronuclear myopathy. Nat Genet 2007; 39: 1134–1139.

76. Bohm J, Yis U, Ortac R, Cakmakci H, Kurul SH, Dirik E, et al. Case report of intrafamilial variability in autosomal recessive centronuclear myopathy associated to a novel BIN1 stop mutation. Orphanet Journal of Rare Diseases 2010; 5: 35.

77. Claeys KG, Maisonobe T, Bohm J, Laporte J, Hezode M, Romero NB, et al. Phenotype of a patient with recessive centronuclear myopathy and a novel BIN1 mutation. Neurology 2010; 74: 519–521.

78. Mejaddam AY, Nennesmo I, Sejersen T. Severe phenotype of a patient with autosomal recessive centronuclear myopathy due to a BIN1 mutation. Acta Myologica: Myopathies and Cardiomyopathies: Official Journal of the Mediterranean Society of Myology/edited by the Gaetano Conte Academy for the Study of Striated Muscle Diseases 2009; 28: 91–93.

79. Bitoun M, Maugenre S, Jeannet PY, Lacene E, Ferrer X, Laforet P, et al. Mutations in dynamin 2 cause dominant centronuclear myopathy. Nat Genet 2005; 37: 1207–1209.

80. Jungbluth H, Zhou H, Sewry CA, Robb S, Treves S, Bitoun M, et al. Centronuclear myopathy due to a de novo dominant mutation in the skeletal muscle ryanodine receptor (RYR1) gene. Neuromuscular Disorders: NMD 2007; 17: 338–345.

81. Bevilacqua JA, Bitoun M, Biancalana V, Oldfors A, Stoltenburg G, Claeys KG, et al. "Necklace" fibers, a new histological marker of late-onset MTM1-related centronuclear myopathy. Acta Neuropathol 2009; 117: 283–291.

82. Toussaint A, Cowling BS, Hnia K, Mohr M, Oldfors A, Schwab Y, et al. Defects in amphiphysin 2 (BIN1) and triads in several forms of centronuclear myopathies. Acta Neuropathol 2011; 121: 253–266.

83. Sewry CA, Quinlivan RC, Squier W, Morris GE, Holt I. A rapid immunohistochemical test to distinguish congenital myotonic dystrophy from X-linked myotubular myopathy. Neuromuscular Disorders: NMD 2012; 22: 225–230.

84. Laporte J, Hu LJ, Kretz C, Mandel JL, Kioschis P, Coy JF, et al. A gene mutated in X-linked myotubular myopathy defines a new putative tyrosine phosphatase family conserved in yeast. Nat Genet 1996; 13: 175–182.

85. de Gouyon BM, Zhao W, Laporte J, Mandel JL, Metzenberg A, Herman GE. Characterization of mutations in the myotubularin gene in twenty six patients with X-linked myotubular myopathy. Hum Mol Genet 1997; 6: 1499–1504.

86. Nishino I, Minami N, Kobayashi O, Ikezawa M, Goto Y, Arahata K, et al. MTM1 gene mutations in Japanese patients with the severe infantile form of myotubular myopathy. Neuromuscul Disord 1998; 8: 453–458.

87. Buj-Bello A, Biancalana V, Moutou C, Laporte J, Mandel JL. Identification of novel mutations in the MTM1 gene causing severe and mild forms of X-linked myotubular myopathy. Hum Mutat 1999; 14: 320–325.

88. Tanner SM, Schneider V, Thomas NS, Clarke A, Lazarou L, Liechti-Gallati S. Characterization of 34 novel and six known MTM1 gene mutations in 47 unrelated X-linked myotubular myopathy patients. Neuromuscul Disord 1999; 9: 41–49.

89. Laporte J, Biancalana V, Tanner SM, Kress W, Schneider V, Wallgren-Pettersson C, et al. MTM1 mutations in X-linked myotubular myopathy. Hum Mutat 2000; 15: 393–409.

90. Tosch V, Vasli N, Kretz C, Nicot AS, Gasnier C, Dondaine N, et al. Novel molecular diagnostic approaches for X-linked centronuclear (myotubular) myopathy reveal intronic mutations. Neuromuscul Disord 2010; 20: 375–381.

91. Trump N, Cullup T, Verheij JB, Manzur A, Muntoni F, Abbs S, et al. X-linked myotubular myopathy due to a complex rearrangement involving a duplication of MTM1 exon 10. Neuromuscular Disorders: NMD 2011. 22(5): 384–388.

92. Laporte J, Kioschis P, Hu LJ, Kretz C, Carlsson B, Poustka A, et al. Cloning and characterization of an alternatively spliced gene in proximal Xq28 deleted in two patients with intersexual genitalia and myotubular myopathy. Genomics 1997; 41: 458–462.

93. Dowling JJ, Gibbs EM, Feldman EL. Membrane traffic and muscle: lessons from human disease. Traffic 2008; 9: 1035–1043.

94. Cowling BS, Toussaint A, Muller J, Laporte J. Defective membrane remodeling in neuromuscular diseases: insights from animal models. PLoS Genetics 2012; 8: e1002595.

95. Clague MJ, Lorenzo O. The myotubularin family of lipid phosphatases. Traffic 2005; 6: 1063–1069.

96. Goryunov D, Nightingale A, Bornfleth L, Leung C, Liem RK. Multiple disease-linked myotubularin mutations cause NFL assembly defects in cultured cells and disrupt myotubularin dimerization. Journal of Neurochemistry 2008; 104: 1536–1552.

97. Dowling JJ, Vreede AP, Low SE, Gibbs EM, Kuwada JY, Bonnemann CG, et al. Loss of myotubularin function results in T-tubule disorganization in zebrafish and human myotubular myopathy. PLoS Genetics 2009; 5: e1000372.

98. Cao C, Laporte J, Backer JM, Wandinger-Ness A, Stein MP. Myotubularin lipid phosphatase binds the hVPS15/hVPS34 lipid kinase complex on endosomes. Traffic 2007; 8: 1052–1067.

 99. Hnia K, Tronchere H, Tomczak KK, Amoasii L, Schultz P, Beggs AH, et al. Myotubularin controls desmin intermediate filament architecture and mito-chondrial dynamics in human and mouse skeletal muscle. The Journal of Clinical Investigation 2011; 121: 70–85.

100. Al-Qusairi L, Weiss N, Toussaint A, Berbey C, Messaddeq N, Kretz C, et al. T-tubule disorganiza-tion and defective excitation-contraction coupling in muscle fibers lacking myotubularin lipid phosphatase. Proc Natl Acad Sci U S A 2009; 106: 18763–18768.

101. Buj-Bello A, Laugel V, Messaddeq N, Zahreddine H, Laporte J, Pellissier JF, et al. The lipid phosphatase myotubularin is essential for skeletal muscle mainte-nance but not for myogenesis in mice. Proc Natl Acad Sci U S A 2002; 99: 15060–15065.

102. Buj-Bello A, Fougerousse F, Schwab Y, Messaddeq N, Spehner D, Pierson CR, et al. AAV-mediated intramuscular delivery of myotubularin corrects the myotubular myopathy phenotype in targeted murine muscle and suggests a function in plasma membrane homeostasis. Hum Mol Genet 2008; 17: 2132–2143.

103. Lawlor MW, Read BP, Edelstein R, Yang N, Pierson CR, Stein MJ, et al. Inhibition of activin recep-tor type IIB increases strength and lifespan in myotubularin-deficient mice. The American Journal of Pathology 2011; 178: 784–793.

104. Durieux AC, Prudhon B, Guicheney P, Bitoun M. Dynamin 2 and human diseases. Journal of Molecular Medicine 2010a; 88: 339–350.

105. Durieux AC, Vignaud A, Prudhon B, Viou MT, Beuvin M, Vassilopoulos S, et al. A centronuclear myopathy-dynamin 2 mutation impairs skeletal mus-cle structure and function in mice. Human Molecular Genetics 2010b; 19: 4820–4836.

106. Pelin K, Hilpela P, Donner K, Sewry C, Akkari PA, Wilton SD, et al. Mutations in the nebulin gene asso-ciated with autosomal recessive nemaline myopathy. Proc Natl Acad Sci U S A 1999; 96: 2305–2310.

107. Nowak KJ, Wattanasirichaigoon D, Goebel HH, Wilce M, Pelin K, Donner K, et al. Mutations in the skeletal muscle alpha-actin gene in patients with actin myopathy and nemaline myopathy. Nature Genetics 1999; 23: 208–212.

108. Laing NG, Wilton SD, Akkari PA, Dorosz S, Boundy K, Kneebone C, et al. A mutation in the alpha tropo-myosin gene TPM3 associated with autosomal domi-nant nemaline myopathy. Nat Genet 1995; 9: 75–79.

109. Donner K, Ollikainen M, Ridanpaa M, Christen HJ, Goebel HH, de Visser M, et al. Mutations in the beta-tropomyosin (TPM2) gene—a rare cause of nemaline myopathy. Neuromuscular Disorders: NMD 2002; 12: 151–158.

110. Johnston JJ, Kelley RI, Crawford TO, Morton DH, Agarwala R, Koch T, et al. A novel nemaline myopa-thy in the Amish caused by a mutation in troponin T1. Am J Hum Genet 2000; 67: 814–821.

111. Agrawal PB, Greenleaf RS, Tomczak KK, Lehtokari VL, Wallgren-Pettersson C, Wallefeld W, et al. Nemaline myopathy with minicores caused by muta-tion of the CFL2 gene encoding the skeletal muscle

actin-binding protein, cofilin-2. American Journal of Human Genetics 2007; 80: 162–167.

112. Sambuughin N, Yau KS, Olive M, Duff RM, Bayarsaikhan M, Lu S, et al. Dominant mutations in KBTBD13, a member of the BTB/Kelch family, cause nemaline myopathy with cores. Am J Hum Genet 2010; 87: 842–847.

113. Wallgren-Pettersson C, Sewry CA, Nowak KJ, Laing NG. Nemaline myopathies. Seminars in Pediatric Neurology 2011; 18: 230–238.

114. Ryan MM, Schnell C, Strickland CD, Shield LK, Morgan G, Iannaccone ST, et al. Nemaline myopa-thy: a clinical study of 143 cases. Ann Neurol 2001; 50: 312–320.

115. Chahin N, Selcen D, Engel AG. Sporadic late onset nemaline myopathy. Neurology 2005; 65: 1158–1164.

116. Sewry CA, Brown SC, Pelin K, Jungbluth H, Wallgren-Pettersson C, Labeit S, et al. Abnormalities in the expression of nebulin in chromosome-2 linked nemaline myopathy. Neuromuscul Disord 2001; 11: 146–153.

117. Dalakas MC, Pezeshkpour GH, Flaherty M. Progressive nemaline (rod) myopathy associated with HIV infection. N Engl J Med 1987; 317: 1602–1603.

118. Nowak KJ, Sewry CA, Navarro C, Squier W, Reina C, Ricoy JR, et al. Nemaline myopathy caused by absence of alpha-skeletal muscle actin. Ann Neurol 2007; 61: 175–184.

119. Pelin K, Donner K, Holmberg M, Jungbluth H, Muntoni F, Wallgren-Pettersson C. Nebulin muta-tions in autosomal recessive nemaline myopathy: an update. Neuromuscul Disord 2002; 12: 680–686.

120. Lehtokari VL, Pelin K, Sandbacka M, Ranta S, Donner K, Muntoni F, et al. Identification of 45 novel mutations in the nebulin gene associated with autoso-mal recessive nemaline myopathy. Human mutation 2006a; 27: 946–956.

121. Laing NG, Dye DE, Wallgren-Pettersson C, Richard G, Monnier N, Lillis S, et al. Mutations and poly-morphisms of the skeletal muscle alpha-actin gene (ACTA1). Hum Mutat 2009; 30: 1267–1277.

122. Anderson SL, Ekstein J, Donnelly MC, Keefe EM, Toto NR, LeVoci LA, et al. Nemaline myopathy in the Ashkenazi Jewish population is caused by a deletion in the nebulin gene. Hum Genet 2004; 115: 185–190.

123. Lehtokari VL, Pelin K, Donner K, Voit T, Rudnik-Schoneborn S, Stoetter M, et al. Identification of a founder mutation in TPM3 in nemaline myopathy patients of Turkish origin. Eur J Hum Genet 2008; 16: 1055–1061.

124. Agrawal PB, Strickland CD, Midgett C, Morales A, Newburger DE, Poulos MA, et al. Heterogeneity of nemaline myopathy cases with skeletal muscle alpha-actin gene mutations. Ann Neurol 2004; 56: 86–96.

125. Lehtokari VL, Pelin K, Sandbacka M, Ranta S, Donner K, Muntoni F, et al. Identification of 45 novel mutations in the nebulin gene associated with autosomal recessive nemaline myopathy. Hum Mutat 2006b; 27: 946–956.

126. Wallgren-Pettersson C, Pelin K, Nowak KJ, Muntoni F, Romero NB, Goebel HH, et al. Genotype-phenotype correlations in nemaline myopathy caused by muta-tions in the genes for nebulin and skeletal muscle alpha-actin. Neuromuscular disorders: NMD 2004; 14: 461–470.

127. Wallgren-Pettersson C, Donner K, Sewry C, Bijlsma E, Lammens M, Bushby K, et al. Mutations in the nebulin gene can cause severe congenital nemaline myopathy. Neuromuscular Disorders: NMD 2002; 12: 674–679.

128. Sparrow JC, Nowak KJ, Durling HJ, Beggs AH, Wallgren-Pettersson C, Romero N, et al. Muscle disease caused by mutations in the skeletal muscle alpha-actin gene (ACTA1). Neuromuscul Disord 2003; 13: 519–531.

129. Jungbluth H, Sewry CA, Counsell S, Allsop J, Chattopadhyay A, Mercuri E, et al. Magnetic resonance imaging of muscle in nemaline myopathy. Neuromuscul Disord 2004; 14: 779–784.

130. Ravenscroft G, Jackaman C, Bringans S, Papadimitriou JM, Griffiths LM, McNamara E, et al. Mouse models of dominant ACTA1 disease recapitulate human disease and provide insight into therapies. Brain 2011; 134: 1101–1115.

131. Ochala J, Lehtokari VL, Iwamoto H, Li M, Feng HZ, Jin JP, et al. Disrupted myosin cross-bridge cycling kinetics triggers muscle weakness in nebulin-related myopathy. FASEB J 2011. 25(6): 1903–1913.

132. Ottenheijm CA, Hooijman P, DeChene ET, Stienen GJ, Beggs AH, Granzier H. Altered myofilament function depresses force generation in patients with nebulin-based nemaline myopathy (NEM2). Journal of Structural Biology 2010; 170: 334–343.

133. Bang ML, Li X, Littlefield R, Bremner S, Thor A, Knowlton KU, et al. Nebulin-deficient mice exhibit shorter thin filament lengths and reduced contractile function in skeletal muscle. The Journal of Cell Biology 2006; 173: 905–916.

134. Clarke NF. Congenital fiber-type disproportion. Seminars in Pediatric Neurology 2011; 18: 264–271.

135. Laing NG, Clarke NF, Dye DE, Liyanage K, Walker KR, Kobayashi Y, et al. Actin mutations are one cause of congenital fibre type disproportion. Ann Neurol 2004; 56: 689–694.

136. Clarke NF, Kidson W, Quijano-Roy S, Estournet B, Ferreiro A, Guicheney P, et al. SEPN1: associated with congenital fiber-type disproportion and insulin resistance. Ann Neurol 2006; 59: 546–552.

137. Clarke NF, Kolski H, Dye DE, Lim E, Smith RL, Patel R, et al. Mutations in TPM3 are a common cause of congenital fiber type disproportion. Ann Neurol 2008; 63: 329–337.

138. Ortolano S, Tarrio R, Blanco-Arias P, Teijeira S, Rodriguez-Trelles F, Garcia-Murias M, et al. A novel MYH7 mutation links congenital fiber type disproportion and myosin storage myopathy. Neuromuscular Disorders: NMD 2011; 21: 254–262.

139. Clarke NF, Smith RL, Bahlo M, North KN. A novel X-linked form of congenital fiber-type disproportion. Ann Neurol 2005; 58: 767–772.

140. Jungbluth H, Sewry CA, Brown SC, Nowak KJ, Laing NG, Wallgren-Pettersson C, et al. Mild phenotype of nemaline myopathy with sleep hypoventilation due to a mutation in the skeletal muscle alpha-actin (ACTA1) gene. Neuromuscul Disord 2001; 11: 35–40.

141. Romero NB, Lehtokari VL, Quijano-Roy S, Monnier N, Claeys KG, Carlier RY, et al. Core-rod myopathy caused by mutations in the nebulin gene. Neurology 2009; 73: 1159–1161.

142. Schoser BG, Frosk P, Engel AG, Klutzny U, Lochmuller H, Wrogemann K. Commonality of TRIM32 mutation in causing sarcotubular myopathy and LGMD2H. Annals of Neurology 2005; 57: 591–595.

143. Foroud T, Pankratz N, Batchman AP, Pauciulo MW, Vidal R, Miravalle L, et al. A mutation in myotilin causes spheroid body myopathy. Neurology 2005; 65: 1936–1940.

144. Schessl J, Zou Y, McGrath MJ, Cowling BS, Maiti B, Chin SS, et al. Proteomic identification of FHL1 as the protein mutated in human reducing body myopathy. The Journal of Clinical Investigation 2008; 118: 904–912.

145. Tajsharghi H, Thornell LE, Lindberg C, Lindvall B, Henriksson KG, Oldfors A. Myosin storage myopathy associated with a heterozygous missense mutation in MYH7. Ann Neurol 2003; 54: 494–500.

146. Meredith C, Herrmann R, Parry C, Liyanage K, Dye DE, Durling HJ, et al. Mutations in the slow skeletal muscle fiber myosin heavy chain gene (MYH7) cause Laing early-onset distal myopathy (MPD1). Am J Hum Genet 2004; 75: 703–708.

147. Wang CH, Dowling JJ, North K, Schroth MK, Sejersen T, Shapiro F, et al. Consensus statement on standard of care for congenital myopathies. Journal of Child Neurology 2012; 27: 363–382.

148. Ryan MM, Sy C, Rudge S, Ellaway C, Ketteridge D, Roddick LG, et al. Dietary L-tyrosine supplementation in nemaline myopathy. J Child Neurol 2008; 23: 609–613.

149. Messina S, Hartley L, Main M, Kinali M, Jungbluth H, Muntoni F, et al. Pilot trial of salbutamol in central core and multi-minicore diseases. Neuropediatrics 2004; 35: 262–266.

150. Arbogast S, Beuvin M, Fraysse B, Zhou H, Muntoni F, Ferreiro A. Oxidative stress in SEPN1-related myopathy: from pathophysiology to treatment. Ann Neurol 2009; 65: 677–686.

151. Nowak KJ, Ravenscroft G, Jackaman C, Filipovska A, Davies SM, Lim EM, et al. Rescue of skeletal muscle alpha-actin-null mice by cardiac (fetal) alpha-actin. The Journal of Cell Biology 2009; 185: 903–915.

Chapter 7

Metabolic Myopathies

Gráinne S. Gorman
Patrick F. Chinnery

ENERGY METABOLISM IN EXERCISING MUSCLE

The main energy substrates used by muscle for energy metabolism are glucose, glycogen, and free fatty acid. Maximal oxygen uptake (VO_2max), exercise economy, the lactate threshold, and critical power are highly correlated with substrate "fuel" and energy metabolism, and endurance exercise performance in exercising muscle (Figure 7–1). During muscle activation, intracellular adenosine 5′-triphosphate (ATP) stores, the molecular unit of intracellular energy transfer, are small (5-6 millimolar (mM)), and are depleted within two seconds of muscle contraction. This results in the activation of other energy substrates and metabolic pathways as

164

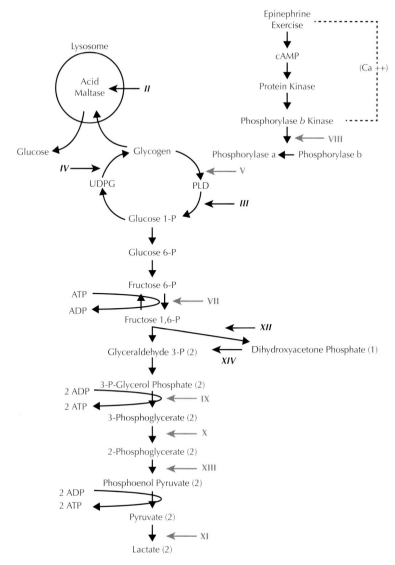

Figure 7–1. Glycolytic pathway showing the generation of high-energy phosphate.

a function of exercise intensity. Two pathways predominate during conversion of fuel substrates to energy in exercising muscle: anaerobic metabolism (without oxygen) and aerobic metabolism (with oxygen). At rest, muscle predominately uses fatty acids as the main energy substrate. During high-intensity, isometric, short-duration exercise, *anaerobic glycolysis* predominates. Carbohydrates are the exclusive substrate for ATP production by this pathway, which produces sufficient energy for short bursts of high-intensity exercise. However, this system rapidly fatigues

linked to the accumulation of lactic acid. Phosphocreatine and lactate become significant contributors to ATP production only at high-energy intensities. The contribution from protein metabolism is zero. Oxidative phosphorylation is characterized by lower maximal power and slow attainment of a steady state in response to increased metabolic demand. This facilitates sustained maximum power for 7 to 10 minutes and a relatively large fraction of the maximal power for significantly longer periods. This is a significant advantage over other systems, which fatigue much faster.

Glycolysis

Glucose is a six-carbon hexagonal molecule and the main substrate of the glycolysis (or glycolytic) pathway. This occurs in the cytosol of the cell and is active during both aerobic and anaerobic conditions. Glucose enters the cell through specific transport proteins; GLUT 1 to 5, which are found in various tissues including all mammalian cells (GLUT1 and GLUT3; responsible for basal glucose uptake), liver and pancreatic β cells (GLUT2; regulates glucose level and accordingly adjusts the rate of insulin secretion), muscle and fat cells (GLUT4; regulated by insulin levels and transporting glucose into muscle and fat cells; increases in muscle membrane in response to endurance exercise training), and small intestine (GLUT5; functions primarily as a fructose transporter). These transporters consist of a single polypeptide chain of approximately 500 residues in length. These glucose transporters mediate the movement of glucose across the plasma membranes of cells, and form part of the tight control of the glycolytic pathway. The first step of glycolysis is facilitated by the enzyme hexokinase, which effectively traps glucose in the cell. This destabilizes glucose in a rate-limiting step that is energy dependent, and causes one of the high-energy phosphate bonds of ATP to be cleaved. This releases a phosphate molecule, which is donated to carbon 6 of the glucose molecule to form glucose-6-phosphate. This intermediary product of the glycolytic pathway can be converted to glycogen, oxidized by the pentose phosphate pathway to form nicotinamide adenine dinucleotide phosphate (NADPH), or structurally modified by phosphoglucose isomerase during glycolysis, and resulting in the formation of a hexagonal molecule, fructose-6-phosphate. A further phosphate is added, facilitated by phosphofructokinase (PFK), forming fructose-1,6-phosphate. This again is an energy-requiring step in the breakdown of glucose. PFK is the most important regulator of the glycolytic pathway in mammals and its activity in the liver is inhibited both by a fall in pH or rise in the ATP:ADP ratio. The inhibition of PFK by H^+ prevents development of an acidotic state due to excessive lactic acid production. Fructose-1,6-bisphosphate, under the influence of aldolase, is broken down into two distinct isomeric molecular structures, dihydroxyacetone phosphate (DHAP) and glyceraldehyde 3-phosphate. DHAP may undergo structural modification to become glyceraldehyde 3-phosphate by the enzyme triphosphate isomerase, and both resulting molecules gain an addition phosphate group and become oxidized to 1,3-diphosphoglycerate. This is the regulatory step in glycolysis. If glycolysis is excessive, DHAP formation is favored, which effectively halts on glycolysis. However, if energy is required, the formation of glyceraldehyde 3-phosphate is favored. The enzyme triphosphate isomerase regulates the balance between the formation of DHAP and glyceraldehyde 3-phosphate, and is dependent on the relative amounts of ATP and ADP. Glyceraldehyde-3-phosphate then loses a phosphate group to form 1,3-bisphosphoglycerate (1,3-BPG), with the resultant release of energy. This molecule has a dual role in that it is not only essential for glycolysis, but is also a precursor to 2,3-bisphosphoglycerate (2,3-BPG), a molecule that regulates hemoglobin's affinity for oxygen in mature red blood cells. Phosphate is then removed from this structure, yielding one molecule of ATP for each molecule of 2,3-BPG, of which there are two, to form 3-phosphoglycerate. Phosphoglyceromutase converts 3-phosphoglycerate into 2-phosphoglycerate. These two molecules of 2-phosphoglycerate then lose water, forming phosphoenolpyruvate; a step regulated by the enzyme enolase. The remaining phosphate group is then lost from each of these molecules, by the action of pyruvate kinase, with the release of a further single ATP molecule to form pyruvate. Pyruvate is the last molecule in the glycolysis pathway and is the substrate of both the Krebs cycle in aerobic conditions, and lactic acid production in anaerobic conditions. Each molecule of glucose produces two molecules of pyruvate with the net production of two ATP molecules per glucose molecule. This pathway is strictly regulated by energy demands and the ATP:ADP ratio; thus when energy is required, glycolysis is promoted.

Although PFK is recognized as the most prominent regulatory enzyme in this pathway, hexokinase is also important, with the inhibition of PFK directly leading to the inhibition of hexokinase activity. This occurs during periods when the cell no longer requires glucose as a preeminent energy source.

Other Fuel Substrates in Glycolysis—Fructose and Galactose

Although glucose is the primary substrate used in glycolysis, fructose and galactose can also be channeled into the glycolytic pathway. Following ingestion of fructose, it is metabolized in the liver via the fructose-1-phosphate pathway. Fructose is phosphorylated by fructokinase to fructose-1-phosphate, which is then split into glyceraldehyde and DHAP, intermediate substrates in glycolysis. Triose kinase then mediates the phosphorylation of glyceraldehyde to glyceraldehyde 3-phosphate. Alternatively, hexokinase can moderate the phosphorylation of fructose to fructose-6-phosphate; however, its affinity for fructose is considerably less than it is for glucose.

Galactose requires conversion into a glucose metabolite to be useful as an energy source. This is regulated by galactokinase, which converts galactose to galactose-1-phosphate which then acquires an uridyl group from uridine diphosphate glucose to form UDP-galactose. This is then epimerized to glucose and glucose-1-phosphate. Subsequent isomerization of glucose-1-phosphate is again regulated by phosphoglucomutase.

Glycogen and Glycogenolysis

Glycogen is a branched polysaccharide and a polymer of glucose residues linked mainly by glycosidic linkages, and is the main storage unit for glucose in liver and skeletal muscle, which may be rapidly mobilized during periods of sudden energy requirement. The first step in glycogen catabolism involves the phosphorlytic cleavage of glycogen to yield release of glucose-1-phosphate, which involves two catalytic enzymes: glycogen phosphorylase and brancher enzymes. Glucose-1-phosphate is the converted into glucose-6-phosphate for further metabolism, catalyzed by phosphoglucomutase, an enzyme also used in galactose metabolism. The remaining glycogen molecule undergoes further degradation, facilitated by a transferase and α-1,6-glucosidase (debranching enzyme). The fate of newly formed glucose-6-phosphate is threefold: it may serve as the initial substrate for glycolysis, enter the pentose phosphate pathway to yield NADPH and ribose substrates,

or be hydrolyzed into glucose by liver-specific glucose-6-phosphatase for release into the bloodstream. This maintains constant glucose levels for use by other tissues.

Lipid Metabolism

Lipid metabolism is closely coupled to carbohydrate metabolism and involves the hydrolysis of lipids to form glycerol and fatty acids. Glycerol is readily metabolized to form dihydroxyacetone phosphate, an intermediate product of glycolysis. It then may undergo one of two fates: Dihydroxyacetone may be converted into pyruvic acid through the glycolytic pathway, or it may be used in gluconeogenesis to make glucose-6-phosphate to maintain blood levels of glucose, pending the energy requirements of the body. In the mitochondria, fatty acids are oxidized to acetyl CoA using the fatty acid spiral and ultimately converted into ATP, CO_2, and H_2O through the citric acid cycle and the electron transport chain.

Metabolic myopathies result from a deficiency or reduced function of any of the catalytic enzymes integral to either aerobic or anaerobic pathways. Disorders of the final common pathway of energy metabolism, the mitochondrial respiratory chain, are considered in chapter 8.

DEFECTS OF GLYCOGEN METABOLISM

Glycogen is a glucose branched-chain polymer and serves as a dynamic reservoir of glucose in skeletal muscle and liver. Glycogen storage disorders (GSD) are a group of inherited metabolic diseases caused by inborn errors of glucose metabolism. To date, 14 different forms of GSD have been described (Table 7–1) manifesting phenotypic and genotypic heterogeneity, and may be classified as either disorders producing *dynamic* symptoms characterized by exercise intolerance, cramps, and myoglobinuria (exercise intolerance) or *static* symptoms (fixed weakness).

The overall incidence of glycogen storage disorders is estimated at one case per 20,000 to 43,000 live births,[1] with genotypic and regional variations reported (Table 7–1). The inheritance of GSD is autosomal recessive for

Table 7–1 Disorders of Carbohydrate Metabolism

Type/ Eponym	Inherit- ance/ Incidence	Enzyme Involved	Diagnosis	Age of Onset	Clinical Features	Genetics	Treatment	Complications
O Lewis' disease	AR	Hepatic glycogen synthase	Raised fasting lactate Hypoglycemia Glycosuria Ketonuria	Infancy/ childhood	Fasting: ketotic hypoglycemia, increased free fatty acids, and low levels of alanine and lactate. Postprandial: hyperglycemia & hyperlactatemia Seizures Muscle cramps after exertion Mild growth retardation	Mutations in GYS1 (muscle) and GYS2 (liver)	*Dietary* Avoidance of fasting Hypoglycemia	Normal growth and intellectual development if episodes of hypoglycemia treated early
Ia Von Gierke's disease	AR 1:100,000	Glucose-6-phosphatase	Clinical features abnormal blood/ plasma parameters Glucagon/ adrenaline stimulation test Molecular genetic testing Liver biopsy (G6Pase)	3–4 months	*At birth* Growth retardation Doll-like face Hepatomegaly Enlarged kidneys Lactic acidosis Hyperuricemia Hyperlipidemia Hypoglycemic seizures Xanthoma Diarrhea Epistaxis	Mutations in G6PC (80%) p.Arg83Cys Arg83His c.378_379dupTA c.648G>T c.79delC, p.Gly188Arg, p.Gln347*	*Dietary* Frequent daytime feedings (complex CHO, high protein, low fat) Nighttime continuous glucose infusion Corn starch	*Long term* Short stature Osteoporosis Delayed puberty Gout Renal disease Pulmonary hypertension Hepatic adenomas Polycystic ovaries Menorrhagia Pancreatitis Neurocognitive
Ib, c, d		glucose-6-phosphate translocase	*See Ia*	*See Ia*	*See Ia;* in addition, chronic neutropenia	Mutations in SLC37A4 (20%)	*See Ia* Prophylactic antibiotics	*See Ia*

Type	Inheritance / Incidence	Deficient enzyme	Diagnosis	Classification (onset)	Clinical features	Molecular genetics	Treatment	Prognosis / long term
II (Pompe disease)	AR 1:14,000 African American; 1:100,000 European descent	acid alpha-glucosidase (GAA)	↑creatine kinase ↑Urinary oligosaccharides Measurement of GAA enzyme activity (skin fibroblasts) Acid alpha-glucosidase protein quantitation Molecular genetic testing	Classic infantile-onset late-onset (childhood, juvenile, adult)	hypotonia, generalized muscle weakness, arrhythmias/HOCM feeding difficulties, failure to thrive, respiratory distress, hearing loss proximal muscle weakness respiratory weakness *without clinically apparent cardiac involvement*	Mutations in *GAA*	*Treatment of manifestations—cardiac* ERT (alglucosidase alfa)	Death within 1 year without treatment Development of antibodies Survival to 5th/6th decade
IIIa/c (liver and muscle) IIIb/d (liver) Cori's disease	AR 1:100,000 (USA) 1:5,400 (North African Jewish descent)	IIIa/b: debranching enzyme nonfunctioning; IIIc/d: debranching enzyme low-functioning	Abnormal blood/plasma parameters Glucagon/ adrenaline challenge Molecular genetic testing	Infancy	*Liver, heart and skeletal muscle* Hepatomegaly Ketotic hypoglycemia Myopathy Cardiomyopathy Raised CK Raised transaminases (ALT/AST) hyperlipidemia *No lactic acidosis or hyperuricemia*	Mutations in *AGL*	*Dietary* High-protein diet & frequent feeds Fructose and galactose Corn starch *Systemic* Liver transplant	*Long term* HOCM Severe hepatic cirrhosis, liver dysfunction, hepatocellular carcinoma Short stature Slowly progressive myopathy Osteoporosis and osteopenia Polycystic ovaries

(continued)

Table 7–1 (Cont.)

Type/ Eponym	Inherit- ance/ Incidence	Enzyme Involved	Diagnosis	Age of Onset	Clinical Features	Genetics	Treatment	Complications
IV Andersen's disease	AR 1:600,000– 1:800,000	transglucosidase	Liver function tests Abdominal ultrasound Glycogen branching enzyme (GBE) activity (fibroblasts) Histopathology of affected tissues (liver, heart, or muscle) Molecular genetic testing	Fatal perinatal neuromuscular subtype In utero	Fetal akinesia deformation sequence (FADS) with decreased fetal movements, polyhydramnios, and fetal hydrops	GBE1 mutations	Liver transplantation Neurologic manifestations Cardiac manifestations Nutritional deficiencies Coagulopathy: FFP	Early fatality by age 4 due to cirrhosis & portal hypertension Arthrogryposis Severe hypotonia Muscular atrophy Mortality in infancy
				Newborn neuromuscular subtype	Profound hypotonia respiratory distress Dilated cardiomyopathy Small stature (2 cases)			
				Classic (progressive) hepatic First 2–3 months	Failure to thrive Hepatomegaly Liver dysfunction and Cirrhosis			Liver transplant; complicated by DCM (death before 5 years)
				Nonprogressive hepatic subtype	Progressive muscle weakness			Good prognosis
				Childhood neuromuscular subtype 2nd decade	Hepatomegaly Liver dysfunction (normalizes) Myopathy Hypotonia Mild to severe myopathy and dilated cardiomyopathy			Mild disease to death by 3rd decade

		Deficient enzyme	Diagnosis	Age of onset	Clinical findings	Molecular testing	Treatment	Complications / Caution
V McArdle disease	AR 1:100,000	Muscle glycogen phosphorylase	Clinical findings Supportive laboratory findings Forearm non-ischemic or ischemic test (↑CK, →lactic acid) Cycle test (*pathognomonic cardiac response*) Myophosphorylase enzyme activity in muscle (↓ absent) Molecular genetic testing	Childhood Infantile form Late onset (6th decade)	Exercise intolerance Muscle stiffness & cramping Muscle weakness Myoglobinuria (50%) Proximal muscle weakness (1/3) *Symptoms relieved by rest* *Second wind phenomenon* Hypotonia, generalized muscle weakness, and progressive respiratory insufficiency Mild proximal muscle weakness	*PYGM* coding region sequence analysis	Creatine monohydrate may improve symptoms Sucrose ingestion Aerobic exercise	Caution with general anesthesia Avoid intense isometric exercise Acute renal failure Rhabdomyolysis Myoglobinuria HyperCKemia Fatal
VI Hers' disease	X-linked 1:100,000	Liver glycogen phosphorylase	Liver Bx Blood enzymatic assay Molecular genetic testing	Childhood	Hepatomegaly Growth retardation Ketotic hypoglycemia (overnight fast) Mild hypoglycemia (prolonged fasting) *Rare cardiac form*	Mutations in *PYGL*	*Dietary* Mild variants: no treatment Frequent small meals Cornstarch	normal life span Cardiac Tx for rare cardiac form

(continued)

Table 7–1 (Cont.)

Type/Eponym	Inheritance/Incidence	Enzyme Involved	Diagnosis	Age of Onset	Clinical Features	Genetics	Treatment	Complications
VII Tarui's disease	AR ≈100 cases	Muscle phosphofructo-kinase	Muscle PFK assay Blood PFK assay	Classic Infantile onset Late onset	Exercise intolerance, muscle and fixed limb weakness most pronounced following exercise Contractures Anemia/jaundice Myoglobinuria Myopathy, psychomotor retardation, cataracts, joint contractures +/-respiratory failure +/-cardiomyopathy Progressive muscle and fixed limb weakness most pronounced following exercise contractures *no myoglobinuria or cramps* +/-IHD, valvular heart disease	Mutations in the gene encoding the M subunit of *PFK*		Death during childhood
IXa	X-linked (liver)	Phosphorylase b kinase		Early childhood	Hepatomegaly Growth retardation Ketotic hypoglycemia	Mutations in *PHKA2*		Symptoms improve with age, relatively benign
IXb	X-linked (muscle)	*See IXa*			Exercise intolerance Myalgia Muscle cramps, myoglobinuria, progressive muscle weakness	Mutations in *PHKA1*		

XI Fanconi-Bickel syndrome	AR	Glucose transporter 2 (GLUT2)		Infantile onset	Failure to thrive Severe renal tubular acidosis Hepatosplenomegaly	Mutations in *SLC2A2*	Symptomatic only	Hypophosphatemic rickets Delayed puberty
XII Red cell aldolase deficiency	AR	Aldolase A			Early muscle weakness and fatigue Rhabdomyolysis Anemia Jaundice Ptosis Cognitive impairment Dysmorphism	Mutations in *ALDOA*		Normal life span
XIII	AR	β-enolase	↑CK ↓enolase 3 activity Reduced protein levels with: focal sarcoplasmic accumulation of glycogen–beta particles (Bx)		Exercise intolerance Increasing myalgia/cramps, fatigue Episodic ↑CK; reduced with rest	Mutations in *ENO3*		Normal life span
XIV Phosphogluco-mutase deficiency type 2	AR 1/1,000,000	Phosphogluco-mutase deficiency type 2	Forearm nonischemic or ischemic test (↑ammonia, ↔lactic acid); CK↑10–20× post exercise Muscle Bx: deficit of muscular *PGM* activity; subsarcolemmal and sarcoplasmic accumulations of glycogen	Childhood	Exercise-induced cramps Rhabdomyolysis post strenuous exertion	Mutations in *PGM1*	Not yet established	Prognosis good

Note. AR = autosomal recessive; CHO = carbohydrates; HOCM = hypertrophic cardiomyopathy; ERT = enzyme replacement therapy; DCM dilated cardiomyopathy.

all forms except VI and IX, which exhibit an X-linked recessive mode of inheritance.

Disorders Producing Dynamic Symptoms (Exercise Intolerance)

GLYCOGEN STORAGE DISEASE TYPE V (GSD V, MCARDLE DISEASE)

GSD V, which results from an inability to mobilize muscle glycogen stores due to the absence of muscle phosphylase,[2] was first described in 1951 by Brian McArdle, when he described a 30-year-old man who presented with muscle weakness and fatigue and antithetical fall in blood lactate following onset of ischemic exercise.[3]

Clinical Features

GSD V is characterized by exercise intolerance with rapid onset muscle pain and cramps, with attacks precipitated by isometric or sustained aerobic exercise and relieved by rest. Myoglobinuria may present in up to 50% of individuals with GSD V, and most, but not necessarily all, may report a "second wind" phenomenon, (although universally present, if patients are exercised in a controlled manner), in which the first phase of exercise is characterized by progressive muscle weakness and fatigue, and rest results in a second adaptive phase of rapid and complete recovery of muscle symptoms facilitating the individual's ability to sustain exercise.[4,5] This adaptation phase results from cardiac, neuronal, and metabolic adaptations to compensate for deficiency of muscle glycogen phosphorylase. The inheritance of GSD V is autosomal recessive, with a reported incidence of 1:100,000. GSDV symptoms classically present in the second and third decades of life and the disorder is associated with a normal life span. Two other muscle phosphorylase deficiency phenotypes are recognized: a fatal infantile form characterized by hypotonia, generalized muscle weakness, and progressive respiratory failure,[6,7] and a late-onset form associated with nonprogressive muscle weakness classically involving proximal musculature.[8]

Clinical Investigations

Diagnosis of GSD V is ultimately confirmed by molecular genetic testing, or the quantitative histochemical or biochemical analysis of a muscle biopsy. However, several clinical investigations support the diagnosis and may be initiated in the outpatient clinic. Serum CK may be raised in the resting state or post isometric or sustained aerobic exercise in the absence of lactic acidosis. Serum electrolytes including potassium, lactate dehydrogenase, renal function, and myoglobin may be increased in cases of suspected rhabdomyolysis. Urine analysis including detection of urinary myoglobin should also be tested if clinically indicated. Nonischemic forearm testing has now superseded ischemic forearm exercise testing in suspected cases of glycolytic defects including GSD V and is characterized by blunted lactate response ("flat lactate curve") to exercise and a reduced postexercise lactate-to-ammonia peak ratio.[9] Plasma lactate concentrations normally increase five- to sixfold above basal values in healthy controls. Incremental exercise testing in GSD V shows a hyperdynamic circulatory response to exercise, sympathetic activation, and increased rate of rise in VO_2 relative to work rate.[10] A pathognomonic heart rate response of the second wind phenomenon in individuals with GSD V can be exploited for diagnostic testing by employing simple heart rate monitoring during moderate constant workload cycle ergometry.[11]

Diagnostic Tests

Muscle biopsy findings characteristically show the absence of myophosphorylase staining on qualitative histochemistry or quantitative biochemical analysis, associated with the subsarcolemmal accumulation of normal glycogen. Phosphorylase-positive fibers have also been described in 19% of muscle biopsies from individuals with GSD V and may explain the second wind phenomenon.[2]

To date, only mutations in the *PYGM* gene are recognized to underlie GSD V. Sequence analysis of the entire coding region of *PYGM* or targeted mutational analyses are performed to diagnose GSDV. It most commonly results from a non-sense mutation at p.Arg50X (previously referred to as p.Arg49X) in exon 1 in North European and Northern American patients.[5,12,13] A second common mutation, p.Gly205Ser, accounts for up to 9% of cases of GSD V in European and American populations.[13]

Treatment

To date, no treatments have been shown to modulate the symptoms of exercise intolerance or ameliorate the risk of myoglobinuria. Dietary manipulation including the ingestion of sucrose pre-exercise has been shown to be effective at improving exercise capacity and well-being [14]. Exploitation of the second wind phenomenon[4] maybe employed to maximize an individual's ability to switch fuel substrates to drive aerobic metabolism. Individuals with GSD V should be advised to avoid isometric and anaerobic exercise as this is likely to result in deleterious muscle damage and increase the risk of rhabdomyolysis and ensuing renal failure. Last, submaximal aerobic exercise training has been shown to be safe and effective in GSD V [15] and aims to improve an individual's metabolic capacity for fatty acid oxidation during exercise, and to circumvent their secondary impairment of oxidative phosphorylation due to lack of pyruvate generation via glycolysis.

GLYCOGEN STORAGE DISEASE TYPE VII (GSD VII, TARUI DISEASE)

GSD VII is a rare metabolic disorder of glycogen metabolism, first reported in 1965[16]; approximately 100 cases[17] have been reported to date. It is transmitted as an autosomal-recessive trait and results from deficiency of muscle phosphofructokinase (PFKM). Mature human muscle exclusively expresses the M4-homotetramer only and patients typically have complete loss of PFKM activity in muscle with only a partial defect in red blood cells. PFK is recognized as the most prominent regulatory enzyme (rate-limiting step) for glycolysis,[18] and PFK catalyzes the conversion of fructose-6-phosphate to fructose-1,6-bisphosphate.

Clinical Features

GSD VII is clinically indistinguishable from McArdle disease, except for the absence of a typical second wind phenomenon[19] and the presence of a compensated hemolysis with increased bilirubin, reticulocytes, and hyperuricemia (myogenic hyperuricemia), which is a pathophysiologic feature of GSD III, V, and VII.[20] Individuals with the classic form of GSD VII present with exercise intolerance and muscle weakness most pronounced following exercise, in addition to joint contractures, anemia, jaundice, and myoglobinuria. Two other forms include a severe infantile presentation with variable multisystem features including myopathy, psychomotor retardation, cataracts, seizures, cortical blindness, joint contractures, encephalopathy, and cortical and cerebellar atrophy, with death usually occurring during early childhood due to respiratory failure or cardiomyopathy[21-27]; and a late-onset presentation with progressive muscle and fixed limb weakness most pronounced following exercise, with contractures but no myoglobinuria or cramps, and also reported in association with ischemic heart disease and valvular heart disease.

Clinical Investigations

Clinical investigations supporting the diagnosis include elevated serum CK. Hyperuricemia with raised bilirubin and reticulocytes may also be detected, which is worsened by exercise and is indicative of a compensated hemolysis associated with GSD VII. Myoglobinuria may occur following intense exercise. Forearm exercise testing typically reveals a blunted lactate response (with a normal ammonia rise).

Diagnostic Tests

A deficiency of phosphofructokinase can be detected in a muscle biopsy (1%–33% residual activity) and the presence of polyglucosan (abnormal glycogen) in muscle may be observed.[28] Molecular genetic testing may reveal mutations in the gene encoding the M subunit of the enzyme.

Treatment

Definitive treatments for GSD VII have not yet been established. Patients should be advised to avoid anaerobic exercise and to aim for increased dietary protein intake. The administration of glucose prior to initiation of exercise has been shown to be detrimental in individuals with GSD VII, and exacerbates exercise intolerance. This is because the metabolic block in PFK deficiency occurs below the entry of glucose into glycolysis and hence glucose cannot be used as a fuel for energy production. Moreover, individuals with GSD VII have been shown to exhibit a decrease in circulating free fatty acids and ketones that are normally used as alternative energy sources in the absence of glucose, referred to as "out of wind phenomenon."[29-31] Myoglobinuria may lead to renal failure and rhabdomyolysis should be managed appropriately. The prognosis is good in the classic form if strenuous exercise is avoided.

MUSCLE FORM OF GLYCOGEN STORAGE DISEASE TYPE IX (GSD IX, PHOSPHORYLASE B KINASE DEFICIENCY)

GSD IX results from a deficiency of the enzyme phosphorylase b kinase (PHK). PHK is a multimeric enzyme that comprises four copies each of four subunits (α, β, γ, and δ).

Clinical Features

This rare form of GSD has two types: liver PHK deficiency, characterized by growth retardation and hepatomegaly with/without fasting hypoglycemia and ketosis; and muscle PHK deficiency, which is extremely rare, and is characterized by exercise intolerance, myalgia, muscle cramps, myoglobinuria, and progressive muscle weakness.[32] Mutations in *PHKA1*, encoding the α subunit, cause this rare X-linked disorder of muscle PHK deficiency, which, to date, has been described only in men, and may present from childhood to adulthood.[33-37]

Clinical Investigations

The serum CK may be above the upper limits of normal in suspected cases of GSD IX. Myoglobinuria may occur following submaximal exercise. Ischemic forearm testing reveals a normal venous lactate rise, suggesting that glycogenolysis is normal under maximal exercise (anaerobic) conditions.[36,38] During submaximal cycle ergometry, there is no change in lactate (blunted glycogenolysis) suggesting that PHK plays a greater role in the activation of muscle glycogen phosphorylase b (myophosphorylase) during submaximal exercise than during maximal exercise.

Diagnostic Tests

Muscle glycogen content is always elevated with normal glycogen structure, and there is modest accumulation of subsarcolemmal glycogen in muscle PHK deficiency. Muscle PHK enzyme activity is markedly reduced, and the activity of glycogen phosphorylase (phosphorylase-a) may also be reduced as PHK also activates muscle glycogen phosphorylase.[32] Molecular genetic testing will reveal mutations in *PHKA1*.

Treatment

A multidisciplinary and multispecialty approach should be undertaken and should include a metabolic disease specialist/biochemical geneticist in addition to a neurologist with interest in neuromuscular disease, a neuromuscular physiotherapist, a genetic counselor, and a metabolic dietician to advise on optimization of blood glucose concentrations based on levels of habitual physical activity and structured exercise.

GLYCOGEN STORAGE DISEASE TYPE X (GSD X, PHOSPHOGLYCERATE MUTASE DEFICIENCY)

GSD X, first reported in 1981, is a rare metabolic myopathy resulting from deficient phosphoglycerate mutase (PAGM) enzyme activity. To date, only 15 individuals have been reported, with this form of glycogen storage disease.[39,40]

Clinical Features

Individuals with PGAM deficiency may often be clinically asymptomatic and then present with exercise-induced cramps and recurrent myoglobinuria.

Clinical Investigations

Serum CK may be above the upper limits of normal in suspected cases of GSD X. Myoglobinuria occurs following brief, strenuous efforts of exercise.

Diagnostic Tests

A striking finding in muscle of patients with PGAM deficiency is tubular aggregates in the skeletal muscle biopsy, originating from the sarcoplasmic reticulum. These are nonpathognomonic pathological findings but among the GSDs are unique to this form of GSD.[41,42] Molecular genetic testing revealed mutations in *PGAM2* in all 15 cases of PGAM deficiency. Of those studied at a molecular level, all African American patients harbored the W78X mutation, supporting a founder effect.[43]

Treatment

Definitive treatments have not yet been established. Generic advice for all forms of GSD, including symptomatic treatment and modulation of habitual physical activity and structured exercise, should be given.

GLYCOGEN STORAGE DISEASE TYPE XIII (GSD XIII)

Clinical Features

GSD XIII is a very rare form of GSD (prevalence unknown), which usually presents in childhood. The disorder is due to β-enolase deficiency, and is characterized by exercise-induced muscle weakness, myalgia, and fatigue. Symptoms improve with rest and prognosis is good, with an expected normal lifespan.[44]

Clinical Investigations

Episodic increases in serum CK may be noted in this form of GSD. No rise of serum lactate is observed in GSD XIII on ischemic forearm exercise testing.

Diagnostic Tests

Enolase-3 activity is low in skeletal muscle and β-enolase protein is dramatically reduced. The focal accumulation of glycogen-β particles may be observed within the sarcoplasm. Identification of mutations in *ENO3* has been reported in GSD XIII.[44]

Treatment

Definitive treatments have not yet been established. Generic advice as all forms of GSD, including symptomatic treatment and modulation of habitual physical activity and structured exercise, should be given.

Disorders Producing Static Symptoms (Fixed Weakness)

GLYCOGEN STORAGE DISEASE TYPE II (GSD II, POMPE DISEASE; ACID MALTASE DEFICIENCY)

GSD II is a multisystem metabolic myopathy, transmitted as an autosomal-recessive trait, resulting from deficient acid-alpha glucosidase (GAA) activity, an enzyme that degrades lysosomal glycogen, giving rise to lysosomal expansion in many tissues but predominantly in cardiac and skeletal muscle. The carrier frequency of GSD II has been estimated at 1 in 40,000,[45] with the incidence of Pompe disease dependent on ethnicity and geographical region evaluated.[46]

Clinical Features

In the most severe forms of GSD II, disease onset is in infancy and characterized by hypotonia, generalized muscle weakness, feeding difficulties, and failure to thrive; death results from cardiac and respiratory failure within the first one or two years of life. Canonical features of the milder late-onset form of GSD II include progressive muscle weakness and respiratory failure (a key distinguishing feature[47]) without clinically apparent cardiac muscle involvement, that results in premature death. Muscle weakness in late-onset GSD II primarily affects proximal and trunk musculature, and affects lower more often than upper limbs.[48]

Clinical Investigations

More than 95% of late-onset cases of GSD II have elevated CK levels[49]; however, individuals with GSD II and CK levels within normal range have been reported. Liver function blood parameters including AST, ALT, and LDH may be elevated in all forms of GSD II. Urine analysis of glucose tetrasaccharide by HPLC is a useful marker for the investigation of patients with GSD II.[50]

Diagnostic Tests

GAA activity is reduced in lymphocytes or leukocytes in GSDII, and can be detected in a dried blood spot. GAA activity is reduced in skeletal muscle, with evidence of vacuolated cells and increased lysosomal glycogen on histological examination. GAA activity is also reduced in skin fibroblasts from individuals with GSD II. Molecular genetic testing will reveal mutations in *GAA*.

Treatment

A multidisciplinary and multispecialty approach should be undertaken and should include a metabolic disease specialist/biochemical geneticist in addition to the specialists dictated by clinical manifestations. These include a neurologist with interest in neuromuscular disease, a pulmonologist, a respiratory physiotherapist, a neuromuscular physiotherapist, a genetic counselor, and a metabolic dietician.[46]

Enzyme replacement therapy (ERT) with recombinant human GAA has proven beneficial in cardiac muscle and infantile forms of GSD II.[51,52] However, the role of ERT in adults has yet to be clarified.[53] Because the benefits of ERT are lessened by the development of antibodies to the enzyme, other approaches are now under development.

GLYCOGEN STORAGE DISEASE TYPE III (GSD III, CORI-FORBES DISEASE; DEBRANCHER ENZYME DEFICIENCY)

GSD III is an autosomal-recessive inborn error of metabolism that primarily affects liver, heart, and skeletal muscle. GSD III was first described in 1928,[54] but it was not until almost four decades later, following Gilbert Forbes's (1953) meticulous description of a third case of the disorder, that the causative metabolic defect relating to debrancher enzyme deficiency was identified.[55,56] GSD III has an incidence ranging from 1:5,400 of individuals of North African Jewish descent to 1:100,000 in the United States. There is marked phenotypic and enzymatic heterogeneity in individuals with GSD III,[57,58] with four subtypes: GSD IIIa and GSD IIId individuals manifest liver and muscle symptoms; those with GSD IIIb have isolated liver involvement; and those with GSD IIIc manifest muscle symptoms only. GSD IIIc and IIId are extremely rare[42,57,59]; the following section refers primarily to GSD IIIa.

Clinical Features

GSD III usually presents in childhood and is characterized by fixed and mostly distal muscle weakness[60] (although it can affect both proximal and distal muscles[48]). The disorder does not affect muscles of respiration but it may cause a cardiomyopathy.[61-64] The simultaneous involvement of muscle and nerve has been reported, potentially explaining why the muscle weakness is fixed from an early stage.[43,65,66]

Laboratory Findings

The serum CK may be raised in cases of GSD III with heart and skeletal muscle involvement.

Hypoglycemia, hyperlipidemia, and abnormal liver function may be detected in children with GSD III. Ischemic forearm testing reveals a blunted lactate response (with a normal ammonia rise). A glucagon administration 2 hours after a carbohydrate-rich meal results in a normal rise in blood sugar, whereas no change in blood glucose occurs following an overnight fast and glucagon challenge.

Diagnostic Tests

Muscle biopsy samples usually demonstrate excessive and structurally abnormal accumulation of glycogen with shorter outer branches and nonfunctioning or low-functioning debranching enzyme activity. Identification of pathogenic mutations in *AGL*, located on chromosome 1p21, has been reported on both alleles.[67]

Treatment

Definitive treatments have not yet been established. Management is primarily symptomatic. A multidisciplinary and multispecialty approach should be undertaken and should include a metabolic disease specialist/biochemical geneticist in addition to the specialists dictated by clinical manifestations, including a neurologist with interest in neuromuscular disease, a cardiologist, a neuromuscular physiotherapist, a genetic counselor, and a metabolic dietician.[48]

GLYCOGEN STORAGE DISEASE TYPE IV (GSD IV, ANDERSEN DISEASE; BRANCHING ENZYME)

Andersen disease is an extremely rare form of glycogen storage disorders that predominates among people of Ashkenazi Jewish descent, with a reported prevalence of 1:600,000 to 1:800,000, and results from deficient glycogen branching enzyme (GBE) activity. This results in the deposition of polyglucosan, an amylopectin-like polysaccharide in various tissues.

Clinical Features

GSD IV is a clinically heterogeneous metabolic disorder with a spectrum of disease manifestations, including the classical hepatic form, with liver cirrhosis and failure requiring solid organ transplantation; progressive muscle weakness resulting in early fatality within the first 5 years of life; and previously underdiagnosed neuromuscular presentations.[43] A fatal, perinatal neuromuscular subtype, characterized by fetal akinesia deformation sequence, with decreased fetal movements, polyhydramnios, and fetal hydrops, has been described; as has a neuromuscular subtype in newborns, with profound hypotonia, respiratory distress, dilated cardiomyopathy in early childhood, and progressive muscle weakness resulting in early fatality within the first 5 years of life.[41,68,69] Two other forms exist: a nonprogressive hepatic form of GSD IV that is characterized by liver dysfunction that normalizes with age and myopathy and is associated with a good prognosis, and a childhood neuromuscular subtype that presents in the second decade of life and is characterized by mild to severe myopathy and dilated cardiomyopathy. Prognosis of this latter form is variable depending on disease severity, with austere manifestations resulting in death by the third decade of life.

Clinical Investigations

The serum CK is usually normal in suspected cases of GSD IV irrespective of the severity of neuromuscular involvement. Hematological studies show evidence of anemia due to coagulopathy or splenic sequestration, prolonged prothrombin time, and activated partial thromboplastin time; reduced fibrinogen; and elevated AST, ALT, GGT, serum alkaline phosphatase, and bilirubin due to liver dysfunction.

Diagnostic Tests

Blood, muscle, or liver biopsy samples demonstrate abnormal glycogen content and deficient *GBE* activity in GSD IV. Cultured skin fibroblasts may also demonstrate abnormal glycogen content in GSD IV. Deficient *GBE* activity in cultured amniocytes and chorionic villi are used in prenatal testing of suspected GSD IV.[70] Another method of prenatal diagnosis may include identification of polyglucosan bodies. Molecular genetic testing reveals pathogenic mutations in *GBE1*, which are the most common cause of GSD IV.

Treatment

To date, treatment for GSD IV is supportive. A multidisciplinary and multispecialty approach should be undertaken and should include a metabolic disease specialist/biochemical geneticist in addition to the specialists dictated by clinical manifestations, including a neurologist with interest in neuromuscular disease, a cardiologist, a neuromuscular physiotherapist, an occupational therapist, a genetic counselor, and a metabolic dietician.

GLYCOGEN STORAGE DISEASE TYPE XII (GSD XII, RED CELL ALDOLASE DEFICIENCY)

GSD Type XII is a very rare form of GSD (prevalence unknown), which is inherited as an autosomal-recessive trait, and results from the deficiency of aldolase A.[71] Aldolase A is an enzyme found in the developing embryo and in abundance in adult muscle, that catalyzes the cleavage of fructose-1,6-diphosphate into triose phosphates (glyceraldehyde 3-phosphate and dihydroxyacetone phosphate).

Clinical Features

GSD XII usually presents in infancy and is characterized by exercise intolerance rhabdomyolysis and hemolytic anemia, with muscle weakness, anemia, and jaundice often triggered by febrile illnesses.[72,73] Dysmorphic features have also been reported including ptosis, short neck, low hairline,[74] short stature, mental retardation, and delayed puberty.[75]

Clinical Investigations

Patients may show hematological evidence of hemolytic anemia, elevated myoglobin, raised blood CK and lactate dehydrogenase levels, and the presence of urinary myoglobin.

Diagnostic Tests.

Identification of mutations in *ALDOA*, which maps to chromosome 16p11.2,[76] has been reported in GSD XII.[71,73]

Treatment

To date, no treatments have been shown to be effective. Supportive measures include avoidance of anaerobic exercise, aggressive treatment of febrile conditions, and red cell transfusions in cases of severe anemia.

GLYCOGEN STORAGE DISEASE TYPE XIV (GSD XIV)

GSD XIV is an extremely rare form of GSD (prevalence = 1:1,000,000), with only two cases reported to date.[31,77] It is transmitted as an autosomal-recessive trait, and results from the deficiency of phosphoglucomutase (PGM). During glycogen metabolism, PGM enzymatic activity is responsible for the switch between glucose-6-phosphate and glucose-1-phosphate. Deficiency of PGM results in metabolic impedance of the glycolytic pathway after glucose-1-phosphate and before glucose-6-phosphate.

Clinical Features

GSD XIV usually presents in childhood, and is characterized by recurrent exercise-induced cramps. Rhabdomyolysis usually only occurs after strenuous exertion. Prognosis is good and GSD XIV is likely associated with a normal lifespan.

Clinical Investigations

Episodic increases in serum CK may be noted in this form of GSD, with a 10- to 20-fold rise post exercise. Ischemic forearm testing can reveal hyperammonemia, and normal elevation of serum lactate may be observed,[77] but a blunted lactate response has been reported.[72]

Diagnostic Tests

A deficit of muscle PGM activity and subsarcolemmal and sarcoplasmic accumulation of glycogen are present in the muscle biopsy. Mutations in *PGM1* has been reported in GSD XIV.

Treatment

Definitive treatments have not yet been established. Generic advice for all forms of GSD should be given, including symptomatic treatment and modulation of habitual physical activity and structured exercise.

DEFECTS OF LIPID METABOLISM

Carnitine Deficiency and Related Disorders

Carnitine is endogenously produced by the liver and kidneys but is also derived from meat and dairy products in the diet. Carnitine plays an essential role in the transfer of long-chain fatty acids into the mitochondrial matrix for beta oxidation (Table 7–2). It binds acyl residues and helps in their elimination from the body in urine. Primary carnitine deficiency results from a deficiency in the plasma membrane carnitine transporter,[78,79] found in kidney and muscle, resulting in systemic carnitine depletion with urinary carnitine wasting. The balance between plasma and tissue concentrations of carnitine is evident when its levels drop below 20% of normal, resulting in clinical manifestations.

Secondary carnitine deficiency may also occur as a result of either inadequate dietary intake, as seen in vegetarians or patients on prolonged total parenteral nutrition, or due to excessive urinary losses of free and acetylated carnitine, as in Fanconi syndrome or patients on renal dialysis.[80,81] Valproic acid may cause secondary carnitine deficiency because it contributes to the formation of acylcarnitine products and the inhibition of carnitine transport in renal cells by acylcarnitines.[82]

Primary deficiency of carnitine is an autosomal-recessive disorder that results in the impairment of transfer of long-chain fatty acids into the mitochondria for beta oxidation with the reduction of energy and ketone body formation. This is associated with the accumulation of acyl CoA esters in the mitochondria, which impacts on the other energy-producing pathways dependent on CoA including amino acid metabolism, the Krebs cycle, and mitochondrial, peroxisomal, and pyruvate oxidation.[83]

The prevalence of primary carnitine deficiency ranges from 1:15,500 to 1:100,000, with no gender predilection observed.[78,79,84]

CLINICAL FEATURES

Carnitine deficiency commonly manifests in the "primary state" as a progressive dilated cardiomyopathy (DCM) presenting at a late age. It is resistant to standard cardiac medications including inotropes and diuretics.[85] Cardiac death ensues if carnitine replacement is not commenced. Secondary carnitine deficiency may also lead to a form of DCM caused by defects in beta-oxidation, including long-chain 3-hydroxyyacyl-CoA dehydrogenase (LCHAD). Primary carnitine deficiency resulting in hypoketotic, hypoglycemic encephalopathy, hepatomegaly, elevated

Table 7–2 Disorder of Lipid Metabolism

Type/ Eponym	Inherit-ance/ Incidence	Enzyme Involved	Diagnosis	Ageo Onset	Clinical Features	Genetics	Treatment
Carnitine deficiency	AR 1/15,500–1/100,000	Plasma membrane carnitine transporter	Clinical investigations Carnitine uptake assay in cultured fibroblasts Tandem mass spectrometry: Newborn screening Molecular genetic testing	Infancy/ chilldhood Adulthood	DCM Metabolic acidosis Hypoketotic hypoglycemia Elevated ammonia Elevated liver enzymes Hyperuricemia Raised CK Lactic acidosis Ketonuria Indolent myopathy, exercise intolerance, myalgia, fatigue	Mutations in OCTN2 gene	*Dietary* L-carnitine supplementation
CPTII	AR 1:100,000	Carnitine palmitoyl-transferase	Clinical investigations ↑creatine kinase ↓glucose Raised liver enzymes Tandem mass spectrometry (C16 peak) Enzymatic activity in fibroblasts/lymphocytes Molecular genetic testing	Neonatal (Day 4) Infantile Adult	*At birth* hypoglycemic seizures Hepatomegaly Liver failure Respiratory failure Cardiomyopathy Neuronal migration brain abnormalities Hypoketotic hypoglycemic seizures and encephalopathy. Hepatomegaly Liver failure Respiratory failure Cardiomyopathy Myoglobinuria Rhabdomyolysis Recurrent muscle pain and weakness	Mutations in CPTII gene	*Dietary* Lipid restriction L-carnitine supplementation Replacement of long-chain with medium-chain triglycerides Avoidance of prolonged fasting and exercise Glucose infusions Triheptanoin (anaplerotic) diet

(continued)

Table 7–2 (Cont.)

Type/ Eponym	Inherit-ance/ Incidence	Enzyme Involved	Diagnosis	Age o Onset	Clinical Features	Genetics	Treatment
MAD	AR	Myoadenylate deaminase	Clinical investigations ↑/→creatine kinase Forearm nonischemic or ischemic test No ammonia production Molecular genetic testing	Early childhood to late adulthood	Exercise-induced cramps, myalgia and early fatigue	Mutations in AMPD1 gene	Dietary D-ribose ingestion
MH	AD		Clinical investigations ↑creatine kinase ↑urine myoglobin Caffeine halothane contracture test Molecular genetic testing	Any stage	Anesthetic-induced core body temperature rise Muscle contraction & rigidity Cardiac arrhythmias Multiorgan failure	Mutations in GAA	Cooling with blankets and antipyretics IV fluids Dantrolene Lidocaine Beta-blockers Avoidance of stimulant drugs, volatile inhalational anaesthetic agents, and succinylcholine
VLCAD	AR 1:12,000	Very-long-chain acyl-coenzyme A dehydrogenase	Clinical investigations Myopathic form: ↑/→creatine kinase (10% always raised) ↑urinary myoglobin (episodic) Tandem mass spectrometry—fasting (C14:1, C14:2, C14, C12:1) Newborn screening Enzymatic activity in fibroblasts Immunoreactive VLCAD protein antigen expression analysis (10% of controls) Molecular genetic testing	Early onset cardiac and multi-organ Hepatic/ hypoketotic hypoglycemia Late onset myopathic (Adolescence to adulthood)	Cardiomyopathy Hepatomegaly intermittent hypoglycemia Myopathy Hepatomegaly Hypoketotic hypoglycemia Exercise intolerance Intermittent myoglobinuria Rhabdomyolysis Renal failure Hypercapnic respiratory failure	Mutations in ACADVL	Dietary Low-fat diet Replacement of long-chain with medium-chain triglycerides Avoidance of prolonged fasting and strenuous exercise IV glucose and hydration/urine alkalisation during acute episodes

	Inheritance/Incidence	Enzyme defect	Clinical investigations	Age of onset	Clinical features	Molecular genetics	Management
LCHADD	AR 1:150–1:90,000 (one case: paternal isodisomy Chrom 2)	Long-chain 3-hydroxyacyl-coenzyme A dehydrogenase	Clinical investigations Plasma carnitine: low Long-chain acylcarnitine levels: ↑ with 3-hydroxydicarboxylic derivatives of C16:0, C18:1, & C18:2 Serum fatty acid analysis Enzymatic activity in fibroblasts Molecular genetic testing Prenatal testing	Early onset Later childhood Adulthood	Hypoketotic hypoglycemia Cardiomyopathy Myopathy Hepatic dysfunction Neuropathy Retinopathy Sudden infant death Muscle pain Rhabdomyolysis Neuropathy Retinopathy Exercise induced pain & rhabdomyolysis 70% of all forms: visual loss	Mutations in *MTP* (G1528C accounts for 90% of mutant alleles)	*Dietary* Low fat diet Replacement of long-chain with medium-chain triglycerides Avoidance of prolonged fasting and strenuous exercise Medium-chain triglyceride oil (MCT oil) L-carnitine Docosahexanoic acid (visual loss)
MCAD	AR 1:4,900–1:17,000	Muscle glycogen phosphorylase	Clinical investigations ↓ glucose ↓ ketones ↑ ammonia Acylcarnitine profile analysis: ↑ C6–C10 (prominent octanoylcarnitine) Urinary organic acids: ↑C6 > C8 > C10; inappropriately low ketones Urinary suberylglycine/acyl-glycine analysis Enzymatic activity in fibroblasts Molecular genetic testing Newborn screening	Early infancy (3–24 months) to adulthood	Hypoketotic hypoglycemia Vomiting Lethargy Hyperammonaemia Liver dysfunction Fatty liver infiltration	Mutations in *ACADM* gene (p.Lys304Glu)	*Dietary* Low fat diet/Avoidance of prolonged fasting, infant formula with medium-chain triglycerides, and vigorous exercise Oral/IV carbohydrate Uncooked corn starch

(continued)

Table 7–2 (Cont.)

Type/ Eponym	Inheritance/ Incidence	Enzyme Involved	Diagnosis	Ageo Onset	Clinical Features	Genetics	Treatment
HADH (SCHAD)	AR extremely rare	3-hydroxyacyl-CoA dehydrogenase deficiency	Clinical investigations ↓ Glucose ↑ Insulin Acylcarnitine profile analysis: ↑ hydroxyl-butyrylcarnitine Urinary organic acids: ↑ 3-hydroxyglutarate Enzymatic activity in fibroblasts, reduced expression and function of HADH enzyme Molecular genetic testing	Infancy/early childhood	Persistent hypoglycemia Hyperinsulinemia Vomiting Diarrhea Lethargy Hypotonia Myopathy Fulminant liver failure Cardiac Seizures Sudden infant death	Mutations in HADH gene	Dietary Protein restriction Diazoxide (↓Glucose) Liver transplantation

Note. AR = autosomal recessive.

liver transaminases, and hyperammonemia frequently occurs in infancy, and attacks are often triggered by viral infections or fasting. If carnitine is not replaced, recurrent episodes of encephalopathy will ensue, resulting in CNS dysfunction and developmental delay.[86-88]

Carnitine deficiency may also present as an indolent or progressive myopathy that manifests in the second and third decade of adult life. This was first described in 1973[89] and is one of the few known lipid metabolism myopathies. Myopathic carnitine deficiency, caused by a defect in the muscle carnitine transporter, is characterized by normal serum concentrations of carnitine but severe depletion of carnitine levels in muscle. Patients typically present with proximal muscle weakness of varying severity, exercise intolerance, muscle fatigue, and myalgia.

CLINICAL INVESTIGATIONS

Clinical investigations include checking for a metabolic acidosis, in addition to blood glucose, urine ketones, elevated ammonia levels, and liver enzymes (which are usually moderately elevated), in addition to raised uric acid, serum CK, and lactic acid.

DIAGNOSTIC TESTS

Carnitine uptake assay in cultured fibroblasts is a confirmatory test for carnitine deficiency. Primary carnitine deficiency is caused by mutations in the *OCTN2* gene.[88] The biochemical basis of the muscle form of the disease is yet to be determined. Tandem mass spectrometry is now employed in extended newborn screening programs in several regions of the United States.

TREATMENT

Oral supplementation with L-carnitine is recognized to improve muscle strength and reduce lipid content in muscle fibers in myopathic carnitine deficiency.

Carnitine Palmitoyltransferase (CPT II) Deficiency

CPT II deficiency is the most common inherited disorder of lipid metabolism affecting adult skeletal muscle, and the most frequent cause of hereditary myoglobinuria. CPT II deficiency is characterized by failure to transport long-chain fatty acids into the mitochondria matrix, where they are a fuel source for energy production. The disorder was first described in 1973 by DiMauro and DiMauro in a familial syndrome of recurrent myoglobinuria[90] with episodes of rhabdomyolysis frequently triggered by prolonged fasting or exercise. Carnitine, which is a natural substance derived from meat and dairy food, mitigates the transport of hydrophobic long-chain fatty acids, harnessing these as an important fuel source for β oxidation. This is catalyzed by three enzymes that form the "carnitine shuttle"[86]: carnitine palmitoyltransferase I (CPT I), carnitine-acylcarnitine translocase, and CPT II, an inner mitochondrial membrane protein that catalyzes the transesterification of palmitoylcarnitine to the activated substrate of β-oxidation, palmitoyl-CoA.[91] This metabolic disorder has an autosomal-recessive pattern of inheritance; it usually presents in early childhood and has male sex predominance.[92]

CLINICAL FEATURES

Three clinical forms of CPTII are recognized, classified based on age of presentation and pattern of symptoms: neonatal, infantile, and adult forms.

The neonatal form is the least prevalent, is characterized by early onset (usually within 4 days of life), and is invariably fatal irrespective of supportive care. Affected babies present with hypoglycemic seizures, hepatomegaly culminating in liver failure, respiratory failure, and cardiomyopathy. Neuronal-migration brain abnormalities have also been reported.

The infantile form classically presents before 1 year of age and is characterized by hypoketotic hypoglycemic seizures and encephalopathy. Hepatomegaly culminating in liver failure, respiratory failure, and cardiomyopathy are also associated with this form of CPT II deficiency. Episodes are frequently triggered by infection, febrile illnesses, and fasting.

The adult form has a purely myopathic phenotype, and presents with myoglobinuria, rhabdomyolysis, and recurrent muscle pain and weakness. Events are classically provoked by exercise, fasting, febrile illnesses, cold, and a diet high in fat. Age of onset is variably between 6 and 20 years, and the clinical course is usually indolent.

CLINICAL INVESTIGATIONS

In the myopathic form, the serum CK level is usually normal between attacks. Approximately 10% of individuals have a persistently elevated serum CK. Total and free carnitine levels are low, and acylcarnitine:free carnitine ratios are high in the disorder. Transaminases are frequently raised during attacks in CPTII deficiency. Myoglobinuria is frequently present during attacks in the myopathic form of CPT II deficiency. In neonatal and infantile forms, hyperammonemia and metabolic acidosis may be present.

DIAGNOSTIC TESTS

Tandem mass spectrometry is usually used to diagnose the disorder, and can be performed on a dried blood spot. This reveals a peak at C16. Enzymatic activity in fibroblasts or lymphocytes may also be used in the diagnosis of CPT II deficiency. Molecular genetic testing is the definitive test for diagnosis. Testing of the *CPT2* gene mapped to chromosomal locus 1p32 reveals the p.Ser113Leu mutation in ~60% of mutant alleles in the adult-onset form.[93,94]

TREATMENT

A multidisciplinary and multispecialty approach should be undertaken and should include a metabolic disease specialist/biochemical geneticist in addition to the specialists dictated by clinical manifestations, including a neurologist with interest in neuromuscular disease, a neuromuscular physiotherapist, an occupational therapist, a genetic counselor, and a metabolic dietician. Treatment includes dietary restriction of lipid intake, replacement of long-chain with medium-chain triglycerides supplemented with L-carnitine, and avoidance of prolonged fasting and exercise. Infusions of glucose during intercurrent infections and adequate hydration to prevent renal failure during episodes of myoglobinuria should be instigated. Avoidance of anesthetic agents and drugs including valproic acid, ibuprofen, and diazepam in high doses pertains to the pediatric form of disease.[94] Recent therapeutic use of a triheptanoin (anaplerotic) diet appears to be an effective treatment in adult-onset CPTII deficiency.[95]

Very-Long-Chain Acyl-Coenzyme A Dehydrogenase Deficiency (VLCAD)

Very long-chain acyl-coenzyme A dehydrogenase deficiency results in an inability to catalyze the first step of mitochondrial beta-oxidation of long-chain (14–20 carbon) fatty acids and is transmitted as an autosomal-recessive trait. The true prevalence of VLCAD is unknown; however, the incidence of short-chain, medium-chain, and very-long-chain acyl-CoA dehydrogenase deficiencies is estimated at approximately 1:12,000.[96]

CLINICAL FEATURES

Three clinical forms of VLCAD are recognized, classified based on age of presentation and pattern of symptoms: severe early-onset cardiac and multiorgan failure, hepatic or hypoketotic hypoglycemic, and later-onset episodic myopathic forms.[97]

The severe early-onset cardiac and multiorgan failure form is the least prevalent and is characterized by early onset, usually within first few months of life, and is often fatal, but may be reversible with early intervention. Affected babies may present with either hypertrophic or dilated cardiomyopathy, in addition to pericardial effusion, and arrhythmias.[98] Systemic features include hypotonia, hepatomegaly, and intermittent hypoglycemia.

The hepatic or hypoketotic hypoglycemic form classically presents in early childhood and is characterized by hypoketotic hypoglycemia and hepatomegaly in the absence of cardiomyopathy. Episodes are frequently triggered by infection, febrile illnesses, and fasting.

The adult form, which is likely the most common phenotype, presents with exercise intolerance characterized by intermittent myoglobinuria and rhabdomyolysis, recurrent muscle pain, and cramps.[99] Events are classically provoked by vigorous exercise, fasting, and a diet high in long-chain fat, as the body changes energy substrate from carbohydrates to fatty acids, especially slow skeletal muscles that use longer chain fatty acid oxidation.[100,101] Age of onset is variably between adolescence to adulthood, and the clinical course is mediated by the risk of ensuing renal failure following bouts of rhabdomyolysis. Hypercapnic respiratory failure has been reported in VLCAD in an isolated case.[102]

CLINICAL INVESTIGATIONS

In the myopathic form, the serum CK level is usually normal between attacks. Approximately 10% of individuals have permanently elevated serum CK. Urinary myoglobinuria is frequently present during attacks in the myopathic form of VLCAD.

DIAGNOSTIC TESTS

Tandem mass spectrometry is usually used to diagnose the disorder, and can be performed on a dried blood spot in the fasting state or during an episode of metabolic stress. This measures C4 to C20 straight-chain acyl-carnitine esters, 3-hydroxy-acyl carnitine esters, and unsaturated acyl-carnitine esters, and most frequently shows abnormalities in C14:1, C14:2, C14, and C12:1.[103] Results may be normal following glucose infusion, in the fed state, or in individuals with a mild phenotype.

Enzymatic activity in fibroblasts and/or lymphocytes and/or skeletal muscle and/or amniocytes may also be used in the diagnosis of VLCAD deficiency. Immunoreactive VLCAD protein antigen expression analysis may also be employed with measured levels below 10% of control specimens indicative of VLCAD. Molecular genetic testing is the definitive test for diagnosis. Testing of the *ACADVL* gene mapped to chromosomal locus 17p13.1 reveals clear correlation between genotype and phenotype in the adult onset form of VLCAD.[105]

TREATMENT

A multidisciplinary and multispecialty approach should be undertaken and should include a metabolic disease specialist/biochemical geneticist in addition to the specialists dictated by clinical manifestations, including a neurologist with an interest in neuromuscular disease, a neuromuscular physiotherapist, an occupational therapist, a genetic counselor, and a metabolic dietician.

Specific treatment includes dietary restriction of high-fat diet, replacement of long-chain with medium-chain triglycerides, and avoidance of prolonged fasting and vigorous exercise. Infusions of glucose during acute episodes and adequate hydration and alkalization of urine to prevent renal failure during episodes of myoglobinuria should be instigated in individuals with VLCAD.

Long-Chain 3-Hydroxyacyl-Coenzyme A Dehydrogenase Deficiency (LCHADD)

Long-chain 3-hydroxyacyl-coenzyme A dehydrogenase forms part of the mitochondrial trifunctional protein.[106] A deficiency of this enzyme results in an inability to use certain dietary fats or stored fats as an energy substrate, precipitating metabolic crises during episodes of prolonged fasting, including overnight sleep, and febrile illnesses, when glycogen stores are deplete.

LCHADD is transmitted as an autosomal-recessive trait, but an unusual case of LCHADD deficiency due to paternal isodisomy of chromosome 2 has been reported[107,108]. The true prevalence of LCHADD is unknown but the carrier rate has been estimated at 1:150 to 1:90,000.

CLINICAL FEATURES

LCHADD is characterized by early onset cardiomyopathy that may be fatal,[109] myopathy, hypoglycemia, hepatic dysfunction,[110,111] neuropathy, and pigmented retinopathy.[106] Sudden infant death syndrome has been reported in LCHADD.[112] Later in childhood, myopathic features including muscle pain, rhabdomyolysis, neuropathy, and retinopathy may predominate; other individuals may present solely with myopathic features of exercise-induced pain and rhabdomyolysis in adulthood.[113] Progressive visual loss may affect up to 70% of those affected by LCHADD.

CLINICAL INVESTIGATIONS

During acute episodes, hypoketotic hypogly-cemia is a metabolic hallmark of LCHADD. Serum CK is usually elevated in addition to ammonia, uric acid, and liver enzymes, and often there is profound lactic acidaemia. Urinary ketones, myoglobinuria, and organic acids are frequently elevated during attacks in the myopathic form of LCHADD.

DIAGNOSTIC TESTS

Plasma carnitine levels are low and long-chain acylcarnitine levels are increased with 3-hydroxydicarboxylic derivatives of the C16:0, C18:1, and C18:2 during acute attacks in indi-viduals with LCHADD. Results may be nor-mal between attacks. Serum fatty acid analysis may be a useful diagnostic tool and may show 3-hydroxylated compounds, even between attacks.

Enzymatic activity in fibroblasts may also be used in the diagnosis of LCHADD deficiency. Molecular genetic testing is the definitive test for diagnosis. Most individuals are homozygous for a guanine-to-cytosine transition at position 1528 (G1528C), involving the alpha subunit of MTP and accounts for about 90% of mutant alleles. Guidelines for prenatal testing for LCHADD have been devised.[114-116]

TREATMENT

A multidisciplinary and multispecialty approach should be undertaken and should include a met-abolic disease specialist/biochemical geneticist in addition to the specialists dictated by clinical manifestations, including a neurologist with an interest in neuromuscular disease, a neuromus-cular physiotherapist, an occupational therapist, a genetic counselor, and a metabolic dietician.

Specific treatment includes dietary restriction of high-fat diet; replacement of long-chain with medium-chain triglycerides; and avoidance of prolonged fasting, intensive exercise, and aggressive treatment of infec-tions. Medium chain triglyceride oil is often used as an energy source in individuals with LCHADD. L-carnitine administration (energy source) and docosahexanoic acid supplementa-tion for prevention of eyesight loss both have been shown to be beneficial in some children with LCHADD.

Medium-Chain Acyl-CoA Dehydrogenase Deficiency (MCAD)

Medium-chain acyl-CoA dehydrogenase defi-ciency (MCAD) results in defective mitochon-drial fatty acid β-oxidation, which fuels hepatic ketogenesis, resulting in metabolic crises when glycogen stores are deplete, with attacks fre-quently precipitated by fasting, vigorous exercise, or febrile illnesses. MCAD is transmitted as an autosomal recessive trait, with the overall preva-lence ranging from 1:4,900 to 1:17,000.[117-122]

CLINICAL FEATURES

MCAD usually presents in early infancy between 3 and 24 months; however, an adult-onset case[123,124] has been reported. Affected children are often normal at birth with attacks frequently precipitated by a common illness. MCAD is characterized by hypoketotic hypo-glycemia, vomiting, and lethargy, and during severe episodes seizures, hepatomegaly, and liver dysfunction (mimicking Reye syndrome) may ensue.[125]

CLINICAL INVESTIGATIONS

Cardinal features of hypoketotic hypoglycemia hyperammonemia, liver dysfunction, and fatty infiltration of the liver are present in individu-als with MCAD deficiency.

DIAGNOSTIC TESTS

In individuals with MCAD deficiency, the acylcarnitine profile analysis is characterized by accumulation of C6 to C10 species, with prominent octanoylcarnitine[126]; however false positives have been reported with secondary carnitine deficiency.[127] Urinary organic acid analysis in symptomatic individuals, is charac-terized by elevated medium-chain dicarboxylic acids (C6 > C8 > C10), and inappropriately low or normal[128] ketones. Urinary suberylg-lycine during acute episodes may aid diag-nosis,[129] whereas urine acylglycine analysis is useful diagnostically immediately after birth.[130] Enzymatic activity in fibroblasts, lymphocytes, skeletal muscle, or amniocytes may also be used in the diagnosis of MCAD deficiency.

Molecular genetic testing is the definitive test for diagnosis. To date, only mutations in the *ACADM* gene are recognized to underlie MCAD, with p.Lys304Glu (985A>G) recognized as the only prevalent causative mutation in individuals of northern European heritage.[125] Newborn screening for MCAD is now readily available and shown to be cost effective.[131]

TREATMENT

A multidisciplinary and multispecialty approach should be undertaken and should include a metabolic disease specialist/biochemical geneticist in addition to the specialists dictated by clinical manifestations, including a neurologist with interest in neuromuscular disease, a neuromuscular physiotherapist, an occupational therapist, a genetic counsellor, and a metabolic dietician.

The mainstay of treatment includes avoidance of prolonged fasting, high-fat diets, infant formulas that contain medium-chain triglycerides as the primary source of fat, and intensive exercise. Administration of carbohydrate by mouth or intravenously is used to ameliorate symptoms of catabolism during acute attacks, and uncooked corn starch at bedtime may ensure adequate blood sugar levels overnight.[132]

3-Hydroxyacyl-CoA Dehydrogenase Deficiency (HADH)

3-Hydroxyacyl-CoA dehydrogenase (HADH, also called short-chain L-3-hydroxyacyl-CoA dehydrogenase [SCHAD]) is an intramitochondrial enzyme that catalyzes the nicotinamide adenine dinucleotide–dependent dehydrogenation of 3-hydroxyacyl-CoA to the corresponding 3-ketoacyl-CoA—the penultimate step of fatty acid β-oxidation[133]—and is caused by beta-cell responsiveness particularly to leucin.[134] HADH deficiency is transmitted as an autosomal-recessive trait and the prevalence of HADH deficiency is unknown, with only a few cases reported worldwide, to date.[135-141] Although fatty acids are recognized to play a pivotal role in insulin secretion, and HADH is highly expressed in pancreatic β-cells, the underlying molecular mechanisms are yet to be elucidated.

CLINICAL FEATURES

Individuals with HADH deficiency usually present in infancy or early childhood with persistent hypoglycemia. HADH is characterized by congenital hyperinsulinism mediated through glutamate dehydrogenase,[142] hypoglycemia, vomiting, diarrhea, lethargy, hypotonia, myopathy, and fulminant liver failure.[134,143,144] Cardiac involvement, seizures and sudden death have also been reported.

CLINICAL INVESTIGATIONS

The defining clinical feature of HADH is congenital hyperinsulinemic hypoglycemia.

DIAGNOSTIC TESTS

In individuals with HADH deficiency the acylcarnitine profile analysis is characterized by raised hydroxybutyrylcarnitine, and urinary organic acid analysis is characterized by raised 3-hydroxyglutarate. Enzymatic activity in fibroblasts may be used in the diagnosis of HADH deficiency, showing decreased expression and function of the HADH enzyme. However, absence of 3-hydroxybutyrylcarnitine and high residual enzyme activity has been reported in two cases.[138,140] Molecular genetic testing is the definitive test for diagnosis with mutations in *HADH* genes recognized to underlie this form of congenital hyperinsulinism.[145]

TREATMENT

A multidisciplinary and multispecialty approach should be undertaken and should include a metabolic disease specialist/biochemical geneticist in addition to the specialists dictated by clinical manifestations, including a neurologist with an interest in neuromuscular disease, a hepatologist, a neuromuscular physiotherapist, an occupational therapist, a genetic counselor, and a metabolic dietician.

The mainstay of specific treatment includes dietary protein restriction in children with HADH. Hypoglycemia appears responsive to diazoxide, as in other forms of congenital hyperinsulinism.[146] In cases of fulminant hepatic failure, liver transplantation should be considered.

OTHER DISORDERS OF MUSCLE METABOLISM

Myoadenylate Deaminase Deficiency (MAD)

Myoadenylate deaminase deficiency (MAD) is a myopathic metabolic disorder characterized by exercise-induced cramps, myalgia, and early fatigue. Adenylate deaminase is an integral factor in the purine nucleotide cycle that produces fumarate, an intermediate substrate of the Krebs cycle; deficiency of this enzyme causes disruption in energy production by this pathway. First recognized in 1978,[147] MAD has been reported in over 200 symptomatic patients, in addition to asymptomatic individuals with enzymatic deficiency. In other individuals it is not clear whether their symptoms are related to MAD deficiency.

CLINICAL FEATURES

There is no gender predeliction of MAD, with men and women equally affected. Symptomatic presentation with exercise-induced cramps, myalgia, and early fatigue may occur during early childhood through late adulthood. Symptoms usually progress during the first few years and then appear to plateau. Multisystem organ involvement has not been reported in patients with MAD, with disease limited to skeletal muscle.

CLINICAL INVESTIGATIONS

The serum creatine kinase may be raised but is often normal. Ischemic forearm testing induces symptoms of pain and cramps but with no ammonia production, the antithesis to healthy skeletal muscle during exercise.

DIAGNOSTIC TESTS

MAD is diagnosed by biochemical detection of myoadenylate deaminase deficiency on muscle biopsy. The majority of patients are homozygous for the C34T mutation in the *AMPD1* gene. Although up to 1% of the Caucasian population harbors a mutation in the causative gene, only a minority of gene mutation carriers develop symptoms. The reasons for this are not yet clear.

TREATMENT

Unfortunately, therapy is very limited and there are few effective treatments. Ingestion of D-ribose, a pentose sugar, may ameliorate immediate symptoms but does not modulate long-term effects of this metabolic disorder. This is because the sugar has a short half-life and is rapidly absorbed from the gut, and thus requires repeated dosing.

Malignant Hyperthermia

Malignant hyperthermia (MH) is transmitted as an autosomal-dominant trait, and may be associated with other muscle disorders including central core disease and multi-minicore myopathy.[148,149]

CLINICAL FEATURES

MH is characterized by anesthesia-induced rise in core body temperature and severe muscle contractions and rigidity, which may be life threatening. Other features include myoglobinuria, exercise-induced myalgia, and cramps, and raised CK during acute episodes of MH.

CLINICAL INVESTIGATIONS

Clinical acumen is perhaps the most useful step in diagnosis. A family history of sudden death following anesthetic or documented family history of MH should be sought in suspected cases. Supportive biochemical evidence includes elevated serum CK and raised urinary myoglobin during an attack. Careful monitoring of renal function, calcium, and phosphate are required to prevent complications during an acute episode.

DIAGNOSTIC TESTS

The caffeine halothane contracture test is the only recognized laboratory test to diagnose MH.[150] Molecular genetic testing to look for defects in the *RYR1* gene may be undertaken in suspected cases of MH.[151-153]

TREATMENT

Immediate complications include cardiac arrhythmias and multi-organ failure including heart, lung, and kidney.[154] Treatment is supportive; untreated episodes maybe fatal. Therapy is targeted at aggressive and timely symptomatic care and includes cooling with blankets and antipyretics to help reduce fever and the risk of serious complications. The additional use of intravenous fluids and the implementation of drugs such as dantrolene, lidocaine, or beta-blockers have been shown to be useful in the acute setting, reducing all-cause mortality of MH.

Genetic screening should be implemented where there is a known family history of MH, or in suspected cases, where there is a family history of dystrophy or muscle disease or previous adverse response to general anesthetic agents. In confirmed or suspected cases of MH, volatile inhalational anesthetic agents and the muscle relaxant succinylcholine should be avoided to prevent triggering life-threatening episodes. Furthermore, avoidance of stimulant drugs such as cocaine, amphetamine, and Estasy is advised, as these agents may also trigger similar episodes, in individuals predisposed to MH.[155]

REFERENCES

1. Ozen H. Glycogen storage diseases: new perspectives. World journal of gastroenterology: 2007;13:2541–2553.
2. Martinuzzi A, Schievano G, Nascimbeni A, Fanin M. McArdle's disease. The unsolved mystery of the reappearing enzyme. The American journal of pathology 1999;154:1893–1897.
3. McArdle B. Myopathy due to a defect of muscle glycogen breakdown. Clin Sci (Lond) 1951;10:13–33.
4. Braakhekke JP, de Bruin MI, Stegeman DF, Wevers RA, Binkhorst RA, Joosten EM. The second wind phenomenon in McArdle's disease. Brain: a journal of neurology 1986;109 (Pt 6):1087–1101.
5. Quinlivan R, Buckley J, James M, et al. McArdle disease: a clinical review. Journal of neurology, neurosurgery, and psychiatry 2010;81:1182–1188.
6. DiMauro S, Hartlage PL. Fatal infantile form of muscle phosphorylase deficiency. Neurology 1978;28:1124–1129.
7. Milstein JM, Herron TM, Haas JE. Fatal infantile muscle phosphorylase deficiency. Journal of child neurology 1989;4:186–188.
8. Felice KJ, Schneebaum AB, Jones HR, Jr. McArdle's disease with late-onset symptoms: case report and review of the literature. Journal of neurology, neurosurgery, and psychiatry 1992;55:407–408.
9. Kazemi-Esfarjani P, Skomorowska E, Jensen TD, Haller RG, Vissing J. A nonischemic forearm exercise test for McArdle disease. Annals of neurology 2002;52:153–159.
10. O'Dochartaigh CS, Ong HY, Lovell SM, et al. Oxygen consumption is increased relative to work rate in patients with McArdle's disease. European journal of clinical investigation 2004;34:731–737.
11. Vissing J, Haller RG. A diagnostic cycle test for McArdle's disease. Annals of neurology 2003;54:539–542.
12. Bartram C, Edwards RH, Clague J, Beynon RJ. McArdle's disease: a nonsense mutation in exon 1 of the muscle glycogen phosphorylase gene explains some but not all cases. Human molecular genetics 1993;2:1291–1293.
13. Arenas J, Martín MA, Andreu AL. Glycogen Storage Disease Type V. 2006 Apr 19 [Updated 2009 May 12]. In: Pagon RA, Adam MP, Bird TD, et al., editors. GeneReviews™ [Internet]. Seattle (WA): University of Washington, Seattle; 1993–2013. Available from: http://www.ncbi.nlm.nih.gov/books/NBK1344/
14. Vissing J, Haller RG. The effect of oral sucrose on exercise tolerance in patients with McArdle's disease. N Engl J Med 2003;349:2503–2509.
15. Quinlivan R, Vissing J, Hilton-Jones D, Buckley J. Physical training for McArdle disease. Cochrane Database Syst Rev 2011(12):CD007931.
16. Tarui S, Okuno G, Ikura Y, Tanaka T, Suda M, Nishikawa M. Phosphofructokinase Deficiency in Skeletal Muscle. A New Type of Glycogenosis. Biochemical and biophysical research communications 1965;19:517–523.
17. Toscano A, Musumeci O. Tarui disease and distal glycogenoses: clinical and genetic update. Acta myologica: myopathies and cardiomyopathies: official journal of the Mediterranean Society of Myology/edited by the Gaetano Conte Academy for the study of striated muscle diseases 2007;26:105–107.
18. Nakajima H, Raben N, Hamaguchi T, Yamasaki T. Phosphofructokinase deficiency; past, present and future. Curr Mol Med 2002;2:197–212.
19. Haller RG, Vissing J. No spontaneous second wind in muscle phosphofructokinase deficiency. Neurology 2004;62:82–86.
20. Mineo I, Kono N, Hara N, et al. Myogenic hyperuricemia. A common pathophysiologic feature of glycogenosis types III, V, and VII. The New England journal of medicine 1987;317:75–80.
21. Moerman P, Lammens M, Fryns JP, Lemmens F, Lauweryns JM. Fetal akinesia sequence caused by glycogenosis type VII. Genet Couns 1995;6:15–20.
22. Swoboda KJ, Specht L, Jones HR, Shapiro F, DiMauro S, Korson M. Infantile phosphofructokinase deficiency with arthrogryposis: clinical benefit of a ketogenic diet. The journal of pediatrics 1997;131:932–934.
23. Spriggs EL, Marles SL, Lacson A, et al. Long-term survival and normal cognitive development in infantile phosphofructokinase-1 deficiency. Clinical genetics 1999;56:235–237.
24. Danon MJ, Carpenter S, Manaligod JR, Schliselfeld LH. Fatal infantile glycogen storage disease: deficiency of phosphofructokinase and phosphorylase b kinase. Neurology 1981;31:1303–1307.
25. Al-Hassnan ZN, Al Budhaim M, Al-Owain M, Lach B, Al-Dhalaan H. Muscle phosphofructokinase deficiency with neonatal seizures and nonprogressive course. Journal of child neurology 2007;22:106–108.

26. Servidei S, Bonilla E, Diedrich RG, et al. Fatal infantile form of muscle phosphofructokinase deficiency. Neurology 1986;36:1465–1470.

27. Amit R, Bashan N, Abarbanel JM, Shapira Y, Sofer S, Moses S. Fatal familial infantile glycogen storage disease: multisystem phosphofructokinase deficiency. Muscle & nerve 1992;15:455–458.

28. Agamanolis DP, Askari AD, Di Mauro S, et al. Muscle phosphofructokinase deficiency: two cases with unusual polysaccharide accumulation and immunologically active enzyme protein. Muscle & nerve 1980;3:456–467.

29. Ono A, Kuwajima M, Kono N, et al. Glucose infusion paradoxically accelerates degradation of adenine nucleotide in working muscle of patients with glycogen storage disease type VII. Neurology 1995;45:161–164.

30. Haller RG, Lewis SF. Glucose-induced exertional fatigue in muscle phosphofructokinase deficiency. The New England journal of medicine 1991;324:364–369.

31. Nakashima H, Suo H, Ochiai J, Sugie H, Kawamura Y. [A case of adult onset phosphoglucomutase deficiency]. Rinsho shinkeigaku [Clinical neurology] 1992;32:42–47.

32. Goldstein J, Austin S, Kishnani P, et al. Phosphorylase Kinase Deficiency. 2011 May 31. In: Pagon RA, Adam MP, Bird TD, et al., editors. GeneReviews™ [Internet]. Seattle (WA): University of Washington, Seattle; 1993–2013. Available from: http://www.ncbi.nlm.nih.gov/books/NBK55061/

33. Bruno C, Manfredi G, Andreu AL, et al. A splice junction mutation in the alpha(M) gene of phosphorylase kinase in a patient with myopathy. Biochemical and biophysical research communications 1998;249:648–651.

34. Wehner M, Clemens PR, Engel AG, Kilimann MW. Human muscle glycogenosis due to phosphorylase kinase deficiency associated with a nonsense mutation in the muscle isoform of the alpha subunit. Human molecular genetics 1994;3:1983–1987.

35. Wuyts W, Reyniers E, Ceuterick C, Storm K, de Barsy T, Martin JJ. Myopathy and phosphorylase kinase deficiency caused by a mutation in the PHKA1 gene. American journal of medical genetics Part A 2005;133A:82–84.

36. Orngreen MC, Schelhaas HJ, Jeppesen TD, et al. Is muscle glycogenolysis impaired in X-linked phosphorylase b kinase deficiency? Neurology 2008;70:1876–1882.

37. Echaniz-Laguna A, Akman HO, Mohr M, et al. Muscle phosphorylase b kinase deficiency revisited. Neuromuscular disorders: NMD 2010;20:125–127.

38. Haller RG. Fueling around with glycogen: the implications of muscle phosphorylase b kinase deficiency. Neurology 2008;70:1872–1873.

39. Salameh J, Goyal N, Choudry R, Camelo-Piragua S, Chong PS. Phosphoglycerate mutase deficiency with tubular aggregates in a patient from Panama. Muscle & nerve 2013;47:138–140.

40. Tonin P, Bruno C, Cassandrini D, et al. Unusual presentation of phosphoglycerate mutase deficiency due to two different mutations in PGAM-M gene. Neuromuscular disorders: NMD 2009;19:776–778.

41. Nolte KW, Janecke AR, Vorgerd M, Weis J, Schroder JM. Congenital type IV glycogenosis: the spectrum of pleomorphic polyglucosan bodies in muscle, nerve, and spinal cord with two novel mutations in the GBE1 gene. Acta neuropathologica 2008;116:491–506.

42. Sugie H, Fukuda T, Ito M, Sugie Y, Kojoh T, Nonaka I. Novel exon 11 skipping mutation in a patient with glycogen storage disease type IIId. Journal of inherited metabolic disease 2001;24:535–545.

43. DiMauro S, Spiegel R. Progress and problems in muscle glycogenoses. Acta myologica: myopathies and cardiomyopathies: official journal of the Mediterranean Society of Myology/edited by the Gaetano Conte Academy for the study of striated muscle diseases 2011;30:96–102.

44. Comi GP, Fortunato F, Lucchiari S, et al. Beta-enolase deficiency, a new metabolic myopathy of distal glycolysis. Ann Neurol 2001;50:202–207.

45. Martiniuk F, Chen A, Mack A, et al. Carrier frequency for glycogen storage disease type II in New York and estimates of affected individuals born with the disease. American journal of medical genetics 1998;79:69–72.

46. Kishnani PS, Steiner RD, Bali D, et al. Pompe disease diagnosis and management guideline. Genetics in medicine: official journal of the American College of Medical Genetics 2006;8:267–288.

47. Mellies U, Lofaso F. Pompe disease: a neuromuscular disease with respiratory muscle involvement. Respiratory medicine 2009;103:477–484.

48. Kishnani PS, Austin SL, Arn P, et al. Glycogen storage disease type III diagnosis and management guidelines. Genetics in medicine: official journal of the American College of Medical Genetics 2010;12:446–463.

49. Ausems MG, Lochman P, van Diggelen OP, Ploos van Amstel HK, Reuser AJ, Wokke JH. A diagnostic protocol for adult-onset glycogen storage disease type II. Neurology 1999;52:851–853.

50. Manwaring V, Prunty H, Bainbridge K, et al. Urine analysis of glucose tetrasaccharide by HPLC; a useful marker for the investigation of patients with Pompe and other glycogen storage diseases. Journal of inherited metabolic disease 2012;35:311–316.

51. van der Ploeg AT, Clemens PR, Corzo D, et al. A randomized study of alglucosidase alfa in late-onset Pompe's disease. The New England journal of medicine 2010;362:1396–1406.

52. van der Ploeg AT. Where do we stand in enzyme replacement therapy in Pompe's disease? Neuromuscular disorders: NMD 2010;20:773–774.

53. Schoser B, Hill V, Raben N. Therapeutic approaches in glycogen storage disease type II/Pompe Disease. Neurotherapeutics: the journal of the American Society for Experimental NeuroTherapeutics 2008;5:569–578.

54. Snappes I VCS. Un cas d'hypoglycemie avec acetonemie chez un enfant. Bull Mem Soc Med Hop (Paris) 1928;52:1315–1317.

55. Forbes GB. Glycogen storage disease; report of a case with abnormal glycogen structure in liver and skeletal muscle. The JOURNAL of pediatrics 1953;42:645–653.

56. Illingworth B, Cori GT, Cori CF. Amylo-1,6-glucosidase in muscle tissue in generalized glycogen storage disease. The Journal of biological chemistry 1956;218:123–129.

57. Van Hoof F, Hers HG. The subgroups of type 3 glycogenosis. European journal of biochemistry / FEBS 1967;2:265–270.

58. Rowland LP, DiMauro S. Glycogen-storage diseases of muscle: genetic problems. Research

publications—Association for Research in Nervous and Mental Disease 1983;60:239–254.

59. Ding JH, de Barsy T, Brown BI, Coleman RA, Chen YT. Immunoblot analyses of glycogen debranching enzyme in different subtypes of glycogen storage disease type III. The journal of pediatrics 1990;116:95–100.

60. DiMauro S, Hartwig GB, Hays A, et al. Debrancher deficiency: neuromuscular disorder in 5 adults. Annals of neurology 1979;5:422–436.

61. Labrune P, Huguet P, Odievre M. Cardiomyopathy in glycogen-storage disease type III: clinical and echographic study of 18 patients. Pediatric cardiology 1991;12:161–163.

62. Miller CG, Alleyne GA, Brooks SE. Gross cardiac involvement in glycogen storage disease type 3. British heart journal 1972;34:862–864.

63. Moses SW, Wanderman KL, Myroz A, Frydman M. Cardiac involvement in glycogen storage disease type III. European journal of pediatrics 1989;148:764–766.

64. Lee PJ, Deanfield JE, Burch M, Baig K, McKenna WJ, Leonard JV. Comparison of the functional significance of left ventricular hypertrophy in hypertrophic cardiomyopathy and glycogenosis type III. The American journal of cardiology 1997;79:834–838.

65. Powell HC, Haas R, Hall CL, Wolff JA, Nyhan W, Brown BI. Peripheral nerve in type III glycogenosis: selective involvement of unmyelinated fiber Schwann cells. Muscle & nerve 1985;8:667–671.

66. Ugawa Y, Inoue K, Takemura T, Iwamasa T. Accumulation of glycogen in sural nerve axons in adult-onset type III glycogenosis. Annals of neurology 1986;19:294–297.

67. Yang-Feng TL, Zheng K, Yu J, Yang BZ, Chen YT, Kao FT. Assignment of the human glycogen debrancher gene to chromosome 1p21. Genomics 1992;13:931–934.

68. Akman HO, Sampayo JN, Ross FA, et al. Fatal infantile cardiac glycogenosis with phosphorylase kinase deficiency and a mutation in the gamma2-subunit of AMP-activated protein kinase. Pediatric research 2007;62:499–504.

69. Raju GP, Li HC, Bali DS, et al. A case of congenital glycogen storage disease type IV with a novel GBE1 mutation. Journal of child neurology 2008;23:349–352.

70. Konstantinidou AE, Anninos H, Dertinger S, et al. Placental involvement in glycogen storage disease type IV. Placenta 2008;29:378–381.

71. Kishi H, Mukai T, Hirono A, Fujii H, Miwa S, Hori K. Human aldolase A deficiency associated with a hemolytic anemia: thermolabile aldolase due to a single base mutation. Proceedings of the National Academy of Sciences of the United States of America 1987;84:8623–8627.

72. Miwa S, Fujii H, Tani K, et al. Two cases of red cell aldolase deficiency associated with hereditary hemolytic anemia in a Japanese family. American journal of hematology 1981;11:425–437.

73. Kreuder J, Borkhardt A, Repp R, et al. Brief report: inherited metabolic myopathy and hemolysis due to a mutation in aldolase A. The New England journal of medicine 1996;334:1100–1104.

74. Beutler E, Scott S, Bishop A, Margolis N, Matsumoto F, Kuhl W. Red cell aldolase deficiency and hemolytic anemia: a new syndrome. Transactions of the Association of American Physicians 1973;86:154–166.

75. Hurst JA, Baraitser M, Winter RM. A syndrome of mental retardation, short stature, hemolytic anemia, delayed puberty, and abnormal facial appearance: similarities to a report of aldolase A deficiency. American journal of medical genetics 1987;28:965–970.

76. Amberger J, Bocchini CA, Scott AF, Hamosh A. McKusick's Online Mendelian Inheritance in Man (OMIM). Nucleic acids research 2009;37:D793–D796.

77. Stojkovic T, Vissing J, Petit F, et al. Muscle glycogenosis due to phosphoglucomutase 1 deficiency. The New England journal of medicine 2009;361:425–427.

78. Koizumi A, Nozaki J, Ohura T, et al. Genetic epidemiology of the carnitine transporter OCTN2 gene in a Japanese population and phenotypic characterization in Japanese pedigrees with primary systemic carnitine deficiency. Human molecular genetics 1999;8:2247–2254.

79. Wilcken B, Wiley V, Sim KG, Carpenter K. Carnitine transporter defect diagnosed by newborn screening with electrospray tandem mass spectrometry. The Journal of pediatrics 2001;138:581–584.

80. Duran M, Loof NE, Ketting D, Dorland L. Secondary carnitine deficiency. Journal of clinical chemistry and clinical biochemistry/Zeitschrift fur klinische Chemie und klinische Biochemie 1990;28:359–363.

81. Bohmer T, Bergrem H, Eiklid K. Carnitine deficiency induced during intermittent haemodialysis for renal failure. Lancet 1978;1:126–128.

82. Van Wouwe JP. Carnitine deficiency during valproic acid treatment. International journal for vitamin and nutrition research/Internationale Zeitschrift fur Vitamin- und Ernahrungsforschung/Journal international de vitaminologie et de nutrition 1995;65:211–214.

83. Roe CR. Inherited disorders of mitochondrial fatty acid oxidation: a new responsibility for the neonatologist. Seminars in neonatology: SN 2002;7:37–47.

84. Wilcken B, Wiley V, Hammond J, Carpenter K. Screening newborns for inborn errors of metabolism by tandem mass spectrometry. The New England journal of medicine 2003;348:2304–2312.

85. Amat di San Filippo C, Taylor MR, Mestroni L, Botto LD, Longo N. Cardiomyopathy and carnitine deficiency. Molecular genetics and metabolism 2008;94:162–166.

86. Stanley CA. Carnitine deficiency disorders in children. Annals of the New York Academy of Sciences 2004;1033:42–51.

87. Karpati G, Carpenter S, Engel AG, et al. The syndrome of systemic carnitine deficiency. Clinical, morphologic, biochemical, and pathophysiologic features. Neurology 1975;25:16–24.

88. Nezu J, Tamai I, Oku A, et al. Primary systemic carnitine deficiency is caused by mutations in a gene encoding sodium ion-dependent carnitine transporter. Nature genetics 1999;21:91–94.

89. Engel AG, Angelini C. Carnitine deficiency of human skeletal muscle with associated lipid storage myopathy: a new syndrome. Science 1973;179:899–902.

90. DiMauro S, DiMauro PM. Muscle carnitine palmityltransferase deficiency and myoglobinuria. Science 1973;182:929–931.

91. Sigauke E, Rakheja D, Kitson K, Bennett MJ. Carnitine palmitoyltransferase II deficiency: a clinical, biochemical, and molecular review. Laboratory investigation; a journal of technical methods and pathology 2003;83:1543–1554.

92. Bonnefont JP, Djouadi F, Prip-Buus C, Gobin S, Munnich A, Bastin J. Carnitine palmitoyltransferases 1 and 2: biochemical, molecular and medical aspects. Molecular aspects of medicine 2004;25:495–520.

93. Wieser T, Deschauer M, Olek K, Hermann T, Zierz S. Carnitine palmitoyltransferase II deficiency: molecular and biochemical analysis of 32 patients. Neurology 2003;60:1351–1353.

94. Wieser T. Carnitine Palmitoyltransferase II Deficiency. 2004 Aug 27 [Updated 2011 Oct 6]. In: Pagon RA, Adam MP, Bird TD, et al., editors. GeneReviews™ [Internet]. Seattle (WA): University of Washington, Seattle; 1993–2013. Available from: http://www.ncbi.nlm.nih.gov/books/NBK1253/

95. Roe CR, Yang BZ, Brunengraber H, Roe DS, Wallace M, Garritson BK. Carnitine palmitoyltransferase II deficiency: successful anaplerotic diet therapy. Neurology 2008;71:260–264.

96. Naylor EW, Chace DH. Automated tandem mass spectrometry for mass newborn screening for disorders in fatty acid, organic acid, and amino acid metabolism. Journal of child neurology 1999;14 Suppl 1:S4–S8.

97. Leslie ND, Tinkle BT, Strauss AW, et al. Very Long-Chain Acyl-Coenzyme A Dehydrogenase Deficiency. 2009 May 28 [Updated 2011 Sep 22]. In: Pagon RA, Adam MP, Bird TD, et al., editors. GeneReviews™ [Internet]. Seattle (WA): University of Washington, Seattle; 1993–2013. Available from: http://www.ncbi.nlm.nih.gov/books/NBK6816/

98. Bonnet D, Martin D, Pascale De L, et al. Arrhythmias and conduction defects as presenting symptoms of fatty acid oxidation disorders in children. Circulation 1999;100:2248–2253.

99. Hoffman JD, Steiner RD, Paradise L, et al. Rhabdomyolysis in the military: recognizing late-onset very long-chain acyl Co-A dehydrogenase deficiency. Military medicine 2006;171:657–658.

100. Orii KO, Aoyama T, Souri M, et al. Genomic DNA organization of human mitochondrial very-long-chain acyl-CoA dehydrogenase and mutation analysis. Biochemical and biophysical research communications 1995;217:987–992.

101. Arnold GL, Van Hove J, Freedenberg D, et al. A Delphi clinical practice protocol for the management of very long chain acyl-CoA dehydrogenase deficiency. Molecular genetics and metabolism 2009;96:85–90.

102. Tong MK, Lam CS, Mak TW, et al. Very long-chain acyl-CoA dehydrogenase deficiency presenting as acute hypercapnic respiratory failure. The European respiratory journal: official journal of the European Society for Clinical Respiratory Physiology 2006;28:447–450.

103. McHugh D, Cameron CA, Abdenur JE, et al. Clinical validation of cutoff target ranges in newborn screening of metabolic disorders by tandem mass spectrometry: a worldwide collaborative project. Genetics in medicine: official journal of the American College of Medical Genetics 2011;13:230–254.

104. Andresen BS, Olpin S, Poorthuis BJ, et al. Clear correlation of genotype with disease phenotype in very-long-chain acyl-CoA dehydrogenase deficiency. American journal of human genetics 1999;64:479–494.

105. Boneh A, Andresen BS, Gregersen N, et al. VLCAD deficiency: pitfalls in newborn screening and confirmation of diagnosis by mutation analysis. Molecular genetics and metabolism 2006;88:166–170.

106. Bertini E, Dionisi-Vici C, Garavaglia B, et al. Peripheral sensory-motor polyneuropathy, pigmentary retinopathy, and fatal cardiomyopathy in long-chain 3-hydroxy-acyl-CoA dehydrogenase deficiency. European journal of pediatrics 1992;151: 121–126.

107. Jackson S, Bartlett K, Land J, et al. Long-chain 3-hydroxyacyl-CoA dehydrogenase deficiency. Pediatric research 1991;29:406–411.

108. Baskin B, Geraghty M, Ray PN. Paternal isodisomy of chromosome 2 as a cause of long chain 3-hydroxyacyl-CoA dehydrogenase (LCHAD) deficiency. American journal of medical genetics Part A 2010;152A:1808–1811.

109. L IJ, Ruiter JP, Hoovers JM, Jakobs ME, Wanders RJ. Common missense mutation G1528C in long-chain 3-hydroxyacyl-CoA dehydrogenase deficiency. Characterization and expression of the mutant protein, mutation analysis on genomic DNA and chromosomal localization of the mitochondrial trifunctional protein alpha subunit gene. The journal of clinical investigation 1996;98:1028–1033.

110. Hagenfeldt L, von Dobeln U, Holme E, et al. 3-Hydroxydicarboxylic aciduria—a fatty acid oxidation defect with severe prognosis. The journal of pediatrics 1990;116:387–392.

111. Tyni T, Palotie A, Viinikka L, et al. Long-chain 3-hydroxyacyl-coenzyme A dehydrogenase deficiency with the G1528C mutation: clinical presentation of thirteen patients. The journal of pediatrics 1997;130:67–76.

112. Wanders RJ, L IJ, Poggi F, et al. Human trifunctional protein deficiency: a new disorder of mitochondrial fatty acid beta-oxidation. Biochemical and biophysical research communications 1992;188: 1139–1145.

113. Spiekerkoetter U, Lindner M, Santer R, et al. Management and outcome in 75 individuals with long-chain fatty acid oxidation defects: results from a workshop. Journal of inherited metabolic disease 2009;32:488–497.

114. Cunniff C. Prenatal screening and diagnosis for pediatricians. Pediatrics 2004;114:889–894.

115. Spiekerkoetter U. Mitochondrial fatty acid oxidation disorders: clinical presentation of long-chain fatty acid oxidation defects before and after newborn screening. Journal of inherited metabolic disease 2010;33:527–532.

116. Autti-Ramo I, Makela M, Sintonen H, et al. Expanding screening for rare metabolic disease in the newborn: an analysis of costs, effect and ethical consequences for decision-making in Finland. Acta Paediatr 2005;94:1126–1136.

117. Sander S, Janzen N, Janetzky B, et al. Neonatal screening for medium chain acyl-CoA deficiency: high incidence in Lower Saxony (northern Germany). European journal of pediatrics 2001;160:318–319.

118. Maier EM, Gersting SW, Kemter KF, et al. Protein misfolding is the molecular mechanism underlying MCADD identified in newborn screening. Human molecular genetics 2009;18:1612–1623.

119. Carpenter K, Wiley V, Sim KG, Heath D, Wilcken B. Evaluation of newborn screening for medium chain acyl-CoA dehydrogenase deficiency in 275 000 babies. Archives of disease in childhood: Fetal and neonatal edition 2001;85:F105–F109.

120. Chace DH, Kalas TA, Naylor EW. The application of tandem mass spectrometry to neonatal screening for inherited disorders of intermediary metabolism. Annual review of genomics and human genetics 2002;3:17–45.

121. Niu DM, Chien YH, Chiang CC, et al. Nationwide survey of extended newborn screening by tandem mass spectrometry in Taiwan. Journal of inherited metabolic disease 2010;33:S295–S305.

122. Shigematsu Y, Hirano S, Hata I, et al. Newborn mass screening and selective screening using electrospray tandem mass spectrometry in Japan. Journal of chromatography B, Analytical technologies in the biomedical and life sciences 2002;776:39–48.

123. Schatz UA, Ensenauer R. The clinical manifestation of MCAD deficiency: challenges towards adulthood in the screened population. Journal of inherited metabolic disease 2010;33:513–520.

124. Raymond K, Bale AE, Barnes CA, Rinaldo P. Medium-chain acyl-CoA dehydrogenase deficiency: sudden and unexpected death of a 45 year old woman. Genetics in medicine: official journal of the American College of Medical Genetics 1999;1:293–294.

125. Matern D, Rinaldo P. Medium-Chain Acyl-Coenzyme A Dehydrogenase Deficiency. 2000 Apr 20 [Updated 2012 Jan 19]. In: Pagon RA, Adam MP, Bird TD, et al., editors. GeneReviews™ [Internet]. Seattle (WA): University of Washington, Seattle; 1993–2013. Available from: http://www.ncbi.nlm.nih.gov/books/NBK1424/

126. Smith EH, Thomas C, McHugh D, et al. Allelic diversity in MCAD deficiency: the biochemical classification of 54 variants identified during 5 years of ACADM sequencing. Molecular genetics and metabolism 2010;100:241–250.

127. Clayton PT, Doig M, Ghafari S, et al. Screening for medium chain acyl-CoA dehydrogenase deficiency using electrospray ionisation tandem mass spectrometry. Archives of disease in childhood 1998;79:109–115.

128. Patel JS, Leonard JV. Ketonuria and medium-chain acyl-CoA dehydrogenase deficiency. Journal of inherited metabolic disease 1995;18:98–99.

129. Gregersen N, Kolvraa S, Rasmussen K, et al. General (medium-chain) acyl-CoA dehydrogenase deficiency (non-ketotic dicarboxylic aciduria): quantitative urinary excretion pattern of 23 biologically significant organic acids in three cases. Clinica chimica acta; international journal of clinical chemistry 1983;132:181–191.

130. Bennett MJ, Rinaldo P, Millington DS, Tanaka K, Yokota I, Coates PM. Medium-chain acyl-CoA dehydrogenase deficiency: postmortem diagnosis in a case of sudden infant death and neonatal diagnosis of an affected sibling. Pediatric pathology/affiliated with the International Paediatric Pathology Association 1991;11:889–895.

131. Pandor A, Eastham J, Beverley C, Chilcott J, Paisley S. Clinical effectiveness and cost-effectiveness of neonatal screening for inborn errors of metabolism using tandem mass spectrometry: a systematic review. Health Technol Assess 2004;8:iii, 1–121.

132. Potter BK, Little J, Chakraborty P, et al. Variability in the clinical management of fatty acid oxidation disorders: results of a survey of Canadian metabolic physicians. Journal of inherited metabolic disease 2012;35:115–123.

133. Agren A, Borg K, Brolin SE, Carlman J, Lundqvist G. Hydroxyacyl CoA dehydrogenase, an enzyme important in fat metabolism in different cell types in the islets of Langerhans. Diabete & metabolisme 1977;3:169–172.

134. Bennett MJ, Weinberger MJ, Kobori JA, Rinaldo P, Burlina AB. Mitochondrial short-chain L-3-hydroxyacyl-coenzyme A dehydrogenase deficiency: a new defect of fatty acid oxidation. Pediatric research 1996;39:185–188.

135. Molven A, Matre GE, Duran M, et al. Familial hyperinsulinemic hypoglycemia caused by a defect in the SCHAD enzyme of mitochondrial fatty acid oxidation. Diabetes 2004;53:221–227.

136. Clayton PT, Eaton S, Aynsley-Green A, et al. Hyperinsulinism in short-chain L-3-hydroxyacyl-CoA dehydrogenase deficiency reveals the importance of beta-oxidation in insulin secretion. The journal of clinical investigation 2001;108:457–465.

137. Hussain K, Clayton PT, Krywawych S, et al. Hyperinsulinism of infancy associated with a novel splice site mutation in the SCHAD gene. The journal of pediatrics 2005;146:706–708.

138. Bennett MJ, Russell LK, Tokunaga C, et al. Reye-like syndrome resulting from novel missense mutations in mitochondrial medium- and short-chain l-3-hydroxy-acyl-CoA dehydrogenase. Molecular genetics and metabolism 2006;89:74–79.

139. Filling C, Keller B, Hirschberg D, et al. Role of short-chain hydroxyacyl CoA dehydrogenases in SCHAD deficiency. Biochemical and biophysical research communications 2008;368:6–11.

140. Kapoor RR, James C, Flanagan SE, Ellard S, Eaton S, Hussain K. 3-Hydroxyacyl-coenzyme A dehydrogenase deficiency and hyperinsulinemic hypoglycemia: characterization of a novel mutation and severe dietary protein sensitivity. The Journal of clinical endocrinology and metabolism 2009;94:2221–2225.

141. Di Candia S, Gessi A, Pepe G, et al. Identification of a diffuse form of hyperinsulinemic hypoglycemia by 18-fluoro-L-3,4 dihydroxyphenylalanine positron emission tomography/CT in a patient carrying a novel mutation of the HADH gene. European journal of endocrinology / European Federation of Endocrine Societies 2009;160:1019–1023.

142. Li C, Chen P, Palladino A, et al. Mechanism of hyperinsulinism in short-chain 3-hydroxyacyl-CoA dehydrogenase deficiency involves activation of glutamate dehydrogenase. The Journal of biological chemistry 2010;285:31806–31818.

143. Bennett MJ, Spotswood SD, Ross KF, et al. Fatal hepatic short-chain L-3-hydroxyacyl-coenzyme A dehydrogenase deficiency: clinical, biochemical, and pathological studies on three subjects with this recently identified disorder of mitochondrial beta-oxidation. Pediatric and developmental pathology: the official journal of the Society for Pediatric

Pathology and the Paediatric Pathology Society 1999;2:337–345.

144. Yang SY, He XY, Schulz H. 3-Hydroxyacyl-CoA dehydrogenase and short chain 3-hydroxyacyl-CoA dehydrogenase in human health and disease. The FEBS journal 2005;272:4874–4883.

145. Kapoor RR, Heslegrave A, Hussain K. Congenital hyperinsulinism due to mutations in HNF4A and HADH. Reviews in endocrine & metabolic disorders 2010;11:185–191.

146. Flanagan SE, Patch AM, Locke JM, et al. Genome-wide homozygosity analysis reveals HADH mutations as a common cause of diazoxide-responsive hyperinsulinemic-hypoglycemia in consanguineous pedigrees. The Journal of clinical endocrinology and metabolism 2011;96:E498–E502.

147. Fishbein WN, Armbrustmacher VW, Griffin JL. Myoadenylate deaminase deficiency: a new disease of muscle. Science 1978;200:545–548.

148. Robinson R, Carpenter D, Shaw MA, Halsall J, Hopkins P. Mutations in RYR1 in malignant hyperthermia and central core disease. Human mutation 2006;27:977–989.

149. Hayes J, Veyckemans F, Bissonnette B. Duchenne muscular dystrophy: an old anesthesia problem revisited. Paediatric anaesthesia 2008;18:100–106.

150. Allen GC, Larach MG, Kunselman AR. The sensitivity and specificity of the caffeine-halothane contracture test: a report from the North American Malignant Hyperthermia Registry. The North American Malignant Hyperthermia Registry of MHAUS. Anesthesiology 1998;88:579–588.

151. MacLennan DH, Duff C, Zorzato F, et al. Ryanodine receptor gene is a candidate for predisposition to malignant hyperthermia. Nature 1990;343:559–561.

152. MacLennan DH. The genetic basis of malignant hyperthermia. Trends in pharmacological sciences 1992;13:330–334.

153. McCarthy TV, Healy JM, Heffron JJ, et al. Localization of the malignant hyperthermia susceptibility locus to human chromosome 19q12–13.2. Nature 1990;343:562–564.

154. Larach MG, Brandom BW, Allen GC, Gronert GA, Lehman EB. Cardiac arrests and deaths associated with malignant hyperthermia in north america from 1987 to 2006: a report from the north american malignant hyperthermia registry of the malignant hyperthermia association of the United States. Anesthesiology 2008;108:603–611.

155. Hopkins PM. Malignant hyperthermia: pharmacology of triggering. British journal of anaesthesia 2011;107:48–56.

Chapter 8

Mitochondrial Myopathy

Gerald Pfeffer
Patrick F. Chinnery

Mitochondrial disorders (also known as mitochondrial myopathies, or mitochondrial encephalomyoapthies) result from a primary defect of the mitochondrial respiratory chain. Most are thought to be genetically determined, although some occur as an adverse response to prescription medication. Mitochondrial dysfunction can be a secondary phenomenon in some common neurological and muscle diseases (e.g., myotonic dystrophy), where the metabolic disturbance may contribute to the pathophysiology—but these disorders are generally not considered to be mitochondrial diseases.

Given the widespread dependence of multiple tissues and organs on mitochondrial function, mitochondrial disorders can present in a variety of different ways, either involving multiple organ systems, or only affecting one organ system. Thus, mitochondrial myopathies can occur either in isolation, or in the context of a multisystem disease. Similarly, a patient with a pure mitochondrial myopathy can have relatives with clinical features affecting other organ systems.

MITOCHONDRIAL BIOLOGY

Mitochondria are organelles present in every nucleated human cell, and they are the primary source of intracellular energy in the form of ATP, which is generated by the final complex (V, ATP synthase) of the respiratory chain. Several characteristics of mitochondria are important to understanding the pathogenesis of these disorders. Mitochondria contain approximately 1,500 proteins,[1,2] which have a dual genetic origin. Thirteen are synthesized from DNA contained within the mitochondria (mtDNA). mtDNA is 16.5 kbp in size, and there are multiple copies of this genome in each mitochondrion. In addition to the polypeptide genes that code for components of complexes I, III, IV and V, mtDNA codes for a critical part of the mitochondrial replicative, transcriptional, and translational machinery. However, the majority of proteins required in mitochondrial biogenesis are synthesized within the cytoplasm from nuclear gene transcripts. As a consequence, mitochondrial disorders can be due to mutations in mtDNA or nuclear DNA (nDNA). Mutations in mtDNA can occur in a proportion of genomes (heteroplasmic) or in all genomes (homoplasmic). The extent to which a tissue is affected by such mutations may depend on the proportion of mutated genomes.

GENERAL PRINCIPLES OF MITOCHONDRIAL MEDICINE

Mitochondrial diseases are among the most common inherited neuromuscular diseases, and have an estimated prevalence in adults and children of > 1:5,000.[3] The clinical presentation of mitochondrial disorders is summarized in Table 8–1. In general, the central or peripheral nervous systems are nearly always affected because of their high energy requirements. Cardiac dysfunction is also often present and frequently subclinical.

In the minority of cases it is possible to identify a well-defined clinical syndrome (Table 8–2). However, many patients do not fit neatly into one of these diagnostic groups, having only some of the features, or having an overlapping clinical syndrome. Carefully documenting these features often suggests a particular genetic diagnosis, leading to specific molecular testing. However, if the genetic diagnosis is not immediately apparent, a systematic clinical and laboratory approach is required to make the diagnosis.

These principles are illustrated by the common mitochondrial phenotype: progressive external ophthalmoplegia (PEO), which may occur as an isolated ocular myopathy (with ptosis and ophthalmoparesis), or in combination with any of the other features, either in a defined disorder such as Kearns-Sayre syndrome (KSS), mitochondrial encephalomyopathy with lactic acidosis and strokelike episodes (MELAS), myoclonic epilepsy with ragged red fibers (MERRF), mitochondrial neurogastrointestinal encephalopathy (MNGIE) disease, and in some of the ataxia-neuropathy syndromes (namely sensory ataxia, neuropathy, dysarthria, ophthalmoplegia [SANDO]), or with a previously unrecognized constellation of features. In this context, patients are given a diagnosis of PEO, or "PEO-plus."[4]

Identical PEO phenotypes may be caused by a broad repertoire of genetic defects, including single large-scale mtDNA deletions, numerous mtDNA point mutations, and a number of nuclear-encoded mitochondrial genes (*POLG1*, *POLG2*, *SLC25A4*, *C10orf2*, *RRM2B*, *TK2* and *OPA1*). Similarly, defects in particular mitochondrial genes or specific mtDNA abnormalities are capable of producing unrelated clinical phenotypes. For example, the m.3243A>G mutation may cause maternally inherited diabetes and deafness, cardiomyopathy, PEO, isolated mitochondrial myopathy, or MELAS syndrome. Likewise, mutations in the gene encoding the mitochondrial DNA polymerase γ, *POLG*, can cause a relatively mild syndrome (PEO) or severe infantile-onset syndromes with mtDNA depletion syndromes or myocerebrohepatopathy (Alpers-Huttenlocher

Table 8–1 Clinical Features and Management of Mitochondrial Disorders

Symptom	Investigation/Abnormality	Treatment
Ocular		
Ophthalmoparesis		For diplopia: prism glasses or strabismus surgery
Ptosis		When visual fields obscured: frontalis slings or levator palpebrae resection.
Optic atrophy		Referral for services as appropriate
Pigmentary retinopathy		for level of visual disability; driving restrictions. Potential benefits from idebenone in LHON
Cataract		Surgical resection
Central neurologic		
Ataxia		
Movement disorder		Symptomatic therapy
Spasticity		Symptomatic therapy
Seizures (generalized, focal, and/or myoclonic)	EEG (epileptiform abnormality)	Anticonvulsants (avoid valproic acid if possible)
Migraine		Analgesics and/or tryptans; prophylactic therapy when appropriate
Encephalopathy	MRI (nonspecific white matter or basal ganglia signal abnormalities) EEG (diffuse slowing)	Supportive therapy Avoidance of precipitating factors or medications
Stroke-like episodes	MRI (High-signal T2 abnormality not conforming to vascular territories, posterior-predominant)	L-arginine may be effective
Peripheral neurologic		
Axonal polyneuropathy	EMG, nerve conduction studies	Symptomatic treatment and mobility aids
Sensory neuronopathy/ ganglionopathy		
Sensorineural hearing loss	Audiography	Auditory aids, cochlear implantation
Autonomic dysfunction	Orthostatic vital signs Clinical history for gastrointestinal dysmotility	Symptomatic treatment of orthostatic hypotension; dietary modification for gastrointestinal dysmotility
Musculoskeletal		
Skeletal myopathy (ocular > axial/ proximal > distal > respiratory)	Pulmonary function testing and/or sleep studies for respiratory muscle weakness CK: normal or mildly elevated (or highly elevated in CoQ10 deficiency myopathy) EMG: myopathic changes	Mobility aids Exercise therapy CPAP/BiPAP for respiratory failure
Smooth muscle myopathy (dysphagia)	Esophageal motility studies	Dietary modification
Cardiac		
Cardiomyopathy	Echocardiogram	ACE blockade
Conduction defects	Electrocardiogram, Holter monitor	Pacemaker, antiarrhythmics
Endocrine		
• Diabetes mellitus		
• Hypothyroidism		
• Hypoparathyroidism		
• Gonadal failure		
• Growth hormone deficiency		

(continued)

Table 8–1 **(Cont.)**

Symptom	Investigation/Abnormality	Treatment
Diabetes mellitus	Fasting glucose, oral glucose tolerance test, HgbA1C	Oral antihyperglycaemics, insulin
Hypothyroidism	TSH, T3, T4	Hormone replacement
Hypoparathyroidism	PTH, serum Ca	
Growth hormone deficiency	GH; GHRH-arginine test or insulin tolerance test	
Gonadal failure	LH, FSH	Hormone replacement in selected cases
Gastrointestinal		
Dysmotility: dysphagia, gastroparesis, diarrhea, constipation, and/or pseudo-obstruction	Swallowing studies: crichopharyngeal achalasia or esophageal dysmotility	Dietary modification, symptomatic therapy
Hepatic failure	Serum liver enzyme elevations, liver biopsy	
Neuropsychiatric		
Cognitive impairment	Mental status testing	Caregiver support, lifestyle modifications, assessment for driving and competency
Fatigue		
Depression	Psychiatric assessment	Antidepressants
Psychosis		Neuroleptics
Other		
Short stature		
Spontaneous abortion		

Note. LHON = Leber hereditary optic neuropathy; EMG = electromyography.

syndrome [AHS]).[5] Specific genetic defects and their associated clinical syndromes are shown in Table 8–2.

CLINICAL INVESTIGATION OF MITOCHONDRIAL DISORDERS

Defining the underlying genetic basis of a mitochondrial disorder is particularly important because ostensibly similar mitochondrial phenotypes can have different inheritance patters and recurrence risks, with maternal, autosomal-dominant, autosomal-recessive, and X-linked forms recognized. Many mitochondrial disorders are sporadic, and some cannot be passed down the paternal line. Defining the inheritance pattern thus has profound implications for genetic counseling and prenatal diagnosis.

The approach to investigation is critically dependent on the clinical presentation and the family history, and the clinician should take the time to collect all relevant information before embarking on often costly and time consuming investigations. Genetic testing may be preferable as an initial investigation when a clear-cut clinical syndrome is present. However, if this is not the case, then a systematic clinical approach should be undertaken aimed at building a complete picture of the multisystem phenotype, and subsequently the demonstration of a biochemical defect of mitochondrial function.

Clinical investigations involve tests for potential complications of mitochondrial diseases, including fasting blood glucose measurements, electro- and echocardiography, nerve conduction studies and electromyography, brain imaging (CT for calcification, or MRI, Figure 8–1), and electroencephalography.

Specific biochemical investigations can also be useful in particular clinical contexts. For example, an elevation of plasma and urine thymidine is seen in the myopathy, neuropathy, gastrointestinal encephalopathy syndrome (aka

Table 8–2 Clinical Syndromes of Mitochondrial Disorders, and Their Associated Molecular Basis

Syndrome	Clinical Symptoms/Signs	V	OM	M	C	S	A/PN	GI	Onset age	Genetics	PM	SD	N
Leber hereditary optic neuropathy (LHON)	Serial monocular visual loss	✓							Adulthood	mtDNA point mutations (m.11778G>A, m.3460G>A, m.14484T>C)	✓		
Progressive external ophthalmoplegia (PEO)	Ptosis, ophthalmoparesis. Proximal myopathy often present. Various other clinical features variably present.	✓	✓	✓			✓		Any age of onset. Typically more severe phenotype with younger onset.	mtDNA single deletions, mtDNA point mutations (including m.3243A>G, m.8344A>G), nDNA mutations (*POLG1, POLG2, SLC25A4, C10orf2, RRM2B, TK2,* and *OPA1*)	✓	✓	✓
Kearns-Sayre syndrome (KSS)	PEO, ptosis, pigmentary retinopathy, cardiac conduction abnormality, ataxia, CSF elevated protein, diabetes mellitus, sensorineural hearing loss, myopathy	✓	✓	✓	✓		✓	✓	<20 years	mtDNA single deletions		✓	
Ataxia neuropathy syndromes (ANS), including MIRAS, SCAE, SANDO, MEMSA	SANDO: PEO, dysarthria, sensory neuropathy, cerebellar ataxia. Other ANS: Sensory axonal neuropathy with variable degrees of sensory and cerebellar ataxia. Epilepsy, dysarthria, or myopathy are present in some.	✓	✓	✓		✓	✓		Teen or adult	nDNA mutations (*POLG, C10orf2, OPA1*)			✓
Myopathy, neurogastrointestinal encephalopathy (MNGIE)	PEO, ptosis, GI dysmotility, proximal myopathy, axonal polyneuropathy, leukodystrophy.	✓	✓	✓			✓	✓	Childhood to early adulthood	nDNA mutations in *TYMP*; MNGIE-like syndromes may occur due to nDNA gene mutations with PEO			✓

(*continued*)

Table 8–2 **(Cont.)**

Syndrome	Clinical Symptoms/ Signs	V	OM	M	C	S	A/ PN	GI	Onset age	Genetics	PM	SD	N
Myopathy, encephalopathy, lactic acidosis, stroke like episodes (MELAS)	Strokelike episodes with encephalopathy, migraine, seizures. Variable presence of myopathy, cardiomyopathy, deafness, endocrinopathy, ataxia. A minority of patients have PEO.	✓	✓	✓	✓	✓	✓		Typically <40 years of age but childhood more common	mtDNA point mutations (m.3243A>G in 80%, m.3256C>T, m.3271T>C, m.4332G>A, m.13513G>A, m.13514A>G)	✓		
Myoclonus, epilepsy, and ragged red fibers (MERRF)	Stimulus sensitive myoclonus, generalized seizures, ataxia, cardiomyopathy. A minority of patients have PEO.		✓	✓	✓	✓	✓		Childhood	mtDNA point mutations (m.8344A>G most common; m.8356T>C, m.12147G>A)	✓		
Mitochondrial myopathy (isolated)	Axial/proximal myopathy. May have other features of mitochondrial disease (ataxia, polyneuropathy).		✓	✓					Any age of onset.	mtDNA point mutations (multiple, including m.3243A>G; m.3302A>G, m.14709T>C) mtDNA single large scale deletions	✓	✓	
Mitochondrial DNA depletion syndrome	Diffuse myopathy, or encephalopathy, or hepatocerebral syndrome			✓	✓			✓	Congenital or infantile presentation, with hypotonia, respiratory weakness, and death within few years of life. Infantile COX-deficiency myopathy occasionally reverses after first year of life.	nDNA mutations (*DGUOK, TK2, C10orf2, POLG, RRM2B, SUCLA2, SUCLG1, MPV17*)			✓

Syndrome	Clinical features	Age of onset	Genetics
Infantile myopathy with COX-deficiency	Diffuse myopathy, lactic acidosis, encephalopathy	Congenital/infantile onset. Fatal in first year, or reversible after first year in some patients.	mtDNA mutation (m.14674T>C) in the reversible form.
Neurogenic weakness with ataxia and retinitis pigmentosa (NARP)	Ataxia, pigmentary retinopathy, weakness	Childhood	*MTATP6* mutation (usually at m.8993)
Leigh syndrome	Encephalopathy precipitated by illness, brainstem and cerebellar dysfunction, neuropathy, cardiomyopathy	Infancy	Recessive or X-linked mutations in nDNA-encoded respiratory chain components, and less commonly mtDNA point mutations (usually *MTATP6*)
Alpers-Huttenlocher syndrome (AHS); childhood myocerebral hepatopathy syndrome (MCHS)	Seizures, developmental delay, hypotonia, hepatic failure	Infancy/childhood	Recessive mutations in *POLG*, or unknown; for AHS; for MCHS mutations in *POLG, c10orf2, MPV17, DGUOK*.
Pearson syndrome	Sideroblastic anaemia, pancreatic failure	Infancy	Single large-scale mtDNA deletions
Maternally inherited diabetes and deafness	Type II diabetes Sensorineural hearing loss	Adulthood	mtDNA point mutations (m.3243A>G, various other point mutations described in isolated reports)
Deafness sensorineural hearing loss	Sensorineural hearing loss	Childhood	mtDNA point mutations (m.1095T>C, m.1555A>G, m.7445A>G, and other mutations from isolated reports)
Mitochondrial cardiomyopathy	Cardiomyopathy (hypertrophic or dilated)	Infancy, childhood or adulthood	mtDNA point mutations (m.3243A>G, m.3260A>G, m.4300A>G, and various other mutations from isolated reports), nDNA mutations *COXI5, SLC25A3*

Note. V = visual findings; OM = ocular myopathy; C = cardiomyopathy or conduction defects; S = seizures or encephalopathy; M = myopathy; C = cardiomyopathy; PM = mtDNA point mutation; SD = mtDNA single large-scale deletion; N = nuclear gene mutation; APN = ataxia or polyneuropathy; GI = gastrointestinal or endocrine dysfunction. A check mark indicates that this feature can be associated with the syndrome.

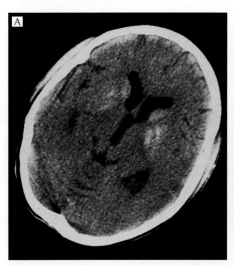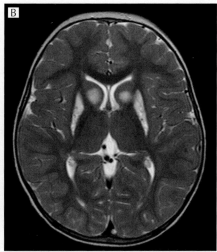

Figure 8–1. Neuroimaging in mitochondrial disorders. A: Brain CT showing basal ganglia calcification in a patient harboring the m.3243A>G MELAS mutation. B: Axial T2 FLAIR MR imaging from a child with Leigh syndrome showing hyperintensity of caudate and putamen (with thanks to Dr. Robert McFarland, University of Newcastle upon Tyne).

MNGIE) due to mutations in *TYMP*. However, blood and even cerebrospinal fluid lactate and pyruvate measurements are nonspecific findings. Although very high levels suggest an underlying mitochondrial disorder, this may also be seen in the context of sepsis or following a prolonged seizure. Conversely, many adults presenting with an indolent phenotype have normal lactate levels. The same applies to serum CK levels, which are often normal in patients with mitochondrial disease, even those with a mitochondrial myopathy. Serum and urine amino acid, organic acid, and carnitine profiles occasionally have nonspecific abnormalities in patients with mitochondrial disorders (respectively elevated alanine, elevated Krebs cycle intermediates, and abnormal fatty acid oxidation). Results of these investigations will vary depending on sample handling as well as the laboratory measurement method.

Serum fibroblast growth factor 21 (FGF-21) measurements have potential diagnostic value in mitochondrial muscle disease.[6] The sensitivity and specificity of FGF21 levels for mitochondrial disease, at least in patients with myopathy phenotypes, appears to be greater than other conventional markers for mitochondrial disease. However, this finding must be replicated in a prospective study before it is incorporated into routine clinical practice.[7]

Noninvasive clinical tests for mitochondrial disorders include exercise testing. There are numerous described protocols for testing using cycle ergometry or treadmill exercise.[8] The specificity[9, 10] and sensitivity[11] of these tests is poor. Venous pO_2 measurement during handgrip testing has high specificity, and is therefore a reasonable screening test,[12,13] but usually when complementing the investigations described above. Functional imaging techniques, such as [31]P- or proton-magnetic resonance spectroscopy, can detect severe mitochondrial myopathy syndromes, but results are often normal in patients with milder syndromes, and can fail to detect lactate elevations in some patients.[14]

If a specific clinical syndrome cannot be diagnosed using molecular genetic testing as the next port of call, the next step is to collect evidence of mitochondrial dysfunction. In general, biochemical and subsequent genetic analysis should be performed on an affected tissue. This usually means a muscle biopsy, but in certain circumstances a liver or cardiac biopsy may be appropriate.[15] In children, investigations usually begin on cultured skin fibroblasts, although these do not always express a biochemical defect.

Muscle Morphology and Histochemistry

Muscle biopsy is typically performed from a limb muscle, such as the quadriceps femoris or deltoid (although in PEO, studies have considered the diagnostic value of levator palpebrae and orbicularis oculi biopsy, which may be useful to avoid a separate procedure for patients who require oculoplastic procedures[16-19]), and is usually snap-frozen in liquid isopentane. In addition to standard histological staining, cryostat sections should undergo a series of histochemical functional assays (see chapter 2). Staining specifically required to demonstrated hallmarks of mitochondrial disease include the Gomori trichrome stain to demonstrate ragged red fibers, which can also be seen on succinate dehydrogenase histochemistry (Figure 8–2).

The major histochemical diagnostic feature is the presence of fibers deficient in cytochrome c oxidase activity (COX; complex IV of the respiratory chain), which represents low COX activity (and is encoded by both mtDNA and nuclear DNA genes). However, COX-negative fibers accumulate with age; therefore an age-dependent threshold must be met to meet criteria for a mitochondrial disorder (>2 % for those under 50, and > 5% for those over 50).[20]

COX-negative fibers are best identified by serially staining muscle for COX followed by SDH, which stains for complex II (and is encoded entirely by nuclear genes). The demonstration of COX-deficient, SDH-positive muscle fibers may have the best sensitivity and specificity for mitochondrial disease, particularly in adults.[21] The subsarcolemmal accumulation of mitochondria is a classic feature of mitochondrial myopathy, and can be demonstrated by SDH histochemistry (ragged blue fibers), or the Gomori trichrome stain (ragged red fibers, or RRF). Again, RRF (< 5%) can be seen in healthy aged individuals. However, the detection of RRF in individuals < 50 years of age, or > 5% RRF at any age is highly suggestive of mitochondrial myopathy. RRF are also seen in sporadic disorders, such as inclusion body myositis, and some inherited disorders, including myotonic dystrophy. The findings on muscle biopsy may provide guidance for appropriate genetic testing. As a general rule, a mosaic appearance of COX-negative fibers suggests a mtDNA mutation (due to the variable degrees of heteroplasmy between muscle

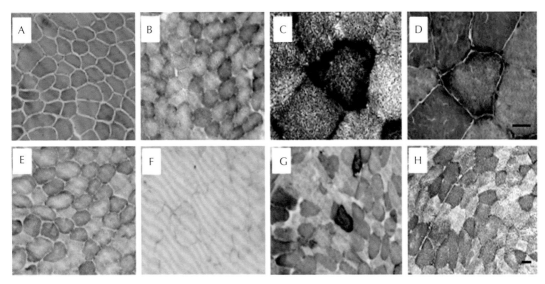

Figure 8–2. Muscle pathology in mitochondrial disorders. 20-μm cryostat sections of quadriceps skeletal muscle. (A) Hematoxylin and eosin, showing increased angulation of the muscle fibers and an increase in the proportion of internal nuclei. (B) Succinate dehydrogenase (SDH) histochemistry in a patient with a heteroplasmic mtDNA defect, showing subsarcolemmal proliferation of mitochondria. (C) Higher power view of SDH histochemistry showing a classical ragged red fiber. (D) Ragged red fiber shown by Gomori trichrome staining. (E) Cytochrome c oxidase (COX) histochemistry in a normal subject. (F) Global reduction in COX activity seen in a patient with a nuclear gene defect. (G) Mosaic COX defect demonstrated by sequential COX-SDH histochemistry in a patient with a heteroplasmic pathogenic mtDNA mutation. (H) COX-SDH histochemistry from an aged subject showing a single COX-deficient muscle fiber. Scale bar for A, B, E, F, G, and H = 50 μm as shown in H. Scale bar for C and D = 25 μm as shown in H (with thanks to Prof. Robert Taylor, Newcastle upon Tyne, based on *Greenfields Pathology*, 9th Edition).

cells), whereas uniformly decreased COX activity suggests a nDNA mutation (which would be equally present in all muscle cells). Other characteristic features include the presence of strongly SDH-positive blood vessels in patients with the m.3243A>G mutation.[22]

Electron microscopy (EM) of muscle may demonstrate enlarged pleiomorphic mitochondria and paracrystalline inclusions. EM provides minor support for the diagnosis of mitochondrial disease because the findings are often nonspecific.[23] It is important to note that muscle histology, histochemistry, and EM may be normal even in genetically proven mitochondrial disorders,[24] particularly early in the disease course, or when the biochemical defect does not involve complex IV (COX).

Respiratory Chain Enzyme Analysis

Respiratory chain enzyme (RCE) analysis must be done either on fresh, or snap-frozen muscle samples. RCE is technically difficult to perform, even in specialist laboratories[25,21,26] and the results should be interpreted in the context of the other investigations. Demonstrating a RCE defect is an important diagnostic step in patients with normal or near-normal muscle histochemistry, particularly children. In conditions such as Leigh syndrome, which is caused by a large array of nuclear gene defects, the demonstration of a specific RCE complex defect can guide the genetic investigations to confirm the diagnosis. However, RCE abnormalities can also occur early in the course of mtDNA depletion syndromes; therefore the presence of a specific complex deficiency does not guarantee that a mutation in a specific complex assembly factor is present. It is important to note that complex V (ATP synthase) is rarely measured in diagnostic laboratories, but a defect of ATP synthase may be the only biochemical abnormality in some patients. It is also important to note that RCE analysis can be normal in some genetically proven mitochondrial disorders.

Diagnostic information can also be obtained from fibroblast cultures, established from a skin biopsy, which can be used for RCE analysis and DNA for genetic studies. However, this tissue has lower sensitivity than muscle, because the RCE defect or molecular genetic defect may not be present in fibroblasts in all patients.[27]

Liver biopsy is appropriate in patients with hepatic disease, providing there is no coagulopathy. In these situations the biopsy is helpful to exclude other disorders and is a tissue source for histological, EM, RCE, and DNA analysis.

Mitochondrial myopathy due to CoQ10 biosynthetic defects can be diagnosed by measuring CoQ10 in muscle tissue, and may be supported by decreased levels in other tissues such as fibroblasts and white blood cells.[26,28] Plasma levels have a broad reference range and may be normal in this condition.[26] RCE analysis on muscle tissue may demonstrate the combination of either complex I and III deficiency, or complex II and III deficiency, since these complexes are CoQ10 dependent.[29]

Molecular Genetic Analysis

Patients presenting with a characteristic clinical phenotype benefit from early genetic testing. The high yield in this context prevents the need for invasive tests. Pathogenic mutations of mtDNA are sometimes (but not always) detectable in leucocyte DNA, and can be used to diagnose MERRF or MELAS syndromes. The percentage level of some point mutations, including the common m.3243A>G that causes MELAS, decreases in blood at an exponential rate during life. As a result, these mutations can be undetectable in blood, despite very high levels in skeletal muscle. Thus, a negative blood test does not necessarily mean that the specific mutation is not causing the disease. These mutations can sometimes be detected in urinary epithelium, spun down from a urine sample, or found in a buccal swab. However, if these tests are negative and the clinical suspicion remains, then it may be necessary to carry out genetic testing on a muscle biopsy. mtDNA deletions cannot be reliably detected in blood, although duplications may be detected and are association with pathogenic deletions of mtDNA. The standard approach is to screen for common mtDNA point mutations using allele-specific assays or targeted sequencing, and to screen for mtDNA deletions using long-range polymerase chain reaction (PCR), or Southern blotting. Real-time PCR can be used to screen for mtDNA deletions, and to determine whether there is depletion (loss) of mtDNA in clinically affected tissues. Mutations in nDNA, when present, are always detectable from leucocyte DNA. Specific clinical syndromes such as the complex neurological phenotype associated with autosomal dominant optic atrophy can be diagnosed this way.

The molecular diagnosis of mitochondrial disorders is rapidly improving. Next-generation sequencing approaches involve the targeted capture of large panels of nuclear genes, and the application of whole exome capture techniques. These techniques have identified new nuclear genes for mitochondrial syndromes[30,31] and have expanded the phenotypic spectrum of other nuclear gene defects.[32] It is conceivable that whole-exome or whole-genome sequencing will become the first test of choice in patients with mitochondrial disease, when costs fall and bioinformatic techniques enable the confident discrimination of pathogenic variants.

CLINICAL MANAGEMENT OF MITOCHONDRIAL DISEASE

Disease Surveillance and the Management of Complications

Cardiac complications are important to identify with electrocardiogram and echocardiogram, and depending on the patient's syndrome, other screening tests may be needed at regular intervals. Patients with KSS, MERRF, and MELAS syndromes (see Table 8–2 for a key to the acronyms) appear to be most likely to develop progressive cardiac disease,[33] although optimal screening recommendations do not exist for these syndromes or others. Cardiac conduction defects can be fatal if untreated, and are addressed with cardiac pacemakers and antiarrhythmics.[34] Cardiomyopathy may be treated with ACE inhibitors and beta-blockers, and cardiac transplantation in selected cases.[35] Ptosis in PEO can become disabling if the eyelids obstruct vision, and surgical treatment include levator palpebrae superioris resection or frontalis slings. Overcorrection of ptosis can cause exposure keratitis. Endocrine investigations may identify diabetes mellitus, hypothyroidism, or growth hormone deficiency, all of which are treatable. Patients with hearing or visual symptoms should be investigated to obtain appropriate aids if required. Cochlear implants can be effective for the deafness of mitochondrial disease.[36] Dysphagia is common in several mitochondrial syndromes[37] and improvement is possible with dietary modification.

Specific Treatments for Mitochondrial Disorders

A recent Cochrane systematic review of all case series and treatment trials in mitochondrial diseases concluded that there were no treatments of proven benefit to influence the outcome of the disorder.[38] As a consequence, the clinical management of mitochondrial disorders concentrates on supportive therapy, and symptomatic management of disease complications, such as those mentioned in the preceding section. Therapeutic agents to date have focused on various nutritional supplements, including carnitine,[39] creatine,[40-42] CoQ10,[43,44] cysteine,[45] dichloroacetate,[43,46-49] dimethyglycine,[50] and the combination of creatine, CoQ10, and lipoic acid,[51] which have been evaluated in controlled trials. Various other agents including ascorbate and menadione, high-fat diet, magnesium, nicotinamide, and succinate have been of benefit in case reports, but further study would be required to indicate whether they are beneficial. Although there are no specific trials showing objective evidence of clinical efficacy, patients with a predominantly myopathic presentation should have muscle CoQ10 measurements performed, because patients with CoQ10 biosynthetic defects may respond to CoQ10 supplementation.[52]

For patients with myopathy, there is evidence that various forms of exercise therapy are beneficial for numerous endpoints, including strength, fatigue, and quality of life. Aerobic,[53,54] endurance,[55,56] and resistance[57] training programs have been studied. Exercise therapy may simply reverse the deconditioning, which is a common feature of many muscle diseases, or it is possible the exercise affects the underlying pathology, or a combination of these.

Data from a single group of investigators suggest L-arginine as therapy for MELAS, for both the acute strokelike episodes, as well as for chronic therapy to prevent further events.[58]

The data should be interpreted with caution because they were not blinded and both studies originate from the same investigators. A separate study suggested L-arginine may be useful in mitochondrial cardiomyopathy.[59] This agent should be studied in a prospective, randomized, blinded, controlled trial.

Last, in patients with MNGIE, platelet transfusions, peritoneal dialysis, transfusions of red blood cells containing entrapped thymidine phosphorylase,[60] and allogeneic stem cell transplantation (SCT)[61] have been shown to reduce the circulating levels of toxic thymidine, but carry high mortality risk.[62] Combination of nonablative SCT with platelet transfusions has also been reported.[63] Consensus guidelines have recently been established to standardize the provision of SCT in carefully selected patients,[64] although evidence demonstrating clinical benefit is limited.[65]

Drug Toxicity in Mitochondrial Disease

Valproic acid interferes with mitochondrial function and can aggravate mitochondrial myopathy symptoms.[66] Valproate-induced hepatotoxicity may be more common in mitochondrial myopathy patients,[67,68] which in some cases is modulated by genetic variation in *POLG*.[69] However, in our clinical experience adult patients with mitochondrial syndromes and seizures may use valproate safely if adequately monitored, and this is appropriate if valproate provides better seizure control.

Antiretroviral agents, particularly nucleotide reverse-transcriptase inhibitors, cause reversible and dose-dependent mitochondrial toxicity.[70] Certain agents have less mitochondrial toxicity[71] and should be used preferentially. Small series have documented the development of PEO-like syndromes in patients on antiretrovirals,[72-74] although whether this is due to an unmasking effect, or whether the disease is caused by cumulative mitochondrial toxicity, requires further study. A recent study hypothesized that HIV and antiretrovirals induced clonal expansion of deleted mtDNA molecules.

Statin medications are thought to interfere with mitochondrial function,[75] although the mechanisms remain unclear. Ten percent of patients who receive statins develop muscle symptoms[76] (chapter 11), and statins have been reported to unmask symptoms in asymptomatic mitochondrial myopathy patients.[77] Statins have been reported in association with syndromes resembling PEO.[78,79] In theory they should be used cautiously in mitochondrial myopathy, but our clinical experience suggests these agents are safe when used with proper monitoring (chapter 11).

The use of anesthetic agents is an unresolved issue in mitochondrial disorders, with case reports documenting adverse reactions. Decisions regarding these agents should be made on a case-by-case basis in consultation with an anesthetist, considering the patient's general condition and specific respiratory and cardiac function.

Genetic Counseling and Prevention

Patients with mitochondrial syndromes should receive genetic counseling. The counseling depends on the underlying genetic diagnosis (chapter 3). Patients with a similar phenotype can have an autosomal-dominant or -recessive or maternally inherited disorder. Some mitochondrial disorders have variable clinical penetrance and expressivity, and some are largely sporadic diseases. When the genetic etiology is known, patients and their family members can make informed decisions regarding whether to have biological children of their own, and if so, whether reproductive technologies will be employed. Available methods include preimplantation genetic diagnosis, and on an experimental basis pronuclear transfer has been achieved,[80] which reduces or may eliminate the risk of transmission of mtDNA defects (see chapter 3).

SPECIFIC SYNDROMES ASSOCIATED WITH MITOCHONDRIAL MYOPATHY

Here we discuss the major clinical syndromes with mitochondrial myopathy. We have not considered other common mitochondrial disorders, such as Leber hereditary optic neuropathy or isolated sensorineural deafness, because myopathy does not form part of the phenotypic spectrum. There is overlap between the various sections, reflecting the clinical and genetic heterogeneity of mitochondrial disorders, and the overlapping disease spectra. It should be stressed that many patients with mitochondrial disease do not neatly fit into these categories, and have an ill-defined multisystem disease that is often associated with muscle weakness.

Progressive External Ophthalmoplegia

PEO is an ocular myopathy characterized by gradual-onset ophthalmoparesis and ptosis. These features can occur in isolation, or with additional features. There is extensive phenotypic variability (may be pure PEO or present with dysfunction in multiple organ systems), variability in onset age (early childhood to late adulthood), and heterogeneity of genetic causes (mtDNA point mutations, single large-scale mtDNA deletions, or nuclear gene defects causing secondary mtDNA defects). To complicate matters further, ocular myopathy is a component of the clinical presentation of various other mitochondrial syndromes (MELAS, MERRF, KSS, MNGIE and the ataxia-neuropathy syndromes, as described in later sections; and other diseases that are not primary respiratory chain disorders, such as dominant optic atrophy due to *OPA1* mutation). In this sense, PEO should be thought of as a syndrome which may occur in isolation, or as a component of other diseases.

Onset of PEO in childhood tends to have more severe phenotype with regard to the ocular myopathy, and is more likely to be complicated by dysfunction in other organ systems, particularly the cardiac system. Many of these cases are caused by single large-scale mtDNA deletions and exist on a phenotypic spectrum with patients having KSS. PEO in adulthood generally has a more slowly progressive ocular myopathy and more benign course, with a milder severity and different pattern of multisystem dysfunction.[51]

On clinical examination patients with PEO have bilateral ptosis, multidirectional ophthalmoparesis, and slow saccades. Other ocular findings depend on etiology, such as pigmentary retinopathy in PEO due to single large-scale deletions, or optic atrophy in PEO due to *OPA1* mutation.[52]

Diagnostic tests include the finding of RRF and COX-negative fibers in most cases on muscle biopsy. Genetic testing for mtDNA defects must be performed on muscle DNA, since the mtDNA abnormalities are usually absent in leucocyte DNA. Testing of mtDNA should include long PCR and Southern blot for mtDNA deletions, mtDNA sequencing for point mutations, and sequencing of nuclear genes including *POLG1*, *POLG2*, *SLC25A4* (*ANT1*), *C10orf2* (*PEO1*), *RRM2B*, *TK2* and *OPA1*. Neuroimaging can incidentally demonstrate volume loss of the extraocular muscles[53] or nonspecific white-matter signal abnormalities.[54] Elevated lactate is occasionally demonstrated on testing of serum at rest and postexercise, or with MR spectroscopy.

Treatment of PEO includes management of secondary complications of the disease. The most disabling component of the ocular myopathy is ptosis, which can be treated (see Disease Surveillance and the Management of Complications section). Cardiac screening with regular echo- and electrocardiograms is recommended particularly for PEO patients with early-onset disease or syndromes resembling KSS, who are at high risk of developing cardiac dysfunction.[55] Adult-onset PEO patients have a low risk of cardiomyopathy or arrhythmia although regular screening is still prudent.[56]

Mitochondrial DNA Deletion Syndromes

These disorders exist on a disease spectrum and include (in decreasing clinical severity): Pearson syndrome, KSS, and some cases of PEO (those caused by single mtDNA deletions).[57] Isolated mitochondrial myopathy can also be caused by single large-scale mtDNA deletions, but like PEO, it is genetically heterogeneous.

KSS includes PEO and pigmentary retinopathy prior to the age of 20, accompanied by cardiac conduction defects, cerebellar ataxia, and/or elevated CSF protein. Various other combinations of organ dysfunction frequently coexist, particularly sensorineural hearing loss and diabetes mellitus. Most cases are caused by single large-scale mtDNA deletions (most frequently, the "common deletion," m.8470-13446del4977).

Genetic testing on mtDNA, as in PEO, should be performed on DNA extracted from muscle. Other diagnostic testing is as for PEO, except that when this syndrome is suspected it should always include further testing to confirm the diagnosis and identify the common treatable complications, specifically electrocardiogram and echocardiogram, fasting glucose, hearing tests, and CSF analysis.

There is no disease-modifying therapy for KSS, and treatment focuses on the management of secondary complications: cardiac manifestations, which may require cardiac pacemakers,[88] antiarrhythmics, ACE inhibitors,[89] or in severe and selected cases, cardiac transplantation.[90]

Pearson syndrome is an infantile-onset disorder including sideroblastic anemia and pancreatic exocrine failure.[91] The condition is usually fatal in infancy, although patients who survive develop a syndrome resembling a severe form of KSS. Bone marrow biopsy is diagnostic and demonstrates ringed sideroblasts and normoblasts with iron deposition within mitochondria. The pancreatic failure causes steatorrhoea. For purposes of genetic testing, leucocyte DNA is suitable because the mtDNA deletion is present at high levels in this tissue in this syndrome.

Mitochondrial Encephalomyopathy with Lactic Acidosis and Strokelike Episodes

MELAS syndrome has a heterogeneous clinical presentation. Onset of symptoms is typically in childhood or early adulthood. Clinical features may include episodes of encephalopathy, proximal myopathy, cardiomyopathy, lactic acidosis, strokelike episodes (preferentially affecting the occipital lobes and not respecting typical vascular distributions), migraine headaches, epilepsy, hearing loss, and endocrinopathy.[92] These comorbidities may cause major disability and shortened lifespan, usually due to cardiac dysfunction or seizures/encephalopathy.[93] The condition is caused by mutations of mtDNA-encoded tRNAs, specifically by the m.3243A>G mutation in 80% of cases.

Diagnosis of MELAS is confirmed by genetic testing, and the mutation can be detected from blood, urine sediment, or muscle. The heteroplasmy level of the m.3243A>G mutation from urine samples may have prognostic significance and correlate with phenotypic severity.[94] Other tests providing evidence for MELAS include muscle biopsy, which characteristically demonstrates RRF and strongly SDH-reactive blood vessels. Respiratory-chain enzyme analysis performed from muscle tissue can be normal or demonstrate nonspecific abnormalities. MRI of the brain during strokelike events may reveal regions of T2 signal abnormality, usually predominantly in the occipital lobes, and not respecting typical vascular boundaries[95] (Figure 8–3).

Management of MELAS includes the identification and treatment of disease complications.[96] There is no proven disease-modifying therapy available, although two nonblinded studies from the same investigators demonstrated benefit of L-arginine for prevention, and acute treatment of strokelike episodes.[58] Genetic counseling is recommended for women with the mutation, who are at risk of transmitting the disease to their offspring.

Myoclonic Epilepsy with Ragged Red Fibers

MERRF classically presents as one of the progressive myoclonic epilepsy (PME) syndromes.

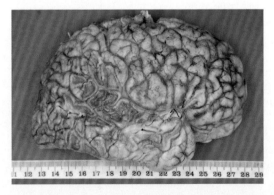

Figure 8–3. Mitochondrial encephalomyopathy with lactic acidosis and strokelike episodes. Extensive cortical ablation/laminar necrosis over the occipital, lateral parietal, and lateral inferior temporal lobes in a fixed right cerebral hemisphere (with thanks to Prof. Robert Perry, Newcastle upon Tyne, Adapted from *Greenfields Pathology*, 9th Edition).

As in the other PMEs, patients have normal early development until the onset of generalized myoclonic jerks, generalized seizures, and other neurologic dysfunction. In the case of MERRF, the syndrome includes myoclonus, generalized epilepsy, ataxia, and RRF on muscle biopsy,[97] and is also extensively clinically heterogeneous.[98] Usually patients also develop other multisystem complications of mitochondrial disease, although cardiac dysfunction deserves special mention because it is common in this syndrome, treatable, and a cause of early morbidity and mortality.[89]

The genetic etiology of about 90% of MERRF cases is mutations of the mitochondrially encoded *TRNK* gene (most often m.8344A>G),[99] and the remainder of cases are caused by other mutations of the mtDNA. The mutation is best detected from muscle DNA but is also detectable from skin biopsy, urine sediment, and leucocyte DNA. Serum lactate is often elevated. Analysis of cerebrospinal fluid can show elevated lactate and/or mildly elevated protein. Muscle biopsy demonstrates RRF and COX-negative fibers. EEG reveals slow background activity, generalized epileptiform abnormalities, and occasionally photoparoxysmal response.[100] MRI is similarly nonspecific and may show generalized cerebral and cerebellar volume loss.

Treatment includes lifelong anticonvulsant therapy with agents that can control both the myoclonic and generalized seizures. There are no trials demonstrating preferred treatment, although there are theoretical contraindications to the use of valproic acid (due to development of carnitine deficiency).[101] However, in our experience valproic acid may be the only agent providing adequate seizure control, and it has not been demonstrated to aggravate MERRF disease symptoms. Notwithstanding this, supplementation with L-carnitine while on therapy with valproic acid has been advocated.[102] Levetiracetam can provide good control of the myoclonic seizures and is an alternative to valproic acid.[103]

Polymerase Gamma–Related Disorders

POLG is a nuclear gene coding for the mtDNA polymerase. Over 160 mutations are associated with a broad clinical spectrum of disease, including autosomal-dominant PEO, autosomal-recessive PEO, ataxia neuropathy spectrum (ANS), MELAS-like syndromes, and the AHS spectrum.

ANS comprises disorders that are typically caused by nuclear gene defects and have been previously designated as spinocerebellar ataxia with epilepsy; myoclonic epilepsy, myopathy, sensory ataxia (MEMSA)[104]; SANDO[105]; and mitochondrial recessive ataxia syndrome (MIRAS).[104] The various syndromes have in common the presence of sensory or sensorimotor neuropathy, cerebellar ataxia, and variable degrees of other central nervous dysfunction, PEO, and involvement of other organ systems.[106] The age of onset, severity, and prognosis is variable, although in general patients with earlier onset, and seizure disorders, tend to have worse outcomes.[107] Seizures are frequently described in patients with MIRAS, and manifest as complex partial, clonic or myoclonic, epilepsia partialis continua, or convulsive status epilepticus. Seizures can be documented on EEG and may trigger strokelike lesions with a posterior predilection, similar to those seen in patients with MELAS.[108]

The pathogenesis of *POLG* disorders is thought to occur through secondary defects in the maintenance of mtDNA (tissue-specific multiple mtDNA deletions, for dominant disorders) or in the replication of mtDNA (mtDNA depletion, for recessive disorders), and patients often have characteristic neuroimaging. The mtDNA depletion syndromes are considered separately in the Mitochondrial DNA Depletion Syndromes section, because only a small proportion of cases are caused by mutations in *POLG*.

Leigh Syndrome

Leigh syndrome has its onset in infancy and is sometimes precipitated by viral illness. Diagnostic criteria have been suggested for this condition,[109] including the presence of progressive disease with brainstem and cerebellar signs (movement disorder, hypotonia, ataxia), elevated lactate in blood or CSF, and characteristic MRI[110] or neuropathologic abnormalities of the basal ganglia and brainstem. Commonly associated features include central respiratory failure, developmental delay, seizures, and pigmentary retinopathy.[111]

Muscle histopathology is of limited value in this condition, although muscle tissue is essential for respiratory chain enzyme analysis. When individual RCE complex defects are identified, it can guide the direction of genetic investigation, which includes a lengthy and expanding list of nDNA defects and mtDNA point mutations.[111] MRI abnormalities are present in most patients and may be visible preclinically with diffusion-weighted imaging.[112] About one-third of cases of Leigh syndrome are caused by mtDNA mutations, and of these mutations in MTATP6 are most common. Prognosis is not predictable based upon the genetic etiology. In most cases the condition is fatal within 1 year of onset, although massive variation in clinical phenotype exists,[113] and presentation can rarely occur even in advanced age.[114]

Neurogenic Muscle Weakness, Ataxia, and Retinitis Pigmentosa Syndrome

NARP syndrome is on a disease spectrum with Leigh syndrome, and these conditions share a common genetic etiology, in the form of mutations in the mitochondrially encoded MTATP6 gene (although the genetic etiology for Leigh syndrome is usually due to one of myriad nDNA defects, as noted in the previous section).[115] NARP is defined by childhood onset of sensorimotor neuropathy, ataxia, and pigmentary retinopathy,[116] accompanied by learning disability and other milder features of Leigh disease such as movement disorder or cardiac dysfunction. Most cases are caused by mutations at position m.8993. Mutations in the MTATP6 gene are part of an even broader disease spectrum that also includes adult-onset spasticity[117] and ataxia.[118,119]

Mitochondrial Neurogastrointestinal Encephalopathy Disease

MNGIE is characterized by diffuse gastrointestinal neuropathy and myopathy, and demyelinating peripheral neuropathy. Age of onset is typically in childhood or early adulthood. The dominant clinical feature of this disease is the presence of severe gastrointestinal dysmotility throughout the gastrointestinal tract, due to atrophy of smooth muscle and autonomic nervous system dysfunction. Patients develop symptoms due to esophageal dysmotility (dysphagia), gastroparesis (nausea, vomiting, early satiety), and intestinal hypomotility (malabsorption, diarrhea, constipation). Symptoms may also be episodic in the form of abdominal pain or pseudo-obstruction.[120] Ultimately cachexia develops as a consequence of the combined gastrointestinal dysfunction, and patients have a shortened lifespan of only 2 to 4 decades after the onset of disease.

The demyelinating sensorimotor peripheral neuropathy affects the distal lower extremities first and most commonly manifests as foot drop, sensory ataxia, and/or neuropathic pain. Myopathy is also a common associated feature, in the form of external ophthalmoplegia and ptosis.

The disease is caused by homozygous or compound heterozygous mutations in thymidine phosphorylase (TYMP), although MNGIE-like syndromes have been described in patients with mtDNA[121] and other nDNA mutations (POLG[122] and RRM2B[123]). Diagnostic testing includes elevations in serum thymidine and deoxyuridine concentrations, a secondary effect of markedly reduced thymidine phosphorylase activity. Muscle biopsy demonstrates RRF and COX-negative fibers. Leukoencephalopathy is present on MRI.

Treatment of MNGIE includes management of secondary complications of the disease and genetic counseling. There is no disease-modifying therapy at present, although experimental interventions to replace thymidine phosphorylase activity are under investigation. Allogeneic bone marrow transplantation corrects the biochemical defects[61] and appears to produce improvement in gastrointestinal symptoms,[65] but carries a high mortality risk,[62] possibly related to the induction phase in already compromised patients. Other possible treatment options that have been trialed in other enzyme deficiency diseases and could be attempted for MNGIE include gene therapy, and various delivery options for ERT.[124] One avenue for the latter option includes encapsulated thymidine phsophorylase enzyme within autologous erythrocytes.[60] Treatment should be decided on a case by case basis with careful attention to patient selection and timing,[64] given the rapidly progressive nature of this disease.

Mitochondrial DNA Depletion Syndromes (Including Alpers-Huttenlocher Syndrome)

The mtDNA depletion syndromes are caused by recessive nuclear gene mutations, and are usually fatal disorders with onset in infancy and severely decreased mtDNA content in cells. The major clinical presentations include two major phenotypes, either severe diffuse myopathy, or a hepatocerebral syndrome (which consists of a disease continuum ranging from more marked cerebral or hepatic involvement, or both; other features such as diffuse myopathy, metabolic derangements, and seizures are often present). The myopathic form is caused by mutations in *TK2* and *RRM2B*,[125,126] whereas hepatocerebral syndromes are caused by mutations in *DGUOK*, *MPV17*, *POLG*, *PEO1*, *SUCLA2*, or *SUCLG1*.[127-130] The common mechanism for all the genetic lesions would appear to be by dysfunction in mtDNA replication and/or maintenance of the mtDNA nucleotide supply. The use of valproic acid is particularly contraindicated in these disorders as it exacerbates hepatic failure (as is also the case for AHS, another hepatocerebral syndrome caused by *POLG* mutations). Death typically occurs in infancy or early childhood, due to liver failure or respiratory failure.

REFERENCES

1. Guda C, Fahy E, Subramaniam S. MITOPRED: A genome-scale method for prediction of nucleus-encoded mitochondrial proteins. Bioinformatics. 2004 Jul 22;20(11):1785–1794.
2. Lopez MF, Kristal BS, Chernokalskaya E, Lazarev A, Shestopalov AI, Bogdanova A, et al. High-throughput profiling of the mitochondrial proteome using affinity fractionation and automation. Electrophoresis. 2000 Oct;21(16):3427–3440.
3. Chinnery PF, Johnson MA, Wardell TM, Singh-Kler R, Hayes C, Brown DT, et al. The epidemiology of pathogenic mitochondrial DNA mutations. Ann Neurol. 2000 Aug;48(2):188–193.
4. Bau V, Zierz S. Update on chronic progressive external ophthalmoplegia. Strabismus. 2005 Sep;13(3):133–142.
5. Horvath R, Hudson G, Ferrari G, Futterer N, Ahola S, Lamantea E, et al. Phenotypic spectrum associated with mutations of the mitochondrial polymerase gamma gene. Brain. 2006 Jul;129(Pt 7):1674–1684.
6. Suomalainen A, Elo JM, Pietiläinen KH, Hakonen AH, Sevastianova K, Korpela M, et al. FGF-21 as a biomarker for muscle-manifesting mitochondrial respiratory chain deficiencies: A diagnostic study. Lancet Neurol. 2011 Sep;10(9):806–818.
7. Suomalainen A. Fibroblast growth factor 21: A novel biomarker for human muscle-manifesting mitochondrial disorders. Expert Opin Med Diagn. 2013 Jul;7(4):313–317.
8. Tarnopolsky M. Exercise testing as a diagnostic entity in mitochondrial myopathies Mitochondrion. 2004 Sep;4(5–6):529–542.
9. Dandurand RJ, Matthews PM, Arnold DL, Eidelman DH. Mitochondrial disease. Pulmonary function, exercise performance, and blood lactate levels. Chest. 1995 Jul;108(1):182–189.
10. Hammaren E, Rafsten L, Kreuter M, Lindberg C. Modified exercise test in screening for mitochondrial myopathies—adjustment of workload in relation to muscle strength. Eur Neurol. 2004;51(1):38–41.
11. Jeppesen TD, Olsen D, Vissing J. Cycle ergometry is not a sensitive diagnostic test for mitochondrial myopathy. J Neurol. 2003 Mar;250(3):293–299.
12. Jensen TD, Kazemi-Esfarjani P, Skomorowska E, Vissing J. A forearm exercise screening test for mitochondrial myopathy. Neurology. 2002 May 28;58(10):1533–1538.
13. Taivassalo T, Abbott A, Wyrick P, Haller RG. Venous oxygen levels during aerobic forearm exercise: An index of impaired oxidative metabolism in mitochondrial myopathy. Ann Neurol. 2002 Jan;51(1):38–44.
14. Gropman AL. Neuroimaging in mitochondrial disorders. Neurotherapeutics. 2013 Apr;10(2):273–285.
15. Mitochondrial Medicine Society's Committee on Diagnosis, Haas RH, Parikh S, Falk MJ, Saneto RP, Wolf NI, et al. The in-depth evaluation of suspected mitochondrial disease. Mol Genet Metab. 2008 May;94(1):16–37.
16. Greaves LC, Yu-Wai-Man P, Blakely EL, Krishnan KJ, Beadle NE, Kerin J, et al. Mitochondrial DNA defects and selective extraocular muscle involvement in CPEO. Invest Ophthalmol Vis Sci. 2010 Jul;51(7):3340–3346.
17. Pfeffer G, Waters PJ, Maguire J, Vallance HD, Wong VA, Mezei MM. Levator palpebrae biopsy and diagnosis of progressive external ophthalmoplegia. Can J Neurol Sci. 2012 Jul;39(4):520–524.
18. Eshaghian J, Anderson RL, Weingeist TA, Hart MN, Cancilla PA. Orbicularis oculi muscle in chronic progressive external ophthalmoplegia. Arch Ophthalmol. 1980 Jun;98(6):1070–1073.
19. Almousa R, Charlton A, Rajesh ST, Sundar G, Amrith S. Optimizing muscle biopsy for the diagnosis of mitochondrial myopathy. Ophthal Plast Reconstr Surg. 2009 Sep-Oct;25(5):366–370.
20. Bernier FP, Boneh A, Dennett X, Chow CW, Cleary MA, Thorburn DR. Diagnostic criteria for respiratory chain disorders in adults and children. Neurology. 2002 Nov 12;59(9):1406–1411.
21. Taylor RW, Schaefer AM, Barron MJ, McFarland R, Turnbull DM. The diagnosis of mitochondrial

muscle disease. Neuromuscul Disord. 2004 Apr;14(4): 237–245.

22. Hasegawa H, Matsuoka T, Goto Y, Nonaka I. Strongly succinate dehydrogenase-reactive blood vessels in muscles from patients with mitochondrial myopathy, encephalopathy, lactic acidosis, and stroke-like episodes. Ann Neurol. 1991 Jun;29(6):601–605.

23. Bernier FP, Boneh A, Dennett X, Chow CW, Cleary MA, Thorburn DR. Diagnostic criteria for respiratory chain disorders in adults and children. Neurology. 2002 Nov 12;59(9):1406–1411.

24. Schaefer AM, Blakely EL, Griffiths PG, Turnbull DM, Taylor RW. Ophthalmoplegia due to mitochondrial DNA disease: The need for genetic diagnosis. Muscle Nerve. 2005 Jul;32(1):104–107.

25. Wibrand F, Jeppesen TD, Frederiksen AL, Olsen DB, Duno M, Schwartz M, et al. Limited diagnostic value of enzyme analysis in patients with mitochondrial tRNA mutations. Muscle Nerve. 2010 May;41(5):607–613.

26. Medja F, Allouche S, Frachon P, Jardel C, Malgat M, Mousson de Camaret B, et al. Development and implementation of standardized respiratory chain spectrophotometric assays for clinical diagnosis. Mitochondrion. 2009 Sep;9(5):331–339.

27. van den Heuvel LP, Smeitink JA, Rodenburg RJ. Biochemical examination of fibroblasts in the diagnosis and research of oxidative phosphorylation (OXPHOS) defects. Mitochondrion. 2004 Sep;4(5–6):395–401.

28. Rotig A, Appelkvist EL, Geromel V, Chretien D, Kadhom N, Edery P, et al. Quinone-responsive multiple respiratory-chain dysfunction due to widespread coenzyme Q10 deficiency. Lancet. 2000 Jul 29;356(9227):391–395.

29. Ogasahara S, Engel AG, Frens D, Mack D. Muscle coenzyme Q deficiency in familial mitochondrial encephalomyopathy. Proc Natl Acad Sci U S A. 1989 Apr;86(7):2379–2382.

30. Wortmann SB, Vaz FM, Gardeitchik T, Vissers LE, Renkema GH, Schuurs-Hoeijmakers JH, et al. Mutations in the phospholipid remodeling gene SERAC1 impair mitochondrial function and intracellular cholesterol trafficking and cause dystonia and deafness. Nat Genet. 2012 Jun 10;44(7):797–802.

31. Galmiche L, Serre V, Beinat M, Assouline Z, Lebre AS, Chretien D, et al. Exome sequencing identifies MRPL3 mutation in mitochondrial cardiomyopathy. Hum Mutat. 2011 Nov;32(11):1225–1231.

32. Tyynismaa H, Sun R, Ahola-Erkkila S, Almusa H, Poyhonen R, Korpela M, et al. Thymidine kinase 2 mutations in autosomal recessive progressive external ophthalmoplegia with multiple mitochondrial DNA deletions. Hum Mol Genet. 2012 Jan 1;21(1):66–75.

33. Wahbi K, Larue S, Jardel C, Meune C, Stojkovic T, Ziegler F, et al. Cardiac involvement is frequent in patients with the m.8344A>G mutation of mitochondrial DNA. Neurology. 2010 Feb 23;74(8):674–677.

34. Polak PE, Zijlstra F, Roelandt JR. Indications for pacemaker implantation in the Kearns-Sayre syndrome. Eur Heart J. 1989 Mar;10(3):281–282.

35. Bhati RS, Sheridan BC, Mill MR, Selzman CH. Heart transplantation for progressive cardiomyopathy as a manifestation of MELAS syndrome. J Heart Lung Transplant. 2005 Dec;24(12):2286–2289.

36. Sinnathuray AR, Raut V, Awa A, Magee A, Toner JG. A review of cochlear implantation in mitochondrial sensorineural hearing loss. Otol Neurotol. 2003 May;24(3):418–426.

37. Read JL, Whittaker RG, Miller N, Clark S, Taylor R, McFarland R, et al. Prevalence and severity of voice and swallowing difficulties in mitochondrial disease. Int J Lang Commun Disord. 2012 Jan-Feb;47(1):106–111.

38. Pfeffer G, Majamaa K, Turnbull DM, Thorburn D, Chinnery PF. Treatment for mitochondrial disorders. Cochrane Database Syst Rev. 2012 Apr 18;4: CD004426.

39. Gimenes AC, Napolis LM, Silva NL, Siquiera GO, Bulle AS, et al. The effect of L-carnitine supplementation on respiratory muscle strength and exercise tolerance in patients with mitochondrial myopathies. [abstract]. Eur Respir J. 2007;51(Suppl):21S[E297].

40. Kornblum C, Schroder R, Muller K, Vorgerd M, Eggers J, Bogdanow M, et al. Creatine has no beneficial effect on skeletal muscle energy metabolism in patients with single mitochondrial DNA deletions: A placebo-controlled, double-blind 31P-MRS crossover study. Eur J Neurol. 2005 Apr;12(4):300–309.

41. Klopstock T, Querner V, Schmidt F, Gekeler F, Walter M, Hartard M, et al. A placebo-controlled crossover trial of creatine in mitochondrial diseases. Neurology. 2000 Dec 12;55(11):1748–1751.

42. Tarnopolsky MA, Roy BD, MacDonald JR. A randomized, controlled trial of creatine monohydrate in patients with mitochondrial cytopathies. Muscle Nerve. 1997 Dec;20(12):1502–1509.

43. Stacpoole PW, Kerr DS, Barnes C, Bunch ST, Carney PR, Fennell EM, et al. Controlled clinical trial of dichloroacetate for treatment of congenital lactic acidosis in children. Pediatrics. 2006 May;117(5):1519–1531.

44. Bresolin N, Doriguzzi C, Ponzetto C, Angelini C, Moroni I, Castelli E, et al. Ubidecarenone in the treatment of mitochondrial myopathies: A multi-center double-blind trial. J Neurol Sci. 1990 Dec;100(1–2): 70–78.

45. Mancuso M, Orsucci D, Logerfo A, Rocchi A, Petrozzi L, Nesti C, et al. Oxidative stress biomarkers in mitochondrial myopathies, basally and after cysteine donor supplementation. J Neurol. 2010 May;257(5):774–781.

46. Kaufmann P, Engelstad K, Wei Y, Jhung S, Sano MC, Shungu DC, et al. Dichloroacetate causes toxic neuropathy in MELAS: A randomized, controlled clinical trial. Neurology. 2006 Feb 14;66(3):324–330.

47. De Stefano N, Matthews PM, Ford B, Genge A, Karpati G, Arnold DL. Short-term dichloroacetate treatment improves indices of cerebral metabolism in patients with mitochondrial disorders. Neurology. 1995 Jun;45(6):1193–1198.

48. Vissing J, Gansted U, Quistorff B. Exercise intolerance in mitochondrial myopathy is not related to lactic acidosis. Ann Neurol. 2001 May;49(5):672–676.

49. Duncan GE, Perkins LA, Theriaque DW, Neiberger RE, Stacpoole PW. Dichloroacetate therapy attenuates the blood lactate response to submaximal exercise in patients with defects in mitochondrial energy metabolism. J Clin Endocrinol Metab. 2004 Apr;89(4):1733–1738.

50. Liet JM, Pelletier V, Robinson BH, Laryea MD, Wendel U, Morneau S, et al. The effect of short-term dimethylglycine treatment on oxygen consumption in cytochrome oxidase deficiency: A double-blind randomized crossover clinical trial. J Pediatr. 2003 Jan;142(1):62–66.

51. Rodriguez MC, MacDonald JR, Mahoney DJ, Parise G, Beal MF, Tarnopolsky MA. Beneficial effects of creatine, CoQ10, and lipoic acid in mitochondrial disorders. Muscle Nerve. 2007 Feb;35(2):235–242.

52. Gempel K, Topaloglu H, Talim B, Schneiderat P, Schoser BG, Hans VH, et al. The myopathic form of coenzyme Q10 deficiency is caused by mutations in the electron-transferring-flavoprotein dehydrogenase (ETFDH) gene. Brain. 2007 Aug;130(Pt 8):2037–2044.

53. Jeppesen TD, Schwartz M, Olsen DB, Wibrand F, Krag T, Duno M, et al. Aerobic training is safe and improves exercise capacity in patients with mitochondrial myopathy. Brain. 2006 Dec;129(Pt 12):3402–3412.

54. Taivassalo T, De Stefano N, Argov Z, Matthews PM, Chen J, Genge A, et al. Effects of aerobic training in patients with mitochondrial myopathies. Neurology. 1998 Apr;50(4):1055–1060.

55. Taivassalo T, Gardner JL, Taylor RW, Schaefer AM, Newman J, Barron MJ, et al. Endurance training and detraining in mitochondrial myopathies due to single large-scale mtDNA deletions. Brain. 2006 Dec;129(Pt 12):3391–3401.

56. Cejudo P, Bautista J, Montemayor T, Villagomez R, Jimenez L, Ortega F, et al. Exercise training in mitochondrial myopathy: A randomized controlled trial. Muscle Nerve. 2005 Sep;32(3):342–350.

57. Murphy JL, Blakely EL, Schaefer AM, He L, Wyrick P, Haller RG, et al. Resistance training in patients with single, large-scale deletions of mitochondrial DNA. Brain. 2008 Nov;131(Pt 11):2832–2840.

58. Koga Y, Akita Y, Nishioka J, Yatsuga S, Povalko N, Tanabe Y, et al. L-arginine improves the symptoms of strokelike episodes in MELAS. Neurology. 2005 Feb 22;64(4):710–712.

59. Arakawa K, Kudo T, Ikawa M, Morikawa N, Kawai Y, Sahashi K, et al. Abnormal myocardial energy-production state in mitochondrial cardiomyopathy and acute response to L-arginine infusion. C-11 acetate kinetics revealed by positron emission tomography. Circ J. 2010 Nov 25;74(12):2702–2711.

60. Moran N, Bax BE, Bain MD. Erythrocyte entrapped thymidine phosphorylase (EE-TP) therapy for mitochondrial neurogastrointestinal encephalomyopathy (MNGIE). Journal of Neurology, Neurosurgery, and Psychiatry. 2012;83(e1):doi:10.1136/jnnp-2011-301993.141.

61. Hirano M, Marti R, Casali C, Tadesse S, Uldrick T, Fine B, et al. Allogeneic stem cell transplantation corrects biochemical derangements in MNGIE. Neurology. 2006 Oct 24;67(8):1458–1460.

62. Filosto M, Scarpelli M, Tonin P, Lucchini G, Pavan F, Santus F, et al. Course and management of allogeneic stem cell transplantation in patients with mitochondrial neurogastrointestinal encephalomyopathy. J Neurol. 2012 Dec;259(12):2699–2706.

63. Hussein E. Non-myeloablative bone marrow transplant and platelet infusion can transiently improve the clinical outcome of mitochondrial neurogastrointestinal encephalopathy: A case report. Transfus Apher Sci. 2013 Feb 12. [epub ahead of print, doi: 10.1016/j.transci.2013.01.014]

64. Halter J, Schupbach WM, Casali C, Elhasid R, Fay K, Hammans S, et al. Allogeneic hematopoietic SCT as treatment option for patients with mitochondrial neurogastrointestinal encephalomyopathy (MNGIE): A consensus conference proposal for a standardized approach. Bone Marrow Transplant. 2011 Mar;46(3):330–337.

65. Sicurelli F, Carluccio MA, Toraldo F, Tozzi M, Bucalossi A, Lenoci M, et al. Clinical and biochemical improvement following HSCT in a patient with MNGIE: 1-year follow-up. J Neurol. 2012 Sep;259(9):1985–1987.

66. Lin CM, Thajeb P. Valproic acid aggravates epilepsy due to MELAS in a patient with an A3243G mutation of mitochondrial DNA. Metab Brain Dis. 2007 Mar;22(1):105–109.

67. Krahenbuhl S, Brandner S, Kleinle S, Liechti S, Straumann D. Mitochondrial diseases represent a risk factor for valproate-induced fulminant liver failure. Liver. 2000 Jul;20(4):346–348.

68. McFarland R, Hudson G, Taylor RW, Green SH, Hodges S, McKiernan PJ, et al. Reversible valproate hepatotoxicity due to mutations in mitochondrial DNA polymerase gamma (POLG1). Arch Dis Child. 2008 Feb;93(2):151–153.

69. Stewart JD, Horvath R, Baruffini E, Ferrero I, Bulst S, Watkins PB, et al. Polymerase gamma gene POLG determines the risk of sodium valproate-induced liver toxicity. Hepatology. 2010 Nov;52(5):1791–1796.

70. Venhoff N, Setzer B, Melkaoui K, Walker UA. Mitochondrial toxicity of tenofovir, emtricitabine and abacavir alone and in combination with additional nucleoside reverse transcriptase inhibitors. Antivir Ther. 2007;12(7):1075–1085.

71. Ananworanich J, Nuesch R, Cote HC, Kerr SJ, Hill A, Jupimai T, et al. Changes in metabolic toxicity after switching from stavudine/didanosine to tenofovir/lamivudine—a staccato trial substudy. J Antimicrob Chemother. 2008 Jun;61(6):1340–1343.

72. Dinges WL, Witherspoon SR, Itani KM, Garg A, Peterson DM. Blepharoptosis and external ophthalmoplegia associated with long-term antiretroviral therapy. Clin Infect Dis. 2008 Sep 15;47(6):845–852.

73. Zannou DM, Azon-Kouanou A, Bashi BJ, Gougounon A, Zinsou R, Ade G, et al. Mitochondrial toxicity: A case of palpebral ptosis in a woman infected by HIV and treated with HAART including zidovudine. Bull Soc Pathol Exot. 2009 May;102(2):97–98.

74. Pfeffer G, Cote HC, Montaner JS, Li CC, Jitratkosol M, Mezei MM. Ophthalmoplegia and ptosis: Mitochondrial toxicity in patients receiving HIV therapy. Neurology. 2009 Jul 7;73(1):71–72.

75. Sirvent P, Bordenave S, Vermaelen M, Roels B, Vassort G, Mercier J, et al. Simvastatin induces impairment in skeletal muscle while heart is protected. Biochem Biophys Res Commun. 2005 Dec 23;338(3):1426–1434.

76. Bruckert E, Hayem G, Dejager S, Yau C, Begaud B. Mild to moderate muscular symptoms with high-dosage statin therapy in hyperlipidemic patients—the PRIMO study. Cardiovasc Drugs Ther. 2005 Dec;19(6):403–414.

77. Baker SK, Vladutiu GD, Peltier WL, Isackson PJ, Tarnopolsky MA. Metabolic myopathies discovered during investigations of statin myopathy. Can J Neurol Sci. 2008 Mar;35(1):94–97.

78. Elsais A, Lund C, Kerty E. Ptosis, diplopia and statins: An association? Eur J Neurol. 2008 Oct;15(10):e90–e91.

79. Fraunfelder FW, Richards AB. Diplopia, blepharoptosis, and ophthalmoplegia and 3-hydroxy-3-methylglutaryl-CoA reductase inhibitor use. Ophthalmology. 2008 Dec;115(12):2282–2285.

80. Craven L, Tuppen HA, Greggains GD, Harbottle SJ, Murphy JL, Cree LM, et al. Pronuclear transfer in human embryos to prevent transmission of mitochondrial DNA disease. Nature. 2010 May 6;465(7294):82–85.

81. Pfeffer G, Sirrs S, Wade NK, Mezei MM. Multisystem disorder in late-onset chronic progressive external ophthalmoplegia. Can J Neurol Sci. 2011 Jan;38(1):119–123.

82. Hudson G, Amati-Bonneau P, Blakely EL, Stewart JD, He L, Schaefer AM, et al. Mutation of OPA1 causes dominant optic atrophy with external ophthalmoplegia, ataxia, deafness and multiple mitochondrial DNA deletions: A novel disorder of mtDNA maintenance. Brain. 2008 Feb;131(Pt 2):329–337.

83. Ortube MC, Bhola R, Demer JL. Orbital magnetic resonance imaging of extraocular muscles in chronic progressive external ophthalmoplegia: Specific diagnostic findings. J AAPOS. 2006 Oct;10(5):414–418.

84. Saneto RP, Friedman SD, Shaw DW. Neuroimaging of mitochondrial disease. Mitochondrion. 2008 Dec;8(5–6):396–413.

85. Aure K, Ogier de Baulny H, Laforet P, Jardel C, Eymard B, Lombes A. Chronic progressive ophthalmoplegia with large-scale mtDNA rearrangement: Can we predict progression? Brain. 2007 Jun;130(Pt 6):1516–1524.

86. Pfeffer G, Mezei MM. Cardiac screening investigations in adult-onset progressive external ophthalmoplegia patients. Muscle Nerve. 2012 Oct;46(4):593–596.

87. DiMauro S, Hirano M. Mitochondrial DNA deletion syndromes. In: Pagon RA, Bird TD, Dolan CR, Stephens K, Adam MP, editors. GeneReviews. Seattle (WA): University of Washington, Seattle; 1993.

88. Polak PE, Zijlstra F, Roelandt JR. Indications for pacemaker implantation in the Kearns-Sayre syndrome. Eur Heart J. 1989 Mar;10(3):281–282.

89. Wahbi K, Larue S, Jardel C, Meune C, Stojkovic T, Ziegler F, et al. Cardiac involvement is frequent in patients with the m.8344A>G mutation of mitochondrial DNA. Neurology. 2010 Feb 23;74(8):674–677.

90. Bhati RS, Sheridan BC, Mill MR, Selzman CH. Heart transplantation for progressive cardiomyopathy as a manifestation of MELAS syndrome. J Heart Lung Transplant. 2005 Dec;24(12):2286–2289.

91. Rotig A, Cormier V, Blanche S, Bonnefont JP, Ledeist F, Romero N, et al. Pearson's marrow-pancreas syndrome. A multisystem mitochondrial disorder in infancy. J Clin Invest. 1990 Nov;86(5):1601–1608.

92. Kaufmann P, Engelstad K, Wei Y, Kulikova R, Oskoui M, Battista V, et al. Protean phenotypic features of the A3243G mitochondrial DNA mutation Arch Neurol. 2009 Jan;66(1):85–91.

93. Majamaa-Voltti K, Turkka J, Kortelainen ML, Huikuri H, Majamaa K. Causes of death in pedigrees with the 3243A>G mutation in mitochondrial DNA. J Neurol Neurosurg Psychiatry. 2008 Feb;79(2):209–211.

94. Whittaker RG, Blackwood JK, Alston CL, Blakely EL, Elson JL, McFarland R, et al. Urine heteroplasmy is the best predictor of clinical outcome in the m.3243A>G mtDNA mutation. Neurology. 2009 Feb 10;72(6):568–569.

95. Ito H, Mori K, Kagami S. Neuroimaging of stroke-like episodes in MELAS. Brain Dev. 2011 Apr;33(4):283–288.

96. Sproule DM, Kaufmann P. Mitochondrial encephalopathy, lactic acidosis, and strokelike episodes: Basic concepts, clinical phenotype, and therapeutic management of MELAS syndrome. Ann N Y Acad Sci. 2008 Oct;1142:133–158.

97. Silvestri G, Ciafaloni E, Santorelli FM, Shanske S, Servidei S, Graf WD, et al. Clinical features associated with the A—>G transition at nucleotide 8344 of mtDNA ("MERRF mutation"). Neurology. 1993 Jun;43(6):1200–1206.

98. Mancuso M, Orsucci D, Angelini C, Bertini E, Carelli V, Comi GP, et al. Phenotypic heterogeneity of the 8344A>G mtDNA "MERRF" mutation. Neurology. 2013 May 28;80(22):2049–2054.

99. Shoffner JM, Lott MT, Lezza AM, Seibel P, Ballinger SW, Wallace DC. Myoclonic epilepsy and ragged-red fiber disease (MERRF) is associated with a mitochondrial DNA tRNA(lys) mutation. Cell. 1990 Jun 15;61(6):931–937.

100. Thompson PD, Hammans SR, Harding AE. Cortical reflex myoclonus in patients with the mitochondrial DNA transfer RNA(lys)(8344) (MERRF) mutation. J Neurol. 1994 Mar;241(5):335–340.

101. Finsterer J, Segall L. Drugs interfering with mitochondrial disorders. Drug Chem Toxicol. 2010 Apr;33(2):138–151.

102. DiMauro S, Hirano M, Kaufmann P, Tanji K, Sano M, Shungu DC, et al. Clinical features and genetics of myoclonic epilepsy with ragged red fibers. Adv Neurol. 2002;89:217–229.

103. Mancuso M, Galli R, Pizzanelli C, Filosto M, Siciliano G, Murri L. Antimyoclonic effect of levetiracetam in MERRF syndrome. J Neurol Sci. 2006 Apr 15;243(1–2):97–99.

104. Rahman S. Mitochondrial disease and epilepsy. Dev Med Child Neurol. 2012 May;54(5):397–406.

105. Van Goethem G, Martin JJ, Dermaut B, Lofgren A, Wibail A, Ververken D, et al. Recessive POLG mutations presenting with sensory and ataxic neuropathy in compound heterozygote patients with progressive external ophthalmoplegia. Neuromuscul Disord. 2003 Feb;13(2):133–142.

106. Kniffin CL. Sensory ataxic neuropathy, dysarthria, and ophthalmoparesis; SANDO. 2011/4/14 [Online resource, accessed 2013/07/16: http://omim.org/entry/607459]

107. Nikali K, Suomalainen A, Saharinen J, Kuokkanen M, Spelbrink JN, Lonnqvist T, et al. Infantile onset spinocerebellar ataxia is caused by recessive mutations in mitochondrial proteins Twinkle and Twinky. Hum Mol Genet. 2005 Oct 15;14(20):2981–2990.

108. Deschauer M, Tennant S, Rokicka A, He L, Kraya T, Turnbull DM, et al. MELAS associated with mutations in the POLG1 gene. Neurology. 2007 May 15;68(20):1741–1742.

109. Rahman S, Blok RB, Dahl HH, Danks DM, Kirby DM, Chow CW, et al. Leigh syndrome: Clinical features and biochemical and DNA abnormalities. Ann Neurol. 1996 Mar;39(3):343–351.

110. Arii J, Tanabe Y. Leigh syndrome: Serial MR imaging and clinical follow-up. AJNR Am J Neuroradiol. 2000 Sep;21(8):1502–1509.

111. Finsterer J. Leigh and Leigh-like syndrome in children and adults. Pediatr Neurol. 2008 Oct;39(4): 223–235.
112. Kumakura A, Asada J, Okumura R, Fujisawa I, Hata D. Diffusion-weighted imaging in preclinical Leigh syndrome. Pediatr Neurol. 2009 Oct;41(4):309–311.
113. Debray FG, Lambert M, Lortie A, Vanasse M, Mitchell GA. Long-term outcome of Leigh syndrome caused by the NARP-T8993C mtDNA mutation. Am J Med Genet A. 2007 Sep 1;143A(17):2046–2051.
114. McKelvie P, Infeld B, Marotta R, Chin J, Thorburn D, Collins S. Late-adult onset Leigh syndrome. J Clin Neurosci. 2012 Feb;19(2):195–202.
115. Holt IJ, Harding AE, Petty RK, Morgan-Hughes JA. A new mitochondrial disease associated with mitochondrial DNA heteroplasmy. Am J Hum Genet. 1990 Mar;46(3):428–433.
116. Ortiz RG, Newman NJ, Shoffner JM, Kaufman AE, Koontz DA, Wallace DC. Variable retinal and neurologic manifestations in patients harboring the mitochondrial DNA 8993 mutation. Arch Ophthalmol. 1993 Nov;111(11):1525–1530.
117. Verny C, Guegen N, Desquiret V, Chevrollier A, Prundean A, Dubas F, et al. Hereditary spastic paraplegia-like disorder due to a mitochondrial ATP6 gene point mutation. Mitochondrion. 2011 Jan;11(1): 70–75.
118. Craig K, Elliott HR, Keers SM, Lambert C, Pyle A, Graves TD, et al. Episodic ataxia and hemiplegia caused by the 8993T->C mitochondrial DNA mutation. J Med Genet. 2007 Dec;44(12):797–799.
119. Pfeffer G, Blakely EL, Alston CL, Hassani A, Boggild M, Horvath R, et al. Adult-onset spinocerebellar ataxia syndromes due to MTATP6 mutations. J Neurol Neurosurg Psychiatry. 2012 Sep;83(9):883–886.
120. Hirano M, Silvestri G, Blake DM, Lombes A, Minetti C, Bonilla E, et al. Mitochondrial neurogastrointestinal encephalomyopathy (MNGIE): Clinical, biochemical, and genetic features of an autosomal recessive mitochondrial disorder. Neurology. 1994 Apr;44(4):721–727.
121. Horvath R, Bender A, Abicht A, Holinski-Feder E, Czermin B, Trips T, et al. Heteroplasmic mutation in the anticodon-stem of mitochondrial tRNA(val) causing MNGIE-like gastrointestinal dysmotility and cachexia. J Neurol. 2009 May;256(5):810–815.
122. Tang S, Dimberg EL, Milone M, Wong LJ. Mitochondrial neurogastrointestinal encephalomyopathy (MNGIE)-like phenotype: An expanded clinical spectrum of POLG1 mutations. J Neurol. 2012 May;259(5):862–868.
123. Shaibani A, Shchelochkov OA, Zhang S, Katsonis P, Lichtarge O, Wong LJ, et al. Mitochondrial neurogastrointestinal encephalopathy due to mutations in RRM2B. Arch Neurol. 2009 Aug;66(8):1028–1032.
124. Lara MC, Valentino ML, Torres-Torronteras J, Hirano M, Marti R. Mitochondrial neurogastrointestinal encephalomyopathy (MNGIE): Biochemical features and therapeutic approaches. Biosci Rep. 2007 Jun;27(1–3):151–163.
125. Bourdon A, Minai L, Serre V, Jais JP, Sarzi E, Aubert S, et al. Mutation of RRM2B, encoding p53-controlled ribonucleotide reductase (p53R2), causes severe mitochondrial DNA depletion. Nat Genet. 2007 Jun;39(6):776–780.
126. Saada A, Shaag A, Mandel H, Nevo Y, Eriksson S, Elpeleg O. Mutant mitochondrial thymidine kinase in mitochondrial DNA depletion myopathy. Nat Genet. 2001 Nov;29(3):342–344.
127. Sarzi E, Bourdon A, Chretien D, Zarhrate M, Corcos J, Slama A, et al. Mitochondrial DNA depletion is a prevalent cause of multiple respiratory chain deficiency in childhood. J Pediatr. 2007 May;150(5):531,4, 534.e1–e6.
128. Spinazzola A, Viscomi C, Fernandez-Vizarra E, Carrara F, D'Adamo P, Calvo S, et al. MPV17 encodes an inner mitochondrial membrane protein and is mutated in infantile hepatic mitochondrial DNA depletion. Nat Genet. 2006 May;38(5):570–575.
129. Ostergaard E, Christensen E, Kristensen E, Mogensen B, Duno M, Shoubridge EA, et al. Deficiency of the alpha subunit of succinate-coenzyme A ligase causes fatal infantile lactic acidosis with mitochondrial DNA depletion. Am J Hum Genet. 2007 Aug;81(2):383–387.
130. Mandel H, Szargel R, Labay V, Elpeleg O, Saada A, Shalata A, et al. The deoxyguanosine kinase gene is mutated in individuals with depleted hepatocerebral mitochondrial DNA. Nat Genet. 2001 Nov;29(3):337–341.

Chapter 9

Muscle Channelopathies

Araya Puwanant
Robert C. Griggs

Skeletal muscle channelopathies are disorders of membrane excitability. Reduced membrane excitability manifests as flaccid paralysis. On the other hand, membrane hyperexcitability manifests as myotonia or paramyotonia. Some muscle channelopathies, such as paramyotonia congenita and hyperkalemic periodic paralysis with myotonia, manifest both. In addition, several neuromuscular disorders have demonstrated abnormal ion channel function as part of their underlying pathophysiology. For example, abnormal chloride channel splicing causes myotonia in both forms of myotonic dystrophy. These

disorders are discussed within the muscular dystrophies in chapter 4. Malignant hyperthermia, another chloride channelopathy, is discussed in chapters 6 and 7. This chapter focuses primarily on two distinct disorders with genetic mutations in ion channels: the periodic paralyses (PPs) and the nondystrophic myotonias.

PERIODIC PARALYSES

The PPs are characterized by episodic attacks of muscle weakness associated with an alteration of serum potassium concentration. Patients may complain of episodic weakness, but often fail to recognize that they are having such episodes. It should be emphasized that patients with episodic weakness often have secondary forms of PP in which the paralysis results from a systemic electrolyte disturbance. These conditions are summarized this chapter, and the major conditions are also noted in chapter 11. Here we focus on the primary PP, caused by specific mutations of the skeletal muscle calcium, sodium, and potassium channels: hypokalemic periodic paralysis (HypoPP), hyperkalemic periodic paralysis (HyperPP), and Andersen-Tawil Syndrome (ATS). Thyrotoxic periodic paralysis (TPP), a muscle channelopathy that manifests similarly to HypoPP but only when the patients are in a thyrotoxic state, will also be discussed.

Classification of Periodic Paralysis

Box 9.1 lists conditions that can be associated with an episode of weakness. Most of these disorders can be recurrent. Only those conditions with either hypokalemia or hyperkalemia are likely to be confused with primary PP. The most frequent secondary disorders that simulate HypoPP are renal tubular acidosis, aldosterone-producing adenomas of the adrenal gland, and villous adenoma of the colon.[1] The only secondary disorders that frequently cause HyperPP are conditions that cause hyporeninemic hypoaldosteronism.[2] This disorder usually occurs in diabetic patients with renal disease and impaired renin production.

Box 9.2 lists the primary PPs, which are divided into three major groups according to

---

Box 9.1 Secondary Causes of Episodic Paralysis

Hypokalemic

Primary hyperaldosteronism (Conn's syndrome)
Renal tubular acidosis
Autosomal-recessive hereditary salt-losing tubulopathy (Bartter and Gitelman's syndrome)
Villous adenoma
Alcoholism
Medications (diruretics, licorice, p-aminoalicylic acid, amphotericin B, corticosteroids)

Hyperkalemic

Potassium load (e.g., oral supplements, salt substitutes)
Potassium-sparing diuretics (spironolactone, triamterene, amiloride)
Hyporeninemic hypoaldosteronism (diabetes mellitus, other renal disease; secondary to indomethacin, ibuprofen)
Addison's disease
Chronic renal failure
Isolated aldosterone deficiency
Chronic heparin therapy
Rhabdomyolysis (e.g., McArdle syndrome)
Ileostomy complicated by tight stoma syndrome

Normokalemic

Guanidine
Sleep paralysis
Myasthenia gravis, Lambert-Eaton myasthenic syndrome, multiple sclerosis
Transient ischemic attacks

Box 9.2 Classification of the Periodic Paralyses

Primary periodic paralyses
Hypokalemic periodic paralysis (types 1 and 2)
Hyperkalemic periodic paralysis
Andersen-tawil syndrome
Thyrotoxic periodic paralysis
Secondary periodic paralysis

the ion channel mutations. A substantial proportion of patients have features that are not typical of any of them. Whether the subdivisions in Box 9.2 are justified remains to be determined by further characterization of the genetic defects. The distinctions between these subgroups listed are useful, however, because there is usually homogeneity within kindred, as well as reproducible, differing responses to provocative and therapeutic modalities.[3,4] In the past, overlap in clinical features between so-called HyperPP and normokalemic PP,[5-7] and between HyperPP with myotonia and the paramyotonias,[8-10] has led to controversy. The fact that certain of these disorders (if not all) are allelic (i.e., involve the same gene) has greatly simplified their nosology.[8-11] Normal function can be restored by treatment for virtually all patients, but each case must be fully evaluated to provide the basis for effective treatment.

All types of the primary PPs have certain similarities (Box 9.3); HypoPP and HyperPP are not mirror images of each other.[4,12] Thus, all PPs are characterized by episodic attacks of

Box 9.3 Similar Clinical Features of the Periodic Paralyses

History

Onset by the second decade
Attacks of limb weakness; sparing of bulbar, ocular, respiratory muscles
Attacks provoked by rest following exercise or certain foods
Greater severity in males
Oliguria preceding and during attacks
Family history (most cases)—autosomal dominant

Clinical findings

Eyelid myotonia
Lid lag
Normal sensation
Normal strength between attacks (for initial 5 to 10 years after onset)
Untreated cases eventually develop "fixed" proximal weakness
Hyporeflexia during attacks

limb weakness; all forms begin by the second decade and are more severe in males in a given family; in all disorders, attacks typically occur after the rest that follows exercise; and in all disorders, strength improves between attacks for the first 5 to 10 years of the disorders, but progressive, proximal "fixed" weakness during attack-free intervals occurs if the attacks are frequent and not treated.[1,13]

Hypokalemic Periodic Paralysis

HypoPP is an autosomal-dominant disorder with reduced penetrance in women. There are two recognized forms of familial HypoPP, type 1 and type 2, with similar phenotypes. HypoPP type 1 results from mutations in the dihydropyridine-sensitive or L-type calcium channel (*CACNA1S*) gene on chromosome 1q. The two most common most commonly reported mutations are R528H and R1239H. A third less common mutation is R1239G. HypoPP type 1 is the more common form and accounts for over two-thirds of the inherited PP. HypoPP type 2 is associated with point mutations of the skeletal muscle sodium channel (*SCN4A*) gene. To date, pathogenic mutations can be identified in at least 70% of cases, but almost one-third of the cases are due to new mutations. Attacks usually begin when patients are in their first or second decade, although rare patients present after age 20. In contrast, HyperPP usually begins within the first decade. Attacks are provoked by cold, carbohydrate ingestion, rest after exercise, alcohol, or emotional stress. Typical attacks of weakness occur on awakening from sleep, especially after strenuous exercise or a large carbohydrate meal the previous day. The weakness may be severe resulting in flaccid quadriplegia with loss of reflexes. The frequency of attacks can vary from once or twice a year to daily. Although some attacks may last only a few hours, most attacks if untreated last longer—up to 24 hours or more in patients with severe disease. Bulbar and respiratory muscles are involved occasionally, but ocular muscles are usually spared. Death from respiratory muscle paralysis and cardiac arrhythmias has been reported but likely relates to injudicious treatment.[14] Fixed proximal muscle weakness is detectable in virtually all patients and may become severe 10 to 15 years after onset of frequent attacks. The potassium level is usually low during attacks (2.0–3.0 mEq/L). This may lead to cardiac arrhythmias if the hypokalemia is profound. Myotonia of the limbs has not been demonstrated by EMG or bedside examination, and its presence of electrical myotonia makes another form of PP more likely. However, lid lag myotonia can be elicited in some patients (Figure 9–1).

Hyperkalemic Periodic Paralysis

HyperPP was initially described in the 1950s and differentiated from HypoPP by either a rise in potassium level during attacks or the induction of weakness with potassium administration. Most HyperPP results from point mutations in the α-subunit of the human skeletal muscle sodium channel (*SCN4A*) gene on chromosome 17q.[15] The most common mutations, T704M and M1592V, account for almost 75% of affected individuals. Other point mutations account for 5% of the

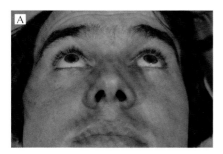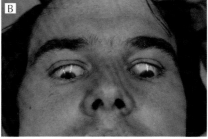

Figure 9–1. Lid lag sign. The patient (A) is instructed to rapidly look down after maintaining sustained upward gaze. (B) The upper eyelid floats for 10 seconds and fails to follow the downward-moving iris.

remainder and 20% of cases remain genetically unidentified, suggesting genetic heterogeneity.[16,17] Many disorders characterized by potassium sensitivity are localized to chromosome 17q and are related to abnormalities of the α-subunit of the sodium channel.[8,15,18] Inheritance is commonly autosomal dominant, but sporadic cases resulting from new mutations have been identified.[19,20] The prevalence is unknown but is considered to be less common than HypoPP. Three variants have been described: HyperPP without myotonia, HyperPP with myotonia, and HyperPP with paramyotonia. This disorder is earlier in onset than HypoPP, and the majority of patients begin to have symptoms within the first decade. Attacks of weakness are brief and mild in most instances, usually lasting from 30 minutes to 4 hours and often in the morning. The frequency of attacks generally lessens in middle age. Attacks of myotonia vary in frequency and severity. Attacks of weakness are precipitated by rest following exercise, fasting, emotional stress, cold, or potassium-rich diet. Weakness is usually in proximal leg or shoulder-girdle muscles, but distal muscles or asymmetrical weakness may be more affected following strenuous activity. During attacks of weakness, involved muscles are flaccid and hyporeflexic. Although Chvostek's sign can often be elicited, and subjective sensory symptoms may be present in the hands or feet, sensory examination is typically normal. Progressive, persistent (interattack) weakness is not as severe or frequent as in HypoPP, but it has been noted in numerous reports.[13,21] Creatine kinase levels are often elevated during attacks of weakness and may be persistently elevated even during interattacks. The potassium level may be normal, elevated, or occasionally even slightly low during attacks of weakness.[22] However, it is often found that potassium level is relatively elevated (while still within the normal range) during attack-free intervals. These findings suggest that mild, recurrent, clinically unapparent attacks may be occurring more than once during the day in patients with HyperPP.[23] Myotonia is prominent on both clinical and EMG evaluation in many patients.[24] Because a myotonic disorder that lacks paralytic attacks is allelic to HyperPP, the differences between these disorders reflect the nature of the sodium channel defect.[18]

Andersen-Tawil Syndrome

ATS is a rare multisystemic disorder characterized by three cardinal features: PP, cardiac arrhythmias, and distinctive facial and skeletal features.[12,25] Paralytic attacks typically starts in the first or second decade and occur in the setting of either low or high potassium. Progressive proximal muscle weakness may develop. Myotonia does not occur in ATS. Cardiac arrhythmias include frequent ectopic ventricular premature beats (most commonly bigeminy or a bidirectional tachycardia), long QT syndrome, ventricular tachycardia, *torsades de pointes*, and cardiac arrest.[25,26] Baseline ECG can be normal or demonstrate U-wave as evidence of hypokalemia (Figure 9–2). Cardiac arrhythmia detected by physical examination or Holter monitoring is often the presenting manifestation of this disorder. The distinctive features include short stature, hypertelorism, low-set ears, micrognathia, broad forehead, mandibular hypoplasia (Figure 9–3A & B), and clinodactyly (Figure 9–3C). Patients may manifest one, two, or all three of the cardinal features; therefore it should be considered in the differential diagnosis of both PP and cardiac arrhythmias. ATS is caused by missense mutations or small deletions in the coding region of the *KCNJ2* gene, which encodes the inward rectifying potassium channel in skeletal and cardiac muscles (Kir 2.1), in 80% to 90% of affected individuals. In reported cases the family history reveals autosomal dominant inheritance, although in certain kindreds the disorder may not be recognized in mildly affected patients. Severe scoliosis is occasionally present (Figure 9–4).[27] The cardiac dysrhythmia and PP can mirror each other's behavior in terms of the response to provocative and therapeutic alteration of potassium level.

Thyrotoxic Periodic Paralysis

TPP is characterized by episodic weakness associated with hypokalemia in patients with thyrotoxicosis. TPP appears to be sporadic but has occurred in families and may reflect an autosomal-dominant susceptibility to the effect of thyrotoxicosis. TPP occurs more frequently in Asian populations, with a higher predilection in males. The overall incidence in Chinese and Japanese populations is close

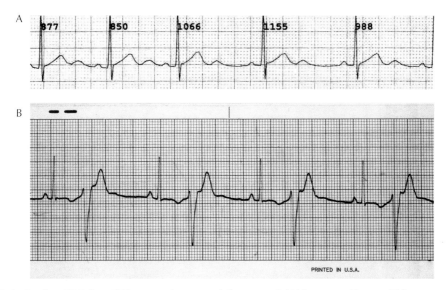

Figure 9–2. Baseline ECG from ATS patients during attack-free interval. (A) Prominent U wave. (B) bigeminy.

to 2%,[28,29] whereas it is less than 0.1% in Caucasians.[30,31] Despite the higher incidence of thyrotoxicosis in women, fewer than 5% of the TPP cases occur in women.[28,32] This disorder resembles HypoPP in clinical features and physiologic ion changes. Acute paralysis manifests only when the patients are in thyrotoxic state, and restores when they are euthyroid. Not surprisingly, the diagnosis of thyrotoxicosis is often clinically inapparent in these patients; those with obvious signs of hyperthyroidism come to medical attention earlier. Attacks of HypoPP presenting in adulthood thus demand thorough evaluation of the patient for occult hyperthyroidism. TPP may be associated with progressive

muscle weakness and with cardiac arrhythmias, probably as a result of the thyrotoxicosis. Recently, six mutations have been identified in an inward rectifying potassium channel (Kir 2.6), encoded *KCNJ18* gene in up to 33% of unrelated TPP patients.[33] The inward rectifying potassium channel is primarily expressed in muscle and transcriptionally regulated by thyroid hormone and is found to be increased during the thyrotoxic state. Muscle fibers of patient with TPP also demonstrates reduced voltage-gated Na^+, inward potassium rectifier, and depolarizing gating pore currents that resembles the membrane changes seen in HypoPP type 1 causing depolarization-induced paralysis.[34]

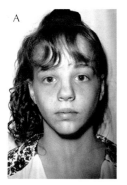
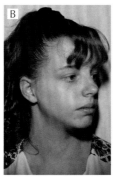
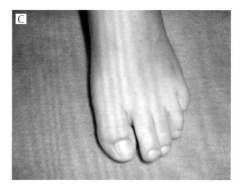

Figure 9–3. Andersen-Tawil syndrome. Distinctive features include low-set ear, hypertelorism, micrognathia (A & B), and clinodactyly (C).

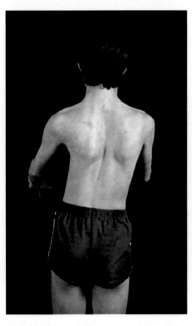

Figure 9–4. Scoliosis can be severe in some ATS patients.

The clinical and electrodiagnostic features of periodic paralyses are summarized in Table 9–1.

Other Disorders That Mimic Primary Periodic Paralyses

In addition to TPP, episodic weakness can be manifested in several neurological disorders. Paramyotonia congenita (autosomal-dominant sodium channelopathy) typically presents in the first decade with muscle stiffness (myotonia) and cold-induced episodic weakness (see the Nondystrophic Myotonias section). Coincidental neuromuscular diseases such as spinal muscular atrophy, muscular dystrophies, or inherited myopathies have been suspected as a cause of permanent or progressive weakness in cases of PP. Whether such weakness is distinct from the characteristic weakness of untreated or inadequately

Table 9–1 Distinguishing Clinical Features and Electrophysiologic Patterns of the Periodic Paralyses

	HypoPP	HyperPP	ATS	TTP
Age of onset	1st–2nd decade	1st decade	1st–2nd decade	2nd–5th decade
Inheritance	AD	AD	AD with variable expression	Sporadic
Mutant channel	Type I: *CACNA1S*, Type II: *SCN4A*	*SCN4A*	*KCNJ2* (Kir 2.1)	*KCNJ18* (Kir 2.6)
Attack duration	Hours to days	Minutes to hours	Minutes to hours	Hours to days
Myotonia	Absent	Present	Absent	Absent
Periodic weakness	Yes	Yes	Yes	Yes
Fixed weakness	Common	Variable	Variable	Absent
Other findings	Lid lag/eyelid myotonia	Lid lag/eyelid	Dysmorphic features, arrhythmias	Thyrotoxicosis signs
Provocative factors	Carbohydrate intake, rest after exercise	Potassium load, rest after exercise fasting	Carbohydrate intake, rest after exercise	Carbohydrate intake, rest after exercise
Potassium level	Low	Normal, high, slightly low	Low-normal	Low
Electrophysiology				
EMG	Normal MUAPs or mild myopathic pattern	Myotonia (50%–75%)	—	—
Long exercise testing	Delayed and persistent decline in CMAP	Initial rise and then fall in CMAP	Variable	Similar to HypoPP
Fournier pattern	V in type I, IV or V in type II	IV	IV or V	V

Note. HypoPP = hypokalemic periodic paralysis, HyperPP = hyperkalemic periodic paralysis, ATS = Andersen-Tawil syndrome, TTP = thyrotoxic periodic paralysis, AD = autosomal dominant, MUAPs = motor unit action potentials.

treated PP is unclear. In our experience, one patient with genetically confirmed HyperPP initially presented with a clinical picture of facioscapulohumeral distribution and vague episodes of periodic weakness. Treatment prevented attacks and improved, but did not totally alleviate, the weakness. Families with episodic ataxia whose intermittent inability to walk resulted from ataxia, not weakness, and responded to acetazolamide, had been misdiagnosed as PP.[35,36]

Evaluation of the Patient with Episodic Weakness

DURING AN EPISODE OF WEAKNESS

Clinical Findings

The clinical findings during an attack of weakness are similar in all types of PP. Weakness is usually proximal and generally symmetric. Weakness precipitated by prolonged rest following exercise may be more marked in the exercised muscles. Sensation is normal. Reflexes are depressed or absent. In certain forms of PP, especially HyperPP, myotonia may be prominent and Chvostek's sign is strongly positive (Box 9.4).

Studies to Obtain

It is important to obtain as much information as possible if the patient is seen during an attack of weakness. Serial electrolyte determinations (every 15–30 minutes) will indicate both the absolute level of potassium and sequential changes. Because potassium levels are often normal in HyperPP and occasionally normal in the hypokalemic form, the direction of serum potassium change during worsening or improving strength is important. Careful quantitation of functional testing, such as the ability to arise from the floor or from a chair, often provides better documentation of weakness than does formal, manual muscle testing. The electrocardiogram should be monitored for cardiac arrhythmias and for T-wave changes characteristic of hypokalemia (flattening, with the appearance of U waves) or hyperkalemia (peaked T waves). Respiratory failure is unusual during attacks, but respiratory function may be reduced, and sequential testing of strength is an excellent means of quantitating duration and severity of the attack.

Body Potassium Distribution and the Regulation of Blood Potassium

The response of patients with PP to provocative and therapeutic agents must be considered

---

Box 9.4 Evaluation of the Patient With Episodic Weakness

Patient seen during episode

Physical examination (special attention to reflexes, myotonia, Chvostek's sign)
Sequential potassium levels (every 15–30 minutes)
Creatine kinase
Electrocardiogram
Sequential tests of respiratory and muscle function
Exclude other disorders—hypercalemia, hypocalcemia, hypermagnesemia; rhabdomyolysis

Patient seen in attack-free episode

Exclude other disorders—thyroid, adrenal
Electromyography and long exercise study—myotonia and decremental pattern of CMAP
Serial serum potassium levels—often elevated in hyperkalemic periodic paralysis
Genetic studies

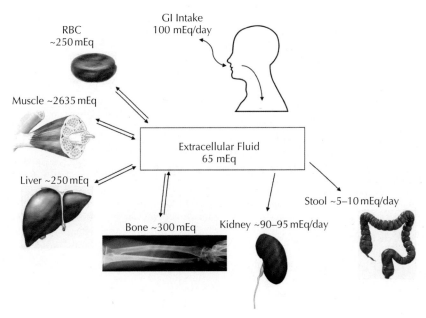

RBC
~250 mEq

GI Intake
100 mEq/day

Muscle ~2635 mEq

Extracellular Fluid
65 mEq

Liver ~250 mEq

Stool ~5–10 mEq/day

Bone ~300 mEq

Kidney ~90–95 mEq/day

Figure 9–5. Body potassium distribution. Plasma or serum potassium is only a small fraction of total body potassium. Red blood cells, muscle, and other tissues are the major repositories of potassium.

in the context of normal potassium distribution and regulation.[37-39] Muscle is the major reservoir of potassium (Figure 9–5). Muscle and other cellular membranes respond to a variety of hormones, substrates, and electrolytes with either potassium uptake or potassium release (Table 9–2) to regulate the plasma potassium (less than 1% of the potassium in the body). Because muscle contains so much potassium, patients with PP who develop atrophy have a decrease in total body potassium that reflects the degree of muscle wasting.[40]

The renin-angiotensin-aldosterone system is a major regulator of renal potassium handling.

Table 9–2 Effects of Hormones, Substrates, and Electrolytes on Plasma Potassium

Lower Potassium	Elevate Potassium
Insulin	Glucagon
Catecholamines	Mannitol
Aldosterone (renin, angiotensin)	Glucose (insulinopenic subjects)
Glucose	Acidosis
Sodium	
Alkalosis	

The kidney produces prostacyclin (prostaglandin I_2),[41] which stimulates renin production by the juxtaglomerular apparatus. Renin, in turn, promotes the formation of angiotensin I in liver, which is then converted to angiotensin II by angiotensin-converting enzyme. Angiotensin II is a potent vasopressor and also stimulates production of aldosterone by the adrenals. Aldosterone regulates extracellular fluid volume and has both renal and extrarenal effects on potassium metabolism. An increase in aldosterone secretion can result in hypokalemia (and resulting weakness), and the administration of potassium stimulates aldosterone secretion.[37,42]

The diagnosis characterization of PP usually depends on evaluation of plasma potassium levels during spontaneous or provoked attacks of weakness. The usual "normal" range of potassium has been defined by many laboratories as approximately 3.5 to 5.5 mEq/L, but many factors can affect routine potassium determinations:[39,42]

- Tourniquet-induced stasis elevates potassium levels or delayed processing of analysis.
- Whole body or forearm exercise elevates potassium levels.
- Morning levels of potassium may be lower than evening levels.

- Food intake affects potassium levels both directly and by stimulating insulin release.
- Hemolysis of erythrocytes can spuriously elevate plasma potassium, but the elevation is not important unless the degree of hemolysis is sufficient to discolor the plasma.

It is likely that a much "tighter" range of normal values is obtained if subjects are studied under controlled conditions. In one study of normal subjects, the range of venous plasma potassium was 3.85 to 4.17 mEq/L (4.01 ± 0.05 mEq/L, mean ± SEM).[43]

Excluding Thyrotoxic Periodic Paralysis

Thyrotoxicosis must be excluded in all patients with HypoPP who have no family history. As already mentioned, the diagnosis is often occult. The free thyroxine (T_4) and thyroid stimulating hormone (TSH) levels should be obtained, and triiodothyronine (T_3) as well (if free thyroxine is normal). T_3 toxicosis, although not common, occurs predominantly in older patients and is usually associated with goiter.

Differential Diagnosis

Patients presenting with an initial attack of weakness may not have a definite history of repeated, spontaneous attacks. For that reason, other causes of acute weakness need to be considered, including hypercalcemia, hypocalcemia, hypophosphatemia, hypermagnesemia, and rhabdomyolysis.[44] In addition, nonneuromuscular neurologic diseases such as multiple sclerosis, spinal cord ischemia, transverse myelitis, and brainstem lesions can produce quadriparesis; however, the sensory symptoms and signs in such patients usually point to a central nervous system origin of paralysis rather than a muscular one.

Conversion disorder and malingering can simulate PP. Psychogenic weakness is usually accompanied by other, nonanatomical findings, however, and is notable for preserved reflexes. The patient with quadriplegia from PP is invariably hyporeflexic or areflexic.

OTHER LABORATORY STUDIES

Muscle biopsy and serum enzyme tests are not very helpful for diagnosis during attacks of paralysis. In severe attacks of all forms of PP, CK level is often elevated, and biopsy may disclose vacuoles within muscle fibers, as well as necrotic fibers. Although electrodiagnostic studies can be abnormal, they are not recommended for acute attack due to nonspecific findings. Sensory nerve conduction studies are normal, but compound motor action potential (CMAP) may be reduced on motor nerve conduction studies. Needle EMG may reveal reduced insertional activity, fibrillation potentials/positive sharp waves, mild myopathic units, or a normal reading, which is not specific for diagnosis.[45] EMG changes are similar in all types of PP with one exception: In patients with HyperPP who have myotonia, the myotonic discharges are evident early in the attack and are of diagnostic importance. The myotonic discharges disappear as weakness increases, and return with clinical recovery.

During Attack-Free Intervals

Most patients with PP present for further evaluation when they are not in acute attacks (see Box 9.4). Their history will usually suggest a diagnosis of PP, and the clinical features may indicate the most likely form. Examination discloses fixed weakness, atrophy, and hyporeflexia only in patients with frequent, untreated, or inadequately treated attacks. Myotonia may be elicited in many patients with HyperPP. In HypoPP, myotonia is confined only to the eyelids.[46] Exercise CMAP study provides guidance for molecular genetic testing. Between attacks, needle EMG may be helpful diagnostically in two respects. First, in patients who develop fixed weakness, a myopathic pattern is observed. Second, the finding of myotonic discharges in a patient with episodic weakness suggests the diagnosis of HyperPP. The other condition associated with episodic weakness and myotonic discharges is paramyotonia congenita. The later condition is relatively easy to characterize because (1) cold provokes attacks; (2) cooling the muscle to 20° C eliminates both myotonic discharges and voluntary activity and results in a fall in evoked CMAP amplitude, and (3) delayed muscle relaxation outlasts myotonic discharges.[47,48]

Confirmatory genetic studies should be indicated if clinical features and/or exercise CMAP study are suggestive, because these studies help to refine specific molecular diagnosis, provide prognosis, and plan for treatment. Specific molecular diagnosis is now commercially available for the majority of patients with PP.[15,33,49,50]

THE EXERCISE TEST

Long Exercise Test

Another approach for evaluating patients with episodic weakness between attacks takes advantage of the changes in CMAP produced after long exercise study. Thus, whereas motor and sensory nerve conduction studies are usually normal between attacks, exercise may provoke diagnostically helpful abnormalities in the evoked CMAP amplitude and area.[51] The test involves supramaximal stimulation of the ulnar motor nerve, taking care to immobilize the hand. The CMAP is recorded with surface electrodes over the belly of the abductor digiti minimi muscle. At least three baseline CMAPs are recorded at 1-minute intervals. Then the patient executes a maximum voluntary contraction (forceful abduction against resistance) for 5 minutes, with brief rest (3–4 seconds) every 15 seconds to avoid ischemia. CMAP is recorded every minute during exercise, and every 2 minutes following the completion of exercise for 40 to 45 minutes or until no change in amplitude is evident for 5 minutes according to the McManis technique.[51] In control subjects, only small CMAP changes occur, in which amplitude increases immediately after exercise (mean 11%, range 0%–27%) and decreases after 5 minutes of recovery (mean 15%, range 0%–30%) in this study. Most patients with PP, on the other hand, show a greater-than-normal increase in CMAP size after exercise. Of 21 patients in whom clinical diagnosis was definitive, the mean increase was 35%, with a range of 0% to 300%. Findings were abnormal on this part of the test for all patients with HyperPP, 7 of 13 with the hypokalemic disorder, and 6 of 9 with secondary paralysis. The subsequent decline in postexercise CMAP amplitude (mean decrease 48%) is maximal during the first 20 minutes after the cessation of exercise (Figure 9–6). An abnormal exercise response occurs in approximately 70% of patients.[51] However, the test doses not help to distinguish between different types of PP.

In clinical practice, the cutoff values for abnormal pattern are slightly different among EMG labs. However, most established labs and clinical studies typically define an abnormal decremental pattern as a greater-than-40% postexercise decline in CMAP amplitude and/or area.[51,52] Long exercise testing is most useful in PP, in which abnormal postexercise decrement in CMAP amplitude is seen in approximately 60% to 70% of patients with PP. McManis' technique has been successfully demonstrated in several studies[52-54] including extensive studies performed in a large patient population with genetically confirmed PP.[53,54] In these studies, patients with HypoPP type 1 generally demonstrate a delayed and persistent decline in CMAP amplitude, reflecting membrane inexcitability, with no increase in CMAP amplitude immediately after postexercise (Figure 9–7D). Interestingly, half of the patients with HypoPP type 2 demonstrate electrophysiologic findings similar to those with HyperPP. Another half of this group demonstrates similar patterns to those with HypoPP type 1. A majority of patients with HyperPP demonstrate an increase in CMAP amplitude in the successive trials of short exercise testing. After long exercise study, there is a transient increase in immediate postexercise CMAP followed by a subsequental decline of CMAP amplitude and area (Figure 9–7C).[53] Patients with ATS can display either pattern depending on whether the attacks are caused by hypokalemia or hyperkalemia (Figure 9–7A & B). Abnormal decremental pattern has been recognized in patients with TPP when they are on thyrotoxic state similar to those with HypoPP type 1.[30]

Short Exercise Test

This technique is developed by Streib and colleagues in 1982 to guide for specific mutations in muscle channelopathies.[55] This test is very useful to provide guidance for further genetic testing in patients with clinically suspected for nondystrophic myotonias.[53,54,56] Short exercise study is carried out by establishing baseline CMAP amplitudes and area with supramaximal stimulation of ulnar nerve at the wrist; participants are asked to exercise their hand with maximal voluntary contraction for a period of 10 seconds. A single supramaximal stimulus is delivered within 2 seconds of completion of exercise, and is repeated every 10 seconds for 50 seconds. The brief exercise test is repeated for two additional times at room temperature with 60 seconds of rest between each trial. During the study, the limb temperature is

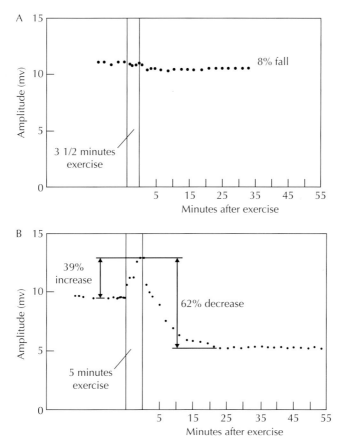

Figure 9–6. The amplitude of compound muscle action potential recorded before, during, and after maximal voluntary contraction of hypothenar muscles. (A) Normal subject. (B) Patient with periodic paralysis. Dots indicate amplitude in response to a single stimulus. (Modified from McManis PG, Lambert EH, and Daube JR. The exercise test in periodic paralysis. *Muscle & Nerve* 1986;9: 704–710, with permission.)

recorded continuously and the skin temperature is maintained above 32° C. Repeated similar procedure after muscle cooling in the contralateral hand provides more information to identify specific genetic defects in muscle channelopathies, particularly those with chloride and sodium channel mutations.[54,56] Abnormal short exercise testing have been classified by Fournier and colleagues.[53,56] Specific details of each pattern will be discussed in electrodiagnostic findings in the Nondystrophic Myotonias section.

Muscle Biopsy Findings

Although muscle biopsy may provide abnormal findings that are characteristic of a specific

diagnosis, it seldom offers a definite diagnosis and is often unnecessary since the molecular diagnosis became widely accessible.

HYPOKALEMIC PERIODIC PARALYSIS

HypoPP is characterized on light microscopy by the presence of distinctive, large, central vacuoles (Figure 9–8A & B). A single vacuole may fill the bulk of the fiber, or multiple vacuoles may be present. The vacuoles are seen more frequently in patients with long-standing weakness,[57] but they can also occur in a large number of fibers in a muscle of normal strength.[58] Muscle fiber necrosis and focal degeneration of myofibers is also noted in some biopsies. The biopsy of muscles that are weak often shows marked atrophy, with angular fibers suggesting chronic denervation.[59]

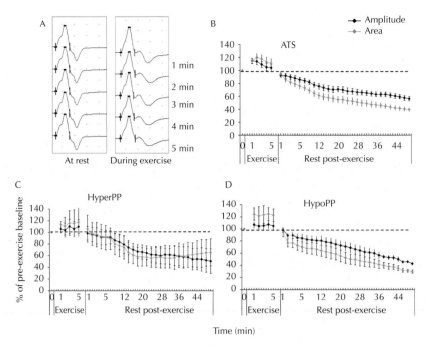

Figure 9–7. The long exercise test in the periodic paralyses. (A) Small after potentials during 5 minutes of exercise in a patient with ATS. (B) The mean CMAP amplitude in ATS patients ($n = 11$). (C) HyperPP ($n = 4$). (D) HypoPP ($n = 4$). Symbols and error bars represent mean ± standard error of the mean. (Modified from Tan SV, Matthews E, Barber M, et al. Refined exercise testing can aid DNA-based diagnosis in muscle channelopathies. *Ann Neurology* 2011;69:328–340, with permission.)

HYPERKALEMIC PERIODIC PARALYSIS

In HyperPP, light microscopy shows vacuolar changes, but the vacuoles are smaller, less numerous, and often peripheral.[57] The extent of fiber necrosis and focal degeneration is similar to that in HypoPP. A spectrum of myopathic changes occurs with long-standing weakness. For ATS, a characteristic biopsy shows numerous tubular aggregates[12] (Figure 9–8C), but vacuoles have not been observed.

Provocative Testing

Provocative testing with oral glucose loading for HypoPP and potassium loading for HyperPP has been used extensively in the past. Challenge tests with these agents may provide information useful for determining treatment. However, this test has become unnecessary for diagnosis because molecular testing is widely available and provides specific diagnosis. In addition, provocative tests require careful monitoring of the patients, ECG, and serial electrolyte testing.

Pathophysiology of Periodic Paralysis

Weakness in all forms of primary PP is produced by prolonged membrane depolarization leading to loss of membrane excitability.[60-62] The mechanism of membrane depolarization in HypoPP type 1 is better understood, although not completely. Mutations in the *CACNA1S* gene alter membrane excitability indirectly by changing the properties of inward rectifier potassium and Na[+] channels.[62-64] Reduced K[+] conductance facilitates membrane depolarization, and a decreased density of Na[+] channels reduces membrane excitability in HypoPP and facilitates depolarization-induced loss of membrane excitability.[65] Reduced density of functional Na[+] channels is characteristic of both HypoPP types 1 type 2.[34,66-68] The low density of Na[+] channels in both forms of HypoPP prevents membrane hyperexcitability from developing with membrane depolarization.[34,66,68] Consequently, myotonia is not present in HypoPP. Recent work has established that the gating pore current is the pathological

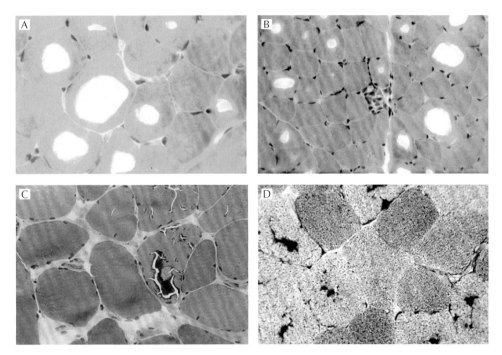

Figure 9–8. Biopsy findings in HypoPP. (A & B) Vacuoles are typical for periodic paralysis; in HypoPP, vacuoles are characteristically large and central (trichrome). (C &D) Representative prominent tubular aggregates in many muscle fibers in trichrome (C) and NADH (D) from muscle biopsy of ATS patient.

depolarizing current in SCN4A encoding the Nav1.4 sodium channel in HypoPP type 2.[69] This finding may imply that similar mutations would produce gating pore current in the L-type calcium channel in HypoPP type 1 given that the voltage-gated sodium and calcium channels are structurally and physiogenetically similar.[65,69,70] However, the origin of the depolarization current and why serum potassium levels drop in order to trigger paralytic attack in HypoPP have remained unknown. In HyperPP, the source of the prolonged membrane depolarization is persistent Na+ currents from impairment of fast- and slow-inactivation of Nav1.4.[71,72] The mechanism of paralysis in ATS may be destabilization of the resting potential. ATS is associated with mutations of Kir2.1, which forms nonfunctional inward rectifier potassium channels.[49,73] When mutant subunits are mixed 1:1 with normal subunits, the Kir current is less than that produced by the normal subunits alone, which indicates that inward rectifier channels containing Kir2.1 subunits are dysfunctional. In TPP, the sodium and inward rectifier potassium currents are reduced in muscle fibers when patient is in thyrotoxic state and normal when euthyroid. The changes of membrane properties in TPP are similar to changes found in HypoPP type 1.[34]

Treatment of Periodic Paralysis

Management of PP is directed toward preventing or decreasing the frequency of attacks and treating major paralytic attack once they occur. All forms of PP are amenable to treatment, and patients' symptoms can usually be alleviated. Emergency treatment is often necessary for acute and severe attacks of HypoPP and TPP but is seldom required for HyperPP. Prophylactic treatment to prevent attacks is indicated for patients with all forms of PP in whom attacks are frequent; as such treatment may prevent progressive myopathy. When persistent proximal muscle weakness has already developed, it can be improved, but severe weakness is seldom completely reversible.

HYPOKALEMIC PERIODIC PARALYSIS

Acute Attacks

The treatment is similar to that of hypokalemia from any cause, except that patients with HypoPP have a pathologically greater uptake of potassium in muscle in response to insulin, catecholamines, and possibly other hormones. This sensitivity of PP muscle to insulin makes the means of potassium administration particularly important.[62] Administration should be oral if at all possible. Only when patients have nausea or vomiting, or are unable to swallow, should intravenous treatment be considered (Box 9.5).

Hazards of Parenteral Potassium Administration

Intravenous potassium administration poses special hazards in PP. In normal subjects, the administration of potassium using glucose or physiologic saline as a diluent is often associated with a fall of plasma potassium.[74] Such a fall, accompanied by greater weakness, has also been observed in patients with PP who were given large doses of intravenous potassium with 5% glucose as a diluent.[75] Use of 5% mannitol

as a diluent for potassium chloride, however, produces a prompt rise in potassium and an improvement in strength.[75] Mannitol also has been shown to increase plasma potassium in normal subjects when given intravenously (see Table 9–2). The potential cardiac hazards of intravenous potassium administration have led us to administer bolus potassium chloride rather than continuous infusions of potassium.

Side Effects

Besides those attributable to diluents used in intravenous treatment, other side effects of potassium administration include gastrointestinal irritation and ulceration with oral potassium preparations, and peripheral vein inflammation and pain with intravenous administration.

Prophylactic Treatment

Patients learn to avoid factors that trigger their attacks through lifestyle and dietary modification. In HypoPP, patients are also advised to avoid strenuous exercise or eating a high-carbohydrate meal or consuming alcohol followed by rest. A low-carbohydrate, low-sodium diet may decrease the severity of attacks but is seldom sufficient to eliminate

---

Box 9.5 Treatment of Acute Attacks of Weakness: Hypokalemic Periodic Paralysis

Preferred

Oral potassium salts (0.25 mEq/kg) until weakness improves, every 30 minutes
Avoid carbohydrate-containing foods
Avoid intravenous fluids

If patient's condition precludes oral potassium administration (e.g., vomiting)

Intravenous potassium—requires serial electrocardiogram monitoring and sequential serum potassium measurements
Potassium dosage must be decreased for patients with impaired renal function
KCl bolus (0.05–0.1 mEq KCl/kg body weight)
KCl in 5% mannitol (20–40 mEq/L)—avoid glucose or NaCl-containing diluents

All patients

Gentle exercise of involved muscle often hastens recovery

them. Most patients require prophylactic therapy to prevent their attacks and the development of progressive interattack muscle weakness (Box 9.6). Only a few randomized, double-blind, placebo-controlled trials have been performed in PP.[76-78] Among those, acetazolamide is the treatment of choice to prevent attacks in HypoPP and is effective in majority of patients.[77,79] Acetazolamide prevents and improves interattack weakness.[58] Some patients, particularly with specific sodium channel mutations, however, not only fail to respond to acetazolamide, but their condition may even be worsened by it.[80] Triamterene has proved effective in such patients.[80] Spironolactone and eplerenone have also been useful in some patients by anecdotal data from Europe. A randomized, double-blind, placebo-controlled trial showed that dichlorphenamide, another carbonic anhydrase inhibitor, is also effective in preventing attacks and may be more effective than acetazolamide in treating persistent interattack weakness.[78,81] Doses can be started at 25 mg by mouth twice daily and slowly increase to 25 to 50 mg two or three times daily. Unfortunately, this agent is not available in the United States.

Acetazolamide is well tolerated. Dosage generally starts at 125 mg orally twice daily, which can be slowly titrated to 250 mg four times daily. Some patients may require a higher dose (up to 1,500 mg daily) to prevent or reduce the severity and frequency of attacks. The toxic effects of acetazolamide include rash and hematologic and hepatic toxicity. These side effects have not been reported in patients with PP but should be considered, particularly as therapy is being introduced. The only common complication of acetazolamide therapy is the formation of renal calculi, which occurs in approximately 10% of patients treated for prolonged periods. Renal failure has never occurred, however, and symptoms related to the calculi are uncommon. Patients taking acetazolamide should be monitored with a baseline and an annual kidney ultrasound for renal calculi, which can be removed by lithotripsy.[82] Slight side effects that are frequent in patients at the beginning of treatment include nausea, anorexia, mild weight loss, and dysgeusia for carbonated beverages. Sulfonamides should not be avoided in patients taking acetazolamide, and allergy to sulfonamide is not a contraindication to acetazolamide or dichlorphenamide.[83]

Box 9.6 Prevention of Attacks: Hypokalemic Periodic Paralysis

Diet

Avoidance of carbohydrate, sodium loads

Oral potassium supplements

0.25–0.5 mEq/kg body weight, taken at bedtime

Prophylactic medications

Carbonic anhydrase inhibitors

Acetazolmide—125–1,000 mg/d
Dichlorphenamide—50–150 mg/d

Patients unresponsive to carbonic anhydrase inhibitors

Triamterene—25–100 mg/d (caution with potassium supplements)
Spironolactone—25–100 mg/d (caution with potassium supplements)

Dichlorphenamide toxicity is, in general, similar to that of acetazolamide, although the number of patients who have been followed on long-term dichlorphenamide therapy is not large enough to indicate the risk of forming renal calculi with chronic use. Some patients (5%–10%) complain of mental clouding.

Bumetanide, the Na-K-2Cl inhibitor, is shown to have benefit in preventing attacks of weakness in HypoPP type 2 in animal model and may be a good candidate for future clinical trials.[84] However, common side effects of this potent loop diuretic (e.g. volume depletion, aggravated hypokalemia, hyperuricemia) are of major concern.

HYPERKALEMIC PERIODIC PARALYSIS

Acute Attacks

Most individual attacks are mild and do not require treatment (Box 9.7). Patients frequently discover that carbohydrate-containing food and fluid promptly improve weakness. Such foods when enriched with potassium (e.g., orange juice, banana) potentially aggravate symptoms, which one would theoretically wish to avoid. The beta-adrenergic agonist salbutamol is effective, and when used as an inhalant, it is convenient and relatively safe.[85] It is important to identify these patients whose condition is associated with ATS or an underlying cardiac arrhythmias, because administration of adrenergic agents is potentially hazardous. In general, oral treatment to lower potassium levels adequately controls mild to moderate attacks (see Box 9.7). The majority of patients with HyperPP do not require intravenous treatment to lower potassium level as a secondary cause of HyperPP unless uncommonly severe attacks. The electrocardiogram must be monitored if patients are receiving intravenous treatment to lower potassium levels.

Prophylactic Treatment

Although individual attacks are characteristically mild, they should be prevented in an effort to forestall permanent weakness (Box 9.8). The beneficial effect of acetazolamide in preventing attacks of PP was first noted in HyperPP, and this drug is occasionally the most effective preventative. However, thiazide diuretics such as hydrochlorothiazide are equally effective, have fewer short-term side effects, and are usually our choice for management. Thiazides are associated with a number of rare, idiosyncratic side effects, including rash, vasculitis, and hematologic and hepatic toxicity. The major side effect encountered with thiazide treatment of HyperPP is the lowering of plasma potassium levels, which result in hypokalemic weakness. Potassium administration improves this weakness. Despite the various concerns about thiazide treatment, it remains the preferred agent. Careful, sequential follow-up of patients with HyperPP is important, because the

---

Box 9.7 Treatment of Attacks of Hyperkalemic Periodic Paralysis

Mild to moderate attacks

Dietary—simple carbohydrate ingestion, avoid potassium-enriched foods
β-adrenergic agents—salbutamol inhalation (contraindication if cardiac arrhythmia present)

Severe attacks[a]

IV treatment of hyperkalemia—sodium bicarbonate, glucose and insulin, calcium gluconate

[a]Uncommon.

Box 9.8 Prevention of Attacks: Hyperkalemic Periodic Paralysis

Hydrochlorothiazide—25–100 mg/d (may require supplemental potassium)
Acetazolamide—125–1,000 mg/d
Dichlorphenamide—50–150 mg/d

---

mildness of attacks often leads patients to ignore them. Such patients may be at risk for progressive interattack weakness that will become irreversible if not recognized and treated relatively early in its course.[1]

ANDERSEN-TAWIL SYNDROME

Treatment of ATS is focused on reducing the risk of cardiac arrhythmias. Patients should avoid sudden intense adrenergic stimulation triggered by any intense emotion or stress. Both cardiac and noncardiac medications that are known to cause prolong QT intervals should be avoided. Beta-adrenergic blockers such as propranolol have been used for long-term management to maintain a maximal heart rate of 130 bpm or less on an exercise treadmill stress test. Doses can be start at 1 mg/kg and titrate to 2 to 3 mg/kg. Occasionally, patients have had an implanted cardiac defibrillator to prevent cardiac arrest. Treatment of the paralytic attacks is similar to the treatment of HypoPP or HyperPP, depending on whether the attacks are associated with elevated or reduced potassium levels.[86] Acetazolamide or dichlorphenamide can be used to prevent attack frequency and severity. These agents lower potassium slightly, but the administration of low-dose potassium supplements appears to prevent the worsening of attacks. Potassium supplementation is also attractive in ATS condition given that elevated potassium level reduces the QT interval, which diminishes cardiac arrhythmias. Progressive muscle weakness has not been documented in this condition.

THYROTOXIC PERIODIC PARALYSIS

TPP treatment involves two steps: treating acute paralytic attacks and preventing further attacks by restoration of euthyroid state. Correction of hypokalemia to avoid cardiac arrhythmias and improve muscle weakness requires urgent treatment. Beta-adrenergic blocking agents such as propranolol are rapidly effective in preventing paralytic attacks and improving persistent interattack weakness in these patients. Conventional management for thyrotoxicosis is the main treatment of TPP. Acetazolamide is not beneficial for attack prevention and is associated with severe side effects.[87] Thyroid ablation by medical or surgical means results in permanent remission of TPP, but overadministration of thyroid hormone for hypothyroidism or recurrence of hyperthyroidism is associated with the return of paralytic attacks.

MECHANISM OF ACTION OF ACETAZOLAMIDE IN PERIODIC PARALYSIS

The basis for acetazolamide action in PP has been the subject of a number of studies.[43,88,89] With all forms of PP, some patients exhibit a paradoxical response to this agent, an observation that suggests some commonality in underlying defect. Acetazolamide is kaliuretic and produces a metabolic acidosis. It lowers plasma potassium in normal subjects and in patients with HypoPP.[43,80] This lowering of potassium may account for the precipitation of hypokalemic paralytic attacks by acetazolamide in approximately 10% of patients with HypoPP, particularly in those with sodium channel mutation.[80] The exact mechanism of acetazolamide to prevent the attacks in PP is unclear but many hypotheses have been raised. One study reports that its therapeutic effect may be produced by metabolic acidosis,[79] as it prevents the intracellular movement of potassium, augments glucose uptake in normal subjects, and may prevent the pathologic ingress of potassium into muscle in patients with HypoPP.

When carbonic anhydrase inhibitor were first recognized to be effective treatment for PP, evidence indicated an absence of carbonic anhydrase (CA) in skeletal muscle.[88] Subsequent study has shown that a sulfonamide-resistant carbonic anhydrase is present in substantial concentrations in skeletal muscle in animals[90] and in humans.[91] Three isozymes (CA I, CA II, and CA III) have been found in skeletal muscle, with CA III constituting up to 20% of noncontractile muscle protein. Diseased muscle may have an alteration in CA enzyme activity. Acetazolamide inhibits only CA I.[91] At this point, therefore, it is unlikely that direct carbonic anhydrase inhibition in muscle contributes to the therapeutic effectiveness of carbonic anhydrase inhibitors in PP and myotonia.

NONDYSTROPHIC MYOTONIAS

Myotonia

CLINICAL FEATURE AND SYMPTOMS OF MYOTONIA

Myotonia has in common the distinctive clinical phenomenon of delayed relaxation of the skeletal muscle following either voluntary contraction or the contraction resulting from muscle percussion (Figure 9–9). Clinical myotonia is both a symptom and a sign, accompanied by repetitive electrical muscle activity reflected as action potentials on EMG. The clinical elicitation of myotonia is discussed in chapters 2 and 4. Because action myotonia and percussion myotonia are not equally expressed in the different myotonic disorders, a specific search for each type of myotonia is necessary. Certain disorders have a characteristic distribution of myotonia. Most notable is myotonic dystrophy, where myotonia is not elicitable in muscles that are clinically less affected.[92]

Slight myotonia is often asymptomatic. Moderate to severe myotonia may cause social embarrassment. For example, eyelid myotonia can cause embarrassment when lid closure produces sustained orbicularis oculi myotonia and a persistent inability to open the eyelids (Figure 9–10). Extraocular muscle myotonia is less common; it may induce double vision or limit eye-hand coordination in sporting events. Bulbar myotonia may interfere with chewing and articulation. Grip myotonia can cause inability to release a handshake. Generalized limb myotonia is often more disabling (Figure 9–11), as sudden muscle contraction may cause "freezing" with virtually complete immobility. Patients may lose balance and fall if they suddenly or unexpectedly initiate activity. Patients with myotonia may complain of "stiffness" but may occasionally describe their symptom as "uncomfortable feeling," "pain," or "cramps." Pain is not usually a feature of myotonia, except in some variant forms of sodium channel myotonia[93] and myotonic dystrophy type 2.[94] A key characteristic of myotonia is its "warmup" phenomenon, a tendency to diminish through repetitive muscle contractions. Good exercise performance is often possible in such patients, however, because of warmup phenomenon, although performance may be severely limited in cold weather. On the other hand, patients with paramyotonia exhibit

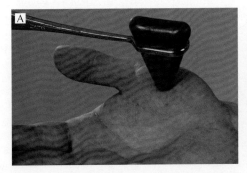
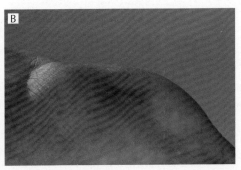

Figure 9–9. Percussion myotonia. (A) After hand relaxation, the thenar eminence is struck with a reflex hammer. (B) A persistent contraction ("dimple") is visible for 10 seconds or longer in this patient with paramyotonia congenita.

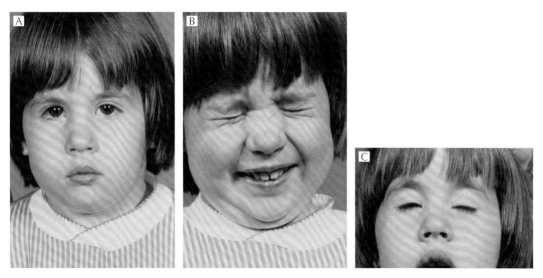

Figure 9–10. Eyelid myotonia. Patient with sodium channel myotonia (A) is instructed to close and open her eyes force-fully (B) and develops difficulty in opening her eyes, which persists for a few minutes after cessation of activity (C).

"paradoxical myotonia" in which muscle relaxation is progressively delayed with repetitive contractions. This important character helps distinguish between different types of myotonic disorders.

Some rare conditions with myotonia-like symptoms do not have electrical myotonia and electrical myotonia is occasionally seen without clinical accompaniment, although in most such instances the abnormal EMG activity is not

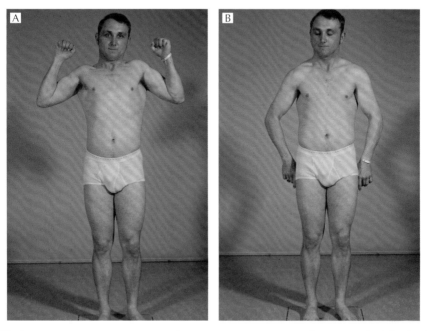

Figure 9–11. Severe action myotonia. A patient with myotonia congenita contracts his arm muscles (A) and is then unable to relax (B).

typical of the classic waxing-waning or "dive bomber" pattern (Box 9.9).

CLASSIFICATION OF MYOTONIA

Box 9.9 lists the major disorders associated with clinical myotonia. Myotonic dystrophy (see chapter 4) is the commonest, outnumbering all other conditions by approximately 12 to 1; it is followed in frequency by the various forms of myotonia congenita.[95]

Myotonic Dystrophy

Myotonic dystrophy (DM1 and DM2), are multisystemic disorders and the most frequent

---

Box 9.9 Classification of Disorders Associated With Myotonia

Clinical and/or electrical myotonia

  Myotonic dystrophy type 1 and type 2
  Nondystrophic myotonias

Chloride-channel defects

  Autosomal dominant (Thomsen's disease)
  Autosomal recessive (Becker's disease)

Sodium-channel defects

  Paramyotonia congenita
  Sodium-channel myotonias
  Myotonia fluctuans
  Myotonia permanans
  Acetazolamide-responsive myotonia
  Hyperkalemic periodic paralysis with myotonia

Electrical myotonia

  Myotubular myopathy
  Polymyositis
  Malignant hyperthermia
  Acid maltase deficiency
  Hypothyroidism
  Severe denervation
  Caveolinopathy
  Drug-induced: 3-hydroxy-3-methylglutaryl-coenzyme (HMG-CoA) reductase inhibitors, clofibrate, colchicine, propranolol, fenoterol, terbutaline, penicillamine, diazocholesterol, monocarboxylic acids, cyclosporine, anthracene-9-carboxylic acid, 2,4-dichlorophenoxyacetate

Myotonia-like symptoms without electrical myotonia

  Schwartz-Jampel syndrome
  Stiff-person syndrome
  Neurogenic muscle cramps
  Isaacs' syndrome: neuromyotonia or myokymia, hyperhidrosis, voltage-gated potassium channel antibodies
  Familial episodic ataxia type 1
  Brody disease

cause of myotonia. The pathogenesis of DM is not a simple channelopathy and therefore has been discussed in detail in chapter 4. Myotonia is helpful in diagnosis but is frequently asymptomatic. Progressive muscle weakness rather than myotonia is usually responsible for clinical presentation and functional impairment, and alleviation of myotonia is seldom helpful in improving function. Myotonia in myotonic dystrophy initially occurs most prominently in muscles that are symptomatically the weakest.[92] On the other hand, as weakness progresses and muscle atrophy occurs, myotonia sometimes can no longer be elicited.

The Nondystrophic Myotonias

The nondystrophic myotonias (NDMs) are a heterogeneous group of rare neuromuscular disorders (prevalence < 1:100,000)[95] caused by mutations in the skeletal muscle chloride and sodium channels with the common clinical features of clinical myotonia and/or electrical myotonia. The NDMs are distinguished from DM by the usual absence of progressive muscle weakness and wasting, extramuscular systemic involvement, and dystrophic changes in muscle biopsy. NDM include the classic diseases of myotonia congenita (MC), paramyotonia congenita (PMC), a group of sodium channel myotonias (SCMs), and hyperPP with myotonia.[8,95-100] Table 9–3 summarizes clinical and electrodiagnostic features of the NDMs.

The Chloride Channelopathies

Chloride channel disorders cause MC, including an autosomal-dominant form (Thomsen's

Table 9–3 Clinical Features and Electrophysiologic Patterns of the Nondystrophic Myotonias

	Dominant MC	Recessive MC	PMC	SCMs
Age of onset	Early 1st decade	Late 1st decade	1st decade	1st decade
Inheritance	AD	AR	AD	AD
Mutant channel	*CLCN1*	*CLCN1*	*SCN4A*	*SCN4A*
Clinical myotonia	Generalized Upper > lower limbs	Generalized Lower > upper limbs	Face, hands, thighs	Proximal > distal
Warmup effect	Present	Present	Absent	Variable
Paradoxical myotonia	Absent	Absent	Present	Variable
Eyelid myotonia	Infrequent	Infrequent	Common	Common
Provocative factors	Exercise after rest, emotional stress	Exercise after rest	Repeated exercise, fasting	Potassium loading, fasting, rest after exercise
Periodic weakness`	Absent	Variable, transient paresis (seconds)	Common, induced by cold or exercise	Absent
Other findings	Muscle hypertrophy	Muscle hypertrophy	No muscle hypertrophy	Painful myotonia
Electrophysiology				
EMG	Generalized myotonic discharges	Generalized myotonic discharges, mild myopathic pattern	Myotonic discharges are distal > proximal	Myotonic discharges are proximal > distal
Fournier pattern	III	II	I	III
Cooling effect	Change to Fournier II	Little effect	Myotonia & fibrillations disappear below 20° C	No effect

Note. MC = myotonia congenita, PMC = paramyotonia congenita, SCMs = sodium channel myotonias, AD = autosomal dominant, AR = autosomal recessive.

disease) and a recessive form (Becker's disease). Both forms arise from similar mutation in the skeletal muscle voltage-gated chloride channel gene (*CLCN1*) on chromosome 7q.[101,102] Several hypotheses have been raised, but the cause for this has remained uncertain, although differential allelic expression may be one of the possible mechanisms. Recent study demonstrates that copy number variation in *CLCN1* may be an important cause of recessive MC. Exon deletions or duplications are an important genetic mechanism in patients with recessive MC.[103]

AUTOSOMAL-DOMINANT MYOTONIA CONGENITA (THOMSEN'S DISEASE)

Clinical Features

This condition was first described by a Danish physician Julius Thomsen in the 19th century.[92,104] Symptoms of myotonia are usually noted in infancy or within the first decade of life, and are more troublesome in males than females. The severity of disease symptoms often lessens when patients reach the third and fourth decade. Patients experience painless muscle stiffness initiated by muscle activation after rest. Lower extremity muscles are more involved than upper extremity and facial muscles. However, myotonia of the grip and eyelid muscle and lid lag phenomenon can be observed. Some patients describe worsening of symptoms in the cold, after prolonged rest, or with emotional surprises. Stiffness usually diminishes through repetitive muscle contraction (the warmup phenomenon). Myotonia is not progressive over time or associated with true muscle weakness. On physical examination, strength is always normal. Muscle bulk is either normal or hypertrophy. Muscle hypertrophy, probably due to the almost constant state of muscle contraction, may develop particularly in the masseter muscles producing a characteristic facial appearance (Figure 9–12), proximal arm muscles, thighs, and calves. The extensor digitorum brevis muscle also is often enlarged. Contractures at the elbows and knees have been observed in some patients. Muscle stretch reflexes and the sensory examination are normal. Prognosis for normal life span is good but disability is lifelong.

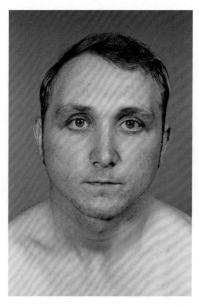

Figure 9–12. Myotonia congenita. Hypertrophy of masseter muscles produces a distinctive facial appearance.

Laboratory Studies

CK level is normal or slightly elevated, possibly because of the enlarged muscle mass.

Muscle Biopsy

There is no evidence of muscle destruction in MC, but a distinctive lack of type 2B fibers has been recognized in both forms of the disease. A generalized enlargement of muscle fibers with or without fiber size variability has also been noted.[105]

Electrodiagnostic Studies

Other than diffuse myotonic discharges, the EMG is usually normal. Even with minimal needle movement or muscle contraction, profuse myotonic discharges may make it difficult to evaluate the motor unit action potentials (MUAPs) in some patients. EMG findings can be temperature dependent. Cooling can induce prolonged myotonic bursts in dominant MC. Low frequency repetitive nerve stimulation, although not typically performed, may provide a CMAP decrement.[92,106] Repetitive short exercise testing has emerged as the most useful tool for providing diagnosis and guidance for further genetic testing. It provides distinctive changes in CMAP amplitude at room temperature and after muscle cooling.[53,54,56] The current recommendations for abnormal short exercise test is greater than 10% amplitude decrement at room temperature[53]; however recent study has shown that using amplitude-only criteria is associated with a high number of false positives in the control group (30%). A suggestion of using concordant amplitude-and-area decrements of > 20% has been raised to improve specificity, particularly when interpreting changes after muscle cooling.[54] The procedure of short exercise testing has been discussed earlier in this chapter. In general, patients with dominant MC demonstrate unchanged CMAP amplitude at room temperature (Fournier pattern III); however, postexercise CMAP amplitude significantly declined after muscle cooling (Fournier pattern II), which helps differentiate it from other NDMs (Figure 9–13). Finally, other family members should be studied to help determine the pattern of inheritance, because asymptomatic family members may have clinical myotonia or myotonic discharges on electrodiagnostic testing.

AUTOSOMAL-RECESSIVE MYOTONIA CONGENITA (BECKER'S DISEASE)

Clinical Features

The autosomal-recessive form of myotonia was fully described by Becker, a German physician, and now bears his name.[107] Although

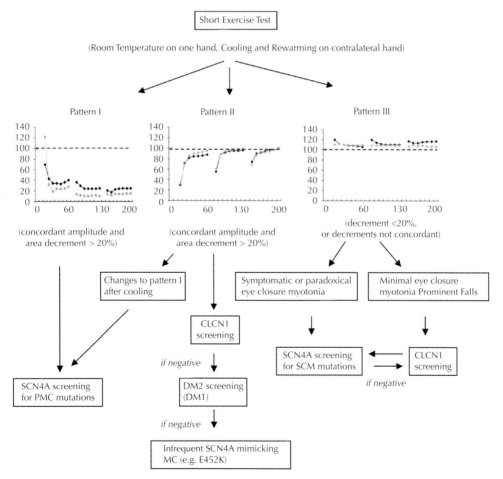

Figure 9–13. Suggested algorithm when using short exercise test for guiding genetic testing in patients with suspected nondystrophic myotonias. (From Tan SV, Matthews E, Barber M, et al. Refined exercise testing can aid DNA-based diagnosis in muscle channelopathies. *Ann Neurology* 2011;69:328–340, with permission.)

clinical features are indistinguishable, Becker's disease is symptomatically more severe than Thomsen's disease and presents later in childhood. Males are typically more affected than females. Patients usually experience symptoms more in the legs, causing abnormal gait or sudden fall. Myotonia can be triggered by cold, prolonged exercise, pregnancy, menstruation, or stress. On clinical examination, muscle hypertrophy is commonly observed in the lower extremity and gluteal muscles. There is both action and percussion myotonia. "Transient paresis" is a unique clinical sign in recessive MC: Patients experience seconds to minutes of true weakness that is triggered after initiating movement after rest.[108] It can be tested at bedside by applying isometric muscle force at the biceps muscle for 5 seconds and determine whether the Medical Research Council score drops below 5.[109] Both transient paresis and clinical myotonia improve with warmup. Although fixed weakness is not a typical feature of MC, slight weakness and atrophy of distal muscles with contractures of distal joints have been observed in some patients with recessive form MC. Prognosis for life span is similar to dominant-form MC but patients usually experience more severe disability. The CK level and muscle biopsy findings are similar to those with dominant-form MC.

Electrodiagnostic Studies

Nerve conduction studies give normal results. MUAPs can be normal or small, short, and polyphasic with early recruitment pattern, consistent with mild myopathy. EMG evidence of myopathy correlates with the moderate weakness that affects many patients with this condition. Myotonic discharges are diffusely present in both proximal and distal muscles. On short exercise testing, recessive MC typically shows Fournier pattern II, in which the first exercise induces a significant drop in CMAP amplitude at room temperature, following which the CMAP amplitude recovers within a minute after exercise cessation, reflecting transient paresis. The decrement of postexercise CMAP amplitude also diminishes with successive trials, reflecting warmup phenomenon.[53] Muscle cooling is not modified changes in CMAP amplitude pattern in this patient group (Figure 9–13). It is important to note that in some patients with

paramyotonia congenita, particularly with Q270K sodium channel mutation, Fournier pattern II can be presented on repeated short exercise test at room temperature, similar to those with recessive MC. However, cold exposure plays an important role as it induces a pattern reversion from pattern II to pattern I that is helpful in distinguishing between these two conditions.[56]

Genetics

Sproadic cases of MC presumably have this recessive form of myotonia. Cases with two or more siblings within one kindred but without affected parents have been identified.[108] It remains unclear whether all sporadic cases represent autosomal recessive myotonia congenita or whether some may be mutations of autosomal-dominant myotonia. Spontaneous mutation of autosomal dominant myotonia occurring *de novo* and exhibiting subsequent transmission consistent with an autosomal-dominant pattern have not yet been documented.

VARIANTS OF MYOTONIA CONGENITA

Both dominant and recessive forms MC are usually painless; however, one autosomal-dominant variant of myotonia congenita, caused by G200R mutation of the human *CLCN1*, is characterized by the long-term fluctuation in the symptoms of muscle stiffness, significant muscle pain, lack of muscle hypertrophy, and later symptomatic onset (typically late in the first decade of life).[110] One of the most striking findings of this variant, fluctuating myotonia congenita, is that the patient will have periods of marked stiffness that alternate with periods of less pronounced stiffness or freedom from symptoms. Each phase lasts several weeks or months, and sometimes years. This phenotype contrasts with the description of myotonia fluctuans, a sodium channelopathy, in that the fluctuations are typically day to day and the patients are very sensitive to potassium challenge. Another variant of autosomal dominant MC, myotonia levoir, is characterized by milder myotonia symptoms and later onset with the absence of muscle pain and hypertrophy.[111] Acetazolamide-responsive myotonia, also known as atypical myotonia congenita, was previously described as a painful variant of MC. It is now classified as one of the variants in SCM due to mutation in the *SCN4A* gene.

THE SODIUM CHANNELOPATHIES

The sodium channelopathies are a varied group of dominantly inherited disorders caused by mutation in the α subunit of Nav 1.4 encoded by the *SCN4A* gene on chromosome 17q23.[71,72,112] Patients with sodium channelopathies present with a diversity of symptoms, including myotonia, pain, and weakness. Disease spectrum also runs from mild myotonia that minimally affects with normal daily activities to severe muscle stiffness causing disability, or frank episodes of paralysis. It is not known why some patients with SCMs experience pain; whereas PMC and the myotonia associated with chloride channelopathies are usually painless. The phenotypic variations associated with many mutations suggest that several unrecognized factors may modify the phenotype.

PARAMYOTONIA CONGENITA

Also known as Eulenburg's disease, PMC is an autosomal-dominant disorder caused by missense mutations in the *SCN4A* gene.[8-10] Among those, Thr1313Met is the most common mutation.[113] Unlike chloride channelopathy, myotonia in these disorders is paradoxical and worsens rather than improves with repeated activity (paramyotonia), to the reverse of the warmup phenomenon. In many instances, myotonia is painless but markedly exacerbated by cold or exercise. Patients with PMC typically present in the first decade with muscle stiffness primarily affecting eyelid, extraocular, bulbofacial, neck, and hand muscles lasting minutes to hours. Cold exposure is the most sensitive trigger resulting in stiffness followed by true flaccid paralysis. However, patients with PMC can also worsen with rest followed by exercise, stress, potassium intake, pregnancy, menstruation, and prolonged fasting.[114,115] The typical physical finding is the inability to immediately open the eyes after repeated sustained eyelid closure or paradoxical eye closure myotonia. This finding is unique and useful to distinct sodium from chloride mutation.[109,113] Eyelid, grip, and percussion myotonia and the lid lag are commonly elicited. Muscle hypertrophy is not a common. PMC has appreciable overlap

in clinical findings with HyperPP has confirmed that they are alleic disorders.[8-11]

Laboratory Studies

CK may be normal or elevated. Potassium level during attacks of weakness may be low. Muscle biopsy often shows nonspecific myopathic features.

Electrodiagnostic Studies

Specific pattern of short exercise test may also help establish the diagnosis of PMC. Most PMC patients with common mutations (T1313M, R1448C, and R1448H) typically demonstrate Fournier pattern I, in which a decline of CMAP amplitude after exercise and muscle cooling that is more pronounced with the successive trials, reflecting flaccid weakness induced by exercise or cold (Figure 9–13).[53] However, PMC with Q270K mutation demonstrates Fournier pattern II at room temperature, imitating MC, but CMAP changes to Fournier pattern I after muscle cooling.[54,56] The shifted pattern was thought to be unique for this mutation. On EMG needle examination, muscle cooling to 20° C may have a profound effect, which is pathognomonic for PMC. Transient dense fibrillation potentials and electrical myotonia become more visible as grip strength declines at first and eventually disappear with cooling below 28° C. As the muscle cools down further, the myotonic discharges completely disappear below 20° C, giving way to muscle paralysis. At this point, the muscle is unexcitable to electrical or mechanical stimulation and goes into a long-lasting electrical silent contracture.[114,116]

SODIUM CHANNEL MYOTONIAS

SCMs, also known as potassium-aggravated myotonias, is a group of pure myotonic disorders caused by an alleic point mutation in the α-subunit of the *SCN4A* gene on chromosome 17q23. They are inherited in an autosomal-dominant fashion. Patients present in childhood or adolescence with episodes of generalized stiffness secondary to myotonia. Distinguishing features include painful myotonia with worsening of symptoms induced by potassium ingestion. The patients do not experience true episodic weakness or paramyotonia, and are not cold sensitive as seen in

PMC. Several variants with distinctive clinical features have been established.

Myotonia Fluctuans

Myotonia flucuans typically presents in the adolescence with fluctuating muscle stiffness. Myotonia may be painful and has a singular feature of being exercise induced, but onset is delayed for several minutes after exercise, which is opposed to PMC in that myotonia occurs immediately after exercise. Muscle stiffness is worsened by the intake of potassium but not by the cold. There is no episodic weakness. Some patients may experience a warmup phenomenon.[117-119] CK levels are elevated in several patients. Muscle pathology illustrates mild myopathic pattern with increased central nuclei and fiber size variability.

Myotonia Permanens

This rare disorder presents in early childhood with severe and unremitting generalized painful myotonia. Patients have neck and shoulder muscle hypertrophy. Worsening of symptoms with potassium intake may be very severe and may affect bulbar and respiratory muscles, resulting in hypoventilation, hypoxemia and respiratory acidosis that can be life threatening.[120,121]

Acetazolamide-Responsive Myotonia

Previously known as atypical MC, acetazolamide-responsive myotonia (ARM) this disorder commonly manifests in early childhood and is characterized by painful myotonia and periodic worsening of muscle stiffness. The myotonia has a predilection for extraocular muscles, axial, and proximal limb muscles. Symptoms are provoked or worsened by fasting, infection, and potassium ingestion. Cold exposure may worsen the myotonia but does not induce paralysis as PMC. Rhabdomyolysis may develop during surgery. Symptoms are markedly relieved with acetazolamide, although mexiletine is also effective.[18,93] Percussion and grip myotonia and paramoytonia of eyelid may be present. Muscle hypertrophy, although is not as common as MC, may be present.[114] ARM can be identified both by the clinical features and by muscle biopsy: Type 2B muscle fibers were present in multiple patients in two separate families,[93] whereas they are absent in the other forms of MC.[105]

Electrodiagnostic Studies

Needle EMG demonstrates diffuse myotonia. On short exercise test, the common mutations of SCMs (G1306A, G1306V, V445M, S804N, and V1293I) typically illustrate Fournier pattern III with no changes after muscle cooling (Figure 9–13). In some patients with A715T and I1310N mutations, cold induces a progressive decrement of CMAP and so the pattern changes from Fournier III to Fournier I after muscle cooling.[53,56]

HYPERKALEMIC PERIODIC PARALYSIS WITH MYOTONIA

HyperPP with myotonia is an autosomal-dominant sodium channelopathy. Patients experience episodes of flaccid paralysis or focal weakness lasting minutes to hours and muscle stiffness secondary to myotonia. Potassium intakes, fasting, rest after exercise, cold, and intense emotional stress can trigger the attacks. Most weakness is more common in lower than upper extremity and mainly proximal. Facial and respiratory muscle involvement is rare. Fixed weakness may develop over time if frequent attacks continue. Although action and percussion myotonia is not as prominent as other NDMs, electrical myotonia is relatively simple to demonstrate. Paramyotonia of eyelid may be observed in some patients. CK is slightly elevated and muscle pathology demonstrates vacuolar myopathy. Short exercise testing is not useful to diagnose this condition. Long exercise testing typically discloses a significant postexercise CMAP amplitude or area decrement over 45-minute rest.[13,116]

Differential Diagnosis and Approach

Numerous other causes of sustained muscle contraction or of impaired muscle relaxation can resemble myotonia (see Box 9.9). All are infrequent and are distinguishable from myotonia on both clinical and electrophysiological evaluation.

A number of common conditions that do not cause myotonia can occasionally be interpreted as suggesting myotonia, based on either history or examination. For example, muscle cramps are painful muscle contractions that result from paroxysmal discharges of nerve. EMG readily distinguishes cramps from myotonia. Increase in muscle tone from central nervous system disease results in spasticity or rigidity on a central basis. Accompanying neurologic signs usually indicate the basis for the abnormal muscle tone. Dystonia, particularly when focal and paroxysmal, is often painless and can suggest a primary muscular rigidity. The sustained postures that are adopted distinguish dystonia clinically from myotonia, and the EMG activity is that of entire motor units, as opposed to muscle fiber hyperactivity.

Patient who demonstrates both clinical and electrical myotonia should be meticulously evaluated for DM type 1 and type 2 due to their much higher prevalence. DM can be distinguished from NDMs using careful bedside evaluation, by the presence of progressive muscle weakness and atrophy, and multisystemic involvement. Genetic testing is also widely available to confirm the diagnosis in DM1 and DM2. If patient shows clinical features suggestive of NDMs, needle EMG and repeated short exercise testing at room temperature on one hand and repeated testing after muscle cooling and rewarming on the contralateral hand are recommended. Clinician should also try to combine distinctive bedside clinical findings and the pattern of short exercise testing in order to guide for molecular genetic testing as shown in the diagnostic approach algorithm (Figure 9–13).

Pathogenesis of Myotonia

The gene lesions responsible for most diseases that cause myotonia have been identified over the past decade. DM1 is caused by an unstable expansion of CTG repeats on chromosome19q13.3 in the untranslated region of the *DMPK* gene[122,123] whereas an expansion of a CCTG repeat in exon 1 of the *CNBP* gene on chromosome 3q21.3, previously known as Zinc Finger Protein 9 (*ZNF9*) is responsible for DM2.[124] Pathogenesis of myotonic dystrophy is discussed in chapter 4. Defects of both the chloride channel[9,102,125] and sodium channel[11,72,118,121,126,127] cause the various forms of MC, PMC, and SCMs.

NONDYSTROPHIC MYOTONIAS

Having reviewed the different syndromes associated with NDMs, we can consider the issue of how dysfunctions of different membrane ion channels can produce similar clinical findings. Myotonia results from membrane excitability and is associated with dysfunction of chloride or sodium channels.[125] Extensive study of myotonic intercostal goat muscle, together with more limited studies in humans, suggests that an abnormal decrease in chloride permeability is a major defect in myotonic muscles.[128,129] The key to understanding myotonia is the fact that low-level depolarization can bring the membrane closer to the threshold for initiating an action potential. Skeletal muscle has a singularly high resting chloride conductance, which serves to stabilize membrane excitability.[130,131] A unique feature of skeletal muscle is the presence of the transverse tubule (T-tubule) system. The T-tubule system is composed of elongated invaginations of the surface membrane, which conduct the action potential inside a muscle fiber to trigger release of calcium from the sarcoplasmic reticulum. The T-tubule system is essential for synchronous activation of myofibrils. An adverse consequence of the T-tubule system is that due to the extremely small volume of the T-tubules, K^+ released during the repolarizing phase of the action potential can accumulate within the T-tubules. Sufficient K^+ accumulates within the T-tubules to depolarize the adjacent surface membrane. The membrane depolarization produced by K^+ accumulation within the T-tubules would trigger repeated action potentials if the membrane were not stabilized by a resting Cl^- conductance.[131,132] Pharmacologically reducing chloride conductance produces myotonia, which can be stopped by mechanically disrupting the T-tubule system have confirmed this predilection.[133,134] This model is also consistent with the observed increase in myotonia predicted by increases in extracellular potassium.[135] Therefore, the high resting membrane Cl^- conductance in skeletal muscle is needed to counter the membrane depolarization produced by K^+ accumulation within the T-tubules. In MC, pathogenesis of myotonia is virtually identical to early experiments in myotonic goats.[129] A marked reduction of chloride conductance from loss-of-function mutations was identified compared with normal individuals, resulting in depolarizing muscle fiber and triggering repetitive, propagated action potentials.[101,130,136] Another way to depolarize the membrane beyond the usual duration of the action potential is to involve gain-of-function sodium channel fast inactivation ($Na_v1.4$).[71,72,112] Fast inactivation is disrupted by all the Na^+ channel point mutations associated with the production of myotonia or paramyotonia. In PMC, muscle cooling in the absence of action will produce repetitive motor unit discharges that reflect cold-induced muscle depolarization.[11] With increased cooling of muscle, myotonia disappears and complete muscle depolarization and paralysis occur.[137] Both mechanisms, reducing Cl^- conductance or impairing Na^+ channel fast inactivation, can result in low-level membrane depolarization, increasing the propensity of the repeated and propagated action potentials, the cardinal feature of myotonia.

Weakness is present in some forms of NDMs. One common feature of skeletal muscle channelopathy-associated weakness is flaccid paresis related with prolonged membrane depolarization producing membrane inexcitability. In PMC and HyperPP, the Na^+ channel point mutations enable altered Na^+ channels to remain open or to repeatedly open, which causes prolonged membrane depolarization.[112,138-140] A key difference in the sodium channel mutations that produce HyperPP or PMC compared with the mutations that produce SCMs is the duration of the membrane depolarization produced by the mutation. The mutations associated with SCMs do not produced prolonged membrane depolarization.[96,141] The brief depolarization produced by some Na^+ channel mutations cause myotonia without weakness, whereas the persistent depolarization produced by other Na^+ mutations can result in initial hyperexcitability followed by depolarization-induced membrane inexcitability.[139,142,143] Interruption of Na^+ channel slow inactivation facilitates the production of a persistent depolarizing Na^+ current, and slow inactivation is disrupted by several of the point mutations associated with HyperPP.[71,139] Disruption of both inactivation processes enables the mutant channels to remain open or to repeatedly open for prolonged periods of time. Slow inactivation is not disrupted by the mutations that produce SCMs.[141] It is not known how reduced temperature induces paralysis in PMC.[144]

Treatment of Myotonic Disorders

NONPHARMACOLOGICAL TREATMENT

Some patients with NDMs have minor complaints that may not need treatment and learn to adjust their activities and lifestyle to reduce symptoms. Many patients, particularly MC, can improve their symptoms with frequent small voluntary movements to succeed a warmup phenomenon. All patients should be instructed to avoid triggers that are specific to their phenotype. Those with PMC should learn to avoid situations such as exposure to the cold coupled with exercise. Unsupervised immersion into cold water should also be discouraged due to potential accidental drowning. Patients with SCMs may reduce their symptoms by avoidance of potassium-rich diets or fasting.

ANESTHETIC CONSIDERATIONS FOR PATIENTS WITH NDMs

Many anesthetic agents are known to aggravate myotonia. Depolarizing ones such as succinylcholine and anticholinesterase agents should be avoided in all forms of NDM and HyperPP with myotonia as they worsen myotonia.[145] Myotonia is not prevented by curare, but is not exacerbated by it either.[146] If muscle relaxation is necessary during anesthesia, d-tubocurarine is preferable. Sevoflurane, a volatile anesthesia, has been used repeatedly in PMC patient without serious adverse effects reported.[147,148] Propofol provides variable responses and its effect is clearly unpredictable. It has been reported to prolong recovery and exacerbate myotonia.[149,150] However, there have been cases where propofol was used successfully during induction and maintenance of anesthesia without adverse events.[151] Therefore, propofol should be used only if indicated and with as minimal a dose as possible. Hyperthermic responses to general anesthesia have been noted in patients with myotonic disorders.[150] It is unclear whether patients with MC or myotonic dystrophy (DM) are likely to develop true malignant hyperthermia.[152,153] Nonetheless, it seems prudent not to use succinylcholine and to avoid general anesthesia when possible. The use of spinal and epidural anesthesia was reported to be safe in these patients.[154,155] Perioperatively and postoperatively, these patients and their intravenous fluid should be kept warm.[156] Because potassium administration exacerbates myotonia,[157] intravenous and oral potassium supplementation should be given only with caution and with careful clinical observation.[156] Ultimately, anesthesiology consultation and ICU facilities should be available whenever a myotonic patient is anesthetized.

PHARMACOLOGICAL TREATMENT

Several medications in various classes have been used successfully in treatment of myotonia (Box 9.10). To date, only few randomized control trials have been conducted to determine the efficacy of antimyotonic medications. Among these medications, mexiletine seems to be the most promising and effective treatment of myotonia in both NDMs and DM. Mexiletine is a class Ib antiarrhythmic medication that works as a high-affinity sodium channel blocker. Mexiletine reduces muscle fiber excitability and enhances fast activation of sodium channels caused by common NDM mutations.[158-161] In a large, multicenter, randomized, double-blind, placebo-controlled two-period crossover study of 59 patients with NDM, mexiletine significantly improves patient-reported outcome of both muscle stiffness scores and quality of life

---

Box 9.10 Treatment of Myotonia

Antiarrhythmic medications

> Mexiletine[a] (450–600 mg/d)
> Tocainide
> Flecanide
> Procainamide

Diuretic

> Acetazolamide[b] (250–750 mg/d)

Antiepileptic medications

> Phenytoin (300–400 mg/d, necessary to achieve a therapeutic level of 10–20 µg/ml)
> Carbamazepine

Antidepressant medications

> Imipramine
> Clomiprimine

Calcium-channel blocker

> Nifedipine
> Verapamil
> Diltiazem

Miscellaneous group

> Quinine
> Dantrolene

[a]First-line drug for all types of myotonia. [b]First-line drug for acetazolamide responsive myotonia.

scores. It also decreases handgrip myotonia on clinical examination.[162] The recommended dose of mexiletine from this study is 200 mg three times daily. It can be taken in a daily basis or intermittently when symptoms are troublesome. Hence, a patient can take mexiletine shortly before engaging in physical activity or when the weather is cold. The common adverse effects are gastrointestinal symptoms, lightheadedness, and unsteady gait. Uncommon adverse effects include tingling, fatigue, depression, chest pain, and palpitations. Although cardiac arrhythmias were not observed in the recent study of 59 patients, patients should have a baseline EKG performed prior to starting medication. In myotonic dystrophy type 1, mexiletine also demonstrates a significant reduction in handgrip relaxation time with no serious adverse events or with prolongation of the PR, QRS duration, or QTc interval from serial electrocardiograms (class I evidence).[163] Mexiletine is now considered as the first choice antimyotonic medication that works in all types of NDMs and myotonic dystrophy.

Acetazolamide, a carbonic anhydrase inhibitor, has been found to be effective in some patients with MC, PCM, and SCMs.[157] Especially in those with ARM, acetazolamide helps dramatically reduce muscle stiffness and pain; hence it is named for its dramatic response.[93,157] Acetazolamide increases urine sodium and potassium and limits potassium influx into muscle.[164] It also has direct effects on *CLC1* by increasing chloride conductance via a process related to intracellular acidification.[165] In some patients with PMC with cold-induced weakness, acetazolamide may provoke the weakness probably by lowering the potassium level.[166] Thus, it is useful to determine whether weakness is temperature dependent because there are clear implications regarding treatment options. When acetazolamide is considered, doses generally begin at 125 mg twice daily, slowly titrating to 250 mg three times daily, as tolerated by the patients. Common side effects include altered taste of carbonated beverages, paresthesia, nephrolithiasis, drowsiness, and rash. Kidney ultrasound is recommended before starting the treatment and periodically thereafter.

When patients do not respond to mexiletine or experience significant adverse effects, other agents in Box 9.10 can be tried for treatment of myotonia. Other antiarrhythmic agents have been studied in treatment of myotonia. Tocainide, a lidocaine derivative that blocks sodium current, has been used in NDM patients who are refractory to mexiletine. However, this agent is no longer available in the United State due to serious side effects of the potential risk for agranulocytosis and interstitial lung disease. Flecanide and quinine have scant data for their benefit as antimyotonic medications. Procainamide demonstrates improved hand opening in a small, randomized, double-blind, crossover study in DM1; however, significant side effects such as agranulocytosis, induction of lupus erythematosis, and *torsades de pointes* are of major concern. Therefore, the oral form of procainamide also is no longer available in the United States. Antiepileptic medications that block sodium channel such as phenytoin and carbamazepine have been used for myotonia treatment. Previous data has shown benefit to reduce grip relaxation time and subjective myotonic symptoms. Side effects are usually not uncommon and patients need to take these medications as a regular basis in order to experience the benefits. Various antidepressants, nifedipine, and dantrolene have been used in myotonia treatment, but data are limited and anti-myotonia effects are relatively slim.

Patients who have HyperPP with myotonia generally do not require antimyotonia medication due to its minor symptom. Majority of these patients suffer from weakness during paralytic attacks and some of them may develop progressive muscle weakness. Treatments in this disorder have been discussed earlier in the periodic paralysis section.

REFERENCES

1. Riggs JE. Periodic paralysis. *Clinical neuropharmacology*. 1989;12(4):249–257.
2. Tan SY, Burton M. Hyporeninemic hypoaldosteronism. An overlooked cause of hyperkalemia. *Archives of internal medicine*. 1981;141(1):30–33.
3. Raja Rayan DL, Hanna MG. Skeletal muscle channelopathies: nondystrophic myotonias and periodic paralysis. *Current opinion in neurology*. 2010;23(5):466–476.
4. Venance SL, Cannon SC, Fialho D, et al. The primary periodic paralyses: diagnosis, pathogenesis and treatment. *Brain: a journal of neurology*. 2006;129(Pt 1):8–17.
5. Poskanzer DC, Kerr DN. A third type of periodic paralysis, with normokalemia and favourable response to sodium chloride. *The American journal of medicine*. 1961;31:328–342.

6. Chinnery PF, Walls TJ, Hanna MG, Bates D, Fawcett PR. Normokalemic periodic paralysis revisited: does it exist? *Annals of neurology.* 2002;52(2):251–252.

7. Vicart S, Sternberg D, Fournier E, et al. New mutations of SCN4A cause a potassium-sensitive normokalemic periodic paralysis. *Neurology.* 2004;63(11):2120–2127.

8. Ptacek LJ, Trimmer JS, Agnew WS, Roberts JW, Petajan JH, Leppert M. Paramyotonia congenita and hyperkalemic periodic paralysis map to the same sodium-channel gene locus. *American journal of human genetics.* 1991;49(4):851–854.

9. Koch MC, Ricker K, Otto M, et al. Linkage data suggesting allelic heterogeneity for paramyotonia congenita and hyperkalemic periodic paralysis on chromosome 17. *Human genetics.* 1991;88(1):71–74.

10. McClatchey AI, Trofatter J, McKenna-Yasek D, et al. Dinucleotide repeat polymorphisms at the SCN4A locus suggest allelic heterogeneity of hyperkalemic periodic paralysis and paramyotonia congenita. *American journal of human genetics.* 1992;50(5): 896–901.

11. Lehmann-Horn F, Rudel R, Ricker K. Membrane defects in paramyotonia congenita (Eulenburg). *Muscle & nerve.* 1987;10(7):633–641.

12. Tawil R, Ptacek LJ, Pavlakis SG, et al. Andersen's syndrome: potassium-sensitive periodic paralysis, ventricular ectopy, and dysmorphic features. *Annals of neurology.* 1994;35(3):326–330.

13. Miller TM, Dias da Silva MR, Miller HA, et al. Correlating phenotype and genotype in the periodic paralyses. *Neurology.* 2004;63(9):1647–1655.

14. Smith W. Periodic paralysis: report of two fatal cases. *J Nerv Ment Dis.* 1939;90(210): 210–215.

15. Fontaine B, Khurana TS, Hoffman EP, et al. Hyperkalemic periodic paralysis and the adult muscle sodium channel alpha-subunit gene. *Science.* 1990;250(4983):1000–1002.

16. Ptacek LJ, Gouw L, Kwiecinski H, et al. Sodium channel mutations in paramyotonia congenita and hyperkalemic periodic paralysis. *Annals of neurology.* 1993;33(3):300–307.

17. Jurkat-Rott K, Lehmann-Horn F. Genotype-phenotype correlation and therapeutic rationale in hyperkalemic periodic paralysis. *Neurotherapeutics: the journal of the American Society for Experimental NeuroTherapeutics.* 2007;4(2):216–224.

18. Ptacek LJ, Tawil R, Griggs RC, Storvick D, Leppert M. Linkage of atypical myotonia congenita to a sodium channel locus. *Neurology.* 1992;42(2):431–433.

19. Fenech FF, Soler NG. Hyperkalemic periodic paralysis starting at age 48. *British medical journal.* 1968;2(5603):472–473.

20. Riggs JE, Moxley RT, 3rd, Griggs RC, Horner FA. Hyperkalemic periodic paralysis: an apparent sporadic case. *Neurology.* 1981;31(9):1157–1159.

21. Bradley WG, Taylor R, Rice DR, et al. Progressive myopathy in hyperkalemic periodic paralysis. *Archives of neurology.* 1990;47(9):1013–1017.

22. Gamstorp I, Wohlfart G. A syndrome characterized by myokymia, myotonia, muscular wasting and increased perspiration. *Acta psychiatrica et neurologica Scandinavica.* 1959;34(2):181–194.

23. Lewis ED, Griggs RC, Moxley RT, 3rd. Regulation of plasma potassium in hyperkalemic periodic paralysis. *Neurology.* 1979;29(8):1131–1137.

24. Van Der Meulen JP, Gilbert GJ, Kane CA. Familial hyperkalemic paralysis with myotonia. *The New England journal of medicine.* 1961;264:1–6.

25. Andersen ED, Krasilnikoff PA, Overvad H. Intermittent muscular weakness, extrasystoles, and multiple developmental anomalies. A new syndrome? *Acta paediatrica Scandinavica.* 1971;60(5):559–564.

26. Sansone V, Griggs RC, Meola G, et al. Andersen's syndrome: a distinct periodic paralysis. *Annals of neurology.* 1997;42(3):305–312.

27. Statland JM, Tawil R, Venance SL. Andersen-Tawil Syndrome. 2004 Nov 22 [Updated 2013 Jan 3]. In: Pagon RA, Adam MP, Bird TD, et al., editors. GeneReviews™ [Internet]. Seattle (WA): University of Washington, Seattle; 1993–2013. Available from: http://www.ncbi.nlm.nih.gov/books/NBK1264/

28. Okinaka S, Shizume K, Iino S, et al. The association of periodic paralysis and hyperthyroidism in Japan. *The journal of clinical endocrinology and metabolism.* 1957;17(12):1454–1459.

29. McFadzean AJ, Yeung R. Periodic paralysis complicating thyrotoxicosis in Chinese. *British medical journal.* 1967;1(5538):451–455.

30. Kelley DE, Gharib H, Kennedy FP, Duda RJ, Jr., McManis PG. Thyrotoxic periodic paralysis. Report of 10 cases and review of electromyographic findings. *Archives of internal medicine.* 1989;149(11): 2597–2600.

31. Ober KP. Thyrotoxic periodic paralysis in the United States. Report of 7 cases and review of the literature. *Medicine.* 1992;71(3):109–120.

32. Shizume K, Shishiba Y, Kuma K, et al. Comparison of the incidence of association of periodic paralysis and hyperthyroidism in Japan in 1957 and 1991. *Endocrinologia japonica.* 1992;39(3):315–318.

33. Ryan DP, da Silva MR, Soong TW, et al. Mutations in potassium channel Kir2.6 cause susceptibility to thyrotoxic hypokalemic periodic paralysis. *Cell.* 2010;140(1): 88–98.

34. Puwanant A, Ruff RL. INa and IKir are reduced in Type 1 hypokalemic and thyrotoxic periodic paralysis. *Muscle & nerve.* 2010;42(3):315–327.

35. Griggs RC, Moxley RT, 3rd, Lafrance RA, McQuillen J. Hereditary paroxysmal ataxia: response to acetazolamide. *Neurology.* 1978;28(12):1259–1264.

36. Livingstone IR, Gardner-Medwin D, Pennington RJ. Familial intermittent ataxia with possible X-linked recessive inheritance. Two patients with abnormal pyruvate metabolism and a response to acetazolamide. *Journal of the neurological sciences.* 1984;64(1):89–97.

37. Greenlee M, Wingo CS, McDonough AA, Youn JH, Kone BC. Narrative review: evolving concepts in potassium homeostasis and hypokalemia. *Annals of internal medicine.* 2009;150(9):619–625.

38. Rabinowitz L. Aldosterone and potassium homeostasis. *Kidney international.* 1996;49(6):1738–1742.

39. Bia MJ, DeFronzo RA. Extrarenal potassium homeostasis. *The American journal of physiology.* 1981;240(4): F257–F268.

40. Griggs RC, Forbes G, Moxley RT, Herr BE. The assessment of muscle mass in progressive neuromuscular disease. *Neurology.* 1983;33(2):158–165.

41. Nadler JL, Lee FO, Hsueh W, Horton R. Evidence of prostacyclin deficiency in the syndrome of hyporeninemic hypoaldosteronism. *The New England journal of medicine.* 1986;314(16):1015–1020.

42. Nardone DA, McDonald WJ, Girard DE. Mechanisms in hypokalemia: clinical correlation. *Medicine.* 1978;57(5):435–446.

43. Riggs JE, Griggs RC, Moxley RT, 3rd, Lewis ED. Acute effects of acetazolamide in hyperkalemic periodic paralysis. *Neurology.* 1981;31(6):725–729.

44. Corbett AJ. Electrolyte disorders affecting muscle. *Semin neurol.* 1983;3(1983):248–257.

45. Engel AG, Lambert EH, Rosevear JW, Tauxe WN. Clinical and electromyographic studies in a patient with primary hypokalemic periodic paralysis. *The American journal of medicine.* 1965;38:626–640.

46. Resnick JS, Engel WK. Myotonic lid lag in hypokalemic periodic paralysis. *Journal of neurology, neurosurgery, and psychiatry.* 1967;30:47–51.

47. Subramony SH, Malhotra CP, Mishra SK. Distinguishing paramyotonia congenita and myotonia congenita by electromyography. *Muscle & nerve.* 1983;6(5):374–379.

48. Thrush DC, Morris CJ, Salmon MV. Paramyotonia congenita: a clinical, histochemical and pathological study. *Brain: a journal of neurology.* 1972;95(3):537–552.

49. Plaster NM, Tawil R, Tristani-Firouzi M, et al. Mutations in Kir2.1 cause the developmental and episodic electrical phenotypes of Andersen's syndrome. *Cell.* 2001;105(4):511–519.

50. Ptacek LJ, Tawil R, Griggs RC, et al. Dihydropyridine receptor mutations cause hypokalemic periodic paralysis. *Cell.* 1994;77(6):863–868.

51. McManis PG, Lambert EH, Daube JR. The exercise test in periodic paralysis. *Muscle & nerve.* 1986;9(8):704–710.

52. Kuntzer T, Flocard F, Vial C, et al. Exercise test in muscle channelopathies and other muscle disorders. *Muscle & nerve.* 2000;23(7):1089–1094.

53. Fournier E, Arzel M, Sternberg D, et al. Electromyography guides toward subgroups of mutations in muscle channelopathies. *Annals of neurology.* 2004;56(5):650–661.

54. Tan SV, Matthews E, Barber M, et al. Refined exercise testing can aid DNA-based diagnosis in muscle channelopathies. *Annals of neurology.* 2011;69(2):328–340.

55. Streib EW SS, Yarkowsky T. Transient paresis in myotonic syndromes. *Muscle & nerve.* 1982;10:603–615.

56. Fournier E, Viala K, Gervais H, et al. Cold extends electromyography distinction between ion channel mutations causing myotonia. *Annals of neurology.* 2006;60(3):356–365.

57. Lehmann-Horn F, Rüdel R, Jurkat-Rott K: Nondystrophic Myotonias and Periodic Paralyses. In Engel AG, franzini-Armstrong C (eds): Myology. McGraw-Hill, New York; 2004, pp 1282–1285.

58. Griggs RC, Engel WK, Resnick JS. Acetazolamide treatment of hypokalemic periodic paralysis. Prevention of attacks and improvement of persistent weakness. *Annals of internal medicine.* 1970;73(1): 39–48.

59. Brooke MH, Engel WK. The histographic analysis of human muscle biopsies with regard to fiber types. 3. Myotonias, myasthenia gravis, and hypokalemic periodic paralysis. *Neurology.* 1969;19(5):469–477.

60. Lehmann-Horn F, Jurkat-Rott K, Rudel R. Periodic paralysis: understanding channelopathies. *Current neurology and neuroscience reports.* 2002;2(1):61–69.

61. Rudel R, Lehmann-Horn F, Ricker K, Kuther G. Hypokalemic periodic paralysis: in vitro investigation of muscle fiber membrane parameters. *Muscle & nerve.* 1984;7(2):110–120.

62. Ruff RL. Insulin acts in hypokalemic periodic paralysis by reducing inward rectifier K+ current. *Neurology.* 1999;53(7):1556–1563.

63. Tricarico D, Capriulo R, Conte Camerino D. Insulin modulation of ATP-sensitive K+ channel of rat skeletal muscle is impaired in the hypokalaemic state. *Pflugers Archiv: European journal of physiology.* 1999;437(2):235–240.

64. Tricarico D, Servidei S, Tonali P, Jurkat-Rott K, Camerino DC. Impairment of skeletal muscle adenosine triphosphate-sensitive K+ channels in patients with hypokalemic periodic paralysis. *The journal of clinical investigation.* 1999;103(5):675–682.

65. Yu FH, Yarov-Yarovoy V, Gutman GA, Catterall WA. Overview of molecular relationships in the voltage-gated ion channel superfamily. *Pharmacological reviews.* 2005;57(4):387–395.

66. Jurkat-Rott K, Mitrovic N, Hang C, et al. Voltage-sensor sodium channel mutations cause hypokalemic periodic paralysis type 2 by enhanced inactivation and reduced current. *Proceedings of the National Academy of Sciences of the United States of America.* 2000;97(17):9549–9554.

67. Ruff RL. Skeletal muscle sodium current is reduced in hypokalemic periodic paralysis. *Proceedings of the National Academy of Sciences of the United States of America.* 2000;97(18):9832–9833.

68. Struyk AF, Scoggan KA, Bulman DE, Cannon SC. The human skeletal muscle Na channel mutation R669H associated with hypokalemic periodic paralysis enhances slow inactivation. *The Journal of neuroscience: the official journal of the Society for Neuroscience.* 2000;20(23):8610–8617.

69. Francis DG, Rybalchenko V, Struyk A, Cannon SC. Leaky sodium channels from voltage sensor mutations in periodic paralysis, but not paramyotonia. *Neurology.* 2011;76(19):1635–1641.

70. Ruff RL. An important piece has been placed in the puzzle of hypokalemic periodic paralysis. *Neurology.* 2011;76(19):1614–1615.

71. Cannon SC, Brown RH, Jr., Corey DP. A sodium channel defect in hyperkalemic periodic paralysis: potassium-induced failure of inactivation. *Neuron.* 1991;6(4):619–626.

72. Lehmann-Horn F, Rudel R, Dengler R, Lorkovic H, Haass A, Ricker K. Membrane defects in paramyotonia congenita with and without myotonia in a warm environment. *Muscle & nerve.* 1981;4(5):396–406.

73. Davies NP, Imbrici P, Fialho D, et al. Andersen-Tawil syndrome: new potassium channel mutations and possible phenotypic variation. *Neurology.* 2005;65(7): 1083–1089.

74. Kunin AS, Surawicz B, Sims EA. Decrease in serum potassium concentrations and appearance of cardiac arrhythmias during infusion of potassium with glucose in potassium-depleted patients. *The New England journal of medicine.* 1962;266:228–233.

75. Griggs RC, Resnick J, Engel WK. Intravenous treatment of hypokalemic periodic paralysis. *Archives of neurology.* 1983;40(9):539–540.

76. Ligtenberg JJ, Van Haeften TW, Van Der Kolk LE, et al. Normal insulin release during sustained hyperglycaemia in hypokalaemic periodic paralysis: role of

the potassium channel opener pinacidil in impaired muscle strength. *Clin Sci (Lond)*. 1996;91(5):583–589.

77. Links TP, Zwarts MJ, Oosterhuis HJ. Improvement of muscle strength in familial hypokalaemic periodic paralysis with acetazolamide. *Journal of neurology, neurosurgery, and psychiatry*. 1988;51(9):1142–1145.

78. Tawil R, McDermott MP, Brown R, Jr., et al. Randomized trials of dichlorphenamide in the periodic paralyses. Working Group on Periodic Paralysis. *Annals of neurology*. 2000;47(1):46–53.

79. Resnick JS, Engel WK, Griggs RC, Stam AC. Acetazolamide prophylaxis in hypokalemic periodic paralysis. *The New England journal of medicine*. 1968;278(11):582–586.

80. Torres CF, Griggs RC, Moxley RT, Bender AN. Hypokalemic periodic paralysis exacerbated by acetazolamide. *Neurology*. 1981;31(11):1423–1428.

81. Dalakas MC, Engel WK. Treatment of "permanent" muscle weakness in familial hypokalemic periodic paralysis. *Muscle & nerve*. 1983;6(3):182–186.

82. Tawil R, Moxley RT, 3rd, Griggs RC. Acetazolamide-induced nephrolithiasis: implications for treatment of neuromuscular disorders. *Neurology*. 1993;43(6):1105–1106.

83. Bendheim PE, Reale EO, Berg BO. beta-Adrenergic treatment of hyperkalemic periodic paralysis. *Neurology*. 1985;35(5):746–749.

84. Sansone V, Tawil R. Management and treatment of Andersen-Tawil syndrome (ATS). *Neurotherapeutics: the journal of the American Society for Experimental NeuroTherapeutics*. 2007;4(2):233–237.

85. Norris FH. Use of acetazolamide in thyrotoxic periodic paralysis. *The New England journal of medicine*. 1972;286:893.

86. Maren TH. Use of inhibitors in physiological studies of carbonic anhydrase. *The American journal of physiology*. 1977;232(4):F291–F297.

87. Riggs JE, Griggs RC, Moxley RT, 3rd. Dissociation of glucose and potassium arterial-venous differences across the forearm by acetazolamide. A possible relationship to acetazolamide's beneficial effect in hypokalemic periodic paralysis. *Archives of neurology*. 1984;41(1):35–38.

88. Jeffery S, Carter ND, Smith A. Immunocytochemical localization of carbonic anhydrase isozymes I, II, and III in rat skeletal muscle. *The journal of histochemistry and cytochemistry*.1986;34(4):513–516.

89. Peyronnard JM, Charron LF, Messier JP, Lavoie J, Faraco-Cantin F, Dubreuil M. Histochemical localization of carbonic anhydrase in normal and diseased human muscle. *Muscle & nerve*. 1988;11(2):108–113.

90. Streib EW. AAEE minimonograph #27: differential diagnosis of myotonic syndromes. *Muscle & nerve*. 1987;10(7):603–615.

91. Trudell RG, Kaiser KK, Griggs RC. Acetazolamide-responsive myotonia congenita. *Neurology*. 1987;37(3):488–491.

92. Suokas KI, Haanpaa M, Kautiainen H, Udd B, Hietaharju AJ. Pain in patients with myotonic dystrophy type 2: a postal survey in Finland. *Muscle & nerve*. 2012;45(1):70–74.

93. Emery AE. Population frequencies of inherited neuromuscular diseases—a world survey. *Neuromuscular disorders: NMD*. 1991;1(1):19–29.

94. Cannon SC. Pathomechanisms in channelopathies of skeletal muscle and brain. *Annual review of neuroscience*. 2006;29:387–415.

95. Fialho D, Schorge S, Pucovska U, et al. Chloride channel myotonia: exon 8 hot-spot for dominant-negative interactions. *Brain: a journal of neurology*. 2007;130(Pt 12):3265–3274.

96. Lehmann-Horn F, Rudel R. Channelopathies: the nondystrophic myotonias and periodic paralyses. *Seminars in pediatric neurology*. 1996;3(2):122–139.

97. Hoffman EP, Wang J. Duchenne-Becker muscular dystrophy and the nondystrophic myotonias. Paradigms for loss of function and change of function of gene products. *Archives of neurology*. 1993;50(11):1227–1237.

98. Sun C, Tranebjaerg L, Torbergsen T, Holmgren G, Van Ghelue M. Spectrum of CLCN1 mutations in patients with myotonia congenita in Northern Scandinavia. *European journal of human genetics: EJHG*. 2001;9(12):903–909.

99. Koch MC, Steinmeyer K, Lorenz C, et al. The skeletal muscle chloride channel in dominant and recessive human myotonia. *Science*. 1992;257(5071):797–800.

100. George AL, Jr., Crackower MA, Abdalla JA, Hudson AJ, Ebers GC. Molecular basis of Thomsen's disease (autosomal dominant myotonia congenita). *Nature genetics*. 1993;3(4):305–310.

101. Raja Rayan DL, Haworth A, Sud R, et al. A new explanation for recessive myotonia congenita: exon deletions and duplications in CLCN1. *Neurology*. 2012;78(24):1953–1958.

102. Thomsen J. Tonische Krampfe in willkurlich beweglichen Muskeln in Folge von ererbter psychischer Disposition. *Arch Psychiatr Nervenkrankheiten*. 1876;6(702–718).

103. Crews J, Kaiser KK, Brooke MH. Muscle pathology of myotonia congenita. *Journal of the neurological sciences*. 1976;28(4):449–457.

104. Gutmann L, Phillips LH2nd. Myotonia congenita. *Semin Neurol*. 1991;11:244–248.

105. Lehmann-Horn F, Rüdel R, Jurkat-Rott K: Nondystrophic Myotonias and Periodic Paralyses. In Engel AG, franzini-Armstrong C (eds). *Myology*. McGraw-Hill, New York; 2004, pp 1261–1262.

106. Sun SF, Streib EW. Autosomal recessive generalized myotonia. *Muscle & nerve*. 1983;6(2):143–148.

107. Trip J, Drost G, Ginjaar HB, et al. Redefining the clinical phenotypes of non-dystrophic myotonic syndromes. *Journal of neurology, neurosurgery, and psychiatry*. 2009;80(6):647–652.

108. Wagner S, Deymeer F, Kurz LL, et al. The dominant chloride channel mutant G200R causing fluctuating myotonia: clinical findings, electrophysiology, and channel pathology. *Muscle & nerve*. 1998;21(9):1122–1128.

109. Lehmann-Horn F, Mailander V, Heine R, George AL. Myotonia levior is a chloride channel disorder. *Human molecular genetics*. 1995;4(8):1397–1402.

110. Cummins TR, Zhou J, Sigworth FJ, et al. Functional consequences of a Na+ channel mutation causing hyperkalemic periodic paralysis. *Neuron*. 1993;10(4):667–678.

111. Trivedi JR, Bundy B, Statland J, et al. Non-dystrophic myotonia: prospective study of objective and patient

reported outcomes. *Brain: a journal of neurology.* 2013;136(Pt 7):2189–2200.

112. Heatwole CR, Statland JM, Logigian EL. The diagnosis and treatment of myotonic disorders. *Muscle & nerve.* 2013;47(5):632–648.

113. Streib EW. Paramyotonia congenita. *Semin Neurol.* 1991;11(3):249–257.

114. Shapiro B, Ruff, R: Disorders of skeletal muscle membrane excitability myotonia congenita, paramyotonia congenita, periodic paralysis and related disorders. In Katirji B, Kaminski H, Preston D, Ruff R, Shapiro B (eds): Neuromuscular disorders in clinical practice. Butterworth-Heinemann, 2002, pp 987–1020.

115. Ricker K, Lehmann-Horn F, Moxley RT, 3rd. Myotonia fluctuans. *Archives of neurology.* 1990;47(3): 268–272.

116. Ricker K, Moxley RT, 3rd, Heine R, Lehmann-Horn F. Myotonia fluctuans. A third type of muscle sodium channel disease. *Archives of neurology.* 1994;51(11):1095–1102.

117. Rudel R, Ricker K, Lehmann-Horn F. Genotype-phenotype correlations in human skeletal muscle sodium channel diseases. *Archives of neurology.* 1993;50(11):1241–1248.

118. Lehmann-Horn F, Rudel R. Hereditary nondystrophic myotonias and periodic paralyses. *Current opinion in neurology.* 1995;8(5):402–410.

119. Colding-Jorgensen E, Duno M, Vissing J. Autosomal dominant monosymptomatic myotonia permanens. *Neurology.* 2006;67(1):153–155.

120. Fu YH, Pizzuti A, Fenwick RG, Jr., et al. An unstable triplet repeat in a gene related to myotonic muscular dystrophy. *Science.* 1992;255(5049):1256–1258.

121. Brook JD, McCurrach ME, Harley HG, et al. Molecular basis of myotonic dystrophy: expansion of a trinucleotide (CTG) repeat at the 3' end of a transcript encoding a protein kinase family member. *Cell.* 1992;69(2):385.

122. Liquori CL, Ricker K, Moseley ML, et al. Myotonic dystrophy type 2 caused by a CCTG expansion in intron 1 of ZNF9. *Science.* 2001;293(5531):864–867.

123. Pusch M. Myotonia caused by mutations in the muscle chloride channel gene CLCN1. *Human mutation.* 2002;19(4):423–434.

124. Ptacek LJ, Tawil R, Griggs RC, et al. Sodium channel mutations in acetazolamide-responsive myotonia congenita, paramyotonia congenita, and hyperkalemic periodic paralysis. *Neurology.* 1994;44(8):1500–1503.

125. Lerche H, Heine R, Pika U, et al. Human sodium channel myotonia: slowed channel inactivation due to substitutions for a glycine within the III-IV linker. *The journal of physiology.* 1993;470:13–22.

126. Mankodi A, Takahashi MP, Jiang H, et al. Expanded CUG repeats trigger aberrant splicing of ClC-1 chloride channel pre-mRNA and hyperexcitability of skeletal muscle in myotonic dystrophy. *Molecular cell.* 2002;10(1):35–44.

127. Wheeler TM, Thornton CA. Myotonic dystrophy: RNA-mediated muscle disease. *Current opinion in neurology.* 2007;20(5):572–576.

128. Bryant SH. Cable properties of external intercostal muscle fibres from myotonic and nonmyotonic goats. *The journal of physiology.* 1969;204(3):539–550.

129. Lipicky RJ, Bryant SH. Sodium, potassium, and chloride fluxes in intercostal muscle from normal goats and goats with hereditary myotonia. *The journal of general physiology.* 1966;50(1):89–111.

130. Bryant SH, Morales-Aguilera A. Chloride conductance in normal and myotonic muscle fibres and the action of monocarboxylic aromatic acids. *The journal of physiology.* 1971;219(2):367–383.

131. Hodgkin AL, Horowicz P. The influence of potassium and chloride ions on the membrane potential of single muscle fibres. *The journal of physiology.* 1959;148:127–160.

132. Adrian RH, Bryant SH. On the repetitive discharge in myotonic muscle fibres. *The journal of physiology.* 1974;240(2):505–515.

133. Ontell M, Paul HS, Adibi SA, Martin JL. Involvement of transverse tubules in induced myotonia. *Journal of neuropathology and experimental neurology.* 1979;38(6):596–605.

134. Kwiecinski H, Lehmann-Horn F, Rudel R. Drug-induced myotonia in human intercostal muscle. *Muscle & nerve.* 1988;11(6):576–581.

135. Durelli L, Mutani R, Fassio F, Delsedime M. The effects of the increase of arterial potassium upon the excitability of normal and dystrophic myotonic muscles in man. *Journal of the neurological sciences.* 1982;55(3):249–257.

136. Adrian RH, Marshall MW. Action potentials reconstructed in normal and myotonic muscle fibres. *The journal of physiology.* 1976;258(1):125–143.

137. Ricker K, Hertel G, Langscheid K, Stodieck G. Myotonia not aggravated by cooling. Force and relaxation of the adductor pollicis in normal subjects and in myotonia as compared to paramyotonia. *Journal of neurology.* 1977;216(1):9–20.

138. Richmond JE, VanDeCarr D, Featherstone DE, George AL, Jr., Ruben PC. Defective fast inactivation recovery and deactivation account for sodium channel myotonia in the I1160V mutant. *Biophysical journal.* 1997;73(4):1896–1903.

139. Cannon SC, Brown RH, Jr., Corey DP. Theoretical reconstruction of myotonia and paralysis caused by incomplete inactivation of sodium channels. *Biophysical journal.* 1993;65(1):270–288.

140. Yang N, Ji S, Zhou M, et al. Sodium channel mutations in paramyotonia congenita exhibit similar biophysical phenotypes in vitro. *Proceedings of the National Academy of Sciences of the United States of America.* 1994;91(26):12785–12789.

141. Mitrovic N, George AL, Jr., Heine R, et al. K(+)-aggravated myotonia: destabilization of the inactivated state of the human muscle Na+ channel by the V1589M mutation. *The journal of physiology.* 1994;478 Pt 3:395–402.

142. Ruff RL. Slow Na+ channel inactivation must be disrupted to evoke prolonged depolarization-induced paralysis. *Biophysical journal.* 1994;66(2 Pt 1):542.

143. Hayward LJ, Brown RH, Jr., Cannon SC. Slow inactivation differs among mutant Na channels associated with myotonia and periodic paralysis. *Biophysical journal.* 1997;72(3):1204–1219.

144. Ruff RL. Effects of temperature on slow and fast inactivation of rat skeletal muscle Na(+) channels. *The American journal of physiology.* 1999;277(5 Pt 1):C937–C947.

145. Thiel RE. The myotonic response to suxamethonium. *British journal of anaesthesia.* 1967;39(10):815–821.

146. Harper PS: Myotonic Dystrophy. WB Saunders. Philadelphia. 1979, pp 54–69.

147. Ay B, Gercek A, Dogan VI, Kiyan G, Gogus YF. Pyloromyotomy in a patient with paramyotonia congenita. *Anesthesia and analgesia*. 2004;98(1): 68–69.

148. Kaneda T, Iwahashi M, Suzuki T. Anesthetic management for subtotal gastrectomy in a patient with paramyotonia congenita. *Journal of anesthesia*. 2007;21(4):500–503.

149. Bouly A, Nathan N, Feiss P. Propofol in myotonic dystrophy. *Anaesthesia*. 1991;46(8):705.

150. Kinney MA, Harrison BA. Propofol-induced myotonia in myotonic dystrophy. *Anesthesia and analgesia*. 1996;83(3):665–666.

151. Johnson GW, Chadwick S, Eadsforth P, Hartopp I. Anaesthesia and myotonia. *British journal of anaesthesia*. 1995;75(1):113.

152. Gronert GA. Myotonias and masseter spasm: not malignant hyperthermia? *Anesthesiology*. 1995;83(6): 1382–1383.

153. Haberer JP, Fabre F, Rose E. Malignant hyperthermia and myotonia congenita (Thomsen's disease). *Anaesthesia*. 1989;44(2):166.

154. Grace RF, Roach VJ. Caesarean section in a patient with paramyotonia congenita. *Anaesthesia and intensive care*. 1999;27(5):534–537.

155. Howell PR, Douglas MJ. Lupus anticoagulant, paramyotonia congenita and pregnancy. *Canadian journal of anaesthesia*. 1992;39(9):992–996.

156. Bandschapp O, Iaizzo PA. Pathophysiologic and anesthetic considerations for patients with myotonia congenita or periodic paralyses. *Paediatric anaesthesia*. 2013;23(9):824–833.

157. Griggs RC, Moxley RT, 3rd, Riggs JE, Engel WK. Effects of acetazolamide on myotonia. *Annals of neurology*. 1978;3(6):531–537.

158. Lehmann-Horn F, Jurkat-Rott K. Voltage-gated ion channels and hereditary disease. *Physiological reviews*. 1999;79(4):1317–1372.

159. Desaphy JF, De Luca A, Tortorella P, De Vito D, George AL, Jr., Conte Camerino D. Gating of myotonic Na channel mutants defines the response to mexiletine and a potent derivative. *Neurology*. 2001;57(10): 1849–1857.

160. Mohammadi B, Jurkat-Rott K, Alekov A, Dengler R, Bufler J, Lehmann-Horn F. Preferred mexiletine block of human sodium channels with IVS4 mutations and its pH-dependence. *Pharmacogenetics and genomics*. 2005;15(4):235–244.

161. Wang GK, Russell C, Wang SY. Mexiletine block of wild-type and inactivation-deficient human skeletal muscle hNav1.4 Na$^+$ channels. *The Journal of physiology*. 2004;554(Pt 3):621–633.

162. Statland JM, Bundy BN, Wang Y, et al. Mexiletine for symptoms and signs of myotonia in nondystrophic myotonia: a randomized controlled trial. *JAMA: the journal of the American Medical Association*. 2012; 308(13):1357–1365.

163. Logigian EL, Martens WB, Moxley RTt, et al. Mexiletine is an effective antimyotonia treatment in myotonic dystrophy type 1. *Neurology*. 2010;74(18): 1441–1448.

164. Cleland JC, Griggs RC. Treatment of neuromuscular channelopathies: current concepts and future prospects. *Neurotherapeutics: the journal of the American Society for Experimental NeuroTherapeutics*. 2008; 5(4):607–612.

165. Eguchi H, Tsujino A, Kaibara M, et al. Acetazolamide acts directly on the human skeletal muscle chloride channel. *Muscle & nerve*. 2006;34(3):292–297.

166. Riggs JE, Griggs RC, Moxley RT. Acetazolamide-induced weakness in paramyotonia congenita. *Annals of internal medicine*. 1977;86(2):169–173.

Chapter 10

Inflammatory Myopathies

Anthony A. Amato
Andrew Mammen

DERMATOMYOSITIS, POLYMYOSITIS, IMMUNE-MEDIATED NECROTIZING MYOPATHY, AND INCLUSION BODY MYOSITIS

Introduction

The inflammatory myopathies are a group of acquired skeletal muscle diseases that include dermatomyositis (DMS), polymyositis (PM), immune-mediated necrotizing myopathy (IMNM), and inclusion body myositis (IBM).[1-5] Although these disorders share the common feature of muscle weakness, they each have distinct clinical features and underlying pathophysiological mechanisms. For example, PM, DMS, and IMNM present with subacute proximal muscle weakness, may involve other organ systems, and are widely accepted to be autoimmune diseases that respond to immunosuppression. In contrast, IBM patients develop insidiously progressive distal and proximal muscle weakness, rarely have significant manifestations outside of skeletal muscle, and do not respond well, if at all, to immunosuppressive therapies.

Historical Perspective

Wagner documented the first case of myositis associated with dermatologic findings in 1863.[6] In 1887, Hans Unverricht reported a similar case with rash, pulmonary involvement, and inflammatory muscle pathology at autopsy[7]; he subsequently coined the term *dermatomyositis* after describing a second case of an inflammatory myopathy with associated skin lesions.[8] Hepp probably reported the first case of PM in 1887 when he described a case of myositis presenting without concomitant skin involvement.[9] Subsequent work by Eaton,[10] Walton and Adams,[11] Rowland,[12] and Pearson and Rose[13] further clarified the clinical and pathologic features of the autoimmune myopathies. In their landmark studies of 1975, Bohan and Peter published diagnostic criteria for DMS and PM that are still widely used today.[1,2]

Whereas most patients with a clinical diagnosis of PM have prominent cellular infiltrates on muscle biopsy, some patients with other characteristic features of PM (e.g., proximal muscle weakness, elevated muscle enzymes, irritable myopathy on electromyography, and response to immunosuppression) have prominent myofiber necrosis with a relative paucity of inflammatory cells. In 2002, Miller and colleagues systematically described seven such patients with autoimmune muscle disease and autoantibodies recognizing the signal recognition particle (SRP); these subjects had necrotizing myopathies without prominent inflammation on biopsy.[14] Similarly, patients with autoimmune myopathy and autoantibodies recognizing HMG-CoA reductase (HMGCR) typically have muscle biopsies with little inflammation, but prominent myofiber necrosis.[15,16] Given its histopathological features and association with specific autoantibodies, IMNM is now considered to be a distinct category of autoimmune myopathy.[17,18]

In 1967, Chou described an elderly male patient with "chronic polymyositis" who had dysphagia, prominent quadriceps weakness, and muscle biopsies revealing intracytoplasmic aggregates of filamentous structures. The term *inclusion body myositis* was first used to

desc... findin... recogn... logicall... and col... that are s...

Section 2: Specific Myopath...

256

Clinical Features

Patients with DMS... cally develop s... greater tha... of weeks... ing f...

Epidemio...

Until recentl... ies utilized re... defined the an... ...am-matory myopath... ...i the range of 0.1 to 1.0 pe... ...person years.[4,19-23] A more recent analysis including millions of US patients indicates that the incidence of inflammatory myopathies may be in excess of 4 cases per 100,000 person years.[24] The largest and most recent studies suggest that the overall prevalence of inflammatory myopathies is in the range of 14 to 32 per 100,000.[24,25]

PM and DMS occur more frequently in women than in men (2:1). Whereas PM occurs almost exclusively in those over the age of 18, DMS may occur in children aged 5 to 15 years and also peaks in those from 45 to 65 years of age.[23] IBM more frequently afflicts men (3:1), who typically present with weakness after the age of 50 years.

The observation that identical twins have a low concordance for inflammatory myopathy (in the 25%–40% range) suggests that environmental exposures trigger disease in genetically susceptible individuals.[23] To date, several environmental exposures have been linked to developing specific forms of autoimmune myopathy. In DMS, for example, convincing evidence indicates that ultraviolet light exposure is associated with disease, with the relative prevalence of DMS compared to PM increasing significantly with geographic latitude.[26] The association of latitude on the development of DMS may be especially strong in women.[27] Similarly, statin exposure is linked to the development of IMNM[15,28,29] and these patients typically have antibodies recognizing HMGCR, the pharmacologic target of statin medications.[16] Last, seasonal patterns of inflammatory myopathy onset suggest that other environmental factors, perhaps infectious in nature, may trigger these autoimmune diseases.[30,31]

, PM, and IMNM typi-
nmetric weakness, proximal
distal, developing over a period
or months. Progressive difficulty ris-
om a chair, ascending steps, and wash-
g one's hair are typical complaints. Scapular
winging is uncommon in autoimmune myopathies, but occurs with some regularity in subjects with IMNM associated with anti-SRP
antibodies.[32] Many subjects also experience
some degree of muscle pain. In severe cases,
subjects may require mechanical ventilation
due to diaphragmatic weakness or placement
of a feeding tube due to dysphagia. In contrast,
the extraocular muscles are spared in subjects
with autoimmune myopathy, even in those with
severe disease.

The tempo and pattern of weakness in subjects with IBM is distinct from that seen in
the other forms of inflammatory myopathy.
The onset is often insidious and progresses
relatively slowly over years. In the upper
extremities, muscles of the forearm flexor compartment are usually most severely affected,
with subsequent weakness of the wrist flexors
and deep finger flexors. Patients may complain
of difficulty opening jars or pulling a trigger.
Although triceps weakness is common, the deltoids and biceps are relatively spared.

In the lower extremities, IBM patients usually have hip flexor weakness, but this may be
overshadowed by selective involvement of the
quadriceps. Patients may experience sudden
falls, with their "knees giving out" while going
down stairs. To compensate for weak quadriceps, patients may walk with locked knees and
hyperextend at this joint with each step. Ankle
dorsiflexion weakness is frequently observed
and, in some cases of IBM, foot drop may be
the initial complaint. Importantly, patients
with IBM often have an asymmetric pattern
of muscle weakness. On careful examination,
weakness of eye closure may be noted even
during the early stages of IBM; this would be
very atypical for patients with DMS, PM, or
IMNM. Dysphagia is another common symptom in IBM and may even be the presenting
manifestation of the disease. It should be noted
that in the more advanced stages of IBM, other
muscle groups, such as the biceps, wrist extensors, and hamstrings, may become involved
as well.

Characteristic dermatologic features usually distinguish subjects with DMS from those
with other forms of inflammatory myopathy.
Two of these, Gottron's papules and the heliotrope rash, are pathognomonic signs of DMS.
Gottron's papules are erythematous lesions
over the extensor surfaces of the metacarpo-
phalangeal, proximal interphalangeal, and/or
distal interphalangeal joints, usually sparing
the spaces in between (Figure 10–1A). The
heliotrope rash is violaceous eruption over
the upper eyelids and may be accompanied by
periorbital edema. In patients with dark skin,
the heliotrope rash may present as hyperpig-
mented lesions in the same location.

DMS patients often have other signs of skin
disease. These include nailfold involvement
with enlarged capillaries, capillary dropout,
and capillary hemorrhage. These pathologic
features, best seen with nailfold capillaroscopy, are also found in patients with scleroderma and other rheumatic diseases.[33] Regions
of hypo- and hyperpigmentation, atrophy,
and telangectasias (e.g., poikiloderma) may
develop on the chest and shoulders. A malar
rash, consisting of erythema over the cheeks
may also be seen in DMS. A similar rash,
when observed on the outer thigh, has been
termed the "holster sign." DMS patients may
have palmar erythema (Figure 10–1B) and/
or hyperkeratotic lesions on the radial surfaces of the fingers known as "mechanic's
hands" (Figure 10–1C). "Mechanic's feet" are
also occasionally appreciated on examination
(Figure 10–1D).

The rash of DMS may precede of follow the
development of muscle weakness. Interestingly,
some patients with typical skin manifestations of DMS never develop overt evidence of
muscle disease. Such patients are said to have
"dermatomyositis sine myositis" or "amyopathic
dermatomyositis." Similarly, some patients
with characteristic DMS muscle biopsy features (see Diagnostic Studies section) never
develop the dermatologic manifestations of the
disease. Frequently misdiagnosed as having
PM, such patients would more appropriately
be designated as having "dermatomyositis sine
dermatitis."

DMS and PM are systemic autoimmune diseases that frequently affect multiple organ systems in addition to muscle and skin. Arthritis,
Raynaud phenomenon, fever, and interstitial lung disease (ILD) may be present and

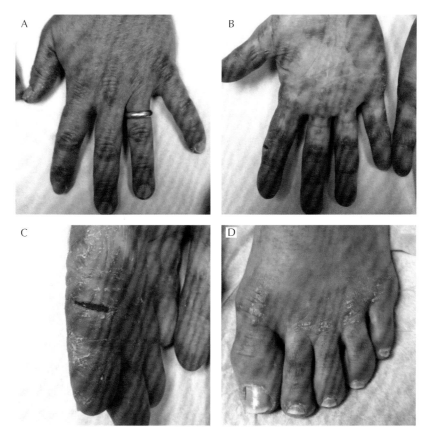

Figure 10–1. Skin manifestations of dermatomyositis. Patients with DM may have Gottron's sign (A), palmar erythema (B), mechanic's hands (C), and/or mechanic's feet (D).

frequently occur together in patients with antibodies recognizing one of the tRNA- synthetases as part of the antisynthetase syndrome[34,35] (see Diagnostic Studies section). Among these, ILD may be the most severe, and often life-threatening, aspect of the disease process. Serious cardiac involvement has been reported in PM and DMS, but is a relatively rare feature of these diseases. In contrast, several reports emphasize more frequent heart involvement in subjects with IMNM associated with anti-SRP autoantibodies.[36-38] In IBM, there may be an increased incidence of length-dependent sensory polyneuropathy.[39-46] Furthermore, in some cases, inflammatory myopathy may be associated with an overlapping rheumatologic condition. For example, lupus, rheumatoid arthritis, or scleroderma may coexist with PM or DMS. Similarly, Sjögren's syndrome is occasionally diagnosed in those with one of the inflammatory myopathies, including IBM.[47]

Numerous studies have demonstrated an increased frequency of malignancy in patients with some forms of inflammatory myopathy. Compared to others in the population, those with PM and DMS have standardized incidence ratios for cancer in the range of 1.3 to 2.0 (PM) and 3.0 to 6.2 (DMS).[48,49] Whereas a variety of cancers are associated with PM and DMS, adenocarcinomas account for approximately 70%. Cancers are detected within the year prior to or after the development of muscle disease, but DMS patients are at an increased risk of malignancy for up to five years after the skin and or muscle disease becomes apparent.[48] In contrast to those with DMS and PM, there does not appear to be a substantially increased risk of cancer in those with IBM. It is currently unclear whether those with IMNM also have an increase risk of malignancy; these patients may have been included in the PM group in prior analyses.

Differential Diagnosis

Patients with DMS usually present to the clinic with progressive symmetric proximal muscle weakness and a characteristic rash that makes diagnoses straightforward. However, in those who present with subacute symmetric proximal muscle weakness without a rash (including those who have dermatomyositis sine dermatitis) the differential is broad. In addition to autoimmune myopathies, other acquired and inherited causes of proximal muscle weakness must be considered.

Medication toxicity is a relatively common cause of acquired myopathy. Among the many medications with myotoxic potential, statin medications are the most widely prescribed. Although up to 10% of patients may have muscle pain or subjective weakness, a significantly smaller number have CK elevations or muscle weakness or both on exam.[50] While statin-associated muscle weakness may rarely be due to an immune-mediated process (see Pathogenesis and Genetics section) most patients will improve over weeks or months once the statin is discontinued. Similarly, myopathies associated with high-dose steroids, amiodarone, colchicine, AZT, and other potential myotoxins will improve once the offending medication is stopped.

Disturbances of the endocrine system may also cause progressive muscle weakness. In Cushing's disease this is typically associated with normal muscle enzymes and muscle biopsies with type 2 fiber atrophy. In contrast, patients with severe hypothyroidism can present with elevated muscle enzymes and a necrotizing muscle biopsy. In addition to the TSH, checking a serum T4 should also be considered because TSH may be normal in cases of central hypothyroidism.

Although many patients with hereditary myopathies are aware of long-standing weakness, some subjects only notice this upon reaching a "tipping point." For example, a patient may become aware of weakness only when they begin to experience falls. Thus, some subjects with inherited myopathy but no significant family history may initially appear to have PM based on their history. In particular, LGMDs, adult-onset Pompe disease, and proximal myotonic myopathy (i.e., DM2) are not infrequently misdiagnosed as PM because these patients may present with late-onset symmetric proximal muscle weakness. Confusion is especially likely when the patient with muscular dystrophy has inflammation on muscle biopsy, as may be seen in those with facioscapulohumeral dystrophy and dysferlinopathy. However, in many cases, the physical exam will reveal distal weakness, scapular winging, calf hypertrophy, clinical or electrophysiologic myotonia/paramyotonia, and/or other helpful features that are typical for certain inherited muscle diseases, but exceedingly uncommon in PM.

The differential diagnosis for IBM includes adult-onset hereditary myopathies presenting with selective weakness of the quadriceps, such as LGMD type 2L. In patients with distal and/or proximal muscle weakness and a muscle biopsy demonstrating rimmed vacuoles, hereditary forms of inclusion body myopathy such as those involving the genes for UDP-N-acetylglucosamine 2-epimerase/N-acetylmannosamine kinase (GNE) or valosin-containing protein (VCP) should be included in the differential. Generally, the hereditary muscle diseases that might be confused with IBM do not typically have inflammatory muscle biopsies. Moreover, these patients often have a pattern of muscle involvement that sets them apart from those with IBM. For example, patients with GNE mutations typically have early, selective weakness of the anterior tibial muscles with relative sparing of the quadriceps. However, patients with VCP mutations may have proximal, distal, or generalized weakness that can mimic IBM.

Because it presents in adulthood with weakness and an inflammatory muscle biopsy that may not include characteristic rimmed vacuoles,[51,52] IBM is frequently misdiagnosed as PM. However, the presence of distal asymmetric weakness in this context should suggest a diagnosis of IBM rather than PM. Making this distinction is of importance because the former rarely, if ever, responds to immunosuppressive therapy.

Diagnostic Studies

On needle exam, patients with an inflammatory myopathy typically have fibrillation potentials, positive sharp waves, and small polyphasic motor units with early recruitment, features that define an irritable myopathy. In patients with IBM, these features may be most prominent in distal muscle groups, such as those of the forearm flexor compartment. It should be noted that some patients with DMS have a nonirritable myopathy due to a lack of the segmental muscle fiber necrosis, which probably underlies spontaneous muscle activity in the inflammatory myopathies. Furthermore, spontaneous discharges may be absent in those who have undergone prior treatment with immunosuppressive agents.

Skeletal muscle MRI reveals areas of active muscle involvement as T2 hyperintensities. In contrast, fatty replacement of muscle tissue is visualized as hyperintense on T1-weighted imaging. Although specific diagnoses cannot usually be made using MRI, some patterns are suggestive of certain conditions[53] (Figure 10–2). For example, fasciitis may be seen as a rim of T2 hyperintensity surrounding a particular muscle and is most commonly seen in DMS (Figure 10–2D). Similarly, selective atrophy, fatty replacement, and edema within the vastus lateralis and medialis muscles with relative sparing of the rectus femoris muscle is characteristic of IBM (Figures 10–2E & 2F).

Serum muscle enzyme levels are elevated in about 80% of patients with autoimmune myopathy.[2,54] However, approximately 20% to 30% of DMS patients may have normal muscle enzymes. Furthermore, muscle enzymes may be normal or only modestly elevated in some patients with IBM, particularly as the disease advances. The most sensitive and specific

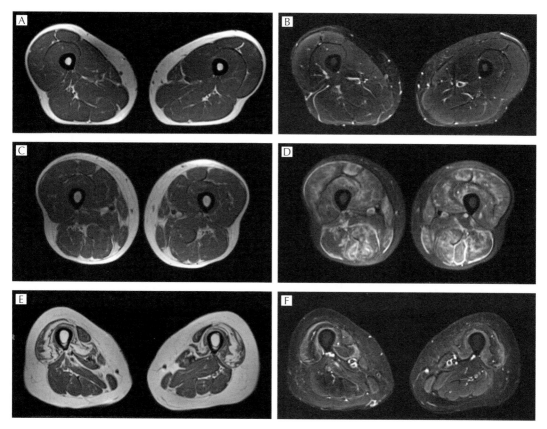

Figure 10–2. Magnetic resonance imaging. A normal subject (A & B), dermatomyositis patient (C & D), and inclusion body myositis patient (E & F) underwent bilateral thigh MRI with T1 (A, C, & D) and STIR (B, C, & D) sequences. The dermatomyositis patient has no fatty replacement (C), but does have significant edema and fasciitis (D). The inclusion body myositis patient has fatty replacement (E) and edema (F) preferentially in the anterior compartment with relative sparing of the rectus femoris.

marker of muscle damage may be the serum CK level. However, some patients with auto-immune myopathy present with normal CK levels and an elevated serum aldolase level.[55] Patients with this laboratory profile tend to have muscle pain, arthralgias, and ILD, but may not have overt weakness on physical exam despite pathology on muscle biopsy.[56] Because both CK and aldolase are found within mature muscle cells, but aldolase is expressed first during muscle fiber regeneration, it has been proposed that the immune response may selectively target regenerating muscle fibers in subjects with isolated aldolase elevations.[57]

In the inflammatory myopathies, the presence of autoantibodies may be diagnostically and prognostically useful as they are associated with distinct clinical phenotypes (Table 10–1). For example, patients with antibodies recognizing one of the aminoacyl tRNA synthetases (e.g., Jo-1) usually have "antisynthetase syndrome." In addition to PM or DMS, those with antisynthetase syndrome usually present with one or more of the following: interstitial lung disease, arthritis, fevers, and hyperkeratotic lesions with a predilection for radial surfaces of the fingers known as "mechanic's hands."

The majority of DMS patients have one of several DMS-specific autoantibodies. Antibodies recognizing the chromatin remodeling enzyme Mi-2 tend to have severe skin disease, but a favorable response to treatment and a low risk of cancer.[38,58-61] Patients with antibodies against MDA5 typically have a predominantly dermatopulmonary phenotype with absent or mild muscle disease, rapidly progressive lung disease, and characteristic cutaneous features including palmar papules.[62-66] Importantly, antibodies recognizing transcription intermediary factor 1γ (TIF1γ) are highly associated with malignancy.[67,68] A recent meta-analysis demonstrated that these antibodies have an 89% sensitivity and 78% specificity for diagnosing cancer-associated DMS.[69]

Table 10–1 Autoantibodies associated with inflammatory myopathies

Antisynthetase Autoantibodies	Autoantigen	Clinical Features
Anti-Jo-1	Histidyl t-RNA synthetase	PM, DMS + ILD
Anti-PL-7	Threonyl t-RNA synthetase	PM, DMS + ILD
Anti-PL-12	Alanyl t-RNA synthetase	ILD > myopathy
Anti-EJ	Glycyl t-RNA synthetase	PM > DMS + ILD
Anti-OJ	Isoleucylt-RNA synthetase	ILD + PM/DMS
Anti-KS	Asparaginyl t-RNA synthetase	ILD > myopathy
Anti-Zo	Phenylalanyl t-RNA synthetase	ILD + myopathy
Anti-Ha	Tyrosyl t-RNA synthetase	ILD + myopathy
Dermatomyositis Autoantibodies		
Anti-Mi-2	Chromatin remodeling enzyme	Severe skin disease Treatment responsive
Anti-MDA5	Melanoma differentiation-associated gene 5	ILD Palmar lesions Rash > myopathy
Anti-TIF1γ	transcriptional intermediary factor 1γ	Cancer-associated dermatomyositis
Anti-NXP-2	nuclear matrix protein	severe muscle weakness
Anti-SAE	small ubiquitin-like modifier-activating enzyme	rapidly progressive ILD rash>myopathy
IMNM Autoantibiodies		
Anti-SRP	SRP	severe, treatment-resistant myopathy cardiac involvement
Anti-HMGCR	HMGCR	statin-associated myopathy
Inclusion body myositis Autoantibody		
Anti-cN1A / anti-Mup44	cytosolic 5'-nucleotidase	Inclusion body myositis

Note. PM = polymyositis, DMS = dermatomyositis, ILD = interstitial lung disease, SRP = signal recognition particle, HMGCR = HMG-CoA reductase, CN1A = cytosolic 5'-nucleotidase

Antibodies recognizing SRP are preferentially found in patients with a rapidly progressive form of IMNM.[14,36-38,70-72] Similarly, anti-HMGCR antibodies are found in patients with statin-triggered IMNM[15,16] but are not found in those with self-limited statin intolerance.[73] Consequently, anti-HMGCR antibodies define another group of patients with myopathy, usually IMNM, who will benefit from immunosuppressive therapy. Note that not all patients with IMNM have either anti-SRP or anti-HMGCR antibodies.

Although IBM is typically refractory to immunosuppressive treatment, the presence of plasma cells[74] and ectopic lymphoid structures in muscle biopsies from these patients suggest the possibility that B cells may play a role in disease pathogenesis. Indeed, recent reports demonstrated that more than half of IBM patients have an autoantibody directed against cytosolic 5'-nucleotidase 1A.[75,76] The presence of this IBM-specific autoantibody is also very specific for IBM may be particularly useful in diagnosing IBM patients early in the course of disease or in those with atypical patterns of weakness.

The muscle biopsy plays an important role in the diagnosis of inflammatory myopathies. In DMS, a predominantly perifascicular distribution of atrophic, degenerating, and regenerating myofibers is pathognomonic for this disease (Figure 10–3A). Similarly, staining for type 1 interferon–inducible proteins including major histocompatibility complex I (MHC-I) may reveal sarcolemmal expression around the edges of fascicles even before there is atrophy. The degree of inflammation varies in DMS, but preferentially localizes to perivascular regions. Where available, staining for CD4 may suggest that many infiltrating cells are helper T cells.[77] However, more recent studies suggest these cells are plasmacytoid dendritic cells[78] (see Pathogenesis and Genetics section). Deposition of the C5b-9 membrane attack complex may be observed on endothelial cells, and capillary dropout may also occur early in the course of disease.[79-81]

It is well accepted that the presence of inflammatory cells surrounding and invading normal-appearing myofibers (i.e., primary inflammation) is a characteristic feature of PM muscle biopsies (Figure 10–3B). Staining for CD8 demonstrates that these are predominantly cytolytic T cells.[77,82,83] Similarly,

most authors agree that s
expression, absent on r
is uniformly upregulat
some authors emphasi.
expression is not absolutely
mune myopathies and may be see.
ditions such as dysferlinopathy.[84] No..
MHC-I expression can be helpful in suppo.
a diagnosis of polymyositis.[85] Although specific for PM, the combined finding of CD8-positive T cells infiltrating MHC-I–expressing myofibers may lack sensitivity for diagnosing this condition.[86]

The characteristic muscle biopsy feature in patients with IMNM is myofiber necrosis with only sparse inflammatory cell infiltrates and the absence of primary inflammation or perifascicular atrophy[17] (Figure 10–3C). Anti-SRP-associated myopathy is the prototypical IMNM. Biopsies from anti-SRP–positive subjects are also characterized by a reduced number of capillaries, enlarged capillaries, and complement deposition on the remaining capillaries.[14,37] Muscle biopsies from those with autoimmune myopathy triggered by statin also have typical features of an IMNM.[29] Indeed, approximately 80% of patients with anti-HMGCR antibodies have an IMNM with little or no inflammation.[16] In contrast to those with anti-SRP, muscle biopsies from anti-HMGCR subjects reveal complement deposition on undamaged myofibers and medium-sized blood vessels.[15] It should be noted that features of IMNM can be found in those with other forms of autoimmune myopathy in the absence of anti-SRP or anti-HMGCR antibodies. For example, some patients with antisynthetase antibodies have muscle biopsies with minimal inflammation and with necrosis as the predominant pathologic feature.[15]

As in PM, muscle biopsies from patients with IBM usually demonstrate CD8-positive T cells surrounding and invading nonnecrotic muscle fibers.[3] An increase in the number of fibers with evidence of mitochondrial dysfunction, such as the presence of RRF and COX fibers, is also frequently observed in IBM[87]. By visualizing Congo red staining under polarized light or using fluorescence techniques, amyloid deposition may be observed in muscle fibers, sometimes within nuclei.[88,89] Last, many patients with IBM have rimmed vacuoles lined with granular material[3,41] (Figure 10–3D). However, because 20% to 30% of patients with clinical features of IBM do not have rimmed

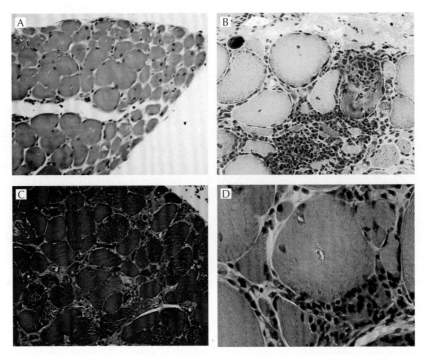

Figure 10–3. Typical inflammatory myopathy muscle biopsies. The hallmark histologic feature of muscle biopsies from DM patients is perifascicular atrophy (A). Patients with a histologic diagnosis of PM have muscle biopsies revealing myofibers surrounded and invaded by lymphocytes (B). Abundant necrosis with little or no lymphocytic infiltration is typical of IMNM (C). Patients with IBM have primary inflammation and, often, rimmed vacuoles on muscle biopsy (D).

vacuoles on muscle biopsy,[51,52] the absence of this feature cannot reliably be used to rule out a diagnosis of IBM.

Pathogenesis and Genetics

The pathogenic mechanisms underlying DMS are poorly understood. In general, it is thought that certain immunogenetic factors render individuals either more or less susceptible to developing the disease.[90] For example, in Caucasian patients, the immunoglobulin gamma heavy-chain Gm 3 23 5,13 polymorphism is associated with DMS.[91] Similarly, certain HLA alleles associated with the 8.1 ancestral haplotype render subjects more or less vulnerable to developing this disease.[92,93] Of note, DMS is also associated with the -308A polymorphism in the tumor necrosis factor (TNF) gene promoter.[94-100] In lupus, this polymorphism is thought to increase vulnerability to skin damage by increasing TNF-α production and thereby triggering keratinocyte apoptosis in response to UV-light exposure.[101] It

has been hypothesized to play a similar role in mediating the sun sensitivity seen in some DMS patients.[96]

Other clues about disease mechanisms in DMS have been obtained by careful study of affected tissues. For example, based on the presence of membrane attack complex (MAC) on blood vessels and the early loss of capillaries, it has been proposed that DMS is predominantly a complement-mediated microangiopathy.[79-81,102] However, the fact that MAC deposition and areas of perifascicular atrophy do not necessarily occur together raises questions about the relationship of microvascular changes to muscle cell pathology.[79,81] Still, why capillaries or medium-sized blood vessels in muscles would be targeted by the immune system remains to be explained.

Several convergent lines of evidence point to a role for interferon (IFN) in DMS pathology. First, it has been shown that DMS muscle tissue contains large numbers of IFN-secreting plasmacytoid dendritic cells.[78] Second, genes known to be induced by IFN are highly upregulated in muscle tissue from patients with DMS.[78,103]

Third, the expression of IFN-inducible genes in the periphery correlates with DMS disease activity.[104,105] Although these observations suggest that dysregulated production of IFN could play a role in disease pathogenesis, it remains to be demonstrated how this might damage blood vessels or muscle cells.

As in DMS, genetic susceptibility plays a role in the development of PM.[90] For example, certain MHC class II alleles confer an increased risk of developing PM.[106,107] Interestingly, an single nucleotide polymorphism within the IFN-γ gene also confers susceptibility to developing this disease.[108] However, how these immunogenetic risk factors predispose patients to developing PM remains unclear.

Although analysis of PM muscle biopsies demonstrates that cytotoxic T cells destroy muscle cells through the perforin pathway,[109] it is unclear what triggers the autoimmune attack. It has been suggested that a viral infection could trigger an attack through molecular mimicry with muscle proteins, but little evidence exists to support this. Others have suggested that MHC-I protein, which is overexpressed on PM muscle fibers, could itself be toxic to muscle fibers. This is supported by an animal model in which targeted expression of MHC-I in mouse muscle results in muscle inflammation[110] activation of a potentially harmful endoplasmic reticulum stress response pathway,[111] and muscle weakness.[112] However, it has not been demonstrated why MHC-I is expressed in PM or whether it plays a direct role in human muscle injury.

As the name implies, subjects with IMNM have marked muscle fiber necrosis in the absence of prominent inflammatory cell exudates. Many patients with this form of muscle disease have antibodies recognizing either SRP or HMGCR, and distinct class II HLA alleles are associated with the presence of each autoantibody.[93,113] For anti-HMGCR–associated IMNM, it appears that most cases are associated with statin exposure.[15,16] Because statins upregulate the expression of HMGCR, we hypothesize that in immunogenetically susceptible individuals, overexpression of the protein leads to aberrant HMGCR proteolytic processing, the generation of novel antigenic epitopes, and loss of tolerance to HMGCR. Once muscle damage has ensued, the presence of high levels of HMGCR in regenerating muscle fibers might then continue to drive the anti-HMGCR

immune response. Although appealing, this model remains to be experimentally validated. Furthermore, even if this model explains anti-HMGCR immunoreactivity, it is not clear that anti-HMGCR antibodies are pathogenic. Indeed, a recent study demonstrating that serum anti-HMGCR antibodies can remain markedly elevated even during disease remission suggests that they are not directly harmful to undamaged muscle cells.[114] In contrast, anti-SRP antibody levels may normalize during periods of disease quiescence, raising the possibility that they could have a more direct pathologic role in damaging muscle cells.[115] Although statins are a clear trigger for disease in anti-HMGCR–associated disease, the mechanisms underlying muscle damage, as well as those through which autoimmunity is initiated and sustained, have yet to be elucidated for any form of IMNM.

Analyses of muscle biopsy specimens from IBM patients have revealed numerous and diverse abnormalities, which have given rise to many different theories of disease pathogenesis.[116] For example, the presence of myofibers being invaded by cytolytic T cells suggest that an antigen-directed T cell response might underlie IBM pathology.[3,52] Similarly, taken together, the observations that B cells mature into plasma cells within IBM muscle, that intramuscular immunoglobulin production is antigen driven,[117] and that many IBM patients make a specific autoantibody not seen in other forms of inflammatory myopathy all suggest that an antigen-driven autoantibody response may play an important role. However, the failure of IBM patients to improve with immunosuppressive therapy raises doubts about the primary role of autoimmunity in this disease.[118]

The presence of congophilic material within muscle cells and the subsequent identification of aggregates (including more than 80 different proteins) have suggested that aberrant protein aggregation may play a role in IBM disease pathology.[119-121] However, it remains to be seen whether these structures are the cause or effect of muscle damage.

It has long been appreciated that IBM muscle fibers have evidence of nuclear degeneration,[122-124] However, more recent studies showing that rimmed vacuoles are lined with nuclear membrane proteins suggest that these pathologic structures may actually be derived from muscle cell nuclei.[125] The observation that the nuclear protein TDP-43 is relocated to the sarcoplasm in IBM muscle cells also suggests that nuclear abnormalities may play a role in the pathology of this disease.[126-129]

Although these and other pathogenic theories have been put forward, the initial events leading to muscle damage and inflammation in IBM have not been determined. Identifying the relevant pathologic pathways is particularly important in IBM because no effective therapies currently exist to treat patients with this debilitating myopathy.

Treatment

Various immunotherapies appear to be beneficial in DMS, PM, and IMNM despite the dearth of support from clinical trials[130-132] (Table 10–2). We do not know which particular therapies are most beneficial, what doses are required to see an effect, the best time to initiate second- or third-line agents, or if specific agents are more effective in different types of myositis. Most cases of IBM, though, do not improve with immunotherapy.

CORTICOSTEROIDS

Corticosteroids are generally considered the first line treatment for DMS, PM, and IMNM.[130-134] There is no consensus regarding the "right way" to treat patients with corticosteriods, but the most common approach is starting prednisone 0.75 to 1.5 mg/kg (up to 60 mg) daily. In patients with severe weakness, we often initiate treatment with a short course of IV Solu-Medrol (1 g daily for 3 days) prior to starting oral prednsione. High-dose prednisone is continued until muscle strength normalizes, improvement in strength has reached a plateau, or there is at least normalization of the serum CK, which usually takes 3 to 6 months. Subsequently, we slowly taper the prednisone by 5 to 10 mg every 2 to 4 weeks. Once the dose is reduced to 20 mg every other day, we taper prednisone no faster than 2.5 mg every 2 weeks. The majority of patients with DMS, PM, and IMNM improve with prednisone treatment, though response may not be complete.

There is equipoise regarding when to initiate treatment with second-line agents (e.g., methotrexate, azathioprine, mycophenolate, or immunoglobulin); clinicians and patients need to weigh the increased risks of immunosuppression versus possible benefits (e.g., faster improvement, steroid-sparing effect). We lean toward starting a second-line agent at the time we initiate treatment with corticosteroids in those patients with severe weakness or other organ system involvement (e.g., myocarditis, interstitial lung disease), those with increased risk of steroid complications (e.g., diabetics, patients with osteoporosis), and those with immune-mediated necrotizing myopathy, as these are much more difficult to manage with prednisone alone. In patients initially treated with prednisone alone, we add a second-line drug in those who fail to improve after 2 to 4 months of treatment or if there is an exacerbation during the subsequent prednisone taper. Most patients should remain on at least a small dose of prednisone (e.g., around 10 mg/day or equivalent) or a second-line agent (e.g., methotrexate) to maintain a sustained remission. Adjustments of prednisone and other immunosuppressive agents are primarily based on the objective clinical examination and not the CK levels or the patient's subjective response. An increasing serum CK can herald a relapse. But without objective clinical deterioration, we do not change treatment, but rather hold the dose or the slow the taper. If no response is noted after an adequate trial of immunotherapy, alternative diagnoses (e.g., IBM or an inflammatory muscular dystrophy) should be considered.

In patients who developed increasing weakness while on corticosteroids, one needs to distinguish if this is caused by a relapse of the myositis or from type 2 muscle fiber atrophy from either disuse or chronic corticosteroids. A steroid myopathy is more likely in a patient with a normal serum CK, EMG, or skeletal muscle MRI. In contrast, flare of myositis is suspected in patients who become weaker during prednisone taper, have increasing serum CK levels, abnormal spontaneous activity on EMG, or increased signal abnormalities on muscle MRI.

CONCURRENT MANAGEMENT

In patients with interstitial lung disease or on prednisone plus another immunosuppressive agent, we usually start Bactrim for pneumocystis prophylaxis. Dual-energy X-ray absorptiometry (DEXA) is obtained at baseline and then

Table 10–2 **Immunosuppressive/Immunomodulating Therapy for Inflammatory Myopathies**

Therapy	Route	Dose	Side Effects	Monitor
First-Line Agents				
Prednisone	p.o.	0.75–1.5 mg/kg/day	Hypertension, fluid and weight gain, hyperglycemia, hypokalemia, cataracts, gastric irritation, osteoporosis, infection, aseptic femoral necrosis	Weight, blood pressure, serum glucose/potassium, cataract formation
Methylprednisone	IV	1 g in 100 mL normal saline over 1–2 hours, daily or every other day for 3–6 doses	Arrhythmia, flushing, dysgeusia, anxiety, insomnia, fluid and weight gain, hyperglycemia, hypokalemia, infection	Heart rate, blood pressure, serum glucose/potassium
Second-Line Agents[a]				
Methotrexate	p.o.	7.5–25 mg weekly, single or divided doses; one day a week dosing	Hepatotoxicity, pulmonary fibrosis, infection, neoplasia, infertility, leukopenia, alopecia, gastric irritation, stomatitis, teratogenicity	Liver enzymes, blood count while adjust dosaging and then every 3 months
	IV/IM	20–50 mg weekly; one day a week dosing	Same as p.o.	Same as p.o.
Azathioprine	p.o.	2–3 mg/kg/day; single a.m. dose	Flu-like illness, hepatotoxicity, pancreatitis, leukopenia, macrocytosis, neoplasia, infection, teratogenicity	Blood count, liver enzymes while adjusting dosage
Mycophenolate mofetil	p.o.	Adults: 1 g BID to 1.5 g BID Children: 600 mg/m²/dose BID No more than 1 g/day in patients with renal failure	Bone marrow suppression, hypertension, tremor, diarrhea, nausea, vomiting, headache, sinusitis, confusion, amblyopia, cough, teratogenicity, infection, neoplasia	Blood counts
Intravenous immunoglobulin	IV	2 g/kg over 2–5 days, then every 4–8 weeks as needed	Hypotension, arrhythmia, diaphoresis, flushing, nephrotoxicity, headache, aseptic meningitis, anaphylaxis, stroke	None routinely
Third-Line Agents				
Rituximab	IV	750 mg/m² (up to 1 g/m²) and repeated in 2 weeks Course is usually repeated every 6–18 months	Infusion reactions (as per IVIG), infection, PML[b]	None routine, though can check B cell count
Tacrolimus	p.o.	0.1–0.2 mg/kg/day in 2 divided doses	Nephrotoxicity, hypertension, infection, hepatotoxicity, hirsutism, tremor, gum hyperplasia, teratogenicity	Blood pressure, creatinine/BUN ratio, liver enzymes, tacrolimus levels

(continued)

Table 10–2 **(Cont.)**

Therapy	Route	Dose	Side Effects	Monitor
Cyclosporine	p.o.	Start at 3–4 mg /kg/day and increase up to –6 mg/kg/day as needed, split into two daily doses	Nephrotoxicity, hypertension, infection, hepatotoxicity, hirsutism, tremor, gum hyperplasia, teratogenicity	Blood pressure, creatinine/ BUN ratio, liver enzymes, cyclosporine levels
Cyclophosphamide	p.o. IV	1.0–2 mg/kg/day as single morning dose; 0.5 to 1 g/m²/month by IV	Bone marrow suppression, infertility, hemorrhagic cystitis, alopecia, infections, neoplasia, teratogenicity	Blood count, urinalysis

Note. Modified with permission from Amato AA, Barohn RJ. Idiopathic inflammatory myopathies. Neurol Clin 1997;15:615-648.
[a]May start at same time as corticosteroids. [b]Progressive multifocal leukoencephalopathy.

yearly while patients are receiving corticosteroids to assess for bone loss. Calcium supplementation (1 g/day) and vitamin D (800 IU/day) are initiated for prevention of steroid-induced osteoporosis. A bisphosphonate may be started for prevention and treatment of osteoporosis, particularly in postmenopausal women. Long-term side effects of bisphosphonates are not known, particularly in children, men, and premenopausal women. We prophylactically treat these individuals only if the DEXA scan is abnormal.

Second-Line Therapies

We start a second-line agent in patients who do not adequately respond to treatment with prednisone alone or along with prednisone at the initiation of treatment in patients with severe weakness or associated comorbidity (i.e., interstitial lung disease, myocarditis), diabetes mellitus (for possible steroid-sparing effect), or in the elderly or those with known osteoporosis (again for possible steroid-sparing effect),as well as in those with immune-mediated necrotizing myopathy. There are no studies that have demonstrated that one agent is necessarily better than another.

METHOTREXATE

Retrospective studies suggest that methotrexate is effective in many patients,[135-138] and it is the most commonly used second-line agent. We usually begin methotrexate orally at 7.5 mg/week given in three divided doses 12 hours apart. The dose is gradually increased by 2.5 mg each week up to 25 mg/week. The dosage needs to be reduced in patients with renal insufficiency. If there is no improvement after one month of 25 mg/week of oral methotrexate, we switch to weekly parenteral (usually subcutaneous) methotrexate and increase the dose by 5 mg every week up to 40 mg/week. The major side effects of methotrexate are alopecia, stomatitis, ILD, teratogenicity, oncogenicity, risk of infection, and pulmonary fibrosis, along with bone marrow, renal, and liver toxicity. We concomitantly treat all patients with folate or folinic acid.

Because methotrexate can cause pulmonary fibrosis, we avoid it in patients with myositis who already have associated ILD and in patients with Jo-1 antibodies. We monitor the complete blood count (CBC) and liver function tests (LFT), including a gamma-glutamyl transpeptidase test, which is important because it is a more reliable indicator of hepatic dysfunction than AST and ALT, which can be elevated from muscle involvement alone.

AZATHIOPRINE

Retrospective studies suggest that azathioprine may help in DMS and PM.[138] A prospective, double-blind study comparing azathioprine (2 mg/kg) in combination with prednisone to placebo plus prednisone found no significant improvement at three months[139]; however, in the open-label follow-up period, patients on the azathioprine combination did better than those on prednisone alone and required lower doses of prednisone.[140] We begin azathioprine at 50 mg daily in adults and increase by 50 mg every 2 weeks up to 2 to 3 mg/kg/day. Approximately 12% of patients develop a systemic reaction characterized by fever, abdominal pain, nausea, vomiting, and anorexia that requires discontinuation of the drug.[141] Other major side effects of azathioprine are bone marrow suppression, hepatic toxicity, pancreatitis, teratogenicity, oncogenicity, and increased risk of infection. Allopurinol should be avoided, because combination with azathioprine increases the risk of bone marrow and liver toxicity. A major drawback of azathioprine is that it may take 6 to 18 months to be effective. CBCs and LFTs are monitored as with methotrexate.

MYCOPHENOLATE MOFETIL

Mycophenylate mofetil inhibits the proliferation of T and B lymphocytes by blocking purine synthesis and is reportedly beneficial in some patients with myositis.[142-145] The starting dose is 1.0 grams twice daily in patients with normal renal function and can be increased to 3 grams daily in divided doses if necessary. Because there is no associated renal or liver toxicity, it is an attractive option to methotrexate and azathioprine. However, we have seen a number of severe infections as a complication.[145] Common side effects include diarrhea, abdominal discomfort, nausea, peripheral edema, fever, and leukopenia.

INTRAVENOUS IMMUNOGLOBULIN

Retrospective series and anecdotes suggest that intravenous immunoglobulin (IVIG) is effective in DMS, PM, and IMNM.[146] A prospective, double-blind, placebo-control study of IVIG in 15 patients with DMS demonstrated significant clinical improvement with IVIG.[147] Whether or not IVIG is effective in PM and IMNM has not been assessed in a clinical trial though our own experiences suggest it can be beneficial in some patients. Given the high cost and lack of studies using IVIG as a monotherapy, we generally use it in patients who do not respond adequately to corticosteroids and usually at least one other second-line agent. Additionally, given our experience with the immune-mediated necrotizing myopathies, which are often quite refractory, we sometimes initiate treatment in patients with severe weakness with IVIG, prednisone, and another second-line agent (e.g., methotrexate).[29,114] We initiate IVIG (2 gm/kg) slowly over 2 to 5 days and repeat infusions at monthly intervals for at least three months. Subsequently, we try to decrease or spread out the dose (2 gm/kg every 2 months or 1 gm/kg per month).

Third-Line Therapies

RITUXIMAB

Rituximab is a monoclonal antibody directed against CD20, thereby leading to depletion B cells. Small series have suggested rituximab may be an effective therapy in DMS,[148] PM,[149] and anti-SRP–associated IMNM.[150] Although a large, prospective, double-blind, placebo-controlled, crossover trial demonstrated no significant benefit (Oddis CV et al., accepted for publication), in our own experience, we have found rituximab to be effective in refractory cases of DMS, PM, and IMNM.[151] The major drawback of rituximab is that there have been rare cases of multifocal progressive leukoencephalopathy associated with its use in other disorders. The dose is 750 mg/m^2 (up to 1 g/m^2) and given once and then repeated in two weeks. The course of rituximab is usually repeated every 6 to 18 months; we have had patients go 2 years or more between courses.

CYCLOSPORINE AND TACROLIMUS

Cyclosporine[152-155] and tacrolimus[156-158] seem to be effective in some patients; however, the cost and side effects (in particular renal toxicity and hypertension) limit their use.

We start cyclosporine at a dose of 3.0 to 4.0 mg/kg/day in two divided doses and gradually increase to 6.0 mg/kg/day as necessary. The cyclosporine dose should initially be titrated to maintain trough serum cyclosporine levels of 50 to 200 mg/ml. Tacrolimus is started at a dose of 0.1 mg/kg and increased up to 0.2mg/kg (in two divided doses daily). The dose is titrated to maintain a trough level of 5 to 15 mg/ml. Blood pressure, electrolytes, and renal function, and trough cyclosporine or tracolimus levels, need to be monitored closely.

CYCLOPHOSPHAMIDE

There are a few reports of patients treated with oral and intravenous cyclophosphamide with mixed results.[159-163] The major side effects are bone marrow toxicity, alopecia, hemorrhagic cystitis, teratogenicity, sterilization, and increased risk of infections and secondary malignancies. Given the increased risks associated with cyclophosphamide, we reserve it for patients who refractory to most other modalities. We usually give cyclophosphamide IV 0.5 to 1 g/m^2/month for 6 to 12 months. Cyclophosphamide can be given orally at a dose of 1.0 to 2.0 mg/kg/day, but there may be greater risk of hemorrhagic cystitis. Urinalysis and CBCs are monitored closely (every 1–2 weeks at the onset of therapy and then at least monthly).

TUMOR NECROSIS FACTOR-ALPHA (TNF-α) BLOCKERS

TNF-α blockers have have had mixed result in PM and DMS; some reports suggest a benefit,[164-170] whereas others have shown no improvement or worsening.[171,172] A small, double-blind, placebo-controlled, pilot study of etanercept in DMS demonstrated no significant significant safety issues although increased rash was seen in some patients.[173] This study was not powered for efficacy, but there did appear to be a steroid-sparing effect.

OTHER THERAPIES

Physical and occupational therapy may help patients retain motor function, improve mobility, prevent contractures that can arise, and decrease side effects of corticosteroids (e.g., type 2 fiber atrophy, weight gain, osteoporosis). Patients with dysphagia or speech disturbance related to inflammation of oropharyngeal or esophageal muscles may benefit from speech/swallow therapy. Cutting food into smaller pieces, alternating food with sips of liquid, and simple maneuvers such as instructing the patient to tuck their chin when they swallow may suffice. Rare patients may need a feeding tube, at least temporarily. Dysphagia is common in IBM patients and may be temporarily improved with esophageal dilatation or cricopharyngeal myotomy.

Future Perspectives

DMS, PM, and IMNM are immune-mediated myopathies currently treated with nonspecific immunosuppressive therapies. Unfortunately, some patients do not have a complete response to treatment. Furthermore, current medication regimens can be complicated by severe side effects. In the case of IBM, no effective therapies exist. Finding novel, targeted therapies in the future will likely require a better understanding of the pathogenic mechanisms that underlie these diseases.

OTHER INFLAMMATORY MYOPATHIES

Focal Myositis

Rarely, patients present with a solitary, painful focus of inflammation in an individual muscle of the legs, arms, abdomen, head, or neck.[174-179] Such lesions are apparent on MRI and may be mistaken for rhabdomyosarcoma.[180] Perhaps because of the limited extent of muscle injury, muscle enzyme levels are typically normal. On muscle biopsy, cellular infiltrates include T cells, macrophages, B cells, and plasmacytoid dendritic cells.[174] Both myopathic and neurogenic features are observed, and MHC-I may be focally overexpressed, but not diffusely as seen in PM.

The specific pathogenic mechanisms of focal myositis are unknown. However, it has been suggested that chronic nerve irritation can cause focal myofiber necrosis with secondary inflammation resulting in muscle pain and MRI findings of muscle hypertrophy and edema.[181] If focal myositis has a neurogenic origin, this might help explain why it only rarely generalizes to include other muscle groups.

Eosinophilic Myositis

Eosinophilic myositis may occur as a focal intramuscular process (focal eosinophilic myositis), diffuse intramuscular process (eosinophilic PM), or perimyositis with eosinophilic infiltrates restricted to the fascia and superficial perimysium.[182-189] These muscle features be found in those with the hypereosinophilic syndrome, characterized by eosinophilia lasting for at least 6 months in the absence of parasitic or other causes of eosinophilia. Patients with this syndrome typically have other manifestations of disease affecting the brain, nerves, lungs, kidneys, gastrointestinal system, and/or lungs. In contrast, patients with diffuse eosinophilic fasciitis (i.e., Shulman's syndrome) often complain of myalgias, arthralgias, and fevers, but do not have other organ system involvement.[190,191] The typical dermatologic feature seen in these patients is the "peau d'orange" sign characterized by thick, dimpled skin.

The CK level may be elevated in focal eosinophilic myositis and eosinophilic PM. In contrast, patients with eosinophilic fasciitis may have an elevated aldolase with a normal CK level. The presence of prominent eosinophilic infiltrates distinguishes the muscle biopsies of patients with eosinophilic myositis from patients with other inflammatory myopathies (Figure 10–4A). However, the presence of eosinophils is not pathognomonic for an autoimmune process, as some patients with LGMD2A (i.e., calpainopathy) or LGMD2C (gamma-sarcoglycanopathy) may present with prominent eosinophilic infiltrates on muscle biopsy.[192,193]

Patients with focal eosinophilic myositis, eosinophilic PM, and eosinophilic perimyositis have a variable response to treatment with corticosteroids and other immunosuppressive agents. In contrast, patients with diffuse eosinophilic fasciitis usually have a brisk response to corticosteroid treatment with improved symptoms, resolution of their skin findings, and a normalization of the peripheral eosinophilia. Occasionally, a steroid-sparing agent such as methotrexate may be required.

Granulomatous Myositis/ Sarcoid Myopathy

Granulomatous myositis is defined by the presence of granulomas and multinucleated giant cells on muscle biopsy (Figure 10–4B). These biopsy features may occur in the context of myasthenia gravis (MG), thymoma, or sarcoidosis.[194-198] In a minority of cases, granulomatous myositis occurs in the absence of an underlying

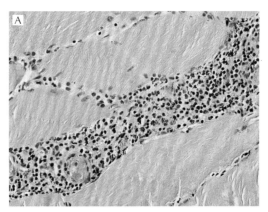

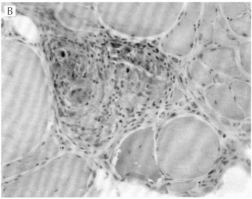

Figure 10–4. Eosinophilic fasciitis (A) and granulomatous inflammation (B).

systemic disease (i.e., isolated granulomatous myositis).[199] Patients with MG often have typical features of that disease (e.g., diplopia, ptosis, bulbar dysfunction, and antibodies recognizing the acetylcholine receptor), whereas those with sarcoidosis typically have predominant pulmonary symptoms and lymphadenopathy. Patients with MG and/or thymoma often have proximal muscle weakness; those with sarcoidosis or isolated granulomatous myositis may have proximal weakness, distal weakness, or no weakness at all. Similarly, CK is usually elevated in those with granulomatous myositis in the context of MG, but may be normal or near-normal in those with sarcoidosis. In contrast to those with sarcoidosis, cardiomyopathy and arrhythmias may be found in those with MG.

Although cell-mediated autoimmunity is thought to underlie these disorders, the precise pathogenic mechanisms have not been defined. While all patients may benefit from treatment with corticosteroids, the response tends to be more robust in those with isolated granulomatous myositis than in those with sarcoid myopathy.[199] Those with granulomatous myositis in the context of MG may also be relatively refractory to treatment and may require treatment with additional agents such as methotrexate.

Infectious Myositis

A variety of viruses, bacteria, fungi, and parasites can be associated with an inflammatory myopathy.

HUMAN IMMUNODEFICIENCY VIRUS

Patients with HIV can present with typical clinical and muscle biopsy features of either PM or IBM.[200-204] In the case of HIV-PM, it is thought that HIV infection triggers a T-cell–mediated immune response against muscle rather than precipitating inflammation through infection of the muscle by the virus. Similarly, immune dysregulation probably plays a role in the pathogenesis of HIV-IBM. Although controlled studies are lacking, we recommend a trial of steroids and/or steroid-sparing medications in HIV positive patients with an inflammatory myopathy. Given the risk of further immunosuppression and the potential for drug interactions in this patient population, treatment with immunosuppressive medications should probably be initiated only in consultation with the treating infectious disease specialist.

HUMAN T-CELL LEUKEMIA VIRUS TYPE 1

Tropical spastic paraparesis (TSP) is the most common neuromuscular complication of human T-cell leukemia virus type 1 (HTLV-1) infection. HTLV-infected patients with or without TSP can also develop proximal muscle weakness, elevated CK levels, upper extremity weakness, and inflammatory muscle biopsies with findings similar to those seen in patients with PM or IBM.[205-209] The pathogenesis of HTLV-1–associated myositis remains to be elucidated and there are no clear guidelines for treating these patients. However, in contrast to the myelopathy, HTLV-1 myopathy may respond to immunosuppressive agents such as corticosteroids.

INFLUENZA VIRUSES

Both adults and children with influenza virus infection can develop a self-limited myositis characterized by severe myalgias, elevated CK levels, muscle tenderness, and muscle swelling.[210-214] In children, calf muscles may be affected alone or along with other muscle groups.[215] Muscle weakness and myoglobinuria are more common in adults, whose muscle biopsies reveal myofiber necrosis with minimal inflammation.[216] In contrast, biopsies from children show a more abundant cellular infiltrate. Patients with influenza-associated myositis can be treated with acetaminophen and aspirin. However, because the symptoms usually resolve within a week, immunosuppressive therapy is not indicated.

BACTERIAL INFECTIONS (PYOMYOSITIS)

Although long considered a disease of the tropics, intravenous drug users, especially those with HIV infection, are also vulnerable to developing focal or multifocal bacterial abscesses.[217-219] The quadriceps, deltoids, and glutei are the most common sites of infection.[220] Patients may present with focal muscle pain and fever, which can progress to life-threatening sepsis if left untreated. Defining the appropriate antibiotic treatment regimen depends upon culturing and identifying the pathogenic organism. Common pathogens include *Staphylococcus aureus*, *Escherichia coli*, *Yersinia*, and *Legionella*.[220-222]

LYME DISEASE (*BORRELIA BURGDORFERI*)

Although myalgias are common in Lyme-infected patients, the presence of myositis associated with weakness, elevated CK levels, and a lymphocytic infiltrate on muscle biopsy is relatively rare.[223-227] Focal muscle involvement is most characteristic of Lyme myositis and can involve various muscle groups, including the orbital muscles.[228,229] However, more diffuse muscle involvement has also been reported.[224,230] Lyme myositis should be treated with appropriate antibiotic therapy.

PARASITIC INFECTIONS[231]

Several days following the ingestion of undercooked meat, *Trichinella spiralis* larvae can invade skeletal muscle after spreading from the gut via the bloodstream and lymphatic system.[232,233] The diaphragm, extraocular muscles, tongue, intercostal muscles, and limb muscles may all be infected. Most cases are subclinical, but muscle invasion can cause pain and weakness along with fever, diarrhea, facial edema, headache, and joint pain.[234,235] In cases where the nematode invades the heart and central nervous system, myocarditis and meningoencephalitis occur. During the acute infection stage, muscle biopsies may reveal prominent infiltration by eosinophils. With persisting infection, parasitic larvae and cysts may be accompanied by a mononuclear cell infiltrate. Fortunately, in most cases this nematodal infection can be treated effectively with a combination of mebendazole and prednisone.

Cysticercosis occurs following ingestion of undercooked meat containing the larva form of the cestode *Taenia solium*. These organisms invade the CNS, where they can cause a variety of neurologic symptoms, including seizure. Although skeletal muscle involvement occurs in 75% of infected patients, this is usually asymptomatic. Symptoms that can occur include myalgias, tenderness, muscle swelling, and weakness. Rarely, solitary soft tissue masses occur[236] and can cause compressive syndromes including nerve entrapment.[237] Biopsy of such lesions reveals the presence of parasitic fragments as well as an inflammatory reaction including eosinophils, neutrophils, lymphocytes, histiocytes, epithelioid cells, and giant cells.[238] Medical management of cysticercosis includes praziquantel or albendazole along with a short course of prednisone.

In immunocompetent subjects, infection with *Toxoplasma gondii* is usually asymptomatic. However, some individuals may experience a clinical syndrome of fever, cervical adenopathy, myalgias, and malaise. In contrast, immunocompromised patients may experience disease involving skeletal muscle as well as the CNS, eyes, and lungs. When skeletal muscles are involved, CK is usually elevated, weakness may occur, and muscle biopsy shows lymphocytes, macrophages, giant cells, and cysts containing the bradyzoite stage of the protozoa.[239-241] Treatment of patients with myositis includes sulfadiazine and pyrimethamine.

REFERENCES

1. Bohan A, Peter JB. Polymyositis and dermatomyositis (first of two parts). N Engl J Med 1975; Feb 13;292(7):344–347.
2. Bohan A, Peter JB. Polymyositis and dermatomyositis (second of two parts). N Engl J Med 1975; Feb 20;292(8):403–407.
3. Griggs RC, Askanas V, DiMauro S, Engel A, Karpati G, Mendell JR, et al. Inclusion body myositis and myopathies. Ann Neurol 1995; Nov;38(5):705–713.
4. Dalakas MC, Hohlfeld R. Polymyositis and dermatomyositis. Lancet 2003; Sep 20;362(9388):971–982.
5. Mammen AL. Dermatomyositis and polymyositis: Clinical presentation, autoantibodies, and pathogenesis. Ann N Y Acad Sci 2010; Jan;1184:134–153.
6. Wagner E. Fall einer seltnen Muskelkrankheit. Dtsch Arch Heilk 1863;4:282.
7. Unverricht H. Polymyositis acuta progressive. Z Klin Med 1887;12:553.
8. Unverricht H. Dermatomyositis acuta. Dtsch Med Wochenschr 1891;17:41.
9. Hepp P. Ueber einen Fall von acuter parenchymatoser Myositis, welche Geschwulste bildete und Fluctuation vortauschte. Klin Wochenschr 1887;24:389.
10. Eaton LM. The perspective of neurology in regard to polymyositis; a study of 41 cases. Neurology 1954; Apr;4(4):245–263.
11. Walton JM, Adams RD. Polymyositis. Edinburgh: E & S Livingstone; 1958.
12. Rowland LP. Muscular dystrophies, polymyositis, and other myopathies. J Chronic Dis 1958; Oct;8(4):510–535.
13. Pearson CM, Rose AS. Myositis: the inflammatory disorders of muscle. Res Publ Assoc Res Nerv Ment Dis 1960;38:422.
14. Miller T, Al-Lozi MT, Lopate G, Pestronk A. Myopathy with antibodies to the signal recognition particle: clinical and pathological features. J Neurol Neurosurg Psychiatry 2002; Oct;73(4):420–428.
15. Christopher-Stine L, Casciola-Rosen LA, Hong G, Chung T, Corse AM, Mammen AL. A novel autoantibody recognizing 200-kd and 100-kd proteins is associated with an immune-mediated necrotizing myopathy. Arthritis Rheum 2010; Sep;62(9):2757–2766.
16. Mammen AL, Chung T, Christopher-Stine L, Rosen P, Rosen A, Doering KR, et al. Autoantibodies against 3-hydroxy-3-methylglutaryl-coenzyme A reductase in patients with statin-associated autoimmune myopathy. Arthritis Rheum 2011; Mar;63(3):713–721.
17. Hoogendijk JE, Amato AA, Lecky BR, Choy EH, Lundberg IE, Rose MR, et al. 119th ENMC international workshop: trial design in adult idiopathic inflammatory myopathies, with the exception of inclusion body myositis, 10–12 October 2003, Naarden, The Netherlands. Neuromuscul Disord 2004; May;14(5):337–345.
18. Mammen AL, Medscape. Autoimmune myopathies: autoantibodies, phenotypes and pathogenesis. Nat Rev Neurol 2011; Jun 8;7(6):343–354.
19. Briani C, Doria A, Sarzi-Puttini P, Dalakas MC. Update on idiopathic inflammatory myopathies. Autoimmunity 2006; May;39(3):161–170.
20. Vargas-Leguas H, Selva-O'Callaghan A, Campins-Marti M, Hermosilla Perez E, Grau-Junyent JM, Martinez

Gomez X, et al. Polymyositis-dermatomyositis: incidence in Spain (1997–2004). Med Clin (Barc) 2007; Nov 24;129(19):721–724.

21. Flachenecker P. Epidemiology of neuroimmunological diseases. J Neurol 2006; Sep;253 Suppl 5:V2–V8.

22. Gaubitz M. Epidemiology of connective tissue disorders. Rheumatology (Oxford) 2006; Oct;45 Suppl 3:iii3–4.

23. Prieto S, Grau JM. The geoepidemiology of autoimmune muscle disease. Autoimmun Rev 2010; Mar;9(5):A330–334.

24. Smoyer Tomic KE, Amato AA, Fernandes AW. Incidence and prevalence of idiopathic inflammatory myopathies among commercially insured, Medicare supplemental insured, and Medicaid enrolled populations: an administrative claims analysis. BMC Musculoskelet Disord 2012; Jun 15;13(1):103.

25. Bernatsky S, Joseph L, Pineau CA, Belisle P, Boivin JF, Banerjee D, et al. Estimating the prevalence of polymyositis and dermatomyositis from administrative data: age, sex and regional differences. Ann Rheum Dis 2009; Jul;68(7):1192–1196.

26. Hengstman GJ, van Venrooij WJ, Vencovsky J, Moutsopoulos HM, van Engelen BG. The relative prevalence of dermatomyositis and polymyositis in Europe exhibits a latitudinal gradient. Ann Rheum Dis 2000; Feb;59(2):141–142.

27. Love LA, Weinberg CR, McConnaughey DR, Oddis CV, Medsger TA,Jr, Reveille JD, et al. Ultraviolet radiation intensity predicts the relative distribution of dermatomyositis and anti-Mi-2 autoantibodies in women. Arthritis Rheum 2009; Aug;60(8):2499–2504.

28. Needham M, Fabian V, Knezevic W, Panegyres P, Zilko P, Mastaglia FL. Progressive myopathy with up-regulation of MHC-I associated with statin therapy. Neuromuscul Disord 2007; Feb;17(2):194–200.

29. Grable-Esposito P, Katzberg HD, Greenberg SA, Srinivasan J, Katz J, Amato AA. Immune-mediated necrotizing myopathy associated with statins. Muscle Nerve 2010; Feb;41(2):185–190.

30. Leff RL, Burgess SH, Miller FW, Love LA, Targoff IN, Dalakas MC, et al. Distinct seasonal patterns in the onset of adult idiopathic inflammatory myopathy in patients with anti-Jo-1 and anti-signal recognition particle autoantibodies. Arthritis Rheum 1991; Nov;34(11):1391–1396.

31. Sarkar K, Weinberg CR, Oddis CV, Medsger TA,Jr, Plotz PH, Reveille JD, et al. Seasonal influence on the onset of idiopathic inflammatory myopathies in serologically defined groups. Arthritis Rheum 2005; Aug;52(8):2433–2438.

32. Matthews E, Plotz PH, Portaro S, Parton M, Elliott P, Humbel RL, et al. A case of necrotizing myopathy with proximal weakness and cardiomyopathy. Neurology 2012; May 8;78(19):1527–1532.

33. Cutolo M, Sulli A, Secchi ME, Paolino S, Pizzorni C. Nailfold capillaroscopy is useful for the diagnosis and follow-up of autoimmune rheumatic diseases. A future tool for the analysis of microvascular heart involvement? Rheumatology (Oxford) 2006; Oct;45 Suppl 4: iv43–46.

34. Yoshida S, Akizuki M, Mimori T, Yamagata H, Inada S, Homma M. The precipitating antibody to an acidic nuclear protein antigen, the Jo-1, in connective tissue diseases. A marker for a subset of polymyositis with interstitial pulmonary fibrosis. Arthritis Rheum 1983; May;26(5):604–611.

35. Marguerie C, Bunn CC, Beynon HL, Bernstein RM, Hughes JM, So AK, et al. Polymyositis, pulmonary fibrosis and autoantibodies to aminoacyl-tRNA synthetase enzymes. Q J Med 1990; Oct;77(282): 1019–1038.

36. Targoff IN, Johnson AE, Miller FW. Antibody to signal recognition particle in polymyositis. Arthritis Rheum 1990; Sep;33(9):1361–1370.

37. Hengstman GJ, ter Laak HJ, Vree Egberts WT, Lundberg IE, Moutsopoulos HM, Vencovsky J, et al. Anti-signal recognition particle autoantibodies: marker of a necrotising myopathy. Ann Rheum Dis 2006; Dec;65(12):1635–1638.

38. Love LA, Leff RL, Fraser DD, Targoff IN, Dalakas M, Plotz PH, et al. A new approach to the classification of idiopathic inflammatory myopathy: myositis-specific autoantibodies define useful homogeneous patient groups. Medicine (Baltimore) 1991; Nov;70(6): 360–374.

39. Carpenter S, Karpati G, Heller I, Eisen A. Inclusion body myositis: a distinct variety of idiopathic inflammatory myopathy. Neurology 1978; Jan;28(1):8–17.

40. Lindberg C, Persson LI, Bjorkander J, Oldfors A. Inclusion body myositis: clinical, morphological, physiological and laboratory findings in 18 cases. Acta Neurol Scand 1994; Feb;89(2):123–131.

41. Lotz BP, Engel AG, Nishino H, Stevens JC, Litchy WJ. Inclusion body myositis. Observations in 40 patients. Brain 1989; Jun;112(Pt 3):727–747.

42. Calabrese LH, Mitsumoto H, Chou SM. Inclusion body myositis presenting as treatment-resistant polymyositis. Arthritis Rheum 1987; Apr;30(4):397–403.

43. Eisen A, Berry K, Gibson G. Inclusion body myositis (IBM): myopathy or neuropathy? Neurology 1983; Sep;33(9):1109–1114.

44. Joy JL, Oh SJ, Baysal AI. Electrophysiological spectrum of inclusion body myositis. Muscle Nerve 1990; Oct;13(10):949–951.

45. Hermanns B, Molnar M, Schroder JM. Peripheral neuropathy associated with hereditary and sporadic inclusion body myositis: confirmation by electron microscopy and morphometry. J Neurol Sci 2000; Oct 1;179(S 1–2):92–102.

46. Arnardottir S, Svanborg E, Borg K. Inclusion body myositis—sensory dysfunction revealed with quantitative determination of somatosensory thresholds. Acta Neurol Scand 2003; Jul;108(1):22–27.

47. Koffman BM, Rugiero M, Dalakas MC. Immune-mediated conditions and antibodies associated with sporadic inclusion body myositis. Muscle Nerve 1998; Jan;21(1):115–117.

48. Hill CL, Zhang Y, Sigurgeirsson B, Pukkala E, Mellemkjaer L, Airio A, et al. Frequency of specific cancer types in dermatomyositis and polymyositis: a population-based study. Lancet 2001; Jan 13;357(9250): 96–100.

49. Buchbinder R, Forbes A, Hall S, Dennett X, Giles G. Incidence of malignant disease in biopsy-proven inflammatory myopathy. A population-based cohort study. Ann Intern Med 2001; Jun 19;134(12):1087–1095.

50. Mammen AL, Amato AA. Statin myopathy: a review of recent progress. Curr Opin Rheumatol 2010; Nov;22(6):644–650.

51. Amato AA, Gronseth GS, Jackson CE, Wolfe GI, Katz JS, Bryan WW, et al. Inclusion body myositis: clinical and pathological boundaries. Ann Neurol 1996; Oct;40(4):581–586.

52. Chahin N, Engel AG. Correlation of muscle biopsy, clinical course, and outcome in PM and sporadic IBM. Neurology 2008; Feb 5;70(6):418–424.

53. Del Grande F, Carrino JA, Del Grande M, Mammen AL, Christopher-Stine L. Magnetic resonance imaging of inflammatory myopathies. Top Magn Reson Imaging 2011; Apr;22(2):39–43.

54. Hochberg MC, Feldman D, Stevens MB. Adult onset polymyositis/dermatomyositis: an analysis of clinical and laboratory features and survival in 76 patients with a review of the literature. Semin Arthritis Rheum 1986; Feb;15(3):168–178.

55. Carter JD, Kanik KS, Vasey FB, Valeriano-Marcet J. Dermatomyositis with normal creatine kinase and elevated aldolase levels. J Rheumatol 2001; Oct;28(10): 2366–2367.

56. Nozaki K, Pestronk A. High aldolase with normal creatine kinase in serum predicts a myopathy with perimysial pathology. J Neurol Neurosurg Psychiatry 2009; Aug;80(8):904–908.

57. Casciola-Rosen L, Hall JC, Mammen AL, Christopher-Stine L, Rosen A. Isolated elevation of aldolase in the serum of myositis patients: a potential biomarker of damaged early regenerating muscle cells. Clin Exp Rheumatol 2012; Jul-Aug;30(4):548–553.

58. Targoff IN, Reichlin M. The association between Mi-2 antibodies and dermatomyositis. Arthritis Rheum 1985; Jul;28(7):796–803.

59. Targoff IN. Laboratory testing in the diagnosis and management of idiopathic inflammatory myopathies. Rheum Dis Clin North Am 2002; Nov;28(4): 859,90, viii.

60. Hengstman GJ, Vree Egberts WT, Seelig HP, Lundberg IE, Moutsopoulos HM, Doria A, et al. Clinical characteristics of patients with myositis and autoantibodies to different fragments of the Mi-2 beta antigen. Ann Rheum Dis 2006; Feb;65(2):242–245.

61. Roux S, Seelig HP, Meyer O. Significance of Mi-2 autoantibodies in polymyositis and dermatomyositis. J Rheumatol 1998; Feb;25(2):395–396.

62. Sato S, Hirakata M, Kuwana M, Suwa A, Inada S, Mimori T, et al. Autoantibodies to a 140-kd polypeptide, CADM-140, in Japanese patients with clinically amyopathic dermatomyositis. Arthritis Rheum 2005; May;52(5):1571–1576.

63. Sato S, Hoshino K, Satoh T, Fujita T, Kawakami Y, Fujita T, et al. RNA helicase encoded by melanoma differentiation-associated gene 5 is a major autoantigen in patients with clinically amyopathic dermatomyositis: Association with rapidly progressive interstitial lung disease. Arthritis Rheum 2009; Jul;60(7): 2193–2200.

64. Nakashima R, Imura Y, Kobayashi S, Yukawa N, Yoshifuji H, Nojima T, et al. The RIG-I-like receptor IFIH1/MDA5 is a dermatomyositis-specific autoantigen identified by the anti-CADM-140 antibody. Rheumatology (Oxford) 2010; Mar;49(3):433–440.

65. Fiorentino D, Chung L, Zwerner J, Rosen A, Casciola-Rosen L. The mucocutaneous and systemic phenotype of dermatomyositis patients with antibodies to MDA5 (CADM-140): a retrospective study. J Am Acad Dermatol 2011; Jul;65(1):25–34.

66. Chaisson NF, Paik J, Orbai AM, Casciola-Rosen L, Fiorentino D, Danoff S, et al. A novel dermatopulmonary syndrome associated with MDA-5 antibodies: report of 2 cases and review of the literature. Medicine (Baltimore) 2012; Jul;91(4):220–228.

67. Targoff IN, Mamyrova G, Trieu EP, Perurena O, Koneru B, O'Hanlon TP, et al. A novel autoantibody to a 155-kd protein is associated with dermatomyositis. Arthritis Rheum 2006; Nov;54(11):3682–3689.

68. Kaji K, Fujimoto M, Hasegawa M, Kondo M, Saito Y, Komura K, et al. Identification of a novel autoantibody reactive with 155 and 140 kDa nuclear proteins in patients with dermatomyositis: an association with malignancy. Rheumatology (Oxford) 2007; Jan;46(1): 25–28.

69. Trallero-Araguas E, Rodrigo-Pendas JA, Selva-O'Callaghan A, Martinez-Gomez X, Bosch X, Labrador-Horrillo M, et al. Usefulness of anti-p155 autoantibody for diagnosing cancer-associated dermatomyositis: a systematic review and meta-analysis. Arthritis Rheum 2012; Feb;64(2):523–532.

70. Reeves WH, Nigam SK, Blobel G. Human autoantibodies reactive with the signal-recognition particle. Proc Natl Acad Sci U S A 1986; Dec;83(24): 9507–9511.

71. Satoh T, Okano T, Matsui T, Watabe H, Ogasawara T, Kubo K, et al. Novel autoantibodies against 7SL RNA in patients with polymyositis/dermatomyositis. J Rheumatol 2005; Sep;32(9):1727–1733.

72. Kao AH, Lacomis D, Lucas M, Fertig N, Oddis CV. Anti-signal recognition particle autoantibody in patients with and patients without idiopathic inflammatory myopathy. Arthritis Rheum 2004; Jan;50(1): 209–215.

73. Mammen AL, Pak K, Williams EK, Brisson D, Coresh J, Selvin E, et al. Rarity of anti-3-hydroxy-3-methylglutaryl-coenzyme A reductase antibodies in statin users, including those with self-limited musculoskeletal side effects. Arthritis Care Res (Hoboken) 2012; Feb;64(2):269–272.

74. Greenberg SA, Bradshaw EM, Pinkus JL, Pinkus GS, Burleson T, Due B, et al. Plasma cells in muscle in inclusion body myositis and polymyositis. Neurology 2005; Dec 13;65(11):1782–1787.

75. Pluk H, van Hoeve BJ, van Dooren SH, Stammen-Vogelzangs J, van der Heijden A, Schelhaas HJ, et al. Autoantibodies to cytosolic 5'-nucleotidase 1A in inclusion body myositis. Ann Neurol 2013;73: 397–407.

76. Larman HB, Salajegheh M, Nazareno R, Lam T, Sauld J, Steen H, et al. Cytosolic 5'-nucleotidase 1A autoimmunity in sporadic inclusion body myositis. Ann Neurol 2013;73:408–418.

77. Arahata K, Engel AG. Monoclonal antibody analysis of mononuclear cells in myopathies. I: Quantitation of subsets according to diagnosis and sites of accumulation and demonstration and counts of muscle fibers invaded by T cells. Ann Neurol 1984; Aug;16(2): 193–208.

78. Greenberg SA, Pinkus JL, Pinkus GS, Burleson T, Sanoudou D, Tawil R, et al. Interferon-alpha/beta-mediated innate immune mechanisms in dermatomyositis. Ann Neurol 2005; May;57(5):664–678.

79. Emslie-Smith AM, Engel AG. Microvascular changes in early and advanced dermatomyositis: a quantitative study. Ann Neurol 1990; Apr;27(4):343–356.

80. Kissel JT, Mendell JR, Rammohan KW. Microvascular deposition of complement membrane attack complex in dermatomyositis. N Engl J Med 1986; Feb 6;314(6):329–334.

81. Kissel JT, Halterman RK, Rammohan KW, Mendell JR. The relationship of complement-mediated microvasculopathy to the histologic features and clinical duration of disease in dermatomyositis. Arch Neurol 1991; Jan;48(1):26–30.

82. Engel AG, Arahata K. Monoclonal antibody analysis of mononuclear cells in myopathies. II: Phenotypes of autoinvasive cells in polymyositis and inclusion body myositis. Ann Neurol 1984; Aug;16(2):209–215.

83. Emslie-Smith AM, Arahata K, Engel AG. Major histocompatibility complex class I antigen expression, immunolocalization of interferon subtypes, and T cell-mediated cytotoxicity in myopathies. Hum Pathol 1989; Mar;20(3):224–231.

84. Fanin M, Angelini C. Muscle pathology in dysferlin deficiency. Neuropathol Appl Neurobiol 2002; Dec;28(6):461–470.

85. Jain A, Sharma MC, Sarkar C, Bhatia R, Singh S, Handa R. Major histocompatibility complex class I and II detection as a diagnostic tool in idiopathic inflammatory myopathies. Arch Pathol Lab Med 2007; Jul;131(7):1070–1076.

86. Dai TJ, Li W, Zhao QW, Zhao YY, Liu SP, Yan CZ. CD8/MHC-I complex is specific but not sensitive for the diagnosis of polymyositis. J Int Med Res 2010; May-Jun;38(3):1049–1059.

87. Rifai Z, Welle S, Kamp C, Thornton CA. Ragged red fibers in normal aging and inflammatory myopathy. Ann Neurol 1995; Jan;37(1):24–29.

88. Askanas V, Engel WK, Alvarez RB. Enhanced detection of congo-red-positive amyloid deposits in muscle fibers of inclusion body myositis and brain of Alzheimer's disease using fluorescence technique. Neurology 1993; Jun;43(6):1265–1267.

89. Mendell JR, Sahenk Z, Gales T, Paul L. Amyloid filaments in inclusion body myositis. Novel findings provide insight into nature of filaments. Arch Neurol 1991; Dec;48(12):1229–1234.

90. O'Hanlon TP, Miller FW. Genetic risk and protective factors for the idiopathic inflammatory myopathies. Curr Rheumatol Rep 2009; Aug;11(4):287–294.

91. O'Hanlon TP, Rider LG, Schiffenbauer A, Targoff IN, Malley K, Pandey JP, et al. Immunoglobulin gene polymorphisms are susceptibility factors in clinical and autoantibody subgroups of the idiopathic inflammatory myopathies. Arthritis Rheum 2008; Oct;58(10):3239–3246.

92. O'Hanlon TP, Carrick DM, Arnett FC, Reveille JD, Carrington M, Gao X, et al. Immunogenetic risk and protective factors for the idiopathic inflammatory myopathies: distinct HLA-A, -B, -Cw, -DRB1 and -DQA1 allelic profiles and motifs define clinicopathologic groups in caucasians. Medicine (Baltimore) 2005; Nov;84(6):338–349.

93. O'Hanlon TP, Carrick DM, Targoff IN, Arnett FC, Reveille JD, Carrington M, et al. Immunogenetic risk and protective factors for the idiopathic inflammatory myopathies: distinct HLA-A, -B, -Cw, -DRB1, and -DQA1 allelic profiles distinguish European American patients with different myositis autoantibodies. Medicine (Baltimore) 2006; Mar;85(2):111–127.

94. Hassan AB, Nikitina-Zake L, Sanjeevi CB, Lundberg IE, Padyukov L. Association of the proinflammatory haplotype (MICA5.1/TNF2/TNFa2/DRB1°03) with polymyositis and dermatomyositis. Arthritis Rheum 2004; Mar;50(3):1013–1015.

95. Chinoy H, Salway F, John S, Fertig N, Tait BD, Oddis CV, et al. Tumour necrosis factor-alpha single nucleotide polymorphisms are not independent of HLA class I in UK Caucasians with adult onset idiopathic inflammatory myopathies. Rheumatology (Oxford) 2007; Sep;46(9):1411–1416.

96. Pachman LM, Liotta-Davis MR, Hong DK, Kinsella TR, Mendez EP, Kinder JM, et al. TNFalpha-308A allele in juvenile dermatomyositis: association with increased production of tumor necrosis factor alpha, disease duration, and pathologic calcifications. Arthritis Rheum 2000; Oct;43(10):2368–2377.

97. Mamyrova G, O'Hanlon TP, Sillers L, Malley K, James-Newton L, Parks CG, et al. Cytokine gene polymorphisms as risk and severity factors for juvenile dermatomyositis. Arthritis Rheum 2008; Dec;58(12):3941–3950.

98. Werth VP, Callen JP, Ang G, Sullivan KE. Associations of tumor necrosis factor alpha and HLA polymorphisms with adult dermatomyositis: implications for a unique pathogenesis. J Invest Dermatol 2002; Sep;119(3):617–620.

99. Lutz J, Huwiler KG, Fedczyna T, Lechman TS, Crawford S, Kinsella TR, et al. Increased plasma thrombospondin-1 (TSP-1) levels are associated with the TNF alpha-308A allele in children with juvenile dermatomyositis. Clin Immunol 2002; Jun;103(3 Pt 1):260–263.

100. Pachman LM, Fedczyna TO, Lechman TS, Lutz J. Juvenile dermatomyositis: the association of the TNF alpha-308A allele and disease chronicity. Curr Rheumatol Rep 2001; Oct;3(5):379–386.

101. Werth VP, Zhang W, Dortzbach K, Sullivan K. Association of a promoter polymorphism of tumor necrosis factor-alpha with subacute cutaneous lupus erythematosus and distinct photoregulation of transcription. J Invest Dermatol 2000; Oct;115(4):726–730.

102. Greenberg SA, Amato AA. Uncertainties in the pathogenesis of adult dermatomyositis. Curr Opin Neurol 2004; Jun;17(3):359–364.

103. Salajegheh M, Kong SW, Pinkus JL, Walsh RJ, Liao A, Nazareno R, et al. Interferon-stimulated gene 15 (ISG15) conjugates proteins in dermatomyositis muscle with perifascicular atrophy. Ann Neurol 2010; Jan;67(1):53–63.

104. Walsh RJ, Kong SW, Yao Y, Jallal B, Kiener PA, Pinkus JL, et al. Type I interferon-inducible gene expression in blood is present and reflects disease activity in dermatomyositis and polymyositis. Arthritis Rheum 2007; Nov;56(11):3784–3792.

105. Baechler EC, Bauer JW, Slattery CA, Ortmann WA, Espe KJ, Novitzke J, et al. An interferon signature in the peripheral blood of dermatomyositis patients is associated with disease activity. Mol Med 2007; Jan-Feb;13(1–2):59–68.

106. Arnett FC, Targoff IN, Mimori T, Goldstein R, Warner NB, Reveille JD. Interrelationship of major histocompatibility complex class II alleles and autoantibodies in four ethnic groups with various forms of myositis. Arthritis Rheum 1996; Sep;39(9):1507–1518.

107. Garlepp MJ. Immunogenetics of inflammatory myopathies. Baillieres Clin Neurol 1993; Nov;2(3):579–597.

108. Chinoy H, Salway F, John S, Fertig N, Tait BD, Oddis CV, et al. Interferon-gamma and interleukin-4 gene polymorphisms in Caucasian idiopathic inflammatory myopathy patients in UK. Ann Rheum Dis 2007; Jul;66(7):970–973.

109. Goebels N, Michaelis D, Engelhardt M, Huber S, Bender A, Pongratz D, et al. Differential expression of perforin in muscle-infiltrating T cells in polymyositis and dermatomyositis. J Clin Invest 1996; Jun 15;97(12):2905–2910.

110. Nagaraju K, Raben N, Loeffler L, Parker T, Rochon PJ, Lee E, et al. Conditional up-regulation of MHC class I in skeletal muscle leads to self-sustaining autoimmune myositis and myositis-specific autoantibodies. Proc Natl Acad Sci U S A 2000; Aug 1;97(16):9209–9214.

111. Nagaraju K, Casciola-Rosen L, Lundberg I, Rawat R, Cutting S, Thapliyal R, et al. Activation of the endoplasmic reticulum stress response in autoimmune myositis: potential role in muscle fiber damage and dysfunction. Arthritis Rheum 2005; Jun;52(6):1824–1835.

112. Salomonsson S, Grundtman C, Zhang SJ, Lanner JT, Li C, Katz A, et al. Upregulation of MHC class I in transgenic mice results in reduced force-generating capacity in slow-twitch muscle. Muscle Nerve 2009; May;39(5):674–682.

113. Mammen AL, Gaudet D, Brisson D, Christopher-Stine L, Lloyd TE, Leffell MS, et al. Increased frequency of DRB1*11:01 in anti-HMG-CoA reductase-associated autoimmune myopathy. Arthritis Care Res (Hoboken) 2012; Aug;64(8): 1233–1237.

114. Werner J, Christopher-Stine L, Ghazarian SR, Pak KS, Kus JE, Daya NR, et al. Antibody levels correlate with creatine kinase levels and strength in anti-HMG-CoA reductase-associated autoimmune myopathy. Arthritis and Rheumatism 2012; Dec;64(12):4087–4093.

115. Benveniste O, Drouot L, Jouen F, Charuel JL, Bloch-Queyrat C, Behin A, et al. Correlation of anti-signal recognition particle autoantibody levels with creatine kinase activity in patients with necrotizing myopathy. Arthritis Rheum 2011; Jul;63(7):1961–1971.

116. Greenberg SA. Pathogenesis and therapy of inclusion body myositis. Curr Opin Neurol 2012; Oct;25(5): 630–639.

117. Bradshaw EM, Orihuela A, McArdel SL, Salajegheh M, Amato AA, Hafler DA, et al. A local antigen-driven humoral response is present in the inflammatory myopathies. J Immunol 2007; Jan 1;178(1): 547–556.

118. Barohn RJ, Amato AA, Sahenk Z, Kissel JT, Mendell JR. Inclusion body myositis: explanation for poor response to immunosuppressive therapy. Neurology 1995; Jul;45(7):1302–1304.

119. Parker KC, Kong SW, Walsh RJ, Salajegheh M, Moghadaszadeh B, et al. Fast-twitch sarcomeric and glycolytic enzyme protein loss in inclusion body myositis. Muscle Nerve 2009; Jun;39(6):739–753.

120. Parker KC, Walsh RJ, Salajegheh M, Amato AA, Krastins B, Sarracino DA, et al. Characterization of human skeletal muscle biopsy samples using shotgun proteomics. J Proteome Res 2009; Jul;8(7): 3265–3277.

121. Doppler K, Lindner A, Schutz W, Schutz M, Bornemann A. Gain and loss of extracellular

molecules in sporadic inclusion body myositis and polymyositis—a proteomics-based study. Brain Pathol 2012; Jan;22(1):32–40.

122. Chous S. Myxovirus-like structures in a case of human chronic polymyositis. Science 1967;158:1453–1455.

123. Yunis EJ, Samaha FJ. Inclusion body myositis. Lab Invest 1971; Sep;25(3):240–248.

124. Carpenter S. Inclusion body myositis, a review. J Neuropathol Exp Neurol 1996; Nov;55(11): 1105–1114.

125. Greenberg SA, Pinkus JL, Amato AA. Nuclear membrane proteins are present within rimmed vacuoles in inclusion-body myositis. Muscle Nerve 2006; Oct;34(4):406–416.

126. Salajegheh M, Pinkus JL, Taylor JP, Amato AA, Nazareno R, Baloh RH, et al. Sarcoplasmic redistribution of nuclear TDP-43 in inclusion body myositis. Muscle Nerve 2009; Jul;40(1):19–31.

127. Olive M, Janue A, Moreno D, Gamez J, Torrejon-Escribano B, Ferrer I. TAR DNA-binding protein 43 accumulation in protein aggregate myopathies. J Neuropathol Exp Neurol 2009; Mar;68(3): 262–273.

128. Weihl CC, Temiz P, Miller SE, Watts G, Smith C, Forman M, et al. TDP-43 accumulation in inclusion body myopathy muscle suggests a common pathogenic mechanism with frontotemporal dementia. J Neurol Neurosurg Psychiatry 2008; Oct;79(10): 1186–1189.

129. Kusters B, van Hoeve BJ, Schelhaas HJ, Ter Laak H, van Engelen BG, Lammens M. TDP-43 accumulation is common in myopathies with rimmed vacuoles. Acta Neuropathol 2009; Feb;117(2): 209–211.

130. Amato AA, Russell JA. Inflammatory Myopathies. Neuromuscular Disorders. 1st ed.McGraw Hill; 2008. p. 681.

131. Amato AA, Barohn RJ. Evaluation and treatment of inflammatory myopathies. J Neurol Neurosurg Psychiatry 2009; Oct;80(10):1060–1068.

132. Gordon PA, Winer JB, Hoogendijk JE, Choy EH. Immunosuppressant and immunomodulatory treatment for dermatomyositis and polymyositis. Cochrane Database Syst Rev 2012; Aug 15;8:CD003643.

133. Bohan A, Peter JB, Bowman RL, Pearson CM. Computer-assisted analysis of 153 patients with polymyositis and dermatomyositis. Medicine (Baltimore) 1977; Jul;56(4):255–286.

134. Tymms KE, Webb J. Dermatopolymyositis and other connective tissue diseases: a review of 105 cases. J Rheumatol 1985; Dec;12(6):1140–1148.

135. Cagnoli M, Marchesoni A, Tosi S. Combined steroid, methotrexate and chlorambucil therapy for steroid-resistant dermatomyositis. Clin Exp Rheumatol 1991; Nov-Dec;9(6):658–659.

136. Giannini M, Callen JP. Treatment of dermatomyositis with methotrexate and prednisone. Arch Dermatol 1979; Oct;115(10):1251–1252.

137. Miller LC, Sisson BA, Tucker LB, DeNardo BA, Schaller JG. Methotrexate treatment of recalcitrant childhood dermatomyositis. Arthritis Rheum 1992; Oct;35(10):1143–1149.

138. Joffe MM, Love LA, Leff RL, Fraser DD, Targoff IN, Hicks JE, et al. Drug therapy of the idiopathic inflammatory myopathies: predictors of response to prednisone, azathioprine, and methotrexate and

a comparison of their efficacy. Am J Med 1993; Apr;94(4):379–387.

139. Bunch TW, Worthington JW, Combs JJ, Ilstrup DM, Engel AG. Azathioprine with prednisone for poly-myositis. A controlled, clinical trial. Ann Intern Med 1980; Mar;92(3):365–369.

140. Bunch TW. Prednisone and azathioprine for poly-myositis: long-term followup. Arthritis Rheum 1981; Jan;24(1):45–48.

141. Kissel JT, Levy RJ, Mendell JR, Griggs RC. Azathioprine toxicity in neuromuscular disease. Neurology 1986; Jan;36(1):35–39.

142. Majithia V, Harisdangkul V. Mycophenolate mofetil (CellCept): an alternative therapy for autoimmune inflammatory myopathy. Rheumatology (Oxford) 2005; Mar;44(3):386–389.

143. Schneider C, Gold R, Schafers M, Toyka KV. Mycophenolate mofetil in the therapy of polymyositis associated with a polyautoimmune syndrome. Muscle Nerve 2002; Feb;25(2):286–288.

144. Tausche AK, Meurer M. Mycophenolate mofetil for dermatomyositis. Dermatology 2001;202(4): 341–343.

145. Rowin J, Amato AA, Deisher N, Cursio J, Meriggioli MN. Mycophenolate mofetil in dermatomyositis: Is it safe? Neurology 2006; Apr 25;66(8):1245–1247.

146. Wang DX, Shu XM, Tian XL, Chen F, Zu N, Ma L, et al. Intravenous immunoglobulin therapy in adult patients with polymyositis/dermatomyositis: a sys-tematic literature review. Clin Rheumatol 2012; May;31(5):801–806.

147. Dalakas MC, Illa I, Dambrosia JM, Soueidan SA, Stein DP, Otero C, et al. A controlled trial of high-dose intravenous immune globulin infusions as treatment for dermatomyositis. N Engl J Med 1993; Dec 30;329(27):1993–2000.

148. Levine TD. Rituximab in the treatment of dermato-myositis: an open-label pilot study. Arthritis Rheum 2005; Feb;52(2):601–607.

149. Mok CC, Ho LY, To CH. Rituximab for refrac-tory polymyositis: an open-label prospective study. J Rheumatol 2007; Sep;34(9):1864–1868.

150. Valiyil R, Casciola-Rosen L, Hong G, Mammen A, Christopher-Stine L. Rituximab therapy for myopathy associated with anti-signal recognition particle antibodies: a case series. Arthritis Care Res (Hoboken) 2010; Sep;62(9):1328–1334.

151. Oddis CV, Reed AM, Aggarwal R, Rider LG, Ascherman DP, Levesque MC, et al.; RIM Study Group. Rituximab in the treatment of refractory adult and juvenile dermatomyositis and adult poly-myositis: a randomized, placebo-phase trial. Arthritis Rheum. 2013;65:314–324.

152. Correia O, Polonia J, Nunes JP, Resende C, Delgado L. Severe acute form of adult dermatomyositis treated with cyclosporine. Int J Dermatol 1992; Jul;31(7):517–519.

153. Lueck CJ, Trend P, Swash M. Cyclosporin in the man-agement of polymyositis and dermatomyositis. J Neurol Neurosurg Psychiatry 1991; Nov;54(11): 1007–1008.

154. Mehregan DR, Su WP. Cyclosporine treatment for dermatomyositis/polymyositis. Cutis 1993; Jan;51(1): 59–61.

155. Pistoia V, Buoncompagni A, Scribanis R, Fasce L, Alpigiani G, Cordone G, et al. Cyclosporin A in the treatment of juvenile chronic arthritis and child-hood polymyositis-dermatomyositis. Results of a preliminary study. Clin Exp Rheumatol 1993; Mar-Apr;11(2):203–208.

156. Oddis CV, Sciurba FC, Elmagd KA, Starzl TE. Tacrolimus in refractory polymyositis with intersti-tial lung disease. Lancet 1999; May 22;353(9166): 1762–1763.

157. Hassan J, van der Net JJ, van Royen-Kerkhof A. Treatment of refractory juvenile dermatomyositis with tacrolimus. Clin Rheumatol 2008; Nov;27(11): 1469–1471.

158. Mitsui T, Kuroda Y, Kunishige M, Matsumoto T. Successful treatment with tacrolimus in a case of refractory dermatomyositis. Intern Med 2005; Nov;44(11):1197–1199.

159. Kono DH, Klashman DJ, Gilbert RC. Successful IV pulse cyclophosphamide in refractory PM in 3 patients with SLE. J Rheumatol 1990; Jul;17(7):982–983.

160. Leroy JP, Drosos AA, Yiannopoulos DI, Youinou P, Moutsopoulos HM. Intravenous pulse cyclophospha-mide therapy in myositis and Sjogren's syndrome. Arthritis Rheum 1990; Oct;33(10):1579–1581.

161. Niakan E, Pitner SE, Whitaker JN, Bertorini TE. Immunosuppressive agents in corticosteroid-refractory childhood dermatomyositis. Neurology 1980; Mar;30(3):286–291.

162. Cronin ME, Miller FW, Hicks JE, Dalakas M, Plotz PH. The failure of intravenous cyclophosphamide therapy in refractory idiopathic inflammatory myopa-thy. J Rheumatol 1989; Sep;16(9):1225–1228.

163. Fries JF, Sharp GC, McDevitt HO, Holman HR. Cyclophosphamide therapy in systemic lupus ery-thematosus and polymyositis. Arthritis Rheum 1973; Mar-Apr;16(2):154–162.

164. Hengstman GJ, van den Hoogen FH, Barrera P, Netea MG, Pieterse A, van de Putte LB, et al. Successful treatment of dermatomyositis and poly-myositis with anti-tumor-necrosis-factor-alpha: pre-liminary observations. Eur Neurol 2003;50(1):10–15.

165. Hengstman GJ, van den Hoogen FH, van Engelen BG. Treatment of dermatomyositis and polymyosi-tis with anti-tumor necrosis factor-alpha: long-term follow-up. Eur Neurol 2004;52(1):61–63.

166. Labioche I, Liozon E, Weschler B, Loustaud-Ratti V, Soria P, Vidal E. Refractory polymyositis respond-ing to infliximab: extended follow-up. Rheumatology (Oxford) 2004; Apr;43(4):531–532.

167. Korkmaz C, Temiz G, Cetinbas F, Buyukkidan B. Successful treatment of alveolar hypoventilation due to dermatomyositis with anti-tumour necro-sis factor-alpha. Rheumatology (Oxford) 2004; Jul;43(7):937–938.

168. Sprott H, Glatzel M, Michel BA. Treatment of myositis with etanercept (Enbrel), a recombinant human soluble fusion protein of TNF-alpha type II receptor and IgG1. Rheumatology (Oxford) 2004; Apr;43(4):524–526.

169. Efthimiou P, Schwartzman S, Kagen LJ. Possible role for tumour necrosis factor inhibitors in the treatment of resistant dermatomyositis and polymyositis: a ret-rospective study of eight patients. Ann Rheum Dis 2006; Sep;65(9):1233–1236.

170. Riley P, McCann LJ, Maillard SM, Woo P, Murray KJ, Pilkington CA. Effectiveness of infliximab in

the treatment of refractory juvenile dermatomyositis with calcinosis. Rheumatology (Oxford) 2008; Jun;47(6):877–880.

171. Dastmalchi M, Grundtman C, Alexanderson H, Mavragani CP, Einarsdottir H, Helmers SB, et al. A high incidence of disease flares in an open pilot study of infliximab in patients with refractory inflammatory myopathies. Ann Rheum Dis 2008; Dec;67(12):1670–1677.

172. Hengstman GJ, De Bleecker JL, Feist E, Vissing J, Denton CP, Manoussakis MN, et al. Open-label trial of anti-TNF-alpha in dermato- and polymyositis treated concomitantly with methotrexate. Eur Neurol 2008;59(3–4):159–163.

173. Muscle Study Group. A randomized, pilot trial of etanercept in dermatomyositis. Ann Neurol 2011; Sep;70(3):427–436.

174. Auerbach A, Fanburg-Smith JC, Wang G, Rushing EJ. Focal myositis: a clinicopathologic study of 115 cases of an intramuscular mass-like reactive process. Am J Surg Pathol 2009; Jul;33(7):1016–1024.

175. Caldwell CJ, Swash M, Van der Walt JD, Geddes JF. Focal myositis: a clinicopathological study. Neuromuscul Disord 1995; Jul;5(4):317–321.

176. Colding-Jorgensen E, Laursen H, Lauritzen M. Focal myositis of the thigh: report of two cases. Acta Neurol Scand 1993; Oct;88(4):289–292.

177. Heffner RR,Jr, Barron SA. Polymyositis beginning as a focal process. Arch Neurol 1981; Jul;38(7):439–442.

178. Moreno-Lugris C, Gonzalez-Gay MA, Sanchez-Andrade A, Blanco R, Basanta D, Ibanez D, et al. Magnetic resonance imaging: a useful technique in the diagnosis and follow up of focal myositis. Ann Rheum Dis 1996; Nov;55(11):856.

179. Moskovic E, Fisher C, Westbury G, Parsons C. Focal myositis, a benign inflammatory pseudotumour: CT appearances. Br J Radiol 1991; Jun;64(762): 489–493.

180. Binesh F, Taghipour S, Navabii H. Focal myositis of the thigh misdiagnosed radiologically as rhabdomyosarcoma. BMJ Case Rep 2011; Apr 1;2011:10.1136/bcr.12.2010.3574.

181. Nielsen M, Lundegaard C, Lund O. Prediction of MHC class II binding affinity using SMM-align, a novel stabilization matrix alignment method. BMC Bioinformatics 2007; Jul 4;8:238.

182. Kobayashi Y, Fujimoto T, Shiiki H, Kitaoka K, Murata K, Dohi K. Focal eosinophilic myositis. Clin Rheumatol 2001;20(5):369–371.

183. Layzer RB, Shearn MA, Satya-Murti S. Eosinophilic polymyositis. Ann Neurol 1977; Jan;1(1):65–71.

184. Moore PM, Harley JB, Fauci AS. Neurologic dysfunction in the idiopathic hypereosinophilic syndrome. Ann Intern Med 1985; Jan;102(1):109–114.

185. Murata K, Sugie K, Takamure M, Fujimoto T, Ueno S. Eosinophilic major basic protein and interleukin-5 in eosinophilic myositis. Eur J Neurol 2003; Jan;10(1):35–38.

186. Serratrice G, Pellissier JF, Roux H, Quilichini P. Fasciitis, perimyositis, myositis, polymyositis, and eosinophilia. Muscle Nerve 1990; May;13(5):385–395.

187. Serratrice G, Pellissier JF, Cros D, Gastaut JL, Brindisi G. Relapsing eosinophilic perimyositis. J Rheumatol 1980; Mar-Apr;7(2):199–205.

188. Dunand M, Lobrinus JA, Spertini O, Kuntzer T. Eosinophilic perimyositis as the presenting feature of a monoclonal T-cell expansion. Muscle Nerve 2005; May;31(5):646–651.

189. Simon HU, Plotz SG, Simon D, Dummer R, Blaser K. Clinical and immunological features of patients with interleukin-5-producing T cell clones and eosinophilia. Int Arch Allergy Immunol 2001; Jan-Mar;124(1–3):242–245.

190. Lakhanpal S, Ginsburg WW, Michet CJ, Doyle JA, Moore SB. Eosinophilic fasciitis: clinical spectrum and therapeutic response in 52 cases. Semin Arthritis Rheum 1988; May;17(4):221–231.

191. Shulman LE. Diffuse fasciitis with eosinophilia: a new syndrome? Trans Assoc Am Physicians 1975;88: 70–86.

192. Baumeister SK, Todorovic S, Milic-Rasic V, Dekomien G, Lochmuller H, Walter MC. Eosinophilic myositis as presenting symptom in gamma-sarcoglycanopathy. Neuromuscul Disord 2009; Feb;19(2):167–171.

193. Krahn M, Lopez de Munain A, Streichenberger N, Bernard R, Pecheux C, Testard H, et al. CAPN3 mutations in patients with idiopathic eosinophilic myositis. Ann Neurol 2006; Jun;59(6):905–911.

194. Pascuzzi RM, Roos KL, Phillips LH,2nd. Granulomatous inflammatory myopathy associated with myasthenia gravis. A case report and review of the literature. Arch Neurol 1986; Jun;43(6):621–623.

195. Namba T, Brunner NG, Grob D. Idiopathic giant cell polymyositis. Report of a case and review of the syndrome. Arch Neurol 1974; Jul;31(1):27–30.

196. Mozaffar T, Lopate G, Pestronk A. Clinical correlates of granulomas in muscle. J Neurol 1998; Aug;245(8):519–524.

197. Silverstein A, Siltzbach LE. Muscle involvement in sarcoidosis. Asymptomatic, myositis, and myopathy. Arch Neurol 1969; Sep;21(3):235–241.

198. Stjernberg N, Cajander S, Truedsson H, Uddenfeldt P. Muscle involvement in sarcoidosis. Acta Med Scand 1981;209(3):213–216.

199. Le Roux K, Streichenberger N, Vial C, Petiot P, Feasson L, Bouhour F, et al. Granulomatous myositis: a clinical study of thirteen cases. Muscle Nerve 2007; Feb;35(2):171–177.

200. Authier FJ, Chariot P, Gherardi RK. Skeletal muscle involvement in human immunodeficiency virus (HIV)-infected patients in the era of highly active antiretroviral therapy (HAART). Muscle Nerve 2005; Sep;32(3):247–260.

201. Cupler EJ, Leon-Monzon M, Miller J, Semino-Mora C, Anderson TL, Dalakas MC. Inclusion body myositis in HIV-1 and HTLV-1 infected patients. Brain 1996; Dec;119(Pt 6):1887–1893.

202. Dalakas MC, Rakocevic G, Shatunov A, Goldfarb L, Raju R, Salajegheh M. Inclusion body myositis with human immunodeficiency virus infection: four cases with clonal expansion of viral-specific T cells. Ann Neurol 2007; May;61(5):466–475.

203. Loutfy MR, Sheehan NL, Goodhew JE, Walmsley SL. Inclusion body myositis: another possible manifestation of antiretroviral-associated mitochondrial toxicity. AIDS 2003; May 23;17(8):1266–1267.

204. Johnson RW, Williams FM, Kazi S, Dimachkie MM, Reveille JD. Human immunodeficiency virus-associated polymyositis: a longitudinal study of outcome. Arthritis Rheum 2003; Apr 15;49(2): 172–178.

205. Matsuura E, Umehara F, Nose H, Higuchi I, Matsuoka E, Izumi K, et al. Inclusion body myositis associated with human T-lymphotropic virus-type I infection: eleven patients from an endemic area in Japan. J Neuropathol Exp Neurol 2008; Jan;67(1): 41–49.

206. Saito M, Higuchi I, Saito A, Izumo S, Usuku K, Bangham CR, et al. Molecular analysis of T cell clonotypes in muscle-infiltrating lymphocytes from patients with human T lymphotropic virus type 1 polymyositis. J Infect Dis 2002; Nov 1;186(9):1231–1241.

207. Caldwell CJ, Barrett WY, Breuer J, Farmer SF, Swash M. HTLV-1 polymyositis. Neuromuscul Disord 1996; May;6(3):151–154.

208. Evans BK, Gore I, Harrell LE, Arnold T, Oh SJ. HTLV-I-associated myelopathy and polymyositis in a US native. Neurology 1989; Dec;39(12):1572–1575.

209. Morgan OS, Rodgers-Johnson P, Mora C, Char G. HTLV-1 and polymyositis in Jamaica. Lancet 1989; Nov 18;2(8673):1184–1187.

210. Mejlszenkier JD, Safran AP, Healy JJ, Embree L, Ouellette EM. The myositis of influenza. Arch Neurol 1973; Dec;29(6):441–443.

211. Middleton PJ, Alexander RM, Szymanski MT. Severe myositis during recovery from influenza. Lancet 1970; Sep 12;2(7672):533–535.

212. Minow RA, Gorbach S, Johnson BL,Jr, Dornfeld L. Myoglobinuria associated with influenza A infection. Ann Intern Med 1974; Mar;80(3):359–361.

213. Morgensen JL. Myoglobinuria and renal failure associated with influenza. Ann Intern Med 1974; Mar;80(3):362–363.

214. Ruff RL, Secrist D. Viral studies in benign acute childhood myositis. Arch Neurol 1982; May;39(5): 261–263.

215. Agyeman P, Duppenthaler A, Heininger U, Aebi C. Influenza-associated myositis in children. Infection 2004; Aug;32(4):199–203.

216. Lorenzoni PJ, Kay CS, Scola RH, Carraro H,Jr, Werneck LC. Muscle biopsy features in critical ill patients with 2009 influenza A (H1N1) virus infection. Arq Neuropsiquiatr 2012; May;70(5):325–329.

217. Antony SJ, Kernodle DS. Nontropical pyomyositis in patients with AIDS. J Natl Med Assoc 1996; Sep;88(9):565–569.

218. Rodgers WB, Yodlowski ML, Mintzer CM. Pyomyositis in patients who have the human immunodeficiency virus. Case report and review of the literature. J Bone Joint Surg Am 1993; Apr;75(4):588–592.

219. Hsueh PR, Hsiue TR, Hsieh WC. Pyomyositis in intravenous drug abusers: report of a unique case and review of the literature. Clin Infect Dis 1996; May;22(5):858–860.

220. Chiedozi LC. Pyomyositis. Review of 205 cases in 112 patients. Am J Surg 1979; Feb;137(2):255–259.

221. Akman I, Ostrov B, Varma BK, Keenan G. Pyomyositis: report of three patients and review of the literature. Clin Pediatr (Phila) 1996; Aug;35(8): 397–401.

222. O'Neill DS, Baquis G, Moral L. Infectious myositis. A tropical disease steals out of its zone. Postgrad Med 1996; Aug;100(2):193,4,199–200.

223. Holmgren AR, Matteson EL. Lyme myositis. Arthritis Rheum 2006; Aug;54(8):2697–2700.

224. Reimers CD, de Koning J, Neubert U, Preac-Mursic V, Koster JG, Muller-Felber W, et al. Borrelia burgdorferi myositis: report of eight patients. J Neurol 1993; May;240(5):278–283.

225. Muller-Felber W, Reimers CD, de Koning J, Fischer P, Pilz A, Pongratz DE. Myositis in Lyme borreliosis: an immunohistochemical study of seven patients. J Neurol Sci 1993; Sep;118(2):207–212.

226. Atlas E, Novak SN, Duray PH, Steere AC. Lyme myositis: muscle invasion by Borrelia burgdorferi. Ann Intern Med 1988; Aug 1;109(3):245–246.

227. Jeandel C, Perret C, Blain H, Jouanny P, Penin F, Laurain MC. Rhabdomyolysis with acute renal failure due to Borrelia burgdorferi. J Intern Med 1994; Feb;235(2):191–192.

228. Seidenberg KB, Leib ML. Orbital myositis with Lyme disease. Am J Ophthalmol 1990; Jan 15;109(1):13–16.

229. Fatterpekar GM, Gottesman RI, Sacher M, Som PM. Orbital Lyme disease: MR imaging before and after treatment: case report. AJNR Am J Neuroradiol 2002; Apr;23(4):657–659.

230. Schoenen J, Sianard-Gainko J, Carpentier M, Reznik M. Myositis during Borrelia burgdorferi infection (Lyme disease). J Neurol Neurosurg Psychiatry 1989; Aug;52(8):1002–1005.

231. El-Beshbishi SN, Ahmed NN, Mostafa SH, El-Ganainy GA. Parasitic infections and myositis. Parasitol Res 2012; Jan;110(1):1–18.

232. Gross B, Ochoa J. Trichinosis: clinical report and histochemistry of muscle. Muscle Nerve 1979; Sep-Oct;2(5):394–398.

233. Davis MJ, Cilo M, Plaitakis A, Yahr MD. Trichinosis: severe myopathic involvement with recovery. Neurology 1976; Jan;26(1):37–40.

234. Murrell KD, Pozio E. Worldwide occurrence and impact of human trichinellosis, 1986-2009. Emerg Infect Dis 2011; Dec;17(12):2194–2202.

235. Akar S, Gurler O, Pozio E, Onen F, Sari I, Gerceker E, et al. Frequency and severity of musculoskeletal symptoms in humans during an outbreak of trichinellosis caused by Trichinella britovi. J Parasitol 2007; Apr;93(2):341–344.

236. Abdelwahab IF, Klein MJ, Hermann G, Abdul-Quader M. Solitary cysticercosis of the biceps/brachii in a vegetarian: a rare and unusual pseudotumor. Skeletal Radiol 2003; Jul;32(7):424–428.

237. Nagaraj C, Singh S, Joshi A, Trikha V. Cysticercosis of biceps brachii: a rare cause of posterior interosseous nerve syndrome. Joint Bone Spine 2008; Mar;75(2): 219–221.

238. Rajwanshi A, Radhika S, Das A, Jayaram N, Banerjee CK. Fine-needle aspiration cytology in the diagnosis of cysticercosis presenting as palpable nodules. Diagn Cytopathol 1991;7(5):517–519.

239. Rowland LP, Greer M. Toxoplasmic polymyositis. Neurology 1961; May;11:367–370.

240. Pollock JL. Toxoplasmosis appearing to be dermatomyositis. Arch Dermatol 1979; Jun;115(6):736–737.

241. Gherardi R, Baudrimont M, Lionnet F, Salord JM, Duvivier C, Michon C, et al. Skeletal muscle toxoplasmosis in patients with acquired immunodeficiency syndrome: a clinical and pathological study. Ann Neurol 1992; Oct;32(4):535–542.

Chapter 11

Myopathies of Systemic Disease and Toxic Myopathies

Michael K. Hehir

Many systemic diseases cause muscle weakness. The management of these disorders varies according to the organ system affected. The myopathies of systemic disease should be distinguished from "primary" disorders of muscle because diagnosis and treatment are directed at the underlying disease; studies of muscle itself are often counterproductive. To avoid simply reiterating information from standard textbooks of medicine, our approach is as follows: (1) to emphasize important points in recognizing clinical manifestations of myopathies in systemic diseases, (2) to note some situations where a myopathy may be suspected but another diagnosis is more likely, and (3) to provide insight into treatment strategies.

There is a major distinction between the constitutional symptoms of fatigue and weakness characterizing common conditions such as chronic heart failure, lung disease, liver disease, and renal disease, and the readily demonstrable muscle weakness justifying the term *myopathy*. Any serious systemic illness causing inactivity and poor nutrition may result in moderate weakness, but patients with such disorders usually demonstrate remarkably good manual muscle strength, muscle function, and motor testing, albeit briefly.

ENDOCRINE MYOPATHIES

Many endocrine disorders are associated with muscle disease.[56,62] However, muscle weakness is infrequently the chief complaint of patients with endocrinopathies.[62] It is important to recognize associated weaknesses, because treatment of the underlying endocrine disorder can improve weakness.

Thyroid Disorders

Myopathies occur in patients with both hyper- and hypothyroidism. In addition to myopathy, myasthenia gravis and thyrotoxic periodic paralysis (discussed in chapter 9) occur in patients with hyperthyroidism.[8,56,62] Graves' ophthalmopathy must also be distinguished from primary ocular MG in the neurology clinic.[62]

HYPERTHYROID MYOPATHY

Thyrotoxicosis can be caused by Graves' disease, by toxic goiter, and occasionally by exogenous thyroid ingestion.[42,56] Neuromuscular disorders occur in up to 67% of patients with hyperthyroidism.[35] However, patients seldom present with a chief complaint of weakness.[35,56] Thyrotoxicosis is most common in women in the fifth decade.[42] The old adage, "motor signs before motor symptoms" applies here. Examination is required, even in patients with major loss of strength.

Clinical Presentation

Patients with thyrotoxicosis often have mild to moderate proximal limb-girdle muscle weakness.[8,38,56,62] Questioning and physical exam should be performed to screen for myopathy in patients with symptoms of hyperthyroidism or known hyperthyroidism. Patients typically describe difficulty rising from a low chair, climbing stairs, or performing activities overhead.[62] Fatigue, muscle pain, and cramps are described in up to 10% of these patients.[35] Respiratory weakness[62] and rhabdomyolysis[75] are rare; rhabdomyolysis may be more common with severe thyrotoxicosis.[8,75] Concurrent MG should be suspected in patients presenting with acute respiratory dysfunction.[56,62]

Physical exam typically reveals mild to moderate weakness (usually MRC grade 4).[35,38,56] Reflexes are often brisk[38,56,62]; some patients also have concurrent tremor.[56] General physical exam may uncover other signs of hyperthyroidism such as tachycardia, atrial fibrillation, brittle nails, goiter, and warm, thin skin.[42]

Diagnosis

Serum CK is typically normal or mildly elevated.[35,62] Free T4 and in some cases T3 levels are elevated, whereas TSH levels are low.[35,56,62] Free T4 levels are typically higher in hyperthyroid patients with weakness than in those with normal strength.[35] EMG is typically normal although rarely patients may show myopathic changes (low-amplitude, short-duration motor units with early recruitment).[35,97] Increased spontaneous activity, fibrillation potentials, and positive waves are uncommon[38,97] Muscle biopsy may be normal or show nonspecific changes, including muscle fiber atrophy, variability in fiber size, increased internal nuclei, scattered necrotic fibers, fatty infiltrate, and decreased glycogen.[38]

Pathology

Although the pathophysiology of thyrotoxic myopathy is unknown, enhanced muscle catabolism due to increased mitochondrial activity and glycogen/ATP depletion are postulated as mechanisms for myopathy/weakness.[8,38] MG observed in these patients is likely the result of autoimmune disease clustering in patients predisposed to autoimmune pathology rather than thyroid hormone exerting a direct effect at the neuromuscular junction.[62]

Treatment/Prognosis

Treatment of hyperthyroidism typically resolves weakness and EMG changes within 3 to 4 months of treatment initiation.[35,97] Resistance training at least twice per week may accelerate recovery of strength in these patients.[16]

GRAVES' OPHTHALMOPATHY

Graves' disease is defined by hyperthyroid goiter, ophthalmopathy, and dermopathy.[56] Patients with Graves' ophthalmopathy typically present with diplopia and associated proptosis. Physical exam reveals proptosis and dysconjugate gaze particularly with upward and lateral gaze.[62] Late corneal and optic nerve involvement can result in vision loss.[56] Ophthalmopathy is the result of inflammatory infiltrate of orbital contents and enlargement of extraocular muscles.[56,62] T4/T3 levels may be high and TSH low in these patients. Orbital MRI and ultrasound can demonstrate enlargement of extraocular muscles and aid in diagnosis.[68,73,115] Graves' ophthalmopathy can occur in euthyroid patients; ancillary imaging studies may be necessary to make the diagnosis.[18,62] MG should be excluded in all patients in whom Graves' ophthalmopathy is considered.

Treatment of Graves' ophthalmopathy typically requires immunosuppression with prednisone.[56] Severe cases may require surgery to preserve vision.[56,62]

HYPOTHYROID MYOPATHY

Thyroid deficiency is typically the result of posttraumatic thyroid ablation or autoimmune thyroiditis.[56] Constitutional symptoms (e.g., alopecia, weight gain, cold intolerance, mental slowing, etc.) are most common. Rare cases present with neuromuscular complaints but many patients with hypothyroidism have symptoms and signs of neuromuscular involvement if evaluated carefully.[8,35,56,62]

Clinical Presentation

Hypothyroid-associated myopathy typically presents in a subacute to chronic timeframe; on average symptoms may be present for 1 year prior to recognition in clinic.[35] Commonly reported neuromuscular symptoms of hypothyroidism include proximal weakness, myalgias, muscle stiffness, and cramps.[35,56,62,63] Manual muscle testing rarely exceeds MRC grade 4 weakness; neck flexors, proximal arms, and pelvic girdle muscles are most involved.[35] Delayed relaxation of tendon reflexes is commonly observed.[62,63] Accentuated mounding of muscle with percussion (myoedema) can be elicited.[56,62,63] A length-dependent, sensory-predominant polyneuropathy also occurs in up to 40% of these patients.[35]

Diagnosis

Patients show the expected pattern of thyroid hormone levels with low T3/T4 and associated elevation of TSH.[56,63] Mild CK elevations, rarely much above 1,000 IU/L, are reported.[35,63] Levels of T3/T4 and CK do not correlate well with the presence or absence of weakness.[35,62] Extremely low levels of T4 (< 20 nmol/L) were associated with increased likelihood of delayed ankle-jerk reflex relation and weakness in one study.[63]

EMG is typically normal but may show myopathic changes (short-duration, low-amplitude motor units with early recruitment) in about 30% of patients.[35,56] Abnormal muscle spontaneous activity (fibrillations and positive waves) is rare and may be associated with concurrent hypothyroid-associated polyneuropathy.[35,56]

Pathology

Lack of thyroid hormone results in slowed metabolic function across many organ systems.[56] Reduced anaerobic and aerobic mitochondrial metabolism with reduction in ATP may account for neuromuscular pathology.[8] Muscle histology can be normal. Nonspecific myopathic findings can be observed, including type 1 fiber predominance, type 2 fiber atrophy, fiber hypertrophy, increased internal nuclei, glycogen accumulation, and mitochondrial abnormalities.[8,40] One case of minicore findings on light microscopy with associated glycogen/lipid accumulation and disarrangement of myofibrils on electron microscopy was reported.[40]

Treatment/Prognosis

The majority of patients improve within 5 to 6 months of initiating thyroid replacement therapy.[35,56,62] Weakness persists after 1 year of thyroid replacement in 10% to 20% of patients.[35]

Parathyroid Disorders

Myopathies are associated with primary and secondary hyperparathyroidism, metabolic bone disease, and hypoparathyroidism. Parathyroid hormone is involved in regulation of calcium and phosphate levels by increasing bone resorption, stimulating conversion of 25-hydroxyvitamin D to 1,25-dihydroxyvitamin D, and increasing renal calcium absorption and phosphate excretion.[8,103]

HYPERPARATHYROID, OSTEOMALACIA, AND MYOPATHY

Primary hyperparathyroidism caused by pituitary adenoma and secondary hyperparathyroidism is typically observed in the setting of chronic renal failure. The presentation of both conditions in muscle is similar, with myopathy reported in 25% to 80% of patients with hyperparathyroidism.[95,103]

Primary Hyperparathyroidism

Clinical Presentation. Patients typically develop fatigue, symmetric proximal upper and lower extremity weakness, muscle atrophy, and muscle stiffness.[95,103] Lower extremity muscles are preferentially involved.[95] Brisk reflexes are typical.[62,95,103] Rare cases of isolated dropped head syndrome are also described.[11,107] Some patients are also described to develop small- and large-fiber sensory loss.[95]

Diagnosis. Serum CK levels are typically normal.[62,103] Increased parathyroid hormone (PTH) is observed with associated hypercalcemia, hypophosphatemia, and elevated 1,25 dihydroxyvitamin D.[62,103] The degree of weakness does not correlate with serum calcium concentration.[62]

EMG typically shows myopathic motor units (low-amplitude, short-duration motor units with early recruitment) without abnormal spontaneous activity (fibrillations and positive waves).[95,103] Neuropathic EMG changes have been observed in some patients with associated normal nerve conduction studies, raising suspicion for anterior horn cell involvement.[95]

Pathology. Type II fiber atrophy is the most common finding on muscle biopsy.[62,95,103] Atrophy of both fiber types and changes suggestive of denervation may also be observed.[95]

The exact mechanism of hyperparathyroid myopathy is unknown. It is postulated that elevated PTH stimulates protein degradation in skeletal muscle through raising intracellular levels of calcium, which activate intracellular proteases.[103] Elevated PTH may also reduce calcium sensitivity of the calcium binding subunit on troponin.[103]

Treatment. Treatment is directed toward the primary cause of hyperparathyroidism. Parathyroidectomy results in resolution of weakness in the majority of cases.[21,95] Cinacalcet, a calcimimetic drug typically employed in secondary hyperparathyroidism, reversed weakness in one case.[107]

HYPERPARATHYRODISM, ALS, AND MYOTONIC DYSTROPHY

Concurrent cases of motor neuron disease and hyperparathyroidism have been described.[95] Despite treatment for hyperparathyroidism, these cases do not improve, which suggests that these conditions are separate entities.[57]

Concurrent cases of myotonic dystrophy and primary hyperparathyroidism have also been reported.[12,31,85,87] Although clinically separate syndromes, in two cases patients experienced some improvement in strength following parathyroidectomy.[85,87] It is important to screen patients with muscular dystrophy for reversible causes of weakness.

SECONDARY HYPERPARATHYROIDISM AND OSTEOMALACIA

Patients with chronic renal failure develop secondary hyperparathyroidism through reduction of 1,25 dihydroxyvitamin D conversion. The clinical presentation of myopathy associated with secondary hyperparathyroidism and osteomalacia is similar to that observed in primary hyperparathyroidism.[77,103,113] Weakness occurs in 50% to 80% of these patients.[77,103,104] EMG is typically myopathic.[103] CK is normal; PTH is high with associated low or normal serum calcium, low serum phosphate, and low 25 dihydroxyvitamin D levels.[8,103] Type II muscle fiber atrophy is the most common muscle biopsy finding.[77] Patients may improve with subtotal parathyroidectomy and vitamin D supplementation.[3,77,103]

HYPOPARATHYROID MYOPATHY

Clinical Presentation

Hypoparathyroidism is associated with many conditions: neck radiation, neck surgery, disease of parathyroid gland, induced by medication, autoimmune disease, and altered levels of magnesium.[24] A true myopathy is rare in hypoparathyroidism.[67,121] The most typical presentation is with tetany; patients describe numbness, carpal-pedal spasms, and diffuse muscle cramping from peripheral nerve hyperexcitability.[8,103,121] Chovstek's sign and Trousseau's sign can be observed.[8,103,121] Peripheral nerve hyperexcitability is related to low serum calcium levels, which moves resting membrane potential closer to threshold. This reduces the current required to elicit an action potential.[8,103]

Diagnosis

Fixed proximal weakness is rare in hypoparathyroidism; patients also show signs of tetany.[67,121] Labs show elevated serum CK, low PTH, low calcium, and high phosphate.[67,121] EMG is normal.[121]

Treatment

Treatment with calcium and vitamin D supplementation typically reverses both peripheral nerve hyperexcitability and muscle weakness.[8,67,103,121] Treatment with magnesium may be needed in patients with concurrent hypomagnesemia.[103]

Adrenal Disorders

CUSHING'S DISEASE

Excess levels of glucocorticoids from pituitary or adrenal tumors and through exogenous administration may cause myopathy. Myopathy due to exogenous administration of glucocorticoids is discussed in the Toxin- and Medication-Associated Myopathies section.

The insidious onset of muscle weakness occurs in 50% to 80% of patients with Cushing's disease.[103] Weakness and atrophy of proximal upper and lower extremities are typical.[8,62,103] Ocular, bulbar, and distal extremity muscles are spared.[8,62,103] Other signs of glucocorticoid excess such as increased adipose tissue and hyperpigmentation are also observed.[8,103]

Diagnosis

Serum CK is normal.[8,62,103] EMG is also typically normal; myopathic motor units (low-amplitude, short-duration motor units with early recruitment) in the absence of fibrillations and positive waves are rarely observed.[103]

Pathology

Muscle biopsy reveals selective atrophy of type 2 muscle fibers.[8,62,103] Accumulation of lipid and mitochondrial changes have been described on electron microscopy.[62,103] Although not fully understood, glucocorticoids may exert their effect on muscle by impairing muscle protein and carbohydrate metabolism as well as by accelerating protein degradation.[103]

Treatment/Prognosis

Recovery is expected within months of removing excess glucocorticoids.[62,103] Surgical resection of pituitary or adrenal mass is often required.[8,103] As discussed under Toxin- and Medication-Related Myopathies, corticosteroids should be tapered in patients with exogenous steroid myopathy.

ADRENAL INSUFFICIENCY

Addison's disease may be accompanied by weakness and generalized fatigue.[8,62] Weakness is likely related to electrolyte abnormalities, particularly hyperkalemia[8,60] rather than a primary myopathic process. Serum CK, EMG, and muscle biopsy are normal.[8] Treatment is corticosteroid replacement.[62]

Diabetes

Diabetes is a common cause of peripheral nervous system dysfunction primarily affecting nerve roots, nerve plexus, and peripheral nerve. Primary diabetic disease of muscle is rare. Painless proximal weakness in the diabetic patient should suggest a coincidental disorder (e.g., ALS, chronic inflammatory demyelinating neuropathy). Diabetic muscle infarction is a cause of proximal lower extremity weakness and pain. The primary differential diagnosis is diabetic lumbosacral radiculoplexus neuropathy (DLRPN, or diabetic amyotrophy).[36] DLRPN is a monophasic microvasculitis of nerve roots/plexus and peripheral nerve in the setting of diabetes that has recently been diagnosed or is very poorly controlled.[36] Patients report the acute onset of proximal and distal asymmetric lower extremity weakness and pain. There is often associated weight loss.[36] Additional diagnostic possibilities include infection, muscle neoplasm, deep vein thrombosis, and inflammatory myopathy.[48,119]

DIABETIC MUSCLE INFARCTION

Diabetic muscle infarction is a rare complication of poorly controlled diabetes. It is more common in women and insulin-dependent diabetes.[14,48,119]

Clinical Presentation

Patients develop the acute onset of unilateral pain, swelling, and reduced range of motion in the thigh.[119] A palpable mass is common.[119] Measurement of thigh circumference reveals increased size of the affected extremity. Range of motion is typically limited rather than frank weakness.[119]

Diagnosis

Serum CK is normal in 75% of cases.[119] EMG can exclude other diagnoses, primarily DLRPN. MRI is the most useful diagnostic technique. Fluid-sensitive fat-suppressed T2 imaging shows high signal intensity, and T1 imaging shows isointense/hypointense signal consistent with edema.[48] Post-gadolinium T1 imaging shows heterogeneous mass-like and peripheral muscle enhancement and areas of diminished or absent enhancement.[48] Ultrasound can be used to exclude DVT. Well-marginated hypoechoic intramuscular lesions may be observed.[48] CT is not as useful to evaluate soft tissue.

Pathology

Muscle biopsy findings are varied and include focal necrosis, perivascular lymphocytic cuffing, hemorrhage, edema, interstitial fibrosis, and proliferation of small vessels in fibrous tissue.[119] Large- and small-vessel atherosclerosis, microvascular disease, and microangiopathy have been proposed as the etiology of diabetic muscle infarction. Vascular findings are not observed in many cases and the true pathogenesis is not understood.[14]

Treatment/Prognosis

Treatment is primarily supportive because in the majority of cases spontaneous resolution occurs. In rare instances the disorder recurs.[14,48,119]

AMYLOID MYOPATHY

Primary systemic amyloidosis results in organ dysfunction through the deposition of amyloid light-chain immunoglobulins. The common manifestations of amyloidosis include nephrotic syndrome, peripheral and autonomic neuropathy, cardiomyopathy, and hepatomegaly.[61,102] Amyloid myopathy is a rare entity and the report of muscle weakness is only infrequently the presenting symptom of primary amyloidosis.[20] Age of onset ranges from 25 to 90 years (mean = 60 years).[20]

Clinical Presentation

Patients with amyloid myopathy typically report progressive weakness of neck, shoulder, and thigh muscles resulting in dysfunction with activities overhead, ascending/descending stairs, and rising from a low chair.[47] Bulbar muscles, respiratory muscles, and distal extremity muscles can be involved.[20] Macroglossia and muscle pseudohypertrophy are classically observed.[20,100] Muscle atrophy is also commonly observed.[47] A case of isolated axial amyloid myopathy with camptocormia (bent spine syndrome) has been described.[44]

Diagnosis

Serum CK is often normal but can be as high as 15,000 IU/L.[20,47] Both lambda and kappa light chains can be observed in serum or urine.[47] Some cases do not show a monoclonal protein. Measurement of serum protein electrophoresis, serum immunofixation, and serum/urine light chains are helpful for diagnosis.

The majority of patients have abnormal nerve conduction studies: Low tibial or peroneal compound motor unit action potentials are most common.[102] EMG typically reveals increased spontaneous activity (fibrillations/ positive waves) in at least one muscle; paraspinal and gluteus medius are most commonly abnormal.[102] Myopathic motor units (low-amplitude, short-duration motor units with early recruitment) are typical in proximal upper and lower extremity muscles.[102]

Many patients have concurrent involvement of myocardium. Echocardiogram demonstrates a concentric or restrictive cardiomyopathy; in some cases, a hyperrefractory or speckled pattern can be observed.[20] All patients with known or suspected amyloidosis should have both a clinical and diagnostic cardiology evaluation.

Pathology

Amyloid deposition in tissue can be observed in abdominal fat pad, skin, peripheral nerve, and muscle. Muscle biopsy typically shows a nonspecific myopathic pattern including variability in fiber size (mixed atrophic and hypertrophic fibers), necrotic and regenerating fibers, and increased internal nuclei.[8] Superimposed changes of denervation can also be observed if there is a concurrent peripheral neuropathy. Congo red staining with the use of polarized light or fluorescent optics reveals amyloid deposition surrounding arterioles and muscle fibers[20] (Figure 11–1). Amyloid deposits will show the classic apple-green birefringence with this method. Congo red staining is not part of the typical battery of stains performed on muscle biopsies in many labs. In one series, amyloid myopathy was missed on initial muscle biopsy in 50% of cases; Congo red stain of the initial biopsy or muscle biopsy at autopsy later showed amyloid deposition.[20] The exact mechanism of muscle dysfunction in the setting of amyloid deposition is unknown.

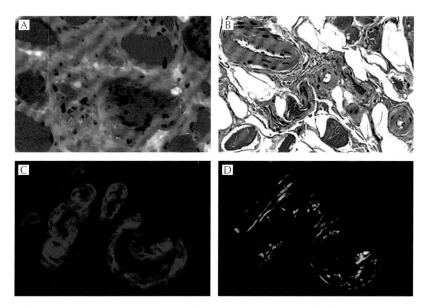

Figure 11–1. Muscle biopsies of amyloid myopathy. (A) Hematoxylin and eosin (H&E)–stained transverse cryosection of skeletal muscle showing peripheral replacement of cytoarchitecture with basophilic granular material and a preserved core ringed with nuclei in some fibers; original magnification × 400. (B) Paraffin-embedded H&E-stained transverse sections reveal subtle thickening of perimysial blood vessels; original magnification × 400. (C) Congo red–stained cryosections viewed under rhodamine fluorescent optics demonstrates marked congophilia of blood vessel walls; original magnification × 200. (D) Same blood vessel and stain as in panel (C) viewed with polarized light revealing the characteristic apple-green birefringence of amyloid protein; original magnification × 200. Reproduced with permission from Chapin JE, Kornfeld M, Harris A. Amyloid myopathy: characteristic features of a still underdiagnosed disease. Muscle and Nerve. 2005;31: 266–272.

Treatment/Prognosis

The prognosis of amyloid myopathy, as in other forms of amyloidosis, is poor. Mean survival from onset of symptoms is 22 months.[20] Some centers are pursuing various chemotherapy regimens to slow progression of disease; their utility in amyloid myopathy is unknown.

MYOPATHY AND ELECTROLYTE ABNORMALITIES

Electrolyte derangements primarily of potassium, phosphorus, magnesium, and calcium can result in weakness. Weakness is caused by direct muscle injury, neuromuscular junction dysfunction, and peripheral nerve dysfunction.

Hypokalemic Myopathy

Hypokalemia (serum K < 3.5 mEq/L) is an uncommon electrolyte abnormality.[122] Hypokalemia is typically observed in patients treated with diuretics, malnutrition, alcoholism, renal tubular acidosis, diarrhea, laxative abuse, and hyperaldosteronism.[122]

Hypokalemia results in skeletal muscle weakness in both familial hypokalemic periodic paralysis (HypoPP; chapter 9) and in primary hypokalemic myopathy. HypoPP is an autosomal-dominant channelopathy related to dysfunction in the calcium (*CACNA1S*) or sodium (*SCN4A*) ion channels.[109] Periodic paralysis occurs in recurrent attacks of flaccid paralysis in the setting of actual or relative potassium deficiency.[109] Hypokalemic myopathy is an acquired acute/subacute myopathy observed in the setting of normal muscle exposed to hypokalemia.[23,65] Myopathy ranges from proximal weakness to rhabdomyolysis.[23]

CLINICAL PRESENTATION

Patients with slight hypokalemia (3–3.5 mEq/L) may develop symptoms of malaise, fatigue, cramps, and muscle weakness.[65] More severe hypokalemia (< 2.5 mEq/L) results in acute to subacute weakness and skeletal muscle injury. Patients develop rapidly progressive proximal upper and lower extremity weakness often with associated myalgia.[17,23,65] Sensory and reflex examinations are typically normal.[23] Polyuria, polydipsia, myoglobinuria, and cardiac conduction abnormalities are described.[23,122]

DIAGNOSTIC STUDIES

Potassium levels are typically below 2.5 mEq/L.[23,65] CK is elevated (600–7,000 IU/L) with associated myoglobinuria.[17,23,122] EMG may show increased insertional activity (fibrillations/positive waves) with associated myopathic motor units (short-duration motor units with early recruitment).[17,23] ECG may show flattened T and U waves.[23]

PATHOLOGY

Scattered necrotic fibers, type 2 muscle atrophy, and muscle fiber vacuoles are observed on muscle biopsy.[17,23,83] The mechanism of muscle fiber injury/weakness is not fully understood but postulated to be the result of a combination of (a) muscle membrane-potential abnormalities due to the change in extracellular potassium concentration, (b) impaired muscle blood flow, (c) protein catabolism in the relative alkalotic state, (d) impaired glycogen synthesis/storage, and (e) muscle necrosis.[65]

TREATMENT/PROGNOSIS

Correction of the underlying hypokalemia typically results in resolution of muscle symptoms within days to months.[23] Patients should be monitored for cardiac conduction abnormalities and provided supportive care to prevent renal failure in the setting of rhabdomyolysis.

Hyperkalemia

The etiology of hyperkalemia (> 5 mEq/L) is varied and includes acute acidemia, potassium-sparing diuretics, catabolic state, renal failure, impaired renin-aldosterone system (e.g., Addison's disease), and renal tubular potassium secretory failure.[29] Hyperkalemic periodic paralysis (Hyper-PP; chapter 9) is an autosomal-dominant muscle channelopathy due to a defect in the muscle sodium (*SCN4A*) channel; it can be associated with clinical and electrical myotonia.[109]

Hyperkalemia is a rare cause of weakness independent from cases of Hyper-PP. Generalized weakness and in some cases respiratory failure have been described in severe hyperkalemia (> 7 mEq/L).[8,51] Chvostek's sign and myotonic lid lag occur and may indicate muscle or peripheral nerve hyperexcitability.[8,51]

DIAGNOSTIC STUDIES

Serum potassium levels are typically greater than 7 mEq/L. Serum CK, EMG, and muscle biopsy are typically normal.[8,51]

PATHOLOGY

Muscle or peripheral nerve hyperexcitability with subsequent inactivation of sodium channels is postulated as the mechanism for muscle weakness.[8]

TREATMENT/PROGNOSIS

Correction of the underlying cause of hyperkalemia typically reverses weakness.[8,51]

Hypophosphatemia

In isolation, hypophosphatemia rarely causes weakness and myopathy. Myopathy associated with hypophosphatemia is well documented in patients with concurrent alcohol withdrawal, refeeding syndrome following a period of starvation, diabetic ketoacidosis, severe diarrhea, and cancer.[65,66] Hypophosphatemic myopathy can present as proximal weakness, rhabdomyolysis with myoglobinuria, and respiratory muscle weakness.[50,65] Serum phosphate is typically between 1 to 2.5 mg/dL in symptomatic patients.[50,65] CK is elevated in cases of rhabdomyolysis. EMG and muscle biopsy findings are not well documented. Patients typically improve with correction of serum phosphate and the underlying concurrent illness.[50,65,66]

Hypermagnesemia

Hypermagnesemia occurs in the setting of magnesium treatment for preeclampsia and overuse of magnesium-containing laxatives.[58] Hypermagnesemia inhibits release of acetylcholine at the neuromuscular junction. Generalized and respiratory muscle weakness can occur at serum magnesium concentrations above 5 mmol/ml.[58] Patients with concurrent neuromuscular disorders, particularly disorders of the neuromuscular junction (MG and Lambert-Eaton syndrome) are at increased risk.[58,88] A true myopathy does not occur in the setting of hypermagnesemia. Weakness typically resolves with correction of serum magnesium levels.[58]

Hypermagnesemia

Hypomagnesemia is associated with neuromuscular irritability, fasciculations, cramps, weakness, and tetany.[65] Tetany typically develops in the setting of concurrent hypocalcemia due to hypoparathyroidism or reduced calcium absorbtion.[65] Isolated muscle fiber necrosis associated with magnesium depletion has been induced in animals.[25] However, myopathy and rhabdomyolysis are usually observed in humans when concurrent with other known myotoxic conditions (e.g. alcoholism, hypokalemia).[65,92] Muscular symptoms typically resolve with treatment.[92]

Disorders of Calcium

Calcium disorders are discussed in the Parathyroid Disorders section.

Disorders of Sodium

Neuromuscular irritability and muscle cramps are described in patients with acute hyponatremia.[65] A true myopathy does not occur in either hypernatremia or hyponatremia.[65]

MYOPATHY ASSOCIATED WITH MALIGNANCY

Malignancy causes dysfunction in multiple locations in the peripheral nervous system that result in neuromuscular weakness. Involvement of nerve root and peripheral nerve are beyond the scope of this chapter.

Neuromuscular junction function is impaired in Lambert-Eaton myasthenic syndrome due to paraneoplastic antibodies directed against the presynaptic voltage-gated calcium channel. In addition, antibody-positive MG is associated with thymoma in about 10% of cases.[60]

Myopathies related to malignancy include inflammatory myopathies (dermatomyositis, polymyositis, necrotizing myopathy), direct tumor invasion of muscle, muscle thrombosis, and cachexia. Inflammatory myopathy is discussed in chapter 10.

Cachexia and Myopathy

Cachexia is a metabolic derangement associated with underlying illness and inflammation that results in severe loss of lean body muscle mass with associated lipolysis, anemia, anorexia, and activation of acute phase reactants.[2,41,117] Cachexia occurs in chronic illnesses such as cancer, HIV, congestive heart failure, sepsis, severe burns, and autoimmune arthritis.[2,117] Cachexia is a common feature of patients with malignancy; 50% of untreated cancer patients lose weight and about one-third lose 5% of original body weight.[117] Weight loss is associated with poor prognosis in cancer patients.[117]

CLINICAL PRESENTATION

Patients with cachectic myopathy present with subacute weight loss, muscle atrophy, and generalized weakness in the setting of another systemic illness.[10,41,117] EMG findings are not well described in this condition. However, one case report of a patient with cachexia and weakness describes an EMG with increased spontaneous activity (fibrillation potentials) in proximal arm muscles and increased spontaneous activity with associated myopathic motor units in proximal and distal lower extremity muscles.[10] CK is normal.

PATHOLOGY

Muscle loss is believed to be related to a combination of reduced protein synthesis and increased protein catabolism.[2] Both processes appear to be mediated by a complex interaction among the cytokines TNF-α, IL-1, IL-6, ciliary neurotrophic factor, and interferon-γ.[2,41,117,118] Tumor cell products including lipid-mobilizing factor and proteolysis-inducing factor are also

involved.[117] Both groups of metabolic products seem to activate the ubiquitin-proteosome proteolytic pathway resulting in protein degradation.[2,117] Animal studies illustrate that myosin heavy chain is preferentially targeted in cachexia in relation to the combination of TNF-α and interferon-γ.[2] In a case report, muscle electron microscopy revealed a preferential loss of myosin heavy chain, and mRNA analysis showed mRNA levels for myosin heavy chain and actin to be 20% to 30% of levels observed in control muscle.[10] Similar loss of myosin heavy chain is observed on light microscopy of patients with critical illness myopathy.[4,28]

TREATMENT/PROGNOSIS

Increased caloric intake is associated with weight gain but not increased muscle mass.[41,117] TNF-α inhibition is not helpful.[118] There is interest in blocking myostatin, a negative regulator of muscle growth that may be helpful in reversing cachectic myopathy based on animal models.[118] Currently there is no treatment beyond treating the underlying illness.

Metastatic and Embolic Myopathy

Diffuse metastatic tumor deposition within muscles is uncommon.[30] Patients develop subacute weakness with associated myopathic motor units on EMG and normal levels of serum CK. Muscle biopsy reveals carcinomatous invasion of the intermyofibrillary network.[30] Direct local invasion of muscle by tumor presenting as painful focal weakness is also described.[51]

Multifocal muscle infarct from nonbacterial, carcinoma associated endocarditis also occurs.[53] Patients develop multifocal muscle pain, swelling, and possibly weakness at varied times of onset.[53] CK may be mildly elevated and EMG is typically normal. Other organs are typically involved. Muscle biopsy shows signs of muscle infarction.[53]

CRITICAL ILLNESS MYOPATHY

Weakness in critically ill patients is a common occurrence and a common cause of increased morbidity and length of hospital stay. A new

Table 11–1 **Differential Diagnosis of Weakness in the Intensive Care Unit**

Central Nervous System
- Stroke
- Acute demyelinating disease
- Spinal cord pathology

Neuromuscular Junction
- Myasthenia gravis
- Myasthenic syndrome
- Botulism
- Aminoglycosides
- Curariform agents

Anterior Horn Cell
- West Nile virus
- Rabies
- Amyotrophic lateral sclerosis

Peripheral Nerve
- Guillain-Barré syndrome
- Chronic inflammatory demyelinating polyneuropathy
- Acute intermittent porphyria
- Critical illness polyneuropathy

Muscle
- Inflammatory myopathies
- Muscular dystrophies
- Critical illness myopathy
- Metabolic myopathies
- Electrolyte abnormalities (K, Ca)

neuromuscular cause of weakness complicates the care of 30% to 80% of critically ill patients.[13,15,70] Causes of weakness in this population are varied (Table 11–1). Critical illness polyneuropathy (CIP) and critical illness myopathy (CIM) are primary disorders of nerve and muscle that result in diffuse limb and diaphragmatic weakness in critical patients. CIP causes diffuse weakness, respiratory weakness, reduced reflexes, sensory loss, and EMG findings supportive of an axonal sensorimotor polyneuropathy.[13,15,72] CIM results in diffuse proximal/distal weakness, depressed reflexes, and myopathic changes on EMG.[13,15,72] CIP and CIM may occur alone or in combination. Other primary causes of neuromuscular weakness, including neuromuscular junction disease, motor neuron disease, inflammatory myopathy, and inflammatory neuropathy should be excluded in cases of suspected CIP and CIM.[13,15,72]

Clinical Presentation

CIM presents as an acute myopathy that develops after the onset of critical illness. CIM is typically the result of loss of myosin heavy chain but both necrotizing myopathy and rhabdomyolysis are rarely described.[15,72] Patients typically exhibit diffuse flaccid weakness (limb, bulbar, neck flexors, and diaphragm muscles) in the absence of sensory dysfunction.[13,15,70,71,72] Weakness often becomes apparent at the time of a failed wean from mechanical ventilation

as critical illness is often associated with diffuse encephalopathy and/or sedation that mask symptoms.[13,15,71,72] CIM is more common in patients treated with steroids and neuromuscular blocking agents for greater than 24 hours.[13,15,55,89] However, CIM is also described outside the setting of these medications; increased severity of illness, renal failure, and hyperglycemia increase risk.[13,15,70] CIM appears more commonly than CIP in the critical population; in one study, 42% of patients with weakness in the ICU had CIM compared to 13% with CIP.[71]

Diagnosis

CIM must be suspected in all critically ill patients. Concurrent medical illness and sedation may prevent some aspects of the neurological exam. Electrodiagnostic testing can be helpful to evaluate for CIP and CIM while excluding other neuromuscular disorders. EMG in CIP is consistent with a primary axonal process (reduced compound motor unit action potentials and sensory nerve action potentials).[13,15,70,72] EMG in CIM shows low-amplitude compound motor unit action potentials, normal sensory-nerve action potentials, and myopathic motor units (short-duration, low-amplitude motor units with early recruitment); in some cases direct muscle stimulation reveals muscle inexcitability.[15,94] In both CIP and CIM, slow repetitive nerve stimulation should be normal to exclude neuromuscular junction pathology. Muscle MRI may be helpful.[82] CK is normal or mildly elevated in CIM; it can be quite elevated in necrotizing myopathy/rhabdomyolysis.[15] Muscle biopsy can show specific changes but may not be indicated in the setting of a clear clinical history and electrodiagnostic testing.

Pathology

Muscle biopsy typically shows diffuse, angular atrophic fibers with associated loss of myosin heavy chain (thick filament) in CIM.[4,28,108] Myosin heavy chain loss can be observed on light microscopy as reduced central staining of type 1 fibers on ATPase and myosin heavy chain stains.[4,28,108] Myosin heavy chain loss can also be demonstrated on electron microscopy[4,28,108]; electron microscopy without typical light microscopy changes should be carried out in all patients in whom CIM is suspected. Similar findings are observed in cachectic myopathy.[2] Rare patients show evidence of a necrotizing myopathy; this carries a poor prognosis.[15]

CIM is directly related to sepsis and the systemic inflammatory response syndrome. Proinflammatory cytokines (TNF-α, INF-γ, interleukins, arachidonic acids) and endogenously produced low-molecular-weight myotoxic factors have been associated with increased proteolysis and activation of the ubiquitin–proteosome proteolytic pathway.[15,45,72] Again, these findings are similar to those observed in cachexia. There is also a component of disuse atrophy in CIM.

Prognosis/Treatment

No specific treatment has been shown to reduce the incidence or frequency of CIP and CIM.[72] Early mobilization and rehabilitation techniques with physical therapists in the ICU may improve some component of disuse atrophy.[72] Most patients with CIM recover within 6 months; severity of weakness is negatively associated with rapidity and completeness of recovery.[72] CIP and patients with combined CIM/CIP and necrotizing myopathy may have worse prognosis.[72] As in cachexia, future therapy may be directed against interrupting the inflammatory cascade.

TOXIN- AND MEDICATION- RELATED MYOPATHIES

Many medications and toxic substances cause potentially reversible myopathies. Suspect a toxic myopathy in patients without preexisting muscle disease who develop weakness, myalgias, myoglobinuria, or rhabdomyolysis that is temporally associated with exposure to a new drug or toxin.[26]

The pathophysiology of toxin-induced myopathies is varied. Other texts classify toxic myopathies by pathological mechanisms including (a) necrotizing myopathy, (b) inflammatory myopathy, (c) thick filament loss myopathy, (d) type 2 muscle atrophy, (e) mitochondrial myopathy, (f) lysosomal storage myopathy, (g) anti-microtubule myopathy, (h) myofibrillar myopathy, and (i) fasciitis.[26] We present the toxic myopathies based on the frequency with which potential offending medications are used (Table 11.2).

Cholesterol-Lowering-Agent Myopathy

HMGCR inhibitors (statins) are commonly prescribed agents that reduce cholesterol levels and reduce the risk of cardiovascular events. Statins are increasingly prescribed at high doses to achieve very low levels of low-density lipoprotein (LDL; < 70–100 mg/dL) for secondary prophylaxis of cardiovascular disease. Statins are typically well tolerated but can result in myotoxicity. The spectrum of statin-induced myopathy ranges from myalgias (least severe) to necrotizing myopathy and rhabdomyolsis (most severe).[26,79,110,116] Not surprisingly, many patients who develop a myopathy on statins have a coincidental myopathy.

PREVALENCE

The use of statin medications exceeds 100 million prescriptions per year, and at least 1.5 million people per year will experience a muscle complaint while on these medications.[110] Severe myotoxicity due to statins is rare; rhabdomyolysis occurs at a rate of 0.44 per 10,000 patient years.[78] Less severe complications (e.g., myalgias, asymptomatic elevations in CK) are estimated to occur at a rate of 9% to 22% of

Table 11–2 Toxin- and Drug-Induced Myopathies

Classification	Medication	Clinical Presentation	Muscle Pathology	Studies
Necrotizing myopathy	• Statin • Acute ETOH • Drugs of abuse • Exercise	Acute/insidious Onset Proximal Weakness Rhabdomyolysis	• Mixed necrotic fibers, normal fibers, regenerating fibers • No inflammation	*EMG:* • Fibrillations/positive waves • Myopathic motor units *Labs:* • Elevated CK
Type 2 fiber atrophy	Corticosteroids	Insidious onset Proximal weakness	• Selective atrophy of type 2B muscle fibers	*EMG:* • Normal *Labs:* • Low creatinine, normal CK
Vacuolar myopathy	• Chloroquine/ hydroxychloroquine	Insidious onset Proximal weakness	• PAS- positive vacuoles • Curvilinear bodies with electron microscopy	*EMG:* • Fibrillations/positive waves • Myotonia • Myopathic motor units *Labs:* • Elevated CK
Vacuolar myopathy	• Colchicine	Chronic proximal weakness	• PAS- positive vacuoles	*EMG:* • Fibrillations/Positive Waves • Myotonia • Myopathic motor units *Labs:* • Elevated CK
Mitochondrial myopathy	• Anti-viral medications • Germanium	Chronic proximal weakness	• Ragged red fibers, COX-negative fibers • Increased Oil red O	*EMG:* • Normal • Mild myopathic motor units *Labs:* • Elevated CK • Elevated lactic acid
Inflammatory myopathy	• D-penicillamine • Alpha interferon	Insidious onset Proximal weakness Elevated CK	• Perivascular/perimysial inflammatory cell infiltrate	*EMG:* • Fibrillations/positive waves • Myopathic motor units *Labs:* • Elevated CK
Myofibrillar myopathy	• Emetin (ipecac)	Acute onset Proximal weakness	• Generalized atrophy • Moth-eaten fibers (NADH stain) • Cytoplasmic inclusions	*EMG:* • Normal *Labs:* • Elevated CK (mild)

Adapted from Amato AA, Russell JA. Toxic Myopathies. In *Neuromuscular Disorders*. McGraw Hill Medical. 2008.[8] and Dalakas MC. Toxic and drug-induced myopathies. *J Neurol Neurosurg Psychiatry.* 2009;80: 832–838.[36]

Box 11.1 Coadministered Drugs Associated With Acute Statin Myopathy

- Other cholesterol-lowering agents
- Cyclosporine, tacrolimus
- Macrolide antibiotics (e.g., erythromycin)
- Warfarin
- Digoxin
- Azole antifungals
- HIV protease inhibitors
- Amiodarone
- Nefazodone

statin users.[79,110,116] About 5% to 10% of statin users will discontinue medications due to less severe complication such as myalgias.[79] Muscle symptoms are more common in patients with diabetes, older age, hypothyroidism, hepatic dysfunction, and concurrent use of some medications (fibrates, corticosteroids, calcium channel blockers, CYP3A4 inhibitors; Box 11.1).[79]

The myotoxicity of statins is variable. The degree of risk for myopathy associated with certain statins varies among different sources. Risk of rhabdomyolysis reported by the FDA is as follows: cerivastatin (32%; no longer available), simvastatin (36%), atorvastatin (12%), pravastatin (12%), lovastatin (7%), and fluvastatin (2%).[26,114] Rosuvastatin has a profile similar to atorvastatin.[79] Statins metabolized by the CYP3A4 (cerivstatin, atorvastatin, simvastatin) may be more likely to cause severe myotoxicity.[79] This may be related to the large number of drugs metabolized by this pathway (50% of available drugs) that may be coadministered with statins.[79] In addition, lipophilic drugs (simvastatin, atorvastatin, lovastatin) may be more likely than hydrophilic agents (pravastatin, rosuvastatin, fluvastatin) to penetrate muscle and induce myotoxicity.[110] Myopathy has been reported with all of the statins. Myalgias are a frequent symptom in patients not taking any medication, and statins are inevitably blamed

for symptoms in some patients where they are innocent.

Higher doses of statins are increasingly required to achieve the stringent low levels of LDL associated with lower cardiovascular risk. However, an increased risk of myopathy is associated with high doses of statins (e.g., simvastatin 80 mg daily). This is particularly true for simvastatin compared to other statin medications.[79] Although one may not be able to achieve stringent levels of LDL with lower doses of statins, there is still cardiovascular benefit to these medications. Given the high number of patients who discontinue these medications (5%–10%) due to muscular complaints, it might be necessary to compromise. Rechallenging patients who experienced muscular side effects with every other day dosing of rosuvastatin has been shown to achieve reasonable LDL control and improve tolerance of the medication.[79]

Pharmacogenomics is becoming increasingly important in medicine. There may be a genetic risk for developing statin-induced myopathy. A recent genome-wide scan identified a single nucleotide polymorphism in the *SLCO1B1* gene on chromosome 12, which is associated with an increased risk of myalgias in patients taking simvastatin[101]; this gene is associated with hepatic uptake. Other candidates may also be identified in the future. Testing for this polymorphism is not currently available.

It is postulated that patients with elevated baseline levels of CK are more likely to develop statin-induced myopathy. However, a study of patients with baseline CK (250–2,500 IU/L) showed no increased risk of myopathic complaints at 4 months.[79] In addition, routine monitoring of CK in asymptomatic patients is not recommended by the American College of Cardiology/American Heart Association/National Heart, Lung, and Blood Institute advisory committee or the National Lipid Association's expert panel.[93,110]

CLINICAL PRESENTATION OF STATIN-INDUCED MYOPATHY

Elevated CK

Statins frequently induce elevations in CK that do not exceed 10 times the upper limits of normal.[26,116] Asymptomatic elevation in CK in a patient taking statins is a common referral to the neuromuscular specialist. Such elevations are unlikely to be clinically significant, and the risk of developing a symptomatic myopathy is not increased in patients with baseline elevated levels of CK.[26,79,116] For these patients, we recommend a good neurological examination and reassurance. If patients remain asymptomatic, following serial CK levels is unnecessary.[26,110]

Myalgias

Myalgias without clinical weakness that influence compliance with statin medications are reported in 9% to 25% of patients.[26,116] This symptom may or may not be associated with elevations in CK and typically resolves within 3 months of discontinuing the medication.[26] Patients can be observed if the myalgia is tolerable or can be rechallenged with an alternative statin or every other day dosing. A muscle biopsy may be indicated in patients in whom myalgias persist despite discontinuing medications.

Muscle Weakness With CK Elevation

Infrequently, acute/subacute proximal weakness (shoulder/hip girdle) is temporally associated with statin administration; hip abduction and flexion weakness is most commonly reported.[116] Muscle biopsy may show a minimal

collection of necrotic fibers, with or without scattered inflammatory cells.[26] Toxin-induced myotonia on needle EMG has been described in symptomatic muscles.[90] Most patients will show resolution of symptoms within 3 months of discontinuing statin medications.

There have been many case reports of statin medications inducing more chronic muscle/anterior horn cell conditions such as IBM, PM, DMS, and ALS.[26,79] It is unclear from the literature whether statins induce or worsen these conditions.[26,79]

Necrotizing Myopathy

There is a subset of patients in whom symptoms do not improve and who worsen despite discontinuing statin medications. Some of these patients have an immune-mediated necrotizing myopathy that appears to be induced by statin administration.[22,49,79] These patients develop progressive proximal weakness with an elevated CK. Muscle weakness can develop during statin administration and has been described up to 20 months after discontinuing therapy.[49] The typical muscle biopsy shows a mixture of necrotic and regenerating muscle fibers without inflammatory infiltrate (Figure 11–2). Patients who develop the necrotizing myopathy have upregulation of HMGCR expression in muscle with associated elevations of anti-HMGCR autoantibodies.[22,80] These autoantibodies are not detected in patients who do not develop the necrotizing myopathy while being treated with statin medications.[80] Treatment often requires multiple simultaneous immunosuppressant agents to reverse the myopathy, despite discontinuing statin therapy.[49]

Acute Rhabdomyolysis

This is a rare complication (< 1/100,000 prescriptions) of statin therapy.[26,91] Patients develop acute weakness, myalgia, myoglobinuria, and CK levels greater than 10 times the upper limits of normal.[26,116] Death can result from hyperkalemia, cardiac arrhythmia, renal failure, and disseminated intravascular coagulation; patients should be managed in an ICU setting.[26,116] The risk of this complication is increased with higher doses of statins and combination of a statin with other drugs (gemfibrizol, fibrates, cyclosporine, macrolide antibiotics, warfarin, digoxin, and azole antifungals).[26] As discussed under Cholesterol-Lowering-Agent Myopathy, this

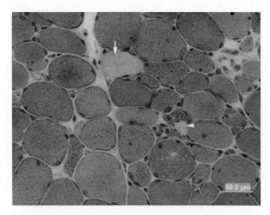

Figure 11–2. Muscle biopsy of statin-associated necrotizing myopathy. Muscle biopsy demonstrates a necrotic muscle fiber (arrow) and myophagocytosis of another necrotic muscle fiber (arrowhead) using modified Gomori trichrome stain. Reproduced with permission from Crable-Esposito P, Katzberg HD, Greenberg SA, Srinivasan J, Katz J, Amato AA. Immune-mediated necrotizing myopathy associated with statins. Muscle and Nerve. 2010;41: 185–190.

complication may be due to interactions with the CYP3A4 system. It may also be related to uncovering a preexisting metabolic myopathy.[26]

Corticosteroid Myopathy

Corticosteroid myopathy is typically associated with chronic administration of high-dose corticosteroids (greater than 30 mg/day prednisone). The myopathy presents as muscle weakness and atrophy of proximal arm/leg muscles; the condition typically spares involvement of bulbar, facial, ocular, and distal extremity muscles.[8,26] Although typically associated with chronic administration of oral medication, corticosteroid myopathy is described within weeks of instituting oral therapy and in patients receiving high-dose intravenous corticosteroids.[8,26]

Muscle biopsies show type 2 muscle fiber atrophy, which is similar to that observed in disuse atrophy.[33] Therefore, there are few other objective findings beyond weakness to indicate this process. Serum CK, nerve conduction studies, and EMG are typically normal.[8,26]

Corticosteroid myopathy typically resolves with discontinuation of the medication or with switching to alternate-day dosing.[26] Because high-dose corticosteroids are often prescribed to treat autoimmune causes of weakness such as chronic inflammatory demyelinating

polyneuropathy, MG, and inflammatory myopathy, it is important to distinguish steroid myopathy from exacerbation of these other conditions. An increase in serum CK and persistence of increased spontaneous activity on EMG in patients with inflammatory myopathy suggest worsening of the underlying process.[7] Persistently abnormal slow repetitive-stimulation nerve-conduction study of a weak muscle in MG may indicate worsening of disease rather than steroid myopathy.[123] However, in many cases, a trial of corticosteroid taper/discontinuation is required to answer this question. Improvement during taper implicates corticosteroid myopathy; worsening suggests worsening of the underlying disease.

Chloroquine/Hydroxychloroquine Myopathy

Chloroquine (CQ) and increasingly hydroxychloroquine (HCQ) are used in the treatment of rheumatic diseases such as systemic lupus erythematosus; these medications are considered to carry less risk of severe side effects compared to other immunosuppressants.[26,69] Both agents have been associated with myopathy, peripheral neuropathy, or both. Myopathy was observed in up to 13% of patients treated with these medications in one prospective study.[19]

Patients typically develop proximal weakness more often than distal.[1,19,69,96] Severe neuromuscular respiratory weakness and cardiomyopathy also occur.[1,69,81,111] EMG typically shows evidence of an irritable myopathy; myotonia has also been observed.[1,69] Muscle pathology resembles that observed in acid maltase deficiency. Light microscopy reveals an acid phosphatase–positive vacuolar myopathy (Figure 11–3). Although vacuolar myopathy is not unique to CQ/HCQ myopathy, curvilinear bodies seen on electron microscopy are specific to CQ/HCQ myopathy[1,19,26,69] (Figure 11–4). Elevation in CK may predate onset of clinical symptoms and EMG changes.[19] In one prospective study of rheumatologic patients treated with CQ and HCQ, all patients with persistent elevated CK showed typical changes of CQ/HCQ myopathy on muscle biopsy electron microscopy, although only 50% of this group showed typical EMG and light microscopy changes.[19] Following serial CK measurements in patients treated with CQ/

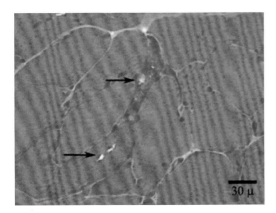

Figure 11-3. Muscle biopsy of hydroxychloroquine myopathy. An hematoxylin-and-eosin–stained cryostat muscle section reveals many myofibers with abnormal punctate basophilia. There are atrophic angular fibers, and occasional myofibers contain rimmed vacuoles (arrows). Reproduced with permission from Abdel-Hamid H, Oddis CV, Lacomis D. Severe hydroxychloroquine myopathy. Muscle and Nerve 2008;38: 1206–1210.

HCQ may be useful to determine which patients are at highest risk for this complication.

The myopathy associated with CQ/HCQ is typically slowly reversible upon discontinuing medications.[1,26,69] This diagnosis must be suspected in patients who develop proximal weakness or shortness of breath while on CQ/HCQ.

Colchicine Myopathy

Colchicine, long used in the symptomatic management of gout, can induce a vacuolar myopathy after several months of use.[26,98,106,112] Patients typically develop slowly progressive proximal weakness accompanied by an elevated CK.[26,112] However, rapidly progressive weakness and rhabdomyolysis are also observed.[6,98] Patient's with renal and hepatic dysfunction are at highest risk to develop colchicine myopathy and are also more likely to exhibit a severe presentation.[34,98] Coadministration of drugs that inhibit colchicine clearance (e.g., erythromycin, cyclosporine) also increase the risk of myopathy.[6,112] EMG typically shows a combination of fibrillation potentials and/or myotonia.[32,106] Muscle biopsy shows a PAS-positive vacuolar myopathy.[112]

The myopathy typically resolves within 4 to 6 weeks of discontinuing colchicine.[26] Colchicine myopathy should be suspected in patients developing weakness while on this therapy; the

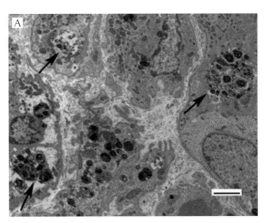

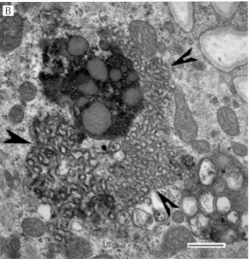

Figure 11-4. EM of hydroxychloroquine myopathy. (A) Low-power electron photomicrograph illustrating myofibers with vacuoles that contain autophagic degradation products, including myeloid bodies (arrows). Myeloid bodies and other types of lamellated electron-dense structures are also seen scattered throughout the sarcoplasm. (B) Higher power magnification reveals curvilinear inclusions (arrowheads) adjacent to a complex lipid structure with globular elements. Reproduced with permission from Abdel-Hamid H, Oddis CV, Lacomis D. Severe hydroxychloroquine myopathy. Muscle and Nerve 2008;38:1206–1210.

patient's medication list and renal/hepatic function should be monitor regularly in patients taking colchicine.

Antiviral Medications

Nucleoside-analog reverse transcriptase inhibitors used in the treatment of HIV and infectious hepatitis can induce a mitochondrial myopathy.[26,27,74,86,112] The HIV medications zidovudine (AZT) and stavudine (d4T) and the hepatitis medication fialuridine (FIAU) are associated with myopathy with accompanying lactic acidosis. The medications are false substrates for mitochondrial DNA polymerase which causes a decrease in mitochondrial DNA and subsequent decline in respiratory chain capacity.[74,112] Zidovudine and stavudine result in a reversible myopathy as they compete with natural thymidine triphosphate and terminate mitochondrial DNA synthesis. FIAU causes an irreversible myopathy as it is an alternate substrate for thymidine triphosphate and is incorporated directly into the mtDNA chain.[26] Nucleoside-analog medications result in selective tissue toxicity due to the varied tissue distribution of phosphorylases necessary to phosphorylate these medications.[74]

Zidovudine myopathy typically occurs within 6 to 12 months after treatment onset. Proximal weakness, myalgia, fatigue, and elevated CK are typical.[26,27,74,112] The myopathy is often accompanied or preceded by elevation in serum lactic acid.[26,74] Muscle histology shows signs of mitochondrial dysfunction, including RRF on trichrome staining, ragged blue fibers on SDH staining, COX-negative fibers on cytochrome C-oxidase staining, and accumulation of lipid on Oil red O staining.[9,26,74] (Figure 11–5A & B). Clinically, this myopathy mimics HIV myopathy. They are distinguished by improvement within 5 weeks of discontinuing medication.[26,112] Stavudine used in combination with a protease inhibitor and an additional reverse transcriptase inhibitor can cause a proximal myopathy with associated lactic acidosis and lipodystrophy.[86] The syndrome is described within 6 to 15 months of instituting therapy; it typically resolves within weeks of discontinuing treatment.[86] FIAU causes a similar but irreversible syndrome of proximal myopathy, lactic acidosis, and lipodystrophy.

D-PENICILLAMINE MYOPATHY

D-penicillamine is associated with the development of inflammatory muscle disease (dermatomyositis) and MG.[26,112] The incidence is estimated at less than 1% of treated patients.[26] The myopathy typically resolves with medication withdrawal but some cases require immunosuppression.[112]

INTERFERON ALPHA

Interferon alpha is used as a treatment for chronic hepatitis and malignancy. Inflammatory myopathy, MG, and systemic lupus erythamatosis have been described in the setting of chronic interferon alpha treatment.[26,112] The cases of inflammatory myopathy resemble PM with CD-8 positive T cells, invasion of nonnecrotic fibers, and increased numbers of RRF on muscle histology.[54] The myopathy typically resolves with discontinuation of interferon.

Myopathy and Drugs of Abuse

ALCOHOL MYOPATHY

Overconsumption of alcohol is associated with both an acute and a chronic myopathy.

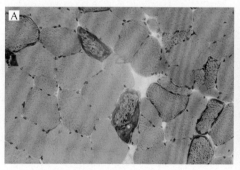
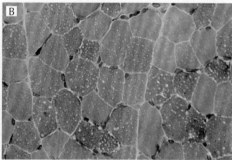

Figure 11–5. Muscle biopsy of HIV-antiviral-associated myopathy. (A) Trichrome stain with ragged red fibers. (B) Oil red O stain with accumulation of lipid.

Acute Alcohol Myopathy

An acute necrotizing myopathy with rhabdomyolysis occurs in up to 2% of alcoholics and typically occurs in the setting of heavy binge drinking.[112] The necrotizing myopathy presents with muscle pain and swelling followed by rhabdomyolysis and myoglobinuria; it typically interrupts a bout of heavy alcohol consumption.[26,112] Muscle biopsy typically shows necrotic muscle fibers among populations of more normal fibers.[112] Muscle strength returns within 10 to 14 days after cessation of alcohol consumption.[112]

Acute hypokalemic myopathy is also associated with alcohol consumption and may be the cause of many cases of acute alcohol myopathy; muscle necrosis leads to autocorrection of hypokalemia. Patients develop painless weakness accompanied by serum potassium levels less than 2.5 mEq.[26] Hypokalemia is the result of potassium redistribution between intra- and extracellular space in this population.[112] The myopathy improves with correction of the underlying hypokalemia.[26]

Chronic Alcoholic Myopathy

Many alcoholics develop chronic muscle weakness involving proximal limb-girdle muscles.[26,112] A second phenotype of elevated CK and mild weakness compared to normal controls occurs in up to 40% of asymptomatic patients.[120] Muscle biopsy findings are varied in this population. Type 2B atrophy is the most prominent finding.[26,112] Other nonspecific findings such as scattered necrosis, variability in fiber size, and moth-eaten fibers occur.[8,112,120] Pathophysiology of weakness is likely multifactorial. Chronic alcohol exposure has been linked to decreased protein synthesis, increased oxidative stress in muscle, induction of skeletal muscle apoptosis, and possibly perturbations in gene expression.[43] Muscle strength typically recovers with abstinence from alcohol or significant reduction in alcohol consumption.[112]

Alcohol-induced dilated cardiomyopathy and arrhythmias can occur following excessive consumption over 10 or more years.[112,120] This condition may be reversible with abstinence.[112]

OTHER DRUGS OF ABUSE

Acute rhabdomyolysis is described in the setting of multiple other drugs of abuse including cocaine,[39,59,112] amphetamine,[26] Ecstasy,[52,105] and heroin.[26] Illicit drugs, including alcohol, are the most common cause of acute rhabdomyolysis; patients with rhabdomyolysis have typically consumed multiple agents.[84] Treatment is primarily supportive care and abstinence.

Dietary Agents

EMETIN (IPECAC)

Emetin is typically consumed by patients with eating disorders to induce vomiting. Use of doses above 500 mg daily for 10 days is associated with an acute proximal myopathy.[8,26] Muscle biopsy resembles myofibrillar myopathy. Light microscopy shows generalized atrophy, moth-eaten fibers with NADH staining, and cytoplasmic inclusions. EM shows many fibers with breakdown of the Z-line and inclusions of compacted myofibrillar derbis.[8] The changes typically resolve slowly after emetin is discontinued.

GERMANIUM

Germanium is used in dietary supplements and natural remedies for conditions such as cancer. Use of these supplements can induce renal failure, anemia, and muscle weakness.[26,112] Muscle biopsy shows muscle vacuoles and increased activity of acid phosphatase.[26,112]

NEEDLE MYOPATHY

Needle insertions into muscle can elicit an inflammatory response in muscle that can persist up to 1 month.[26] When obtaining a muscle biopsy, one should avoid muscles recently examined by needle EMG due to this reaction, especially in patients in whom inflammatory myopathy is suspected.

EXERTIONAL RHABDOMYOLYSIS

Rhabdomyolysis is a potential complication of overexertion and exercise.[5,37,46,64,76,84] Many cases are associated with concurrent exercise and another potential cause of rhabdomyolysis (dehydration, myotoxic agents such as alcohol or illicit drugs, etc.). Some cases are due to exercise alone.[37] Many cases are observed in the setting of military training; an incidence of 22/100,000 trainees is reported in one study.[5]

The increasing popularity of militarylike commercial exercise programs may result in more cases in the general population. The recurrence of isolated exercise-induced rhabdomyolysis is low (0.08% per patient year).[5] Therefore, management is supportive and return to exercise postrecovery is typically safe. In cases of recurrent exercise-induced rhabdomyolysis, a search for an underlying metabolic myopathy (e.g. McArdle's disease, carnitine palmitoyltransferase II deficiency) is indicated.[37,99]

REFERENCES

1. Abdel-Hamid H, Oddis CV, Lacomis D. Severe hydroxychloroquine myopathy. *Muscle and Nerve.* 2008;38: 1206–1210.
2. Acharyya S, Ladner KJ, Nelsen LL, Damrauer J, Reiser PJ, et al. Cancer cachexia is regulated by selective targeting of skeletal muscle gene products. *The Journal of Clinical Investigation.* 2004;114(3): 370–378.
3. Adeniyi O, Agaba EI, King M, Servilla KS, Massie L, Tzamaloukas AH. Severe proximal myopathy in advanced renal failure. Diagnosis and treatment. *Afr J Med.* 2004; 33: 385–388.
4. Al-Lozi MT, Pestronk A, Yee WC, Flaris N, Cooper J. Rapidly evolving myopathy with myosin-deficient muscle fibers. *Ann Neuro.* 1994; 35(3): 273–279.
5. Alpers JP, Jones LK. Natural history of exertional rhabdomyolysis: a population based cohort. *Muscle and Nerve* 2010;42: 487–491.
6. Altman A, Szyper-Kravitz M, Shoenfeld Y. Colchicine induced rhabdomyolysis. *Clin Rheumatol.* 2007;26: 2197–2199.
7. Amato AA, Barohn RJ. Evaluation and treatment of inflammatory myopathies. *J Neurol Neurosurg Psychiatry.* 2009;80: 1060–1068.
8. Amato AA, Russell JA. Toxic Myopathies. In *Neuromuscular Disorders.* McGraw Hill Medical. 2008.
9. Arnaudo E, Dalakas M, Shanske S, Moraes CT, DiMauro S, Schon EA. Depletion of muscle mitochondrial DNA in AIDS patients with zidovudine-induced myopathy. *Lancet.* 1991;337(8740): 508–510.
10. Banduseela V, Ochala J, Lamberg K, Kalimo H, Lassson L. Muscle paralysis and myosin loss in a patient with cancer cachexia. *Acta Myologica.* 2007 26: 136–144.
11. Beekman R, Tijssen CC, Visser LH, Schellens RLLA. Dropped head syndrome as the presenting symptom of primary hyperparathyroidism. *J Neurol.* 2002;249: 1738–1739.
12. Bell E, Lorimer AR, Hinnie J. Assoiciation between myotonic dystrophy and primary hyperparathyroidism. *The Journal of International Medical Research.* 1994 22: 296–298.
13. Bird SJ. Diagnosis and management of critical illness polyneuropathy and critical illness myopathy. *Current Treatment Options in Neurology.* 2007;9: 85–92.
14. Bjornskov EK, Carry MR, Katz FH, Lefkowitz J, Ringel SP. Diabetic muscle infarction: a new perspective of pathogenesis and management. *Neuromusc Disorders.* 1995;5(1): 39–45.
15. Bolton CF. Neuromuscular manifestations of critical illness. *Muscle and Nerve.* 2005;32: 140–163.
16. Bousquet-Santos K, Vaisman M, Barreto ND, Cruz-Fihlo RA, Salvador BA, et al. Resistance training improves muscle function and body composition in patients with hyperthyroidism. *Arch Phys Med Rehabil.* 2006;87: 1123–1130.
17. Budka H, Finsterer J, Hess B, Jarius C, Mamoli B, Stollberger C. Malnutrition-induced hypokalemic myopathy in chronic alcoholism. *Journal of Toxicology: Clinical Toxicology.* 1988;36(4): 369.
18. Cakir M. Euthyroid Grave's ophthalmopathy with negative autoantibodies. *Journal of the National Medical Association.* 2005;97(11): 1547–1549.
19. Casado E, Gratacos J, Tolosa C, Martinez JM, Ojanguren I, et al. Antimalarial myopathy: an underdiagnosed complication? Prospective longitudinal study of 119 patients. *Ann Rheum Dis.* 2006;65: 385–390.
20. Chapin JE, Kornfeld M, Harris A. Amyloid myopathy: characteristic features of a still underdiagnosed disease. *Muscle and Nerve.* 2005;31: 266–272.
21. Chou FF, Lee CH, Chen JB. General weakness as an indication for parathyroid surgery in patients with secondary hyperparathyroidism. *Arch Surg.* 1999;134: 1108–1111.
22. Christopher-Stine L, Casciola-Rosen LA, Hong G, Chung T, Corse AM, Mammen AL. A novel autoantibody recognizing 200-kd and 100-kd proteins in associated with an immune mediated necrotizing myopathy. *Arthritis and Rheumatism.* 2010;62(9): 2757–2766.
23. Comi G, Testa D, Cornelio F, Comola M, Canal N. Potassium depletion myopathy: a clinical and morphological study of six cases. *Muscle and Nerve.* 1985;8: 17–21.
24. Cooper MS. Disorders of calcium metabolism and parathyroid disease. *Best Practice and Research Clinical Endocrinology and Metabolism.* 2011;25(6): 975–983.
25. Cronin RE, Ferguson ER, Shannon WA, Knochel JP. Skeletal muscle injury after magnesium depletion in the dog. *American Journal of Physiology.* 1982;24(2): F113–F120.
26. Dalakas MC. Toxic and drug-induced myopathies. *J Neurol Neurosurg Psychiatry.* 2009;80: 832–838.
27. Dalakas MC, Illa I, Pezeshkpour GH, Laukaitis JP, Cohen B, Griffin JL. Mitochondrial myopathy caused by long-term zidovudine therapy. *NEJM.* 1990;322(16): 1098–1105.
28. Danon MJ, Carpenter S. Myopathy with thick filament (myosin) loss following prolonged paralysis with vecuronium during steroid treatment. *Muscle and Nerve.* 1991;14: 1131–1139.
29. DeFronzo RA, Bia M, Smith D. Clinical disorders of hyperkalemia. *Ann Rev Med.* 1982;33: 521–554.
30. Doshi R, Fowler T. Proximal myopathy due to discrete carcinomatous metastases in muscle. *Journal of Neurology, Neurosurgery, and Psychiatry.* 1983;46: 358–360.
31. Downie A, Jepson E,. Hyperparathyroidism in a patient with myotonic dystrophy. *Journal of the Royal Society of Medicine.* 1990;83: 58.
32. Duarte J, Cabezas C, Rodriguez F, Claveria LE, Palacin T. Colchicine induced myopathy with myotonia. *Muscle and Nerve.* 1998;21(4): 550
33. Dubowitz V, Sewry CA. *Muscle Biopsy: a practical approach 3rd Ed.* Saunders Elsevier, 2007.

34. Dupont P, Hunt I, Goldberg L, Warrens A. Colchicine myoneuropathy in a renal transplant patient. *Transpl Int*. 2002;15: 374–376.

35. Duyff RF, Van den Bosch J, Laman M, Potter van Loon BJ, Linseen WHJP. Neuromuscular findings in thyroid dysfunction: a prospective clinical and electrodiagnostic study. *J Neurol Neurosurg Psychiatry*. 2000;68: 750–755.

36. Dyck PJB, Windebank AJ. Diabetic and nondiabetic lumbosacral radiculoplexus neuropathies: new insights into pathophysiology and treatment. *Muscle and Nerve*. 2002;25: 477–491.

37. Elsayed EF, Reilly RF. Rhabdomyolysis: a review, with emphasis on the pediatric population. *Pediatric Nephrology*, 2009;25: 7–18.

38. Engel AG. Neuromuscular manifestations of Grave's disease. *Mayo Clin Proc* 1976;47: 919–925.

39. Enriquez R, Palacios FO, Gonzalez CM, Amoros FA, Cabezuelo JB, Hernandez F. Skin vasculitis, hypokalemia, and acute renal failure in rhabdomyolysis associated with cocaine. *Nephron*. 1991;59: 336–337.

40. Evans RM, Watanabe I, Singer PA. Central changes in hypothyroid myopathy; a case report. *Muscle and Nerve* 1990;13: 952–956.

41. Evans WJ. Skeletal muscle loss: cachexia, sarcopenia, and inactivity. *Am J Clin Nutr*. 2010;91(suppl): 1123S–1127S.

42. Franklyn JA, Boelaert K. Thyrotoxicosis. *Lancet*. 2012;379: 1155–1166.

43. Fernandez-Sola J, Preedy VR, Lang CJ, Gonzalez-Reimers E, Arno M, et al. Molecular and cellular events in alcohol induced muscle disease. *Alcohol Clin Exp Res*. 2007;31(12): 1953–1962.

44. Friedman Y, Paul JT, Turley J, Hazrati LN, Munoz D. Axial myopathy due to primary amyloidosis. *Muscle and Nerve*. 2007;36: 542–546.

45. Friedrich O, Fink RHA, Hund E. Understanding critical illness myopathy: approaching the pathomechanism. *J Nutr*. 2005;135: 1813s–1817s.

46. Galvez R, Stacy K, Howley A. Exertional rhabdomyolysis in seven division-1 swimming athletes. *Clin J Sport Med*. 2008;18: 366–368.

47. Gertz MA, Kyle RA. Myopathy in primary systemic amyloidosis. *Journal of Neurology, Neurosurgery, and Psychiatry*. 1996;60: 655–660.

48. Glauser SR, Gluaser J, Hatem SF. Diabetic muscle infarction: a rare complication of advanced diabetes mellitus. *Emerg Radiol*. 2008;15: 61–65.

49. Grable-Esposito P, Katzberg HD, Greenberg SA, Srinivasan J, Katz J, Amato AA. Immune-mediated necrotizing myopathy associated with statins. *Muscle and Nerve*. 2010;41: 185–190.

50. Gravelyn TP, Brophy N, Sigert C, Peters-Golden M. Hypophosphatemia-associated respiratory muscle weakness in a general inpatient population. *The American Journal of Medicine*. 1988;84: 870–876.

51. Griggs RC, Mendell JR, Miller RG. Myopathies of systemic disease. In *Evaluation and Treatment of Myopathies* F.A. Davis, 1995.

52. Hall AP, Henry JA. Acute toxic effects of Ecstasy (MDMA) and related compounds: overview of pathophysiology and clinical management. *British Journal of Anesthesia* 2006;96(6): 678–685.

53. Heffner RR. Myopathy of embolic origin in patients with carcinoma. *Neurology*. 1971;21: 840–846.

54. Hengstman GJ, Vogels OJ, ter Laak HJ, de Witte T, van Engelen BG. Myositis during long-term interferon-alpha treatment. *Neurology*, 2000;54(11): 2186.

55. Hirano M, Ott BR, Raps EC, Minetti C, Lennihan L, et al. Acute quadriplegic myopathy: a complication of treatment with steroids, nondepolarizing blocking agents, or both. *Neurology*. 1992;42: 2082–2087.

56. Horak HA, Pourmand R. Endocrine myopathies. *Neurologic Clinics*. 2000;18(1): 203–213.

57. Jackson CE, Amato AA, Bryan WW, Wolfe GI, Sakhaee K, Barohn RJ. Primary hyperparathyroidism and ALS: Is there a relation? *Neurology*. 1998;50(6): 1795–1799.

58. James MFM. Magnesium in obstetrics. *Best Practice and Research Clinical Obstetrics and Gynecology*. 2010;24: 327–337.

59. Jandreski MA, Bermes EW, Leischner R, Kahn SE. Rhabdomyolysis in a case of free base cocaine (crack) overdose. *Clin Chem*. 1989;35(7): 1547–1549.

60. Juel VC and JM Massey. Myasthenia gravis. *Orphanet Journal of Rare Diseases*. 2007;2: 1–13.

61. Karacostas D, Soumpourou M, Mavromatis I, Karkavelas G, Pouios I, Milonas I. Isolated myopathy as the initial manifestation of primary systemic amyloidosis. *J Neurol*. 2005;252: 853–854.

62. Kendall-Taylor P, Turnbul DM. Endocrine myopathies. *British Medical Journal*. 1983;287: 705–708.

63. Khaleeli AA, Griffith DG, Edwards RHT. The clinical presentation of hypothyroid myopathy and its relationship to abnormalities in structure and function of skeletal muscle. *Clinical Endocrinology*. 1983;19: 365–376.

64. Kiberd M, Campbell F. Delayed-onset rhabdomyolysis after intense exercise. *CMAJ*. 2011;183(16): E1222.

65. Knochel JP. Neuromuscular manifestations of electrolyte disorders. *The American Journal of Medicine*. 1982;72: 521–535.

66. Knochel JP. The clinical status of hypophosphatemia. *NEJM*. 1985;313(7): 447–449.

67. Kruse K, Scheunemann W, Baier W, Schaub J. Hypocalcemic myopathy in idiopathic hypoparathyroidism. *Eur J Pediatr*. 1982;138: 280–282.

68. Kvetny J, Puhakka KB, Rohl L. Magnetic resonance imaging determination of extraocular eye muscle volume in patients with thyroid-associated ophthalmopathy and proptosis. *Acta Ophthalmologica Scandinavica*. 2006;84: 419–423.

69. Kwon JB, Kleiner A, Ishida K, Godown J, Ciafaloni E, Looney RJ. Hydroxychloroquine-induced myopathy. *J Clin Rheumatol*. 2010;16: 28–31.

70. Lacomis D, Zochodne D, Bird SJ. Critical illness myopathy. *Muscle and Nerve*. 2000;23: 1785–1788.

71. Lacomis D, Petrella JT, Giuliani MJ. Causes of neuromuscular weakness in the intensive care unit: a study of ninety-two patients. *Muscle and Nerve*. 1998;21: 610–617.

72. Latronico N, Bolton CF. Critical illness polyneuropathy and myopathy: a major cause of muscle weakness and paralysis. *Lancet Neurol*. 2011;10: 931–941.

73. Lennerstrand G, Tian S, Isberg B, Hogbeck IL, Bolzani R, et al. Magnetic resonance imaging and ultrasound measurements of extraocular muscles in thyroid-associated ophthalmopathy at different stages of the disease. *Acta Ophthalmologica Scandinavica*. 2007;85: 192–201.

74. Lewis W, Dalakas MC. Mitochondrial toxicity of antiviral drugs. *Nature Medicine*. 1995;1(5): 417–422.

75. Lichtstein DM, Arteaga RB. Rhabdomyolysis associated with hyperthyroidism. *The American Journal of the Medical Sciences*. 2006;332(2): 103–105.

76. Lin ACM, Lin CM, Wang TL, Leu JG. Rhabdomyolysis in 119 students after repetitive exercise. *Br J Sports Med*, 2005;39: e3.

77. Mallette LE, Patten BM, Engel WK. Neuromuscular disease in secondary hyperparathyroidism. *Annals of Internal Medicine*. 1975;82: 474–483.

78. Mammen AL. Autoimmune myopathies: autoantibodies, phenotypes, and pathogenesis. *Nat. Rev. Neurol.* 2011;7: 343–354.

79. Mammen AL, Amato AA. Statin myopathy: a review of recent progress. *Current Opinion in Rheumatology*. 2010;22: 644–650.

80. Mammen AL, Chung T, Christopher-Stine L, Rosen P, Rosen A, et al. Autoantibodies against 3-hydroxy-3-methylglutaryl-coenzyme A reductase in patients with statin associated autoimmune myopathy. *Arthritis and Rheumatism*. 2011;63(3): 713–721.

81. Mateen FJ, Keegan BM. Severe, reversible dysphagia from chloroquine and hydroxychloroquine myopathy. *Can J. Neurol. Sci.* 2007;34: 377–379.

82. Matsuda N, Kobayashi S, Tanji Y, Hasegawa A, Tase C, Ugawa Y. Widespread muscle involvement in critical illness myopathy revealed by MRI. *Muscle and Nerve*. 2011;44(5): 842–844.

83. Martin JB, Craig JW, Eckel RE, Munger J. Hypokalemic myopathy in chronic alcoholism. *Neurology*. 1971;21: 1160–1167.

84. Melli G, Chaudhry V, Cornblath DR. Rhabdomyolysis: an evaluation of 475 hospitalized patients. *Medicine* 2005;84: 377–385.

85. Middleton PG, Posen S. Hyperparathyroidism in a patient with myotonic dystrophy. *Journal of the Royal Society of Medicine*. 1989;82: 227.

86. Miller KD, Cameron M, Wood LV, Dalakas MC, Kovacs JA. Lactic acidosis and hepatic steatosis associated with use of stavudine: report of four cases. *Ann Intern Med*. 2000;133: 192–196.

87. Molina M, Lara JI, Riobo P, Guijarro S, Moreno A, et al. Primary hyperthyroidism and associated hyperparathyroidism in a patient with myotonic dystrophy. *The American Journal of the Medical Sciences*. 1996;311(6): 296–298.

88. Muecksch JN, Stevens WA. Undiagnosed myasthenia gravis masquerading as eclampsia. *International Journal of Obstetric Anesthesia*. 2007;16: 379–382.

89. Murray MJ, Brull SJ, Bolton CF. Brief review: nondepolarizing neuromuscular blocking drugs and critical illness myopathy. *Can J Anesth*. 2006;53(11): 1148–1156.

90. Nakahara K, Kuriyama M, Sonoda Y, Yoshidome H, Nakagawa H, et al. Myopathy induced by HMG-CoA reductase inhibitors in rabbits: a pathological, electrophysiological, and biochemical study. *Toxicology and Applied Pharmacology*, 1998;152: 99–106.

91. Omar MA, Wilson JP. FDA adverse event reports of statin-associated rhabdomyolysis. *Ann Pharmacother* 2002;36: 288–295.

92. Pall HS, Williams AC, Heath DA, Sheppard M, Wilson R. Hypomagnesemia causing myopathy and hypocalcemia in an alcoholic. *Postgraduate Medical Journal* 1987;63: 665–667.

93. Pasternak RC, Smith SC, Bairey-Merz CN, Grundy SM, Cleeman JL, Lenfant C. ACC/AHA/NHLBI clinical advisory on the use and safety of statins. *J. Am Coll Cardiol*. 2002;40: 567–572.

94. Pati S, Goodfellow JA, Iyadurai S, Hilton-Jones D. Approach to critical illness polyneuropathy and myopathy. *Postgrad Med*. 2008;84: 354–360.

95. Patten BM, Bilezikian JP, Mallette LE, Prince A, Engel WK, Aurbach GD. Neuromuscular disease in primary hyperparathyroidism. *Annals of Internal Medicine*. 1974;80: 182–193.

96. Posada C, Garcia-Cruz A, Garcia-Doval I, San Millan B, Teijeira S. Chloroquine-induced myopathy. *Lupus*. 2011;20: 773–774.

97. Ramsay ID. Electromyography in thyrotoxicosis. *Quarterly Journal of Medicine* 1965;135: 255–267.

98. Rana SS, Giuliani MJ, Oddic CV, Lacomis D. Acute onset of colchicine myoneuropathy in cardiac transplant recipients: case studies of three patients. *Clinical Neurology and Neurosurgery*. 1997;99: 266–270.

99. Rigante D, Bersani G, Compagnone A, Zampetti A, DeNisco A, Sacco E, Marrocco R. Exercise-induced rhabdomyolysis and transient loss of deambulation as outset of partial carnitine palmityl transferase II deficiency. *Rheumatol Int*. 2011;31:805–807.

100. Ringel SP, Claman HN. Amyloid associated muscle pseudohypertrophy. *Arch Neurol* 1982;39: 413–417.

101. Romaine SPR, Bailey L,, Hall SD, Balmforth AJ. The influence of SLCO1B1 (OATP1B1) gene polymorphisms on response to statin therapy. *The Pharmacogenomics Journal* 2010;10: 1–11.

102. Rubin DI, Hermann RC. Electrophysiologic findings in amyloid myopathy. *Muscle and Nerve*. 1999;22: 355–359.

103. Ruff RL, Weissmann J. Endocrine myopathies. *Neurologic Clinics*. 1988;6(3): 575–592.

104. Russell JA. Osteomalacic myopathy. *Muscle and Nerve*. 1994;17: 578–580.

105. Rusyniak DE, Tandy SL, Hekmatyar SL, Mills E, Smith DJ, et al. The role of mitochondrial uncoupling in 3,4-methylenedioxymethamphetamine-mediated skeletal muscle hyperthermia and rhabdomyolysis. *The Journal of Pharmacology and Experimental Therapeutics*. 2005;313(2): 629–639.

106. Rutkove SB, De Girolami U, Preston DC, Freeman R, NardinR, et al. Myotonia in colchicine myoneuropathy. *Muscle and Nerve* 1996;19: 870–875.

107. Rymanowski JV, Twydell PT. Treatable dropped head syndrome in hyperparathyroidism. *Muscle and Nerve*. 2009;39(3): 409–410.

108. Sander HW, Golden M, Danon MJ. Quadriplegic arreflexic ICU illness: selective thick filament loss and normal nerve histology. *Muscle and Nerve*. 2002;26: 499–505.

109. Saperstein DS. Muscle channelopathies. *Seminars in Neurology* 2008;28(2): 260–269.

110. Sathasivam S, Lecky B. Statin induced myopathy. *BMJ* 2008;337: 1159–1162.

111. Siddiqui AK, Huberfeld SI, Weidenheim KM, Einberg KR, Efferen LS. Hydroxychloroquine-induced toxic myopathy causing respiratory failure. *Chest* 2007;131: 588–590.

112. Sieb JP, Gillessen T. Iatrogenic and toxic myopathies. *Muscle and Nerve* 2003;27: 142–156.

113. Smith R, Stern G. Muscular weakness in osteomalacia and hyperparathyroidism. *Journal of the Neurological Sciences* 1969;8(3): 511–520.

114. Staffa JA, Chang J, Green L. Cerivastatin and reports of fatal rhabdomyolysis. *NEJM*. 2002;346(7): 539–540.

115. Tachibana S, Murakami T, Noguchi H, Nogushi Y, Nakashima A, et al. Orbital magnetic resonance imaging combined with clinical activity score can improve the sensitivity of detection of disease activity and prediction of response to immunosuppressive therapy for Grave's ophthalmopathy. *Endocrine Journal*. 2010;57(10): 853–861.

116. Thompson PD, Clarkson P, Karas RJ. Statin associated myopathy. *JAMA*. 2003;289(13): 1681–1690.

117. Tisdale MJ. Cachexia in cancer patients. *Nature Reviews Cancer*. 2002;2: 862–870.

118. Tisdale MJ. Reversing cachexia. *Cell*. 2002;142: 511–512.

119. Umpierrez GE, Stiles RG, Kleinbart J, Krendel DA, Watts NB. Diabetic muscle infarction. *The American Journal of Medicine* 1996;101: 245–250.

120. Urbano-Marquez A, Estruch R, Navarro-LopezR, Grau JM, Mont L, Rubin E. The effects of alcoholism on skeletal and cardiac muscle. *NEJM* 1989;320(7): 409–415.

121. Van Offel JF, De Gendt CM, De Clerck LS, Stevens WJ. High bone mass and hypocalcemic myopathy in a patient with idiopathic hypoparathyroidism. *Clin Rheum*. 2000;19: 64–66.

122. Weiner ID, Wingo CS. Hypokalemia—consequences, causes, and correction. *Journal of the American Society of Nephrology*. 1997;8(7): 1179–1188.

123. Zinman L, D Baryshnik, V Bril. Surrogate therapeutic outcome measures in patients with myasthenia gravis. *Muscle and Nerve*. 2008;37: 172–176.

General Strategies of Clinical Management

Chapter 12

Muscle Pain and Fatigue

Michael R. Rose
Patrick Gordon

INTRODUCTION

Muscle pain and fatigue are recognized in most cases as part of normal life experience. The most common cause of muscle pain is trauma or unaccustomed exercise. However, when these symptoms are considered to be outside of the normal experience and reach medical attention, it may be assumed that they indicate an underlying muscle condition. Although certain muscle conditions may be considered, most often there is no specific muscle disease. Instead, alternative nonmuscle disease diagnoses may apply, such as remote or even systemic diseases causing muscle pain, connective tissue diseases, fibromyalgia, and chronic fatigue syndrome. When presented with such cases, the key decisions are whether there is or is not a muscle disease, how far to take investigations looking for an underlying muscle disease, the extent to which it is likely that a muscle disease might still be possible when clinical assessment and investigations are unrewarding, and whether an alternative nonmuscle diagnosis can be suggested.

Paradoxically, whereas the vast majority of patients who present with myalgia and excessive fatigue do not turn out to have muscle disease, the roles that pain and fatigue do play in the lives of those with proven muscle disease are frequently underappreciated even by muscle specialists.

In this chapter, therefore, we outline the physiologic basis for muscle pain and fatigue, provide a framework for evaluating patients with these symptoms, and suggest strategies for management. We highlight those muscle diseases for which pain may be a symptom and the nonmuscle disease diagnoses that require consideration in the differential for myalgia and fatigue. We also discuss the role of pain and fatigue in proven muscle disease.

PATHOGENESIS OF MUSCLE PAIN

Painful stimuli from skeletal muscle are transmitted by small afferent nerve fibers, which are either thinly myelinated (group ID or A delta) or unmyelinated. These nerve endings are distributed throughout skeletal muscle. particularly in tendons and fascia. There are generally two types of pain receptors within muscle, and these are receptive either to chemical change or to mechanical alteration. Some of these nociceptors respond only to a variety of chemical stimuli, whereas others respond to chemical, thermal, and mechanical stimuli. The activity of these receptors is influenced by histamine, potassium ion, hydrogen ions, bradykinin, 5-hydroxytryptamine, TNF, and various lymphokines. Aspirin reduces their responsiveness. These same receptors are also important in modulating cardiovascular responses during exercise and in regulating motor unit discharge frequencies.

Intense muscle exertion can produce pain due to:

- ischemia during sustained high-intensity muscle contraction;
- tearing muscle fibers ("a pulled muscle");
- rupturing a muscle tendon;
- inducing a true muscle cramp;
- claudication of muscle in individuals with impaired circulation from vascular disease; and
- exhausting fuel supply and producing contracture in patients with metabolic defects in glycogen, beta-oxidation, or mitochondrial pathways.

During most types of exercise there is little muscle pain, which is surprising when one considers that blood flow declines to a nadir when the force of a sustained muscle contraction exceeds 40% of the maximum voluntary contraction.[1-3] In normal muscle, ischemia probably accounts for much of the pain that occurs during high-intensity exercise. The precise mechanisms underlying this type of pain are not entirely clear. Ischemia alone produces relatively little muscle pain unless it is very long standing. Similarly, pre-exercise ischemia does not influence muscular endurance during ischemia. Accumulating metabolites appear to play a major role in the production of ischemic pain, but the belief that lactic acid is the major cause of ischemic pain is no longer tenable. Patients with myophosphorylase deficiency experience substantial pain during ischemic exercise and have no lactic acid buildup. Similarly, the clearance of lactic acid is much slower than the resolution of pain during the recovery period after ischemic exercise. Recent evidence suggests that lymphokines may contribute to this pain and that changes in potassium ions, hydrogen ions, and possibly other substances also may be important.

Pain After Exercise

After unaccustomed exercise, normal individuals often have pain and soreness of muscles, especially during active movement. This pain begins after a delay of several hours and persists from 12 hours up to 5 days.[4] The muscles are tender to palpation and may be uncomfortable at rest. Demonstrable weakness[4,5] and evidence of muscle destruction[6,7] accompany the pain and soreness, particularly after vigorous training.

Eccentric Versus Concentric Muscle Contraction

The nature of the muscle contraction is an important determinant of the extent of muscle pain and damage. Muscle contraction can occur as the muscle shortens (concentric contraction) or as it lengthens (eccentric contraction). The difference in stress placed on muscle fibers in concentric compared with eccentric contraction is clinically important. Eccentric contraction is more likely than concentric contraction to produce muscle soreness,[4] histologic evidence of muscle damage,[7] and abnormalities of CK level.[6] Indeed, even brief periods (20 minutes) of eccentric leg exercise can produce 10- to 100-fold elevations of CK levels.[5] Thus walking down a mountain is more likely to provoke muscle pain and elevated CK level than walking up the mountain. Eccentric contraction may be especially damaging to diseased muscle.[8] The basis for postexertional muscle soreness may be an increase in intramuscular fluid pressure caused by muscle fiber breakdown and edema.[9]

Muscle Cramp

Muscle cramps are defined as intense pain of acute onset and short duration resulting in a strong, hard, palpable muscular contraction that is immediately relieved by stretching the muscle. The cramp may be preceded by muscle twitching and can occur at rest or following trivial activity. Although itself of short duration, it can, sometimes after a delay of more than 12 hours, result in soreness and swelling of the muscle peaking at 48 to 72 hours. Some residual discomfort can persist for up to 2 weeks. During the actual muscle cramp there is direct activation of muscle nociceptors, causing damage to the muscle fibers with elevated CK level and, in severe cases, myoglobinuria. The persistent pain that follows is the result of sensitization of the nociceptors by vasoneuroactive substances.[10] EMG during cramp shows high-voltage, high-frequency motor unit discharges.

Muscle cramps are a common phenomenon, which in various series have been experienced by 37% to 50% of the normal population surveyed.[11-13] They are more common in older people and in women. They commonly occur in the legs and most often during the night. For most they are occasional phenomena, but for some they are a repeated, distressing problem. Cramps have been strongly associated with peripheral vascular disease,[11] intermittent claudication,[12] arthritis,[11] and/or angina[12] and not with heart failure, hypertension, diabetes mellitus, or stroke.[11] Despite the strong association with angina and intermittent claudication, further analysis showed that these two factors only described 12% of the variance in cramp, suggesting that their role was limited.[12]

Cramps in normal people may be associated with exercise, pregnancy, acute extracellular volume depletion, and electrolyte disturbances. Cramps may also been seen in systemic diseases such as cirrhosis, uremia (and dialysis treatment), hypothyroidism, Cushing's disease, and adrenal insufficiency. Toxins such as excess alcohol and organophosphates, and drugs such as pyridostigmine, beta-agonists like terbutaline and salbutamol, nifedipine, cimetidine, clofibrate, cyclosporin, penicillamine, and diuretics have been blamed for cramps. One study, however, showed no positive association between cramp and commonly prescribed drugs including diuretics.[11]

Lower motor neuron disease can result in cramps, sometimes with fasiculations as seen in ALS, where brisk denervation can also lead to an elevated CK level. Cramps can also occur with other lower motor disorders such as spinal stenosis, radiculopathy, plexopathy, polyneuropathy multifocal motor neuropathy, or proximal diabetic neuropathy. Such cramps are often in unusual places and not just in the legs as seen with isolated cramp. In most cases clinical features of a lower motor neuron lesion are seen together with EMG features of fasciculations, denervation, and reinnervation.

Families with autosomal-dominant cramps have been described in the 1990s with EMG and muscle biopsy evidence for neurogenic origin. In some families, nerve conduction studies have suggested an axonal neuropathy. Whether there is a specific genetic explanation for these cases is unclear.[14-16] Rare cramp syndromes include Flier's syndrome, in which muscle cramps coexist with acanthosis nigracans and insulin resistance and which may respond to phenytoin,[17,18] and Satoyoshi's syndrome, featuring muscle cramps with alopecia and diarrhea.[19]

Differential Diagnosis for Cramps

The term *cramp* is often misapplied to other neurological phenomenon such as contracture, tetany, spasticity, rigidity, dystonia, myotonia, neuromyotonia, and Brody's disease.

TETANY

Hypocalcemia- and hyperventilation-induced tetany can resemble ordinary muscle cramps and need consideration in the differential of cramps, especially as the hyperventilation may not be a presenting symptom.

SPASTICITY

Patients with well-characterized upper motorneuron disorders such as multiple sclerosis occasionally complain of severe muscle pain. The neurologic findings of spasticity, hyperreflexia, Babinski reflex, or other pathologic reflexes indicate the presence of central nervous system disease.

DYSTONIAS

Focal dystonias may cause pain and may be labeled as cramp (e.g., "writer's cramp") but none of the dystonias exhibit the true characteristics of cramp. The onset of such focal dystonias is usually task specific, and is therefore provoked by specific activity, usually of more gradual onset and described as aching rather than the intense pain experienced with cramp.

MYOTONIA

The delayed relaxation of muscle that is the hallmark of the myotonic conditions is more often described as stiffness rather than painful or cramping. It generally follows muscle contraction rather than occurring spontaneously as do cramps. Paradoxical myotonia refers to myotonia worsening rather than improving with exercise, and such myotonia may be provoked by cold rather than by muscle contraction. Rarely, severe myotonia may be both spontaneous and painful, but such cases are unlikely to be confused with a cramp syndrome especially when EMG shows profuse myotonic discharges.[20] A family with potassium-aggravated myotonia was described as having familial cramp, but this refered to the family's description of their symptoms rather than being at all like true cramps clinically or electrophysiologically.[21] (For more detailed consideration, see chapter 9).

NEUROMYOTONIA

This usually presents with various combinations of muscle stiffness, cramps, twitching, weakness, and delayed muscle relaxation, sometimes resulting in muscle hypertrophy. The twitching is associated with doublet or triplet motor unit discharges on EMG.[22] An extreme generalized form results in Isaac's syndrome.[23] The association of neuromyotonia with other autoimmune conditions and its response to plasma exchange predicted that this would be an antibody-mediated disorder, and in a proportion of cases antibodies to the voltage-gated potassium channel have been detected.[24]

BRODY'S DISEASE

Brody's disease is a rare inherited disorder characterized by a lifelong history of exercise-induced impairment of skeletal muscle relaxation (pseudomyotonia), stiffness, and cramps. The lack of intense pain and the silent EMG distinguish this from true muscle cramps. It is caused by a dysfunction of SERCA1, a fast-twitch skeletal-muscle sarcoplasmic reticulum Ca^{2+} ATPase.[25,26] In some but not all cases this can be linked to autosomal-recessive inherited mutations of its encoding gene *ATP2A1*, suggesting genetic heterogeneity.[27] Diagnosis is usually confirmed by immunostaining of skeletal muscle to detect the loss of SERCA1 protein, but the genetic heterogeneity may mean that this will not detect cases where there is a functional rather than structural abnormality of SERCA1. Calcium handling in Brody's disease has been studied in culture muscle cells, and the abnormalities in calcium ion handling disappeared with administration of dantrolene or verapamil concomitantly with acetylcholine.[28] A literature and clinical review found that the usual presenting symptoms were cramps, myalgia, muscle stiffness, and fatigue with later complaints of delayed muscle relaxation and exercise-induced muscle stiffness and muscle weakness.[29] Muscle stiffness and delayed muscle relaxation most frequently affected the hands, legs, and toes rather than being generalized. Myalgia, predominantly felt in legs and arms, and muscle cramp, most often in fingers and toes, can be present at rest or after exercise. Those cases with Brody's disease (reduced SERCA1 function with mutation in *ATP2A1*) were more likely to have autosomal-recessive inheritance, earlier onset, more generalized symptoms, and delayed relaxation after repetitive contraction of the elbow flexors. By contrast myalgia was a more common symptom for those with Brody's syndrome (reduced SERCA1 function without mutation in *ATP2A1*).[29] Symptoms usually progress over the years, curtailing sporting activities and often work, with more than half needing to use a wheelchair or mobility scooter. Contrary to experimental studies only a few patients found dantrolene or verapamil helpful, and many had to stop these drugs either because of side effects or lack of benefit. Clonazepam or etoricoxib helped a few, whereas simple analgesics or nonsteroidal anti-inflammatory drugs were of limited benefit.

CRAMP-FASCICULATION SYNDROME

Cramp-fasciculation syndrome is a heterogenous condition encompassing a number of etiologies. The association of cramps with fasciculation is rare in the general population as compared with the commonality of fasciculations and cramp separately.[12] The muscle twitching that can be seen in those with muscle cramp may be either fasciculations or myokymia. These two phenomena may be distinguishable clinically in that the former are spontaneous muscle twitches, whereas myokymia results in continuous rippling or undulating of the muscle surface. Such muscle undulation should be distinguished from that seen in rippling muscle disease, in which mechanical stimuli provoke electrically silent contractions, causing characteristic balling of muscle (myoedema) and transversely rolling waves of muscle contraction across large muscle groups. Rippling muscle disease can be acquired with autoimmune associations or genetically associated with caveolin mutations.[30-34] On EMG fasciculations show as single motor-nerve discharges, whereas myokymia is associated with spontaneous repetitive discharges. Cramp associated with myokymia may be a manifestation of a neuromyotonia syndrome (see Neuomyotonia section). Cramps associated with fasciculations are usually benign with no clinical evidence for muscle wasting or weakness and with no EMG abnormality other than the fasciculations. However, in rare cases there is evidence for varying degrees of motor neuron loss.[35-38]

EXERTIONAL MUSCLE PAIN

Patients with differential diagnosis of myalgia can be usefully aided by dividing them into those who have constant pain and those whose pain is exercise related.

The presentation of pain or fatigue after exercise often prompts suspicion of muscle disease, especially the possibility of a metabolic myopathy. However, it is instructive to examine the true presentation of metabolic myopathies to better appreciate when these are likely to be a cause. Such metabolic myopathies include disorders of glucose and carbohydrate metabolism, disorders of lipid metabolism, and mitochondrial disorders. The archetypal glycogenolytic defect of McArdle disease, also the commonest suspected metabolic myopathy in this scenario, may present late in life, but patients have usually had their symptoms since their teens or early adulthood. They most often complain of severe pain within minutes of initiating exercise that, if continued, can lead to painful muscle contractures with muscle swelling persisting for hours. These episodes are invariably accompanied by myoglobinuria with high CK. Isometric exercise is more likely to trigger such episodes. However in one series 22% of those with McArdle did not report a second wind phenomenon, and 38% had never had myoglobinuria.[39] Examination can be normal with only a proportion showing muscle hypertrophy and with weakness more usual in older subjects if at all. Where there is weakness, it affects shoulder girdle and upper limbs and not lower limbs—a very different presentation from that more often obtained from those referred with a complaint of exertional muscle pain. In many such cases the problem is of late onset with no retrospective history of any muscle symptoms or impaired muscle performance. The relationship of the pain to the exercise is often not so suggestive of a metabolic muscle disease when this is probed more fully. More often the complaint is of muscle pain that comes on with activity that is not necessarily vigorous or so different from the usual. Such pain is usually of delayed onset, typically occurring the day after activity, and is of prolonged duration, persisting for days. In most cases of an underlying metabolic muscle disease, there are symptoms of myoglobinuria, weakness on examination, high CK, myopathic EMG, or muscle biopsy abnormalities. The lipid disorders and mitochondrial diseases may have normal CK and EMG. Muscle biopsy is abnormal in most cases of mitochondrial disease, especially where muscle symptoms predominate, but not so for lipid disorders, where evidence for lipid accumulation may be absent. However, lipid disorders usually cause muscle pain in the setting of intense and prolonged physical exertion or during intercurrent illness. This is usually accompanied by myoglobinuria. A personal or family history of encephalopathy, hepatic failure, and cardiomyopathy may be evidence for the multisystem manifestations of a beta-oxidation defect. Similarly, there would be a range of associated nonmuscle features that would support a diagnosis of mitochondrial disease.

Tubular Aggregates and Cylindrical Spirals

In some patients exertional muscle pain has been associated with the finding of numerous tubular aggregates in the muscle biopsy.[40-42] Small numbers of tubular aggregates are a nonspecific finding in many normal subjects and in many different diseases.[43,44] Large numbers are not common, however, and the larger numbers found in these cases suggest that they may be related to the muscle pain, although the mechanism remains unknown. In several cases tubular aggregates occurred in association with cylindrical spirals, further distinguishing this subset of patients with muscle pain.[40,42]

DRUG-INDUCED MUSCLE PAIN

Many drugs produce myalgia, and it is always worth getting a detailed drug history of current and recent past medications used, including over-the-counter and herbal remedies, so that these can be checked for any propensity for causing muscle pain. For some drugs the mechanism by which they cause pain is partially understood, such as those causing hypokalemia including diuretics, carbenoxalone, purgatives, licorice, and amphotericin A. For other drugs, such as clofibrate, heroin, cimetidine, emetine, vincristine, etretinate, zidovudine (AZT), phencyclidine, antirheumatic drugs including colchicine and (hydroxy)chloroquine, and cardiovascular drugs such as amiodarone and perhexiline, the precise mechanism for the myalgia is unknown.

Two forms of toxicity-induced myalgia deserve particular mention.

Alcohol-Related Myopathy

This can result in both acute muscle symptoms and a more chronic myopathy. Episodes of painful muscle swelling particularly of the thighs or gastrocnemius muscles can occur most often in male adults who binge-drink. This may be aggravated by poor nutritional status. In some cases there is hypokalemia. The CK can be high. However, muscle pathology findings can be quite sparse, sometimes with just a few necrotic fibers. It is worth bearing in mind that muscle symptoms might actually be worse with sudden alcohol withdrawal rather than necessarily relating to toxic alcohol levels.

Statin Myopathy

Although not a strictly defined term, it covers a number of scenarios occurring in patients taking not just statins but also other treatments for lowering cholesterol levels. It should be appreciated that statins have a major benefit by reducing death and vascular events such as stroke and myocardial infarction. According to large, randomized, controlled trials of statins, muscle symptoms were uncommon and serious complications were extremely rare. Guidelines on the use of statins therefore do not suggest that baseline CK levels should be obtained before starting such treatments. This recommendation can cause problems with management when muscle symptoms do occur. In fact, muscle-related problems seem more common in clinical practice than in the original studies, so much so that statins may be underused, with only 50% of those who should use them doing so and with many patients stopping statins—25% at 6 months and 60% at 2 years.[45] The true incidence of muscular symptoms in an unselected population varies between 9% and 20%.

The risk of muscle complications with statins may be dose related but not necessarily related to the degree to which the cholesterol has been lowered. The risk is higher in older people, women, and those who are more physically active. Hypothyroidism, renal or hepatic insufficiency, diabetes, and excessive alcohol increase risk. Taking other drugs that increase the serum concentration of statin also increases risk. Hinting at a possible genetic predisposition, statin-related myopathies are also more common in patients with a family history of similar problems and in those who have had muscle symptoms with other drugs such as bisphosphonate or diuretics. Some statins may be less toxic than others; in the PRIMO study, percentage risk for mild to moderate symptoms such as muscle pain and cramps was least for fluvastatin (5.1%), pravastatin (10.9%), and atorvostatin (14.9%), and greatest for simvastatin (18.2%).[46]

The muscle problems that can arise from statin treatment include (a) myalgia with normal CK, (b) asymptomatic or symptomatic high CK; (c) myopathy with normal CK, (d) myoglobinuria, and (e) inflammatory necrotizing myopathy.[47-49]

There is no consensus on the mechanism of statin myopathies, with several theories advanced.[50-52] Patients may sometimes have myalgia when first starting a statin, but this may resolve after 2 weeks, so it is worth persisting with treatment for at least that period of time if the symptoms are not too troublesome. The commonest myalgia symptom is unaccustomed symmetrical burning sensations particularly after exercise. The differential diagnosis of statin-related myalgia includes myalgia caused by hormonal and vitamin deficiencies and other drug toxicity, as described in the Systemic Disorders Causing Muscle Pain section of this chapter as well as pain syndromes related to musculoskeletal or neurogenic causes.

Myalgia that resolves on cessation of statins and recurs on statin rechallenge, however, is likely to be related to the statin. Adverse drug interactions that may have triggered statin symptoms should be checked; these include prescription drugs that increase statin blood levels such as erythromycin, clarithromycin, antifungal agents, calcium channel blockers; recreational drugs like heroin and cocaine; over-the-counter drugs such as ipecacuanha and vitamin E; and foods such as grapefruit and red yeast rice (which contains lovastatin). Drugs and excess alcohol causing synergistic myotoxicity should be watched for and discontinued where possible. If there is persistence of symptoms despite cessation of statin, then a drug holiday of 6 weeks from all lipid-lowering treatment may be required. In this situation, some people advocate use of CoQ10 and fish oil, though the evidence base for these is uncertain.

If there is persisting myalgia on resumption of treatment with other factors and causes excluded, then there should be a reassessment of the lipid treatment goals or vascular risk, balancing the necessity for statin against the symptoms it provokes. This risk profile assessment may lead to the acceptance of either no statin treatment or less stringent targets for cholesterol-level lowering that allow a lower, asymptomatic dose of statin to be used. (See NIH National Heart, Lung and Blood Institute, Risk Assessment Tool for Estimating Your 10-Year Risk of Having a Heart Attack: http://cvdrisk.nhlbi.nih.gov/calculator.asp.) Alternative statins with a longer duration of action or less dependence on cytochrome P450 metabolism such as pravastatin may avoid symptoms. Using a more potent statin such as rosuvostatin in alternate-day or in a once or twice a week regime may also avoid symptoms. Alternative treatments such as ezetimibe or fibrate may be an option but may not necessarily avoid muscle symptoms and do not have the evidence base for reduction in cardiovascular risk independent of their cholesterol-lowering action, which characterises the statins.

If muscle symptoms with or without raised CK levels fail to resolve with cessation of statin, this may mean that there is an undiagnosed underlying myopathy or that the statin has triggered an inflammatory myopathy. In some cases where there is a persistently raised CK with no actual muscle symptoms, there are alternative benign explanations for the elevated creatine kinase (e.g., African ancestry). In such situations a pretreatment CK level would be useful. There are reports of statin treatment unmasking preexisting muscle disease that was either asymptomatic or with symptoms that were not appreciated at the time treatment was started. In the elderly, who commonly start statins for secondary prevention, inclusion body myositis is a common diagnosis. There have been cases reported where there has been persistent myopathy with muscle biopsy showing necrotizing myopathy increased expression of major histocompatibility complex I. These patients had proximal weakness and elevated CK levels and sometimes needed quite aggressive immunosuppressive treatment.[52-54]

A question that arises regards the advisability of using statins in those with diagnosed muscle disease. In one small series, seven patients with known neuromuscular disorders including minicore myopathy, myotonic dystrophy, postpolio syndrome, McArdle disease, and spinal muscular atrophy were treated with either statin or fibrate. Some of these did show a rise in creatine kinase, but this seemed related to physical exertion and did not require stopping the lipid therapy. None developed rhabdomyolysis.[55] It is reasonable to give statins where clearly indicated with vigilance for new or worsening muscle symptoms. It remains unclear how helpful monitoring CK is in such people. Patients should be told the risk benefit considerations and should be suitably educated to the possibility of myoglobinuria so that they recognize it and seek urgent advice.

Rarely statins may induce an autoimmune necrotizing myopathy which persists after cessation of statin therapy. This syndrome is associated with antibodies to 3-hydroxy-3-methylglutaryl-coenzyme A reductase which is upregulated in regenerating muscle fibers.[56]

SYSTEMIC DISORDERS CAUSING MUSCLE PAIN

Thyroid Disease

Hypothyroidism is frequently associated with muscle pain as well as proximal muscle weakness. In one prospective cohort of 24 hypothyroid patients, 42% complained of muscle cramps, with weakness on manual muscle testing in 54%.[57] Raised CK was found in 37.5% and myopathic electrophysiology in 33%. On examination patients may have pseudomyotonia (electrically silent slowing of muscle relaxation), and delayed tendon relaxation after reflex testing. Hypothyroid patients with true weakness often have myotonic dystrophy (DM2; see chapter 11).

Although muscle weakness is commoner in hyperthyroid than hypothyroid patients (62% vs. 37.5%), muscle cramps are less frequent, occurring in approximately 10% of patients.[57] Muscle recovery also tends to be faster in hyperthyroid disease with a median time to resolution of muscle symptoms of 3.6 months compared to 6.9 months in one small study.[57] In this study, none of the hyperthyroid patients had raised CK and only 10% had a myopathic EMG (see chapter 11).

Thyrotoxic periodic paralysis (TPP) is a rare complication of hyperthyroidism found predominantly in Asian populations with an incidence of 1.9% in thyrotoxic Japanese compared to 0.1% to 0.2% in thyrotoxic North Americans.[58] It occurs typically in men between 20 to 40 years of age with attacks usually precipitated by a heavy carbohydrate load, exercise, or alcohol. The attacks vary from weakness to flaccid paralysis with complete recovery between attacks. Muscle pain may occur as a prelude to the attacks. They are characterized by hypokalemia due to an intracellular shift of potassium. Acute emergency treatment consists of cautious potassium supplementation as rebound hyperkalemia may subsequently occur once the intracellular flux of potassium is reversed. Intravenous or oral propranolol IV or orally may also reverse the paralysis acutely. Long-term treatment consists of treatment of the underlying hyperthyroidism, as the condition does not occur once a euthyroid state is attained. Recent work has identified a mutation of the potassium channel Kir2.6 in some patients with TPP (see chapter 9).

Parathyroid Disease and Vitamin D

Hypoparathyroid disease may present with cramping or tetany causing pain and a raised CK. A rare painful myopathy secondary to hypoparathyroidism has also been described.[59]

Primary hyperparathyroidism is asymptomatic in 70% to 80% of patients, although a myopathy with atrophy on biopsy may occur with severe bone disease.[60]

Osteomalacia is characterized by delayed bone mineralization with an osteoid volume greater than 10%, usually as a result of a low calcium:phosphorus ratio. Osteomalacia causes musculoskeletal pain generally involving the spine, pelvis, shoulder girdle, and rib cage. A myopathy with a "waddling" gait occurs in almost a quarter of patients with biopsy-proven osteomalacia.[61] This is generally a proximal weakness, although distal weakness may also occur. Histology mainly shows type 2 fiber atrophy with some reversibility following vitamin D supplementation in vitamin D–deficient subjects.[62] Several studies have shown an association between vitamin D levels and physical function in subjects over 60 years old,[62] suggesting an important role for vitamin D in muscle function beyond the context of overt osteomalacia. Although there has been some literature suggesting a role of low vitamin D in chronic pain syndromes, including fibromyalgia, overall the evidence for this is poor[63] (see chapter 11).

Adrenal and Pituitary Disease

Cushing's syndrome due to endogenous or exogenous glucocorticoid therapy may cause a proximal myopathy, affecting particularly the pelvic girdle, usually with an insidious onset. Pain is either absent or mild. Generally but not always patients will have other clinical features of Cushing's syndrome. Endogenous steroid therapy is the commonest cause and is more likely to occur with the use of fluorinated corticosteroids than nonfluorinated corticosteroids such as prednisolone. It is unusual to develop steroid myopathy at a dose of prednisolone below 10 mg daily, whereas approximately 65% of patients on a prednisolone dose of over 40 mg will have evidence of weakness on manual muscle testing.[64] Muscle enzymes are not generally raised and there is no relationship between muscle enzyme levels and muscle strength or corticosteroid dose.[64] Muscle biopsy findings are nonspecific with type 2b fiber atrophy, variation in fiber size with central nuclei, and (rarely) muscle necrosis[65] (see chapter 11).

Adrenal insufficiency can frequently cause muscle fatigability. Notably in patients on long-standing corticosteroid therapy, as the therapy is reduced patients frequently suffer from musculoskeletal pain and fatigue. In primary hyperaldosteronism, muscle disease occurs as a result of hypokalaemia with proximal weakness. In acromegaly there is frequently a mild proximal weakness despite muscle hypertrophy.

Diabetes

Muscle infarction is a painful complication of long-standing poorly controlled diabetes. It usually occurs in patients in their forties with established diabetic vasculopathy, both retinopathy and nephropathy.[66] It itself is thought to be a microvascular disease complication with ischemic reperfusion.[66] It presents as sudden-onset pain and swelling of the affected muscle. Vastus lateralis, the thigh adductors, and biceps femoris are the most commonly affected muscles, although involvement of calf, upper limb, and abdominal musculature has been described.[67,68] At the acute presentation CK is usually raised as is the erythrocyte sedimentation rate. However, a normal creatine kinase does not exclude the diagnosis particularly if there has been a delay in the diagnosis. Generally diabetic muscle infarction has a good short-term prognosis with conservative therapy. The overall long-term outcome for the patient is extremely poor, however, with a 1-year survival of 55% in a small cohort of six patients, and five out of six patients dying after a minimum 4-year follow-up in another cohort[66] (see chapter 11).

Vasculitis

Muscle can be affected in systemic vasculitis presenting with muscle pain. This is a classical presentation of the medium-sized vessel vascultitis, polyarteritis nodosa, where muscle pain is one of the items on the American College of Rheumatology Classification Criteria. However, muscle vasculitis can occur in many other vasculitides.

In one retrospective study of 24 patients with a biopsy-proven vasculitic neuropathy who also had a muscle biopsy, 46% had evidence of a coexistent muscle vasculitis.[69] The diagnoses in this study included Wegener's granulomatosis, polyarteritis nodosa, rheumatoid vasculitis, microscopic polyangiitis, hepatitis B and C, Sjögren's syndrome, undifferentiated connective tissue disease, and systemic Sclerosis. In another review of 40 cases of biopsy-proven skeletal muscle vasculitis, the diagnoses included rheumatoid arthritis, Churg-Strauss syndrome, hepatitis B and/or C, Sjögren's syndrome, and scleroderma.[70] The finding of vasculitis in a muscle biopsy should lead to a careful assessment of the extent of organ involvement of the vasculitis, including renal disease, to make a firm diagnosis and ensure early recognition of life-threatening disease.

MUSCLE PAIN ARISING FROM BONE AND JOINT DISORDERS

Muscle pain is common even when the actual cause is a joint, bone, or tendinous disorder. Nonmuscular disorders may present with muscle pain because of a misperception of the location of pain. A misleading complaint of "muscle pain" may make localization of the site of pathology very difficult, and this may be compounded by the fact that muscular atrophy may develop because nonmuscular pain hinders exercise or daily activities. For example, with polymyalgia rheumatica (PMR), despite typical complaints of "muscle pain and stiffness" in the shoulder or hip-girdle musculature, radionuclide scanning shows inflammation of the joints and increased joint fluid, suggesting that the pain arises from joints rather than muscles.[71] Examples of contiguous joint or bone diseases that produce muscle atrophy and muscle pain are listed in Box 12.1. Failure to recognize the underlying condition may result in a mistaken diagnosis

---

Box 12.1 Important Causes of Muscle Pain of Nonmuscular Origin

Joint Disease

> Rheumatoid arthritis
> Systemic lupus erythematosus
> Scleroderma
> Polymyalgia rheumatic
> Gout

Joint hypermobility syndromes (common)

> Ehlers-Danlos syndrome (relatively uncommon)

Bone Disease

> Osteomalacia
> Primary and secondary hyperparathyroidism

Myeloproliferative disorders

of myopathy. Coincidental abnormalities of muscle may also point to the wrong location. Pain associated with certain conditions, especially metabolic bone disease and rheumatoid arthritis, lead to disuse and visible muscle atrophy as well as abnormal muscle histological and electrophysiological findings. These biopsy and electromyographic (EMG) changes result from two factors: (1) coincidental but not necessarily important abnormalities of nerve and (2) changes in the muscle resulting from disuse. Such findings as atrophy of type 1 or type 2 muscle fibers, moth-eaten fibers (multifocal loss of oxidative enzyme staining in individual muscle fibers), inflammatory cell infiltrates, and small angular fibers that appear dark on staining with NADH-tetrazolium reductase are frequent and nonspecific. These abnormalities do not cause the muscle pain but rather result from underlying joint or bone disease.[72,73]

Pain in Inflammatory Muscle Disease and the Other Connective Tissue Diseases

Myalgia is relatively common in patients with inflammatory myositis (approximately 60% of patients).[74] In addition to polymyositis and dermatomyositis, inflammatory muscle disease can occur in other connective tissue diseases including systemic lupus erythematosus, systemic sclerosis, mixed connective tissue disease, and Sjögren's syndrome. Our group assessed 95 patients with idiopathic inflammatory myopathy (polymyositis and dermatomyositis) under long-term follow-up in three London teaching hospitals and asked them to rank seven major symptoms (fatigue, difficulty in daily function, pain or discomfort, weakness, sleep disturbance, problems with memory or concentration, and stomach or digestive problems) in terms of their impact on their health status. Whereas the greatest proportion of patients (25%) rated fatigue as the greatest symptom impacting their health status, pain was next most frequently cited (20%). In contrast, only 10% ranked weakness as the top symptom impacting on their health status.[75] In a multivariate model assessing predictors of fatigue, the strongest contributions came from depression and pain, with disease activity, damage, and strength showing much

weaker predictive value.[76] The patients in this study were under long-term follow up with predominantly low disease activity, and as such this study does suggest that even in patients with well-controlled disease, pain is a common problem.

Muscle pain may also occur secondary to calcinosis. Calcinosis is relatively rare in adult idiopathic inflammatory myopathies, but occurs in approximately 20% of juvenile dermatomyositis patients.[77] Risk factors for the development of calcinosis in the pediatric population include cumulative length of active disease[77] and testing positive for anti-NXP antibodies.[78]

Apparent Muscle Pain in Nonmuscle Diseases

Many conditions may masquerade as muscle disease and present with "muscular pain" as a prominent feature: PMR, fibromyalgia, chronic fatigue syndrome, avascular necrosis, arthritis of the hip or shoulder, and rotator cuff disease of the shoulders. Notably none of these conditions has true muscle weakness, although in the situation where there is a lot of pain this can be difficult to assess. In eosinophilic fasciitis and macrophagic fasciitis, the inflammation is focused on the fascia rather than muscle, but causes pain that appears muscular.

Fibromyalgia

Fibromyalgia is a common syndrome of chronic diffuse pain, with cognitive and sleep disturbances affecting 2% to 5% of the adult population. To fulfil the 1990 classification criteria of the American College of Rheumatology, there must be widespread pain combined with at least 11 out of 18 positive trigger points (defined in Figure 12–1) for a period of at least 3 months. For a trigger point to be considered positive, digital pressure of approximately 4 kg applied to it should cause pain. To be considered as being widespread, the pain must:

- present on both the left and right sides of the body, *and*
- both above and below the waist, *and*
- must involve the axial skeleton (cervical, thoracic, lower back, or anterior chest).

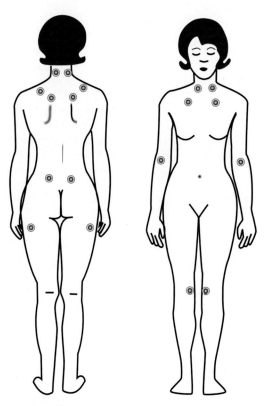

Figure 12–1. Tender Points from the 1990 American College of Rheumatology Fibromyalgia Classification Criteria Fibromyalgia tender point localizations:
- Suboccipital
- Cervical: the C5–C7 transverse processes
- Upper trapezius border midpoint
- Supraspinatus medially in the supraspinous fossa
- Lateral to the second rib costochondral junction
- 2 cm below the lateral epicondyle
- Upper lateral quadrant of the gluteal region
- Greater trochanter
- Proximal to the joint line of the medial femur

Modified from the American College of Rheumatology Fibromyalgia Classification Criteria, Arthritis & Rheumatism, 1990;33(2):160–172. Image courtesy of Wikipedia.

However, in recognition of the variation in positive trigger points over time in patients with fibromyalgia, a further complementary set of diagnostic criteria were released in 2010 that do not depend on trigger points. Rather, the patient needs to score sufficiently highly on two scores: the widespread pain score and the symptom severity scale (see Box 12.2) in the absence of an alternative explanation for the symptoms. Both criteria require symptoms to have been present for at least 3 months. Beyond the classification criteria there is no diagnostic test for fibromyalgia, and it is important to assess for

other possible causes of this constellation of symptoms, including connective tissue disease, thyroid disease, and osteomalacia. More than 20 years after the original classification criteria were produced there remains some debate as to whether fibromyalgia is a truly unique syndrome separate from other pain syndromes. Certainly it is frequently associated with other central sensitization syndromes such as chronic fatigue syndrome, temporomandibular joint pain, and irritable bowel syndrome.

Secondary fibromyalgia frequently occurs in the context of inflammatory conditions such as rheumatoid arthritis and systemic lupus erythematosus when pain persists despite the control of inflammatory disease. In systemic lupus erythematosus the incidence has been reported as high as 22%, with a further 23% having features of fibromyalgia but not fulfilling the 1990 classification criteria.[79]

There is evidence of central sensitization in fibromyalgia. A stimulus of a sufficient level to cause pain in fibromyalgia patients but not controls produces different patterns of central nervous system activation on functional MRI in the patients versus the controls.[80] There is evidence of abnormalities in central pain mechanisms affecting both the ascending and descending pathways in fibromyalgia.

Pharmacological therapies that have an evidence base in relieving fibromyalgia include pregabalin and the serotonin norepinephrine reuptake inhibitors, duloxetine and milnacipran.[81] In addition, there is a good evidence base for the benefit of cognitive behavioral therapy (CBT).

Polymyalgia Rheumatica

PMR is an inflammatory condition of the elderly. It is associated with an inflammatory response and proximal muscle pain and stiffness affecting the shoulder and pelvic girdles. The diagnosis is clinical with a characteristic rapid response to oral prednisolone at a starting dose of 15 mg daily, often within 24 hours.

Despite the prominent muscle symptoms, there is no evidence of muscle pathology and no detectable muscle weakness in PMR. However, glenohumeral synovitis, subdeltoid bursitis, biceps tenosynovitis, hip synovitis, and

Box 12.2 Proposed Criteria for Primary Fibromyalgia

Major Criteria

1. Three or more areas of pain, aching, or stiffness lasting 3 months or longer

2. Exclusion of other causes of muscle pain

3. Tender points (5 or more specific proposed areas; see Figure 12-1)

Minor Criteria

1. Exercise-related symptoms

2. Subjective subcutaneous swelling

3. Areas of cutaneous numbness

4. Change in symptoms with weather

5. Aggravation in symptoms by anxiety or stress

6. Disturbed sleep

7. Fatigue or tiredness

8. Anxiety

9. Chronic headache

10. Irritable bowel syndrome

Presence of 3 major and at least 3 of the minor criteria supports the diagnosis (modified from Yunus[123]).

---

trochanteric bursitis are demonstrable by ultrasound in the majority of patients. Peripheral synovitis may also occur making it difficult to differentiate from a polymyalgic presentation of rheumatoid arthritis. Temporal arteritis often has polymyalgic symptoms, and as such it is important to make patients aware of the symptoms of temporal arteritis (e.g., temporal headache and tenderness, jaw claudication, visual disturbance), their significance, and seriousness. In approximately 30% of subjects who have pure PMR clinically, vascular uptake can be detected on fluorodeoxyglucose positive emission tomograpy, indicating an element of vasculitis.

The recently published classification criteria for PMR use a scoring system of morning stiffness for more than 45 minutes (2 points), hip pain/limited range of motion (1 point), absence of rheumatoid factor and/or anti-citrullinated protein antibodies (2 points), and absence of peripheral joint pain (1 point). A score of 4 or higher had 68% sensitivity and 78% specificity for discriminating all comparison subjects from PMR.[82]

MYOPATHIES ASSOCIATED WITH MUSCLE PAIN

Some of the myopathies considered earlier in this volume may produce pain (Box 12.3). The suggested diagnostic approach to the patient with muscle pain is outlined in Box 12.4. In one series, roughly one-third of patients with muscle pain had an alternative definable cause of the pain.[83]

Box 12.3 2010 American College of Rheumatology Fibromyalgia Diagnostic Criteria

A patient satisfies diagnostic criteria for fibromyalgia if the following 3 conditions are met:

1. Widespread pain index (WPI) ≥7 and symptom severity (SS) scale score ≥5 or WPI 3–6 and SS scale score ≥9.

2. Symptoms have been present at a similar level for at least 3 months.

3. The patient does not have a disorder that would otherwise explain the pain.

Scoring for the WPI and SS scale

1. Note the number areas in which the patient has had pain over the last week. In how many areas has the patient had pain? Score will be between 0 and 19.

Shoulder girdle, left	Hip (buttock, trochanter), left	Jaw, left	Upper back
Shoulder girdle, right	Hip (buttock, trochanter), right	Jaw, right	Lower back
Upper arm, left	Upper leg, left	Chest	Neck
Upper arm, right	Upper leg, right	Abdomen	
Lower arm, left	Lower leg, left		
Lower arm, right	Lower leg, right		

2) SS scale score:

Fatigue
Waking unrefreshed
Cognitive symptoms

For the each of the 3 symptoms above, indicate the level of severity over the past week using the following scale:

0 = no problem
1 = slight or mild problems, generally mild or intermittent
2 = moderate, considerable problems, often present and/or at a moderate level
3 = severe: pervasive, continuous, life-disturbing problems

Considering somatic symptoms in general, indicate whether the patient has:[a]

0 = no symptoms
1 = few symptoms
2 = a moderate number of symptoms
3 = a great deal of symptoms

(continued)

Box 12.3   2010 American College of Rheumatology Fibromyalgia Diagnostic Criteria (cont.)

The SS scale score is the sum of the severity of the 3 symptoms (fatigue, waking unrefreshed, cognitive symptoms) plus the extent (severity) of somatic symptoms in general. The final score is between 0 and 12.

ªSomatic symptoms that might be considered: muscle pain, irritable bowel syndrome, fatigue/tiredness, thinking or remembering problem, muscle weakness, headache, pain/cramps in the abdomen, numbness/tingling, dizziness, insomnia, depression, constipation, pain in the upper abdomen, nausea, nervousness, chest pain, blurred vision, fever, diarrhea, dry mouth, itching, wheezing, Raynaud's phenomenon, hives/welts, ringing in ears, vomiting, heartburn, oral ulcers, loss of/change in taste, seizures, dry eyes, shortness of breath, loss of appetite, rash, sun sensitivity, hearing difficulties, easy bruising, hair loss, frequent urination, painful urination, and bladder spasms.
Adapted from Arthritis Wolfe F, Clauw DJ, Fitzcharles MA, Goldenberg DL, Katz RS, Mease P, Russell AS, Russell IJ, Winfield JB, Yunus MB. The American College of Rheumatology preliminary diagnostic criteria for fibromyalgia and measurement of symptom severity. Arthritis Care Res (Hoboken). 2010 May;62(5):600–610.

Box 12.4   Occurrence of Muscle Pain in Myopathies

Muscular dystrophies

　　Facioscapulohumeral—stretch injuries
　　Limb girdle, Becker's, myotonic—extertional pain
　　Others (less common)—muscle damage secondary to overuse

　　Inflammatory myopathies (seldom a presenting complaint except in childhood dermatomyositis)
　　Metabolic myopathies (e.g., deficiency of myophosphorylase [McArdle's disease]; phosphofructokinase deficiency)
　　Mitochondrial myopathies
　　Myotonia congenita

X-Linked Myalgia and Cramp

X-linked familial cases of myalgia have been described where there may be no weakness but often pseudohypertrophy of the calves and an elevated CK.[84-87] Cases can have weakness, exertional fatigue or weakness, and episodes of myoglobinuria in various combinations even within the same family.[86] The muscle biopsy may be normal or show dystrophic changes. Immunostaining for dystrophin is normal but western blot shows reduced dystrophin levels; a variety of in-frame mutations in the dystrophin gene have been described. It is therefore suggested that dystrophin western blotting for gene analysis be done in cases of familial myalgia, especially in childhood. Although the condition may be rare, its existence raises the possibility that some patients with unexplained muscle pain may represent undefined allelic variants of a muscular dystrophy or other hereditary myopathy.

Eosinophilic Myopathies

A small number of patients with constant and diffuse muscle pains but normal strength have eosinophilic infiltrates of muscle.[88,89] Peripheral eosinophilia is not necessarily present. Disorders include eosinophilic polymyositis, diffuse fasciitis with eosinophilia, and the eosinophilia myalgic syndrome with ingestion of tryptophan.

Eosinophilic fasciitis is a rare condition first described in 1974. It usually occurs in the third to sixth decade of life. Its onset is associated with an intense period of exertion in up to half the patients.[90] The cutaneous manifestations comprise of skin edema of the distal extremities, which progresses to a peau d'orange appearance and then to induration over time. The majority of patients develop joint contractures and approximately 40% of patients develop an inflammatory arthritis.[90] However, internal organ disease is rare and, unlike systemic sclerosis, it is not associated with Raynaud's. In a minority there is an associated hematological disorder including aplastic anaemia, myeloproliferative disorders, myelodysplastic disorders, lymphoma, and leukemia. The majority of patients have a peripheral eosinophilia. The diagnosis is confirmed by a full-thickness skin-to-muscle biopsy; inflammation is focused on the panniculus and deep fascia, with the infiltrate comprising eosinophils and lymphocytes.[91] The mainstay of therapy is corticosteroids.

Macrophagic Myofasciitis

Macrophagic myofasciitis generally presents with diffuse myalgia with a proportion of patients presenting with arthralgia, fever, and muscle weakness.[92] A raised CK or erythrocyte sedimentation rate, and/or a myopathic EMG may be found. It is characterized by macrophage infiltration of the muscle connective tissues on biopsy. On ultrastructure the macrophages have aggregates of dense spicules secondary to the deposition of phosphate crystals, which originate from the use of aluminium as an adjuvant in intramuscular vaccines. Steroid therapy has been reported as beneficial in the majority of cases.[92]

OTHER NEUROLOGIC CONDITIONS WITH MUSCLE PAIN

Restless Legs Syndrome

Patients with this condition usually present after age 30 and may have a positive family history.[93] Patients experience an intensely uncomfortable feeling in their legs especially the calf muscles and hamstrings. Symptoms develop almost exclusively during sitting or lying down and may be described as "painful," although patients seldom seek or respond to analgesic medication. Activity relieves the abnormal sensation. Detailed studies of peripheral nerve histology and function usually show no consistent pathology, although similar symptoms have been described in association with neuropathies of known cause such as uremia. Symptoms can be alleviated by opiates, phenothiazines, or clonazepam, but chronic use of neuroleptics should be avoided if possible because of the frequent occurrence of side effects. In severe cases dopaminergic agents such as bromocritpine or L-dopa may be effective and appropriate.[94-97]

Intermittent Claudication

Both spinal and vascular claudication may present with muscle pain. Clues to this diagnosis are the relationship to walking and that the symptoms are confined to the legs. With spinal claudication radicular signs may be absent and critical review of the spinal imaging may be required.

Assessment of Fatigue in the Neuromuscular Clinic

Patients may be referred to neuromuscular clinics complaining of fatigue, weakness, or heaviness in the limbs, using these terms interchangeably. Care providers also sometimes fail to appreciate what patients mean by fatigue, confusing this with fatigability or excessive daytime sleepiness (EDS). Terms such as *objective, subjective, physical, mental, central, peripheral, physiological,* and *experienced fatigue* lead to further confusion about what is being discussed. Fatigue is an intrusive and unpleasant symptom that is not alleviated by rest or sleep. Fatigability is the clinically detectable weakening of muscle strength with repetitive muscle use and is a feature of neuromuscular transmission defects, and sometimes mitochondrial disease. EDS is not as intrusive or unpleasant as fatigue and is alleviated by rest, meaning that subjects do have a refreshing sleep. EDS may reflect nocturnal hypoventilation resulting from neuromuscular respiratory weakness and may also result from primary hypersomnolence as seen in myotonic dystrophy. EDS can result from obstructive sleep apnea (OSA) occurring as a primary disorder or as seen in a neuromuscular disease, particularly those affecting bulbar musculature. OSA is a condition with rising incidence in part due to the obesity epidemic. Not only may EDS be mistaken for or associated with fatigue, but there also may be concern regarding an underlying myopathy, because a proportion of those with OSA do have a high CK that normalizes with treatment of the OSA.[98]

Fatigue can be studied as a physiological phenomenon and this is sometimes referred to as objective or physical fatigue. However physical fatigue also has an alternate meaning as described in the next paragraph. During sustained maximal voluntary contraction there is a steady decline in muscle force generated. A fatigue index can therefore be calculated as the ratio between the area under the actual muscle force–time curve and the area that would be obtained if peak force were maintained for the same time period. Alternatively, the objective fatigue can be assessed during repetitive muscle contractions, usually at 50% of maximum force, whereupon there is a decline in the force generated with increasing repetitions. It could be argued that fatigue shown during repetitive contractions is closer to the physiological situation, as sustained maximum force is rarely used in everyday activities. A component of the fatigue seen in these laboratory situations is centrally mediated, involving the processes of cortical activation, motivation, and conduction down both the upper and lower motor neuron pathways, with the sensory and other feedback systems participating in this pathway. Insight into the central component of fatigue can be obtained by comparing the muscle force generated by transcranial magnetic stimulation compared with that obtained voluntarily. A component of the fatigue will be peripheral, involving processes within the muscle itself—that is, beyond the neuromuscular junction. Insight into this peripheral component of fatigue can be obtained by the process of twitch interpolation, whereby an electrical stimulus is delivered to the muscle or nerve to evoke a maximum force, which again can be compared with voluntary force.[99] These techniques have been applied to neurological conditions such as multiple sclerosis and Parkinson's disease and to neuromuscular diseases such as ALS and post-polio syndrome. In the latter two diseases, objective fatigue is greater than that seen in normal controls, with a mixed central and peripheral component.[100,101] By contrast one study of Duchenne muscular dystrophy showed that fatigue seen during a 4-minute sustained maximum voluntary contraction was no different to that seen in controls and with similar if not better central and peripheral mechanisms in play.[102] The relationships between these physiologic fatigue parameters and fatigue as a symptom are unclear, but they are probably not related, as has been shown for some muscle diseases.[103]

Fatigue as a symptom rather than a physiological process is a common feature of many systemic and long-term illnesses both non neurological (including cardiac, pulmonary, and renal disorders; blood dyscrasias of all types; and cancer) and neurological (including ALS, multiple sclerosis and Parkinson syndrome). It has become the focus of more attention of late as it makes an important adverse contribution to quality of life (QoL). Fatigue often has a physical and mental component. Physical fatigue in this particular context (rather than as a synonym for objective fatigue) is that provoked by physical exertion usually causing physical symptoms, and is the sort that most often raises the suspicion of a neuromuscular disorder, particularly neuromuscular junction defects or metabolic myopathies. Mental fatigue is that provoked by cognitive activities such that sufferers will describe fatigue trying to read a newspaper or watch a television program to the extent that they become unable to do such activities. In some cases physical exertion will also impact cognitive abilities and vice versa. Mental fatigue is unlikely to be a presenting feature of a neuromuscular disease. In most cases physical and mental fatigue coexist, thus making a primary neuromuscular condition less likely. Subjective fatigue being a patient experience is assessed by way of patient-reported questionnaires with many examples being available.[104] There is no consensus as to which of the many fatigue measures should be used for muscle disease. Many of the measures were developed and hence validated, to differing degrees, in patient populations other than those with muscle disease. Some questionnaires include questions that assess fatigue in terms of physical activities that would be affected more by muscle weakness than any fatigue, emphasizing one reason for the need to validate any proposed fatigue measure in a muscle disease population. Some work assessing certain fatigue scales has been undertaken for myotonic dystrophy.[105]

THE ROLE OF PAIN AND FATIGUE IN ESTABLISHED MUSCLE DISEASE

Patients who present with fatigue rarely have muscle disease as a cause. However, even though most patients with muscle disease do not present with a complaint of fatigue, it is in fact an important underrecognized symptom. Semistructured interviews with muscle disease subjects used to construct a QoL questionnaire specific to muscle disease revealed that both pain and fatigue were significant symptoms affecting QoL alongside symptoms of weakness and myotonia (for those with myotonic conditions).[106] Kalkman et al. found that 61% of those with FSHD and 74% of those with myotonic dystrophy were severely fatigued and had more problems with physical and social functioning, with the fatigued FSHD patients also having more associated bodily pain.[103]

Pain is also an underappreciated symptom in those with established muscle disease. In one series of patients with neurogenic and myopathic neuromuscular disease, 83% had some pain, with 54% rating it as moderate to very severe and impacting their QoL.[107] A smaller sample confined to those with various muscle diseases and with myotonic dystrophy type 2 (DM2) in particular found that

pain affected 75% of the muscle group and 96% of the DM2 patients.[108] Seventy-three percent of 119 patients with muscle diseases reported pain, with 27% of these reporting that this pain was severe.[109] Muscle pain has been described as the presenting feature in four cases of genetically proven FSHD, with two cases having a family history of FSHD and all four cases having obvious weakness compatible with FSHD.[110] The nature of the pains described and their distribution are widespread and various including musculoskeletal and myalgic pains. Descriptions such as *deep, tiring, dull, aching, sharp,* and *excruciating* have been used. Some muscle diseases are said to have distinctions, with DM2 more likely to be described as *dull, stabbing,* and *tender* and with a long mean duration of 10 hours, compared with 5 hours for other muscle diseases.[108] Pain in muscle disease adversely affects QoL and sleep quality and is also associated with fatigue.[107,109,111] Rose et al. confirmed that fatigue and pain did affect QoL in those with muscle disease but more for psychosocial than physical QoL domains.[112] Furthermore, the pain and fatigue symptoms did not relate that well with disease severity.

It therefore seems that the factors influencing pain and fatigue in muscle disease are similar and overlapping. Some aspects of pain may be myalgic but also musculoskeletal in origin, affecting sleep quality and thus lead to fatigue, while other aspects of both fatigue and pain, and the degree to which they impact on QoL have psychosocial elements. This is a pattern mirrored by many long-term chronic conditions in which pain and fatigue do not relate just to disease severity and are in some cases more likely to relate to psychosocial factors. Lower physical activity in part related to muscle weakness, pain, and sleep disturbance was found to contribute to fatigue severity.[113] The management of these symptoms can be proactive and helpful especially if one realizes that they are not an inexorable effect of an untreatable myopathy and their reduction can significantly improve QoL. Management of pain and fatigue in muscle disease requires a holistic approach to tackle the musculoskeletal elements of pain, improve sleep quality, increase activity levels, and also to change attitudes to the long-term condition that is muscle disease. A good stretching regime can alleviate many myalgic and joint-related pains and can be active or passive as required. Maintenance of good posture is also very helpful. This means considering appropriately chosen and sized walking aids, good wheelchair truncal and limb support, and adequate mattress support with provision for turning during the night for those unable to do so for themselves. Submaximal, low-impact exercise such as walking, swimming, or cycling can improve pain and fatigue. Patients can be reassured that exercise performed sensibly for conditioning, rather than in an attempt to build up diseased muscle, is not harmful, as evidenced by several studies.[114,115] Judicious use of simple analgesia, nonsteroidal anti-inflammatories, and the tricyclic antidepressant and antiepileptic drugs used for neurogenic pain relief may contribute to pain management. Modafanil has been advocated for fatigue management in neurological disease and by extension in muscle disease, but is unproven, and its variable efficacy should not divert attention from the more holistic nondrug approaches to fatigue management.

Chronic Fatigue Syndrome

Chronic fatigue syndrome (CFS) is a syndrome of chronic fatigue and disability that is frequently associated with self-reported poor concentration, poor memory, sleep disturbance, and musculoskeletal pain. Medical and psychiatric conditions including depression, dementia, pyschosis, organic brain disease, chronic inflammatory disease, chronic infections, organ failure, morbid obesity, major neurological disorders, endocrine disorders, and primary sleep disorders, which can cause this constellation of symptoms, need to be excluded before a diagnosis can be made. Various medications, substance and alcohol abuse, and treatments such as radiotherapy may also cause this constellation of symptoms and also need to be considered.

There are many sets of definition criteria currently in use for CFS, however, the most frequently used is the Centers for Disease Control and Prevention 1994 criteria.[116] These criteria require clinically evaluated, unexplained persistent or relapsing fatigue of at least 6 months' duration that is not a result of exertion, is not substantially relieved by rest, is of new or a clear time of onset, and causes significant reduction in social, educational, work or personal activity.

In addition, four of the eight following associated symptoms must be present for at least six months: (1) self-reported impairment in short-term memory or concentration; (2) sore throat; (3) tender cervical or axillary lymph nodes; (4) muscle pain; (5) polyarthralgia without joint swelling or erythema: (6) headaches of a new pattern, type or severity: (7) postexertional malaise lasting more than 24 hours; and (8) unrefreshing sleep. There is no diagnostic test or consensus on the pathogenesis of CFS.

Patients with CFS may suggest a muscle disease expecially in naive cases where myalgia and poor muscle performance are prominent. In fact, even in such cases muscle energetics are normal.[117-120] Clues to the possibility of CFS are that any postexertional weakness and pain are also accompanied by additional complaints of subjective and mental fatigue. This should then prompt direct questioning for other features of CFS. The results of physical and neurologic examinations of such patients are usually normal. Laboratory tests including serum CK and lactate levels, thyroid function, blood counts, and metabolic screen should be normal. EMG studies often demonstrate low-frequency discharge of motor units with intermittent recruitment, a pattern most often seen with incomplete voluntary effort. Muscle biopsies may be normal or show nonspecific findings, especially type 2 fiber atrophy commonly seen with muscle underuse. Abnormal investigation results, especially elevated CK, EMG, and muscle biopsy abnormalities suggest an alternative cause and require a critical assessment as to their role in causing the widespread symptoms that are unlikely to have muscle disease as a sole unifying diagnosis. However, those with established muscle disease can exhibit features of CFS, as was the case in 40% of patients in one series with McArdle disease.[39] Perhaps such additional features may result from a prolonged period with unrecognized or misrepresented muscle symptoms. These so-called secondary CFS cases make confident exclusion of underlying muscle disease a challenge in some patients.

Although various medications, including monoamine oxidase inhibitors, hydrocortisone, thyroxine, and antivirals, have been advocated as treatments for CFS, the evidence base for pharmacological therapy is poor and is not recommended by the authors. Notably, it is specifically recommended by the National Institute of

Clinical Excellence, a UK governmental agency, that these agents not be used (http://www.nice.org.uk/nicemedia/live/11824/36193/36193.pdf).[121]

There is, however good evidence, for the benefits of both graded exercise therapy (GET) and cognitive behavioral therapy (CBT) when added to specialist medical care. In particular, the PACE study was a large, randomized trial of 614 subjects with CFS randomized to GET, CBT, or adaptive pacing therapy (APT).[122] At 52 weeks, fatigue scores as measured by the Chalder Fatigue Questionnaire, and physical function as assessed by the physical function subscale of the short form 36 questionnaire (SF-36), were significantly improved in both the GET and CBT group compared to the APT and standard medical therapy alone group.

REFERENCES

1. Boska MD, Moussavi RS, Carson PJ, Weiner MW, Miller RG. The metabolic basis of recovery after fatiguing exercise of human muscle. Neurology 1990;40:240–244.
2. Griggs RC, Matthews SM, Rennie MJ. The metabolic response to graded isometric forearm exercise in over-night fasted man. J Physiol 1982;332:39P.
3. Taylor DJ, Styles P, Matthews PM, et al. Energetics of human muscle: exercise-induced ATP depletion. Magn Reson Med 1986;3:44–54.
4. Newham DJ, Mills KR, Quigley BM, Edwards RH. Pain and fatigue after concentric and eccentric muscle contractions. Clin Sci (Lond) 1983;64:55–62.
5. Davies CT, White MJ. Muscle weakness following eccentric work in man. Pflugers Arch 1981;392:168–171.
6. Newham DJ, Jones DA, Edwards RH. Large delayed plasma creatine kinase changes after stepping exercise. Muscle Nerve 1983;6:380–385.
7. Newham DJ, McPhail G, Mills KR, Edwards RH. Ultrastructural changes after concentric and eccentric contractions of human muscle. J Neurol Sci 1983;61:109–122.
8. Weller B, Karpati G, Carpenter S. Dystrophin-deficient mdx muscle fibers are preferentially vulnerable to necrosis induced by experimental lengthening contractions. J Neurol Sci 1990;100:9–13.
9. Friden J, Sfakianos PN, Hargens AR. Muscle soreness and intramuscular fluid pressure: comparison between eccentric and concentric load. J Appl Physiol 1986;61:2175–2179.
10. Mense S. Nociception from skeletal muscle in relation to clinical muscle pain. Pain 1993;54:241–289.
11. Abdulla AJ, Jones PW, Pearce VR. Leg cramps in the elderly: prevalence, drug and disease associations. Int J Clin Pract 1999;53:494–496.
12. Jansen PH, van Dijck JA, Verbeek AL, Durian FW, Joosten EM. Estimation of the frequency of the muscular pain-fasciculation syndrome and the muscular

cramp-fasciculation syndrome in the adult population. Eur Arch Psychiatry Clin Neurosci 1991;241:102–104.
13. Naylor JR, Young JB. A general population survey of rest cramps. Age Ageing 1994;23:418–420.
14. Lazaro RP, Rollinson RD, Fenichel GM. Familial cramps and muscle pain. Arch Neurol 1981;38:22–24.
15. Ricker K, Moxley RT, 3rd. Autosomal dominant cramping disease. Arch Neurol 1990;47:810–812.
16. Chiba S, Saitoh M, Hatanaka Y, et al. Autosomal dominant muscle cramp syndrome in a Japanese family. J Neurol Neurosurg Psychiatry 1999;67:116–119.
17. Flier JS, Young JB, Landsberg L. Familial insulin resistance with acanthosis nigricans, acral hypertrophy, and muscle cramps. New England Journal of Medicine 1980;303:970–973.
18. Minaker KL, Flier JS, Landsberg L, et al. Phenytoin-induced improvement in muscle cramping and insulin action in three patients with the syndrome of insulin resistance, acanthosis nigricans, and acral hypertrophy. Arch Neurol 1989;46:981–985.
19. Satoyoshi E. A syndrome of progressive muscle spasm, alopecia, and diarrhea. Neurology 1978;28:458–471.
20. Nicole S, Topaloglu H, Fontaine B. 102nd ENMC International Workshop on Schwartz-Jampel syndrome, 14-16 December, 2001, Naarden, The Netherlands. Neuromuscul Disord 2003;13:347–351.
21. Orrell RW, Jurkat-Rott K, Lehmann-Horn F, Lane RJ. Familial cramp due to potassium-aggravated myotonia. J Neurol Neurosurg Psychiatry 1998;65:569–572.
22. Hart IK, Newsom-Davis J. Neuromyotonia (Isaac's syndrome). In: Lane RJM, ed. Handbook of muscle disease. New York: Marcel Dekker, 1996: 355–363.
23. Isaacs H. A syndrome of continuous muscle fibre activity. J Neurol NeurosurgPsychiatry 1961;24:319–325.
24. Newsom-Davis J, Buckley C, Clover L, et al. Autoimmune disorders of neuronal potassium channels. Ann NY Acad Sci 2003;998:202–210.
25. Brody I. Muscle contracture induced by exercise: a syndrome attributable to decreasing relaxing factor. New Eng J Med 1969;281:187–192.
26. Karpati G, Charuk J, Carpenter S, Jablecki C, Holland P. Myopathy caused by a deficiency of Ca2+-adenosine triphosphatase in sarcoplasmic reticulum (Brody's disease). Annals of Neurology 1986;20:38–49.
27. Odermatt A, Barton K, Khanna VK, et al. The mutation of Pro789 to Leu reduces the activity of the fast-twitch skeletal muscle sarco(endo)plasmic reticulum Ca2+ ATPase (SERCA1) and is associated with Brody disease. HumGenet 2000;106:482–491.
28. Benders AA, Veerkamp JH, Oosterhof A, et al. Ca2+ homeostasis in Brody's disease. A study in skeletal muscle and cultured muscle cells and the effects of dantrolene and verapamil. J Clin Invest 1994;94:741–748.
29. Voermans NC, Laan AE, Oosterhof A, et al. Brody syndrome: A clinically heterogeneous entity distinct from Brody disease: A review of literature and a cross-sectional clinical study in 17 patients. Neuromuscul Disord 2012.
30. Ansevin CF, Agamanolis DP. Rippling muscles and myasthenia gravis with rippling muscles. Archives of Neurology 1996;53:197–199.
31. Ansevin CF, Vorgerd M, Malin JP, Mortier W, Kubisch C. Phenotypic variability in rippling muscle disease. Neurology 2000;54:273.

32. Ashok Muley S, Day JW. Autoimmune rippling muscle. Neurology 2003;61:869–870.
33. Betz RC, Schoser BG, Kasper D, et al. Mutations in CAV3 cause mechanical hyperirritability of skeletal muscle in rippling muscle disease. Nat Genet 2001;28: 218–219.
34. Van den Bergh PY, Gerard JM, Elosegi JA, Manto MU, Kubisch C, Schoser BG. Novel missense mutation in the caveolin-3 gene in a Belgian family with rippling muscle disease. J Neurol Neurosurg Psychiatry 2004;75:1349–1351.
35. de Carvalho M, Swash M. Fasciculation-cramp syndrome preceding anterior horn cell disease: an intermediate syndrome? J Neurol Neurosurg Psychiatry 2011;82:459–461.
36. Fleet WS, Watson RT. From benign fasciculations and cramps to motor neuron disease. Neurology 1986;36: 997–998.
37. Finsterer J, Stollberger C. Quinine-responsive muscle cramps in X-linked bulbospinal muscular atrophy Kennedy. J Neurol 2009;256:1355–1356.
38. Harding AE, Thomas PK, Baraitser M, Bradbury PG, Morgan-Hughes JA, Ponsford JR. X-linked recessive bulbospinal neuronopathy: a report of ten cases. J Neurol Neurosurg Psychiatry 1982;45:1012–1019.
39. Quinlivan R, Buckley J, James M, et al. McArdle disease: a clinical review. J Neurol Neurosurg Psychiatry 2010;81:1182–1188.
40. Danon MJ, Carpenter S, Harati Y. Muscle pain associated with tubular aggregates and structures resembling cylindrical spirals. Muscle Nerve 1989;12:265–272.
41. Lazaro RP, Fenichel GM, Kilroy AW, Saito A, Fleischer S. Cramps, muscle pain, and tubular aggregates. Arch Neurol 1980;37:715–717.
42. Niakan E, Harati Y, Danon MJ. Tubular aggregates: their association with myalgia. J Neurol Neurosurg Psychiatry 1985;48:882–886.
43. Beyenburg S, Zierz S. Chronic progressive external ophthalmoplegia and myalgia associated with tubular aggregates. Acta Neurol Scand 1993;87:397–402.
44. Jacques TS, Holton J, Watts PM, Wills AJ, Smith SE, Hanna MG. Tubular aggregate myopathy with abnormal pupils and skeletal deformities. J Neurol Neurosurg Psychiatry 2002;73:324–326.
45. Jackevicius CA, Mamdani M, Tu JV. Adherence with statin therapy in elderly patients with and without acute coronary syndromes. JAMA 2002;288:462–467.
46. Bruckert E, Hayem G, Dejager S, Yau C, Begaud B. Mild to moderate muscular symptoms with high-dosage statin therapy in hyperlipidemic patients—the PRIMO study. Cardiovasc Drugs Ther 2005;19:403–414.
47. Thompson PD, Clarkson P, Karas RH. Statin-associated myopathy. JAMA 2003;289:1681–1690.
48. Fernandez G, Spatz ES, Jablecki C, Phillips PS. Statin myopathy: a common dilemma not reflected in clinical trials. Cleve Clin J Med 2011;78:393–403.
49. Phillips PS, Haas RH, Bannykh S, et al. Statin-associated myopathy with normal creatine kinase levels. Ann Intern Med 2002;137:581–585.
50. Baker SK. Molecular clues into the pathogenesis of statin-mediated muscle toxicity. Muscle & Nerve 2005;31:572–580.
51. Mammen AL, Amato AA. Statin myopathy: a review of recent progress. Curr Opin Rheumatol 2010;22:644–650.
52. Needham M, Fabian V, Knezevic W, Panegyres P, Zilko P, Mastaglia FL. Progressive myopathy with

up-regulation of MHC-I associated with statin therapy. Neuromuscul Disord 2007;17:194–200.
53. Wahl D, Petitpain N, Frederic M, Bour S, Kaminsky P, Trechot P. Myopathy associated with statin therapy. Neuromuscul Disord 2007;17:661–662.
54. Hilton-Jones D. Myopathy associated with statin therapy. Neuromuscul Disord 2008;18:97–98.
55. Leung NM, Ooi TC, McQueen MJ. Use of statins and fibrates in hyperlipidemic patients with neuromuscular disorders. Ann Intern Med 2000;132:418–419.
56. Mammen AL, Chung T, Christopher-Stine L, Rosen P, Rosen A, Doering KR, Casciola-Rosen LA. Autoantibodies against 3-hydroxy-3-methylglutaryl-coenzyme A reductase in patients with statin-associated autoimmune myopathy. Arthritis Rheum. 2011 Mar;63(3):713–721.
57. Duyff RF, Van den Bosch J, Laman DM, van Loon BJ, Linssen WH. Neuromuscular findings in thyroid dysfunction: a prospective clinical and electrodiagnostic study. J Neurol Neurosurg Psychiatry 2000;68:750–755.
58. Kung AW. Clinical review: Thyrotoxic periodic paralysis: a diagnostic challenge. J Clin Endocrinol Metab 2006;91:2490–2495.
59. Nora DB, Fricke D, Becker J, Gomes I. Hypocalcemic myopathy without tetany due to idiopathic hypoparathyroidism: case report. Arq Neuropsiquiatr 2004;62:154–157.
60. Fraser WD. Hyperparathyroidism. Lancet 2009;374: 145–158.
61. Reginato AJ, Falasca GF, Pappu R, McKnight B, Agha A. Musculoskeletal manifestations of osteomalacia: report of 26 cases and literature review. Semin Arthritis Rheum 1999;28:287–304.
62. Ceglia L. Vitamin D and skeletal muscle tissue and function. Mol Aspects Med 2008;29:407–414.
63. Straube S, Andrew Moore R, Derry S, McQuay HJ. Vitamin D and chronic pain. Pain 2009;141:10–13.
64. Bowyer SL, LaMothe MP, Hollister JR. Steroid myopathy: incidence and detection in a population with asthma. J Allergy Clin Immunol 1985;76:234–242.
65. Pereira RM, Freire de Carvalho J. Glucocorticoid-induced myopathy. Joint Bone Spine 2011;78:41–44.
66. Chow KM, Szeto CC, Wong TY, Leung FK, Cheuk A, Li PK. Diabetic muscle infarction: myocardial infarct equivalent. Diabetes Care 2002;25:1895.
67. Chawla J. Stepwise approach to myopathy in systemic disease. Front Neurol 2011;2:49.
68. Iyer SN, Drake AJ, 3rd, West RL, Tanenberg RJ. Diabetic muscle infarction: a rare complication of long-standing and poorly controlled diabetes mellitus. Case Report Med 2011;2011:407921.
69. Bennett DL, Groves M, Blake J, et al. The use of nerve and muscle biopsy in the diagnosis of vasculitis: a 5 year retrospective study. J Neurol Neurosurg Psychiatry 2008;79:1376–1381.
70. Prayson RA. Skeletal muscle vasculitis exclusive of inflammatory myopathic conditions: a clinicopathologic study of 40 patients. Hum Pathol 2002;33: 989–995.
71. O'Duffy JD, Wahner HW, Hunder GG. Joint imaging in polymyalgia rheumatica. Mayo Clin Proc 1976;51: 519–524.
72. Brooke MH, Kaplan H. Muscle pathology in rheumatoid arthritis, polymyalgia rheumatica, and polymyositis: a histochemical study. Arch Pathol 1972;94: 101–118.

73. Telerman-Toppet N, Bacq M, Khoubesserian P, Coers C. Type 2 fiber predominance in muscle cramp and exertional myalgia. Muscle Nerve 1985;8:563–567.

74. Kao AH, Lacomis D, Lucas M, Fertig N, Oddis CV. Anti-signal recognition particle autoantibody in patients with and patients without idiopathic inflammatory myopathy. Arthritis Rheum 2004;50:209–215.

75. Campbell R, Scott D, Kiely P, Gordon P. Fatigue in idiopathic inflammatory myopathy (IIM): Prevalence, impact and association with quality of life. Arthritis Rheum 2011;63:S89.

76. Campbell R, Scott D, Kiely P, Gordon P. Predictors of experienced fatigue in idiopathic inflammatory myopathy (IIM): Psychological factors and pain are more predictive than disease activity, damage or strength. Arthritis Rheum 2011;63:S90.

77. Ravelli A, Trail L, Ferrari C, et al. Long-term outcome and prognostic factors of juvenile dermatomyositis: a multinational, multicenter study of 490 patients. Arthritis Care Res (Hoboken) 2010;62:63–72.

78. Gunawardena H, Wedderburn LR, Chinoy H, et al. Autoantibodies to a 140-kd protein in juvenile dermatomyositis are associated with calcinosis. Arthritis Rheum 2009;60:1807–1814.

79. Middleton GD, McFarlin JE, Lipsky PE. The prevalence and clinical impact of fibromyalgia in systemic lupus erythematosus. Arthritis Rheum 1994;37:1181–1188.

80. Gracely RH, Petzke F, Wolf JM, Clauw DJ. Functional magnetic resonance imaging evidence of augmented pain processing in fibromyalgia. Arthritis Rheum 2002;46:1333–1343.

81. Choy E, Marshall D, Gabriel ZL, Mitchell SA, Gylee E, Dakin HA. A systematic review and mixed treatment comparison of the efficacy of pharmacological treatments for fibromyalgia. Semin Arthritis Rheum 2011;41:335–345 e336.

82. Dasgupta B, Cimmino MA, Kremers HM, et al. 2012 Provisional classification criteria for polymyalgia rheumatica: a European League Against Rheumatism/American College of Rheumatology collaborative initiative. Arthritis Rheum 2012;64:943–954.

83. Mills KR, Edwards RH. Investigative strategies for muscle pain. Journal of the Neurological Sciences 1983;58:73–78.

84. Gospe SM, Jr., Lazaro RP, Lava NS, Grootscholten PM, Scott MO, Fischbeck KH. Familial X-linked myalgia and cramps: a nonprogressive myopathy associated with a deletion in the dystrophin gene. Neurology 1989;39:1277–1280.

85. Minetti C, Bonilla E. Mosaic expression of dystrophin in carriers of Becker's muscular dystrophy and the X-linked syndrome of myalgia and cramps. N Engl J Med 1992;327:1100.

86. Sanchez-Arjona MB, Rodriguez-Uranga JJ, Giles-Lima M, et al. Spanish family with myalgia and cramps syndrome. Journal of Neurology, Neurosurgery, and Psychiatry 2005;76:286–289.

87. Ishigaki C, Patria SY, Nishio H, Yabe M, Matsuo M. A Japanese boy with myalgia and cramps has a novel in-frame deletion of the dystrophin gene. Neurology 1996;46:1347–1350.

88. Serratrice G, Pellissier JF, Roux H, Quilichini P. Fasciitis, perimyositis, myositis, polymyositis, and eosinophilia. Muscle Nerve 1990;13:385–395.

89. Sladek GD, Vasey FB, Sieger B, Behnke DA, Germain BF, Espinoza LR. Relapsing eosinophilic myositis. J Rheumatol 1983;10:467–470.

90. Lakhanpal S, Ginsburg WW, Michet CJ, Doyle JA, Moore SB. Eosinophilic fasciitis: clinical spectrum and therapeutic response in 52 cases. Semin Arthritis Rheum 1988;17:221–231.

91. Bischoff L, Derk CT. Eosinophilic fasciitis: demographics, disease pattern and response to treatment: report of 12 cases and review of the literature. Int J Dermatol 2008;47:29–35.

92. Gherardi RK, Coquet M, Cherin P, et al. Macrophagic myofasciitis: an emerging entity. Groupe d'Etudes et Recherche sur les Maladies Musculaires Acquises et Dysimmunitaires (GERMMAD) de l'Association Francaise contre les Myopathies (AFM). Lancet 1998;352:347–352.

93. Walters A, Hening W, Cote L, Fahn S. Dominantly inherited restless legs with myoclonus and periodic movements of sleep: a syndrome related to the endogenous opiates? Adv Neurol 1986;43:309–319.

94. Garcia-Borreguero D, Stillman P, Benes H, et al. Algorithms for the diagnosis and treatment of restless legs syndrome in primary care. BMC Neurol 2011; 11:28.

95. Managing patients with restless legs. Drug and Therapeutics Bulletin 2003;41:81–83.

96. Holmes R, Tluk S, Metta V, et al. Nature and variants of idiopathic restless legs syndrome: observations from 152 patients referred to secondary care in the UK. J Neural Transm 2007;114:929–934.

97. Martinez C, Finnern HW, Rietbrock S, Eaton S, Chaudhuri KR, Schapira AH. Patterns of treatment for restless legs syndrome in primary care in the United Kingdom. Clin Ther 2008;30:405–418.

98. Lentini S, Manka R, Scholtyssek S, Stoffel-Wagner B, Lüderitz B, Tasci S. Creatine phosphokinase elevation in obstructive sleep apnea syndrome: An unknown association?. Chest 2006;129:88–94.

99. Lou JS. Approaching fatigue in neuromuscular diseases. [Review] [49 refs]. Physical Medicine & Rehabilitation Clinics of North America 16(4): 1063–1079, xi 2005.

100. Sharma KR, Miller RG. Electrical and mechanical properties of skeletal muscle underlying increased fatigue in patients with amyotrophic lateral sclerosis. Muscle Nerve 1996;19:1391–1400.

101. Sharma KR, Kent-Braun J, Mynhier MA, Weiner MW, Miller RG. Excessive muscular fatigue in the postpoliomyelitis syndrome. Neurology 1994;44:642–646.

102. Sharma KR, Mynhier MA, Miller RG. Muscular fatigue in Duchenne muscular dystrophy. Neurology 1995;45:306–310.

103. Kalkman JS, Zwarts MJ, Schillings ML, van Engelen BG, Bleijenberg G. Different types of fatigue in patients with facioscapulohumeral dystrophy, myotonic dystrophy and HMSN-I. Experienced fatigue and physiological fatigue. Neurol Sci 2008;29 Suppl 2:S238–S240.

104. Dittner AJ, Wessely SC, Brown RG. The assessment of fatigue: a practical guide for clinicians and researchers. J Psychosom Res 2004;56:157–170.

105. Laberge L, Gagnon C, Jean S, Mathieu J. Fatigue and daytime sleepiness rating scales in myotonic dystrophy: a study of reliability. Journal of Neurology, Neurosurgery, and Psychiatry 2005;76:1403–1405.

106. Vincent KA, Carr AJ, Walburn J, Scott DL, Rose MR. Construction and validation of a quality of life questionnaire for neuromuscular disease (INQoL). Neurology 2007;68:1051–1057.

107. Abresch RT, Carter GT, Jensen MP, Kilmer DD. Assessment of pain and health-related quality of life in slowly progressive neuromuscular disease. Am J Hosp Palliat Care 2002;19:39–48.

108. George A, Schneider-Gold C, Zier S, Reiners K, Sommer C. Musculoskeletal pain in patients with myotonic dystrophy type 2. Arch Neurol 2004;61: 1938–1942.

109. Jensen MP, Abresch RT, Carter GT, McDonald CM. Chronic pain in persons with neuromuscular disease. Arch Phys Med Rehabil 2005;86:1155–1163.

110. Bushby KM, Pollitt C, Johnson MA, Rogers MT, Chinnery PF. Muscle pain as a prominent feature of facioscapulohumeral muscular dystrophy (FSHD): four illustrative case reports. Neuromuscul Disord 1998; 8:574–579.

111. Padua L, Aprile I, Frusciante R, et al. Quality of life and pain in patients with facioscapulohumeral muscular dystrophy. Muscle Nerve 2009;40:200–205.

112. Rose MR, Sadjadi R, Weinman J, et al. The role of disease severity, illness perceptions and mood on quality of life in muscle disease. Muscle & Nerve 2012:;46(3):351–359.

113. Kalkman JS, Schillings ML, Zwarts MJ, van Engelen BG, Bleijenberg G. The development of a model of fatigue in neuromuscular disorders: a longitudinal study. J Psychosom Res 2007;62:571–579.

114. Arnardottir S, Alexanderson H, Lundberg IE, Borg K. Sporadic inclusion body myositis: pilot study on the effects of a home exercise program on muscle function, histopathology and inflammatory reaction. J Rehabil Med 2003;35:31–35.

115. Alexanderson H, Stenstrom CH, Lundberg I. Safety of a home exercise programme in patients with polymyositis and dermatomyositis: a pilot study. Rheumatology (Oxford) 1999;38:608–611.

116. Fukuda K, Straus SE, Hickie I, Sharpe MC, Dobbins JG, Komaroff A. The chronic fatigue syndrome: a comprehensive approach to its definition and study. International Chronic Fatigue Syndrome Study Group. Ann Intern Med 1994;121:953–959.

117. Barnes PR, Taylor DJ, Kemp GJ, Radda GK. Skeletal muscle bioenergetics in the chronic fatigue syndrome. J Neurol Neurosurg Psychiatry 1993;56:679–683.

118. Byrne E, Trounce I. Chronic fatigue and myalgia syndrome: mitochondrial and glycolytic studies in skeletal muscle. J Neurol Neurosurg Psychiatry 1987;50: 743–746.

119. Lloyd AR, Gandevia SC, Hales JP. Muscle performance, voluntary activation, twitch properties and perceived effort in normal subjects and patients with the chronic fatigue syndrome. Brain 1991;114 (Pt 1A): 85–98.

120. Lloyd AR, Hales JP, Gandevia SC. Muscle strength, endurance and recovery in the post-infection fatigue syndrome. J Neurol Neurosurg Psychiatry 1988;51:1316–1322.

121. National Collaborating Centre for Primary Care (UK). Chronic Fatigue Syndrome/Myalgic Encephalomyelitis (or Encephalopathy): Diagnosis and Management of Chronic Fatigue Syndrome/Myalgic Encephalomyelitis (or Encephalopathy) in Adults and Children [Internet]. London: Royal College of General Practitioners (UK); 2007 Aug. (NICE Clinical Guidelines, No. 53.) Available from: http://www.ncbi.nlm.nih.gov/books/NBK53577/

122. White PD, Goldsmith KA, Johnson AL, et al. Comparison of adaptive pacing therapy, cognitive behaviour therapy, graded exercise therapy, and specialist medical care for chronic fatigue syndrome (PACE): a randomised trial. Lancet 2011;377: 823–836.

123. Yunus M, Masi AT, Calabro JJ, et al: Primary fibromyalgia (fibrositis): Clinical study of 50 patietns with matched normal controls. Semin Arthritis Rheum 1982;11:151.

Chapter 13

Prevention and Management of Systemic Complications of Myopathies

Wendy M. King
Robert C. Griggs

RESPIRATORY MANAGEMENT

Normal Respiratory Muscle Function

The lungs fill with air and the chest expands by contraction of the inspiratory muscles. The principal muscle of inspiration is the diaphragm, assisted by the external intercostal, parasternal intercartilaginous, sternocleidomastoid, and scalene muscles. The muscles of expiration are passive during normal quiet breathing but become active during talking, singing, and coughing. The muscles of expiration are the internal intercostals, the internal and external obliques, the rectus abdominis, and the transverse abdominis. Normal respiration is also dependent on the many muscles of deglutition (muscles of the tongue, soft palate, suprahyoid and infrahyoid, larynx, and pharynx) so that choking and aspiration do not occur.

Abnormalities of Respiratory Function

Evidence of respiratory dysfunction can be found in many patients with myopathies. (Table 13–1). Abnormalities include:

- decreased respiratory muscle strength, either generalized or selective;
- impaired glottic function, leading to an ineffective cough;
- impaired central nervous system ventilatory drive;
- upper airway obstruction during sleep; and
- abnormal swallowing function leading to recurrent aspiration.

In addition, chest wall stiffness and kyphoscoliosis can complicate neuromuscular diseases and further increase the work of breathing.[1,2] Generalized respiratory muscle weakness produces restrictive lung disease with a reduction in vital capacity, a decrease in total lung volume, and a decrease in lung compliance. The earliest detectable abnormality is a reduction in static pressures. Maximum expiratory pressure (MEP) is reduced to a greater extent than maximum inspiratory pressure (MIP; also referred to as negative inspiratory pressure).[3,4]

If the diaphragm is selectively involved prior to other muscles becoming weak, vital capacity is reduced to a much greater extent when the patient is supine causing orthopnea.[5]

ROUTINE SURVEILLANCE AND TREATMENT

Patients with myopathies in which respiratory involvement is frequent should have an annual assessment of lung function beginning at the time of diagnosis.[5] Patients with a low vital capacity or whose disease is rapidly progressive should be assessed more frequently. MEP and MIP are useful to detect early respiratory muscle involvement and peak cough flow (PCF) is valuable to monitor expiratory function. The clinician should measure daytime oxygen saturation (SpO_2) in patients with respiratory symptoms and in those with a forced vital capacity (FVC) < 1.5 L.[7] Certain myopathies, most notably acid maltase deficiency, may present with respiratory failure as the first sign of an underlying muscle disease (Box 13–1). These disorders must be considered in patients with unexplained respiratory failure.

Conversely, respiratory muscle weakness leading to respiratory failure seldom affects patients with other specific myopathies. Severe pulmonary symptoms in patients with these disorders are usually the result of coincidental illness. However, respiratory involvement can occur with any myopathic disorder, and therefore baseline pulmonary function testing is prudent following the diagnosis of a muscle disease.[2]

Diaphragm function can be measured by several means. Bedside assessment by percussion and stethoscope auscultation are rapidly being replaced by ultrasonography. Diaphragmatic ultrasound and phrenic nerve conduction are noninvasive methods for evaluation of patients with neuromuscular disease.[8]

Recognition of Impending Respiratory Failure

SYMPTOMS

Acute respiratory failure is usually precipitated by a readily recognized event such as pneumonitis, bronchitis, atelectasis, aspiration,

Table 13–1 **Respiratory Involvement in the Myopathies**

Condition	Respiratory Involvement
DMD	Inevitable, usually in teenage years
BMD	Less known, can occur with disease progression
DM1	Common, due to:
	Sleep-disordered breathing
	Respiratory muscle weakness & myotonia
	Alveolar hypoventilation
	Aspiration pneumonia
FSHD	Respiratory involvement only in severe disease
LGMD1	Can occur due to scoliosis, spinal rigidity
LGMD2	
LGMD2A (calpainopathy)	Late involvement
LGMD2C (γ sarcoglycanopathy)	Common
LGMD2D (α sarcoglycanopathy)	Common
LGMD2E (β sarcoglycanopathy)	Common
LGMD2F (δ sarcoglycanopathy)	Common
LGMD2H	Reported
LGMD2I	Common
LGMD2J	Late onset
EDMD	Occurs in association with skeletal deformities
OPMD	Aspiration pneumonia and sleep disordered breathing reported
Autosomal-dominant distal myopathies	
Laing	
Welander	
Markesbery-Griggs-Udd	Common
Autosomal-recessive distal myopathies	
Nonaka	Rare
Miyoshi	Rare
Myofibrillar myopathy with abnormal desmin	
Inflammatory myopathies	Rare
Dermatomyositis	Rare
Polymyositis	Common
Metabolic myopathies	
Glycogenosis type II (AMD)	
Infantile	Interstitial lung disease
Childhood/adults	Interstitial lung disease
Glycogenosis type V (McArdle's)	Common
Fatty acid metabolism disorders	Common
Carnitine transporter deficiency	Respiratory failure with acidosis reported
LCHAD deficiency	Uncommon unless severe rhabdomyolysis
SCAD deficiency	Occasionally
Mitochondrial disorders	Common
	Occasional
	Can present with:
	Respiratory muscle weakness
	Hyperventilation syndrome secondary to acidosis
	Central hypoventilation

(continued)

Table 13–1 **(Cont.)**

Condition	Respiratory Involvement
Congenital myopathy	
Nemaline myopathy	
Infantile/childhood	Inevitable
Adult	Common
Central core disease	Rare
Myotubular/centronuclear myopathy	
Congenital fiber-type proportion	Inevitable
Reducing body myopathy	
Cap myopathy	Occasional
Congenital muscular dystrophy (CMD)	Common
	Common
	Variable

Note. AMD, acid maltase deficiency; BMD, Becker muscular dystrophy; DMD, Duchenne muscular dystrophy; DM1, myotonic dystrophy type 1; EDMD, Emery-Dreifuss muscular dystrophy; FSHD, facioscapulohumeral muscular dystrophy; LCHAD, long chain 3-hydroxyacyl-CoA deficiency; LGMD1, autosomal-dominant limb-girdle muscular dystrophy; LGMD2, autosomal-recessive limb-girdle muscular dystrophy; OPMD, oculopharyngeal muscular dystrophy; SCAD, short-chain acyl-CoA dehydrogenase deficiency.
Adapted from Shahrizaila N, Kinnear WJM, Wills AJ. Respiratory involvement of inherited primary muscle conditions. J Neurol Neurosurg Psychiatry 2006;77:1108–1115; Amato AA, Russell JA. Neuromuscular Disorders. McGraw-Hill, New York, 2008; Guglieri M, Bushby K. In Neuromuscular Disorders. Edited by Yawil R and Venance S. Oxford: Wiley-Blackwell, 2011.

Box 13.1 Myopathies Commonly *Presenting* With Respiratory Failure

Myotonic dystrophy (DM1 >> DM2)
Acid maltase deficiency
Limb-girdle muscular dystrophy type 2I
Centronuclear myopathy
Nemaline myopathy
Myofibrillar myopathy (titin mutations)

---

pneumothorax, or congestive heart failure. *Chronic* respiratory failure, however, usually presents insidiously with symptoms of nocturnal oxygen desaturation, such as frequent nighttime arousals, morning headache, excessive daytime sleepiness, anxiety, depression, and lethargy. Generalized fatigue, unexplained weight loss, or cough should raise the suspicion of respiratory failure in a patient with neuromuscular disease. Chronic hypoxia increases pulmonary vascular resistance, which may in turn lead to symptoms of cor pulmonale: ankle edema, nocturia, and orthopnea.

Dyspnea is uncommon as a presenting symptom.

Disorders affecting swallowing may predispose to aspiration, with symptoms of coughing or dyspnea during or following meals. Patients with selective diaphragmatic weakness often experience severe orthopnea.[5,9]

PHYSICAL FINDINGS

Signs of respiratory compromise include tachypnea, tachycardia, and use of accessory respiratory muscles (the external intercostal, parasternal intercartilaginous, sternocleidomastoid, and scalene muscles).[2] Examination of the chest of patients with respiratory insufficiency usually shows (a) diminished breath sounds and atelectatic (paninspiratory) rales at lung bases; (b) diminished diaphragmatic excursion as detected by percussion of the chest, comparing diaphragm descent from *maximum* expiration to maximum inspiration; and (c) decreased effectiveness of the cough. Signs of cor pulmonale, such as cardiomegaly, hepatomegaly, distended neck veins, and papilledema may be present. Many patients, particularly those with DMD, learn the trick of glossopharyngeal "frog" breathing, in which rapid cycling of the tongue muscles forces air into the lungs. This maneuver enables patients to cough more effectively and to speak more loudly. It can increase the measured FVC substantially. If the diaphragm is selectively weakened, a seemingly paradoxical breathing pattern occurs during which the patient's abdomen flattens or moves inward during inspiration.

ROUTINE TESTING OF PULMONARY FUNCTION

Spirometry should be used to determine forced vital capacity. Other measurements, such as forced expiratory volume in one second, PCF, or flow volume loop may be obtained depending on the specific information needed and the capability of the individual being assessed.[10,11] In patients with symptoms, signs, or laboratory tests (e.g., elevated hematocrit) suggesting respiratory failure, the vital capacity should be measured with the patient supine as well as seated. Static pressures (MEP and MIP) are the most sensitive indicators of respiratory muscle weakness.[4] They are extremely helpful in evaluating the patient with muscle weakness and unexplained respiratory symptoms. *If static pressures are normal, respiratory symptoms are not the result of muscle weakness.*

If the assessment of inspiratory muscle strength is believed to be clinically relevant, both the noninvasive combination of maximal inspiratory mouth pressure and sniff nasal pressure should be performed.[12] O_2 saturation should be monitored in patients with respiratory signs or symptoms or if the FVC is < 1.5 L.[7] Evaluation of pulmonary function can also include (a) chest roentgenogram to assess heart size, diaphragmatic position, and evidence of atelectasis; (b) electrocardiography to search for signs of cor pulmonale (abnormal P waves, right axis deviation, right ventricular hypertrophy); (c) hematocrit, to detect an elevation that may indicate chronic hypoxia; and (d) electrolyte determination, to look for an elevation in bicarbonate, which would indicate metabolic compensation for chronic hypercapnia.

In patients with respiratory symptoms or signs or in patients with a reduced vital capacity who are not feeling well, additional studies may be indicated, including determination of arterial blood gas levels. Levels of arterial blood gases should also be determined when signs indicate cor pulmonale. According to one review, arterial blood gases should be checked when the vital capacity falls below 40% to 50% predicted, or when MIP falls below 30%. A *single normal arterial oxygen value does not exclude intermittent hypoxia.* Noninvasive overnight monitoring of oxygenation with ear lobe or digit oximetry is often necessary.

Prevention of Respiratory Complications

At the recommended age, all neuromuscular patients should receive a one-time prophylactic immunization for pneumococcal infections,[13] and annual immunization should be given for influenza viral infection.[14]

Respiratory muscle exercises may be considered, although such exercises are not recommended in DMD.[15] In general, inspiratory exercises should emphasize improving the chest wall elasticity by gentle range of motion exercises. Antibiotics should be administered for respiratory infections to prevent secondary infection. Such therapy has been shown to be effective against disorders such as chronic bronchitis.[16] Adequate hydration must also be maintained to ensure easy mobilization of secretions. This can be a problem for individuals who need toileting assistance, as these persons may judiciously limit their fluid intake to avoid asking for help. Keeping the urine specific gravity between 1.010 and 1.015 usually accomplishes this goal. The patient and family can check specific gravity daily and encourage adequate fluid intake accordingly.

Weight control can be difficult in weak patients (see Dietary Management section), but obesity must be avoided; if possible, dietary counseling should be offered. In those myopathies with bulbar involvement, inability of clear airway secretions can impair breathing. Anticholinergic medication, botulinum toxin injections, and surgical interventions are potential treatments for sialorrhea (see Swallowing Abnormalities section).

ACUTE RESPIRATORY FAILURE

Anticipation of Respiratory Failure

When the FVC falls below 40% to 50% of normal in patients with DMD and in other myopathies associated with severe compromise of respiratory function, both patient and family should be informed of the risk of both acute and chronic ventilatory failure, and the management of acute and chronic respiratory failure should be discussed. The opinions and wishes of patient and family should be considered, and a plan of action (or inaction) charted. If the topics of a living will and durable power of attorney for health care have not yet been addressed, they should be openly talked about now. *When such discussions are not held, decisions concerning respiratory supportive measures are often made by strangers* such as emergency medical technicians or emergency department physicians.

Precipitating Factors

The sudden appearance of respiratory symptoms in myopathy usually results from an acute, often reversible illness and is seldom due to muscle weakness alone.[17-19] The events most commonly precipitating respiratory failure are shown in Box 13.2. The recognition of the causative event is often difficult because of preexisting abnormalities of chest examination, pulmonary function tests, chest roentgenogram, and ECG. Diagnosis is facilitated if these have been monitored regularly. *Atelectasis is the precipitating factor in most patients.* Chest roentgenograms in a patient who has acute respiratory symptoms from atelectasis often show no interval change, particularly if they are obtained shortly after the onset of symptoms. Roentgenographic findings of atelectasis often appear following subsequent intravenous hydration.

Management

For patients who are obtunded and for dyspneic patients whose arterial blood determinations show hypoxia and hypercapnia, emergency endotracheal intubation may be necessary. If hypoxia alone is present and the patient is alert, oxygen at low flow rates (< 1 L/min) may correct hypoxia without causing hypercapnia. Special

---

Box 13.2 Precipitating Factors Leading to Acute Respiratory Failure or Symptoms in Myopathy

Frequent

Atelectasis
Pneumonitis
Obstructive lung disease (> age 40)
Congestive heart failure

Infrequent

Pulmonary thromboemboli
Fat emboli
Pneumothorax
Bronchospasm (e.g., marijuana use, allergic reactions)

equipment is often necessary for providing such low flow rates. If oxygen is administered, it is essential to obtain blood gas determinations frequently enough to exclude developing hypercapnia. *Patients with neuromuscular disease are often intermittently or persistently hypercapneic, and the administration of oxygen often depresses ventilatory drive and exacerbates hypoventilation.*[20]

Noninvasive positive pressure ventilation (NPPV) should usually be tried initially if control of secretions and cough assistance is successful.[21,22] Whether intubation or NPPV is utilized, patients with some myopathies can be weaned following the precipitating respiratory crisis; others may require ventilation assistance indefinitely.[20]

CHRONIC VENTILATORY FAILURE

In the last two decades, expert committees have recommended noninvasive positive ventilation over tracheostomy for chronic ventilatory failure due to myopathies and other restrictive respiratory diseases.[11,23,24] Mechanical in/exsufflators have also been utilized for those individuals without an effective cough.[25,26]

The Decision to Have Long-Term Respiratory Support

Appropriately managed patients and families will have been made aware of the risk of respiratory failure and options for support in advance of an acute deterioration. A gradual deterioration in respiratory function with symptoms or signs of hypoxia should prompt consideration of the elective institution of respiratory support. The use of NPPV during sleep and during daytime is now the standard method of mechanical ventilation for myopathies. DMD patients can survive with NPPV support alone for many years.[27,28] However, NPPV is contraindicated in some instances, including in those patients with copious secretions, cognitive impairment, or lack of caregiving support.[2,29] In these instances, ventilation may be more easily managed with tracheostomy and positive-pressure ventilation.

Initiation of chronic respiratory support poses major ethical responsibilities for the clinician. Full discussion is beyond the scope of this chapter. Whereas many patients are content on long-term support, others are not, and the expense and personal toll borne by family members must also be considered. Patients who are deciding about respiratory support are helped by discussing the procedure with others who are receiving such support. Family members and friends who will be involved can discuss home management with care providers at the same time. Competent patients have the right to accept or refuse life-sustaining therapies, and withdrawing life support and refraining from initiating life support are considered equivalent from an ethical point of view.[30]

Sleep-Related Breathing Complications

Sleep increases the susceptibility to breathing disruptions.[31] If a patient with a muscle disease has symptoms of respiratory impairment during the day, it is likely he or she is also having difficulties at night also. As previously noted, the clinician must regularly probe for hints of sleep-related breathing abnormalities (frequent nighttime arousals, daytime sleepiness, weight loss). One study reported 42% of patients with neuromuscular population had sleep-disordered breathing.[32]

The etiology of sleep-disordered breathing is multifactorial and depends on the specific myopathy. If the patient has demonstrated diaphragmatic weakness, is obese, or has scoliosis, sleep abnormalities are likely. In DM1 sleep apnea can be both central and obstructive.[33,34] Further investigation with nighttime oximetry or a polysomnogram is recommended when inspiratory pressure is below 30 cm H_2O, FVC is less than 55% predicted,[34,31] or if the patient has any other risk factors.

CARDIAC MANAGEMENT

Cardiac involvement occurs in most myopathies (Table 13–2). Symptomatic heart disease is uncommon in patients with muscle disease, but ECG, echocardiogram, Holter monitoring, and MRI detect myocardial involvement more frequently than clinical signs indicate.[35,36] Dilated cardiomyopathy, conduction defects,

Table 13–2 **Cardiac Disease in the Myopathies**

Congestive heart failure, dilated cardiomyopathy	DMD; BMD; female carriers of DMD, BMD; laminin A/C; LGMD 1A, 1B, 1D, 1E, 2C, 2D, 2E, 2F, 2G, 2I, 2M; CMD ; myofibrillar myopathies; multi-minicore myopathy; nemaline myopathy; hyaline body myopathy; acid maltase deficiency (infantile and juvenile; GSD III, IV, VII, VIII—rare); primary carnitine deficiency; MERRF; MELAS; polymyositis; dermatomyositis
Arrthymias, heart block	DMD; BMD; DM1; DM2; LGMD 1A, 1B, 1E; EDMD 2; female carriers of X-linked EDMD; FSHD; Bethlem myopathy; MFM; acid maltase deficiency (adult); KSS; ATS
Cardiomegaly/hypertrophic, cardiomyopathy	acid maltase deficiency (infancy; GSD type II), VLCAD deficiency, primary carnitine deficiency, Danon disease

Note. ATS = Anderson-Tawil syndrome; BMD, Becker muscular dystrophy; CMD, congenital muscular dystrophy; DMD, Duchenne muscular dystrophy; DM1, myotonic dystrophy type 1; DM2, myotonic dystrophy type 2; EDMD, Emery-Dreifuss muscular dystrophy; FSHD, facioscapulohumeral muscular dystrophy; GSD, glycogen storage disorder; HAD, 3 hydroxyacyl-CoA dehydrogenase deficiency; KSS = Kearns-Sayre syndrome; LGMD1, autosomal-dominant limb-girdle muscular dystrophy; LGMD2, autosomal-recessive limb-girdle muscular dystrophy; MELAS; mitochondrial encephalomyopathy with lactic acidosis and strokelike episodes; MERRF, myoclonic epilepsy with ragged red fibers; MFM, myofibrillar myopathy; OPMD, oculopharyngeal muscular dystrophy; VLCAD, very long chain acyl-coenzyme A dehydrogenase deficiency.

and arrhythmias are the most common cardiac abnormalities found, but a few disorders (desmin myopathy, nemaline myopathy) may display hypertrophic cardiomyopathy.[37] Not infrequently, individuals demonstrate combinations of more than one type of cardiomyopathy.[38] Certain myopathies may *present* with cardiac manifestations (Table 13–3).

Cardiac Symptoms and Signs

Symptoms of cardiomyopathy include insomnia, cough, poor appetite, abdominal pain, nausea, or ankle swelling. Fatigue, orthopnea, and dyspnea seldom occur as an early sign of heart failure in the myopathies. Because individuals with skeletal muscle weakness cannot exercise normally, exercise intolerance is seldom a complaint. (Exceptions are some metabolic and mitochondrial myopathies.) Patients may complain of dizziness or syncope if arrhythmias are present.[39] Respiratory failure with resulting hypoxia can lead to signs of heart failure when intrinsic cardiomyopathy is not present. In such patients (e.g., cor pulmonale) correction of the hypoxia reverses signs of heart failure.

Monitoring of weight, examination for ankle edema, and auscultation of the chest all aid the clinician in the early detection of heart failure. Congestive heart failure from cardiomyopathy develops insidiously; early signs are cough, pedal edema, and late inspiratory rales. Noncardiac, dependent edema is frequent in wheelchair patients, but its presence should still prompt consideration of heart failure, especially in the young. Pulmonary rales are frequent in all patients with respiratory muscle weakness but are usually paninspiratory (atelectatic).[40] *Late-inspiratory rales suggest heart failure.*[40] More florid signs of congestive heart failure include tachycardia, right or

Table 13–3 **Myopathies Commonly *Presenting* with Cardiac Disease**

Congestive heart failure	
Muscular dystrophy	Myotonic, limb-girdle, dystrophinopathy
Metabolic	Acid maltase, carnitine, and CPT deficiencies
Inflammatory	Polymyositis
Arrhythmias	
Muscular dystrophy	Myotonic dystrophy, limb-girdle, Emery-Dreifuss
Metabolic	Kearns-Sayre syndrome, hyperkalemic periodic paralysis
Inflammatory	Polymyositis

Note. CPT = carnitine palmitoyltransferase.

left ventricular enlargement, gallop rhythm, pulsus alternans, hepatomegaly, and neck vein distention.

Laboratory Evaluation

The ECG often helps with both diagnosis and management. The ECG shows distinctive changes in the dystrophinopathies (DMD, BMD), EDMD, some LGMDs, DM1 and DM2,[38] and infantile acid maltase deficiency[41] (see individual diseases in earlier chapters). The presence of first-degree heart block should prompt consideration and careful follow-up for more severe cardiac conduction disorders. Severe myocardial disease in which there is replacement fibrosis of myocardium is characterized by a loss of QRS-complex voltage in anterior leads and poor P wave progression.[42] The appearance of Q waves in inferior leads may also accompany fibrosis.[42] Echocardiography is used routinely and can suggest a specific myopathy.[38]

Because technical problems can interfere with echocardiograms in obese and scoliotic patients, cardiac magnetic resonance imaging has been used for DMD, DM and some LGMD patients.[43-46] Late gadolinium enhancement has also been used in conjunction with cardiac magnetic resonance imaging.[36,47]

B-type natriuretic peptide in heart failure in the general population has not yet been found to be useful as a marker for cardiac disease in DMD.[48-50] The cardiac isoform troponin-I (cTnI) is the most informative biomarker to detect cardiac ischemia in sporadic inclusion body myositis[51] and other myopathies.

Routine Surveillance and Treatment

Current guidelines for DMD recommend ECGs and echocardiograms at time of diagnosis or by 6 years of age, repeated every 2 years until the age of 10 and then performed annually.[52] The same surveillance has been recommended for individuals with the LGMDs that have cardiac involvement.[53-55] Cardiac involvement varies considerably in the CMDs, but ECG, Holter monitoring, and echocardiogram should be obtained for all CMD patients at diagnosis.[37] Individuals with myopathies associated

with conduction defects or arrhythmias should have annual ECGs and consideration of Holter monitoring. Prophylactic prevention of sudden cardiac death with an implantable cardioverter defibrillator should be considered for those with *LMNA* mutations.[53,54] The decision to place a pacemaker in patients with DM1 is a class 2 indication according to the American Heart Association.[56] Although some investigators recommend pacemakers in patients with MD, it was not found to decrease the risk of sudden death in DM1 in a large multicentered observational study. In that study, severe ECG abnormalities and atrial tachyarrhythmia predicted sudden death.[57] Dilated cardiomyopathy and conduction defects can occur less commonly in DM2.[58]

In the inflammatory myopathies, an ECG is recommended upon the diagnosis of DM or PM but not asymptomatic sIBM.[59,51] Echocardiography and MRI have been utilized to assess abnormalities, but standard practice parameters have not been established. Any abnormalities on the ECG, however, should prompt additional investigation. Endomyocardial biopsies have been performed to confirm myocardial involvement in patients with DM or PM.[59]

Angiotensin-converting enzyme inhibitors are now recommended in DMD and BMD at the first indication of cardiac abnormality.[39] Beta blockers are being investigated also,[60] as is the philosophy of initiating cardiac medications as prophylactic agents in the dystrophinopathies. Furthermore, any patient with a suspected or confirmed myopathy should have thorough cardiac and respiratory evaluations prior to undergoing anesthesia. Specific anesthetic agents may be contraindicated for certain neuromuscular disorders, and the ability to be weaned from a respirator can also be influenced.[54]

Carriers of X-linked muscle disorders (DMD, BMD, EDMD) are at risk for cardiomyopathy. Current recommendations for these individuals call for echocardiograms at least every 5 years beginning by age 16.[38,61,62]

Patients who are being treated with corticosteroids for skeletal muscle weakness have added complications: weight gain, increased blood pressure, and fluid retention. The impact of corticosteroids specifically on the heart in the myopathies is inconsistent. Various studies have shown beneficial effects of steroids on the heart in DMD,[63,64] but there are conflicting reports regarding corticosteroid therapy and their effect on cardiac abnormalities in DM and PM.[59, 65]

Heart transplants are being performed on individuals with muscular dystrophy and other myopathies,[66] and one retrospective report concluded that clinical outcomes were similar to those observed in patients without muscular dystrophy.[67]

Recent studies have suggested that particular deletions in the dystrophin gene responsible for DMD and BMD may lead to an earlier risk of cardiomyopathy.[68-70]

The respiratory status of patients with cardiomyopathy must be monitored. Noninvasive assisted ventilation (such as BiPap) and mechanically-assisted cough devices can decrease cardiac workload.[71] CK testing and determination of CK-MB (see chapter 2) does not help to identify patients with myocardial disease in the presence of an underlying myopathy.[72,73] Troponin values are more helpful.

Patients in whom cardiomyopathy has resulted in congestive heart failure can develop pulmonary and systemic emboli.[74,75] In such circumstances, anticoagulation therapy is indicated.[76] We also treat patients with heart failure from cardiomyopathy with measures used in other primary myocardial diseases, including diuretics, after-load reduction, and positive inotropic agents.[42,77] Digitalis is generally ineffective and may increase the incidence of arrhythmias, particularly in patients who have cor pulmonale.

The use of kaliuretic diuretics, such as thiazides, which cause reduction in blood and total body potassium, pose a special problem in patients with muscle wasting, in whom hypokalemia may exacerbate weakness.[4,78] At the same time, potassium must be replaced cautiously because tolerance to potassium decreases because of muscle wasting.[79]

PREVENTION OF EDEMA

Dependent foot, ankle, and leg edema occurs frequently in patients who spend the majority of time in a wheelchair. Such edema should prompt a search for clinical signs of (a) respiratory failure and cor pulmonale, (b) cardiomyopathy, or (c) a coincidental illness, particularly in young patients. In most patients, however, only the lack of muscle-pumping action of the legs can be identified as the cause.

Edema interferes with function because of its mechanical effect and because it increases weight. It also predisposes to skin infection and ulceration. Edema can be diminished by elevating the legs periodically (with elevating leg rests attached to a wheelchair in manual wheelchair patients, or by a tilt in space option on a motorized chair) and by reducing dietary sodium. Pressure stockings, either over the counter or custom made, are often helpful; patients almost always require assistance to put them on. Intermittent diuretic therapy often helps, although the use of potassium-sparing and potassium-depleting diuretics poses risks. Agents such as beta-adrenergic blocking agents, nonsteroidal anti-inflammatory agents, and calcium channel blockers may cause severe edema, precluding their use in many wheelchair-bound patients with myopathies.[79,80]

DIETARY MANAGEMENT: COMPLICATIONS OF OBESITY AND WEIGHT LOSS

Obesity is a common problem for many with myopathies. As muscle weakness progresses, it becomes more and more difficult for individuals to remain physically active. Decreased mobility (spending less time moving against the force of gravity) and immobility (spending most or all waking hours in a motorized wheelchair or bed) result in fewer calories burned. Unless such a person severely reduces his or her caloric input, weight gain will occur.

Most of the literature on obesity in muscle disease addresses DMD. Weight issues in DMD have been noted for decades.[81] Overeating and reduced energy expenditure were hypothesized as causes. Complicating the picture, individuals with DMD have reduced muscle mass.[82] Their actual weight, then, is artificially low in terms of their ideal weight, as they have a higher proportion of fat mass (fat is less dense than muscle) compared to those who do not have DMD.

The use of corticosteroids in DMD has further complicated this issue. DMD patients on the recommended daily prednisone dose of 0.75 mg/kg demonstrate excessive weight gain compared to placebo groups.[83] Deflazacort, another corticosteroid not available by prescription in the United States, has a lesser weight gain profile,[84] but still encourages weight gain compared to nontreated DMD individuals.

Most clinicians advise low sodium, low simple sugar, and reduced caloric diets for their muscle disease patients on chronic corticosteroid therapy.[85-87] Metformin therapy resulted in weight loss in a randomized, placebo-controlled trial that included boys with DMD.[88] Topiramate has also been used.[89] Ultimately, it becomes a perpetual battle for patients to maintain an ideal weight.

Cachexia is the other complication that occurs when a myopathic patient expends more energy that the nutrients taken in. Generally, this only happens in patients with impaired swallowing. Sometimes the work of breathing contributes to weight loss. Ventilatory assistance to reduce energy expenditure and supplemental caloric intake may be necessary. This often means insertion of a nasogastric tube or percutaneous endoscopic gastrostomy for indefinite use, as the work of self-feeding or mastication becomes profoundly exhausting.[90]

SWALLOWING ABNORMALITIES

Abnormalities of swallowing function (deglutition) occur in many myopathies (Box 13.3) and may occasionally be the presenting feature, although neuromuscular junction disorders should be considered in such patients. Impaired function of pharyngeal muscles may result in pooling of secretions in the hypopharynx, choking, and aspiration. Atelectasis and pneumonia may result if weakness of respiratory and glottic muscles impairs cough. Several myopathies present with different degrees of involvement. For example, individuals with FSHD can develop such severe facial muscle weakness that they cannot move food in their mouth or chew effectually,[91] whereas many patients with OPMD and inflammatory myopathies initially present with swallowing difficulties, coughing, and hoarseness. The tongue can also be involved with muscle fiber loss and fatty infiltration demonstrated by MRI or CT in individuals with OPMD.[92]

Symptoms and Recognition

Patients with abnormalities of deglutition usually recognize the problem and localize the

---

Box 13.3 Myopathies With Abnormal Deglutition

Muscular dystrophies
   Myotonic dystrophy: DM1 >> DM2
   Oculopharyngeal
   Oculopharyngodistal
   Duchenne (rarely)

Congenital
   Myofibrillar myopathies
   Congenital myopathies (most)

Inflammatory
   Dermatomyositis
   Polymyositis
   Inclusion body myositis

Mitochondrial

difficulty themselves. Patients with diseases of the muscles initiating deglutition, such as OPMD or DMS indicate that the submental and glottic regions are the site of obstruction. These disorders affect the upper one-third of the esophagus, which is striated muscle. Patients localize the problem by indicating a "sticking" of food in the suprasternal region. If the problem is localized to the lower portions of the esophagus and affects smooth muscle (as in scleroderma), the patient will point to the substernal region as the site of obstruction or pain.

Patients with swallowing abnormalities often fail to recognize that their symptoms are caused by weakness of the muscles of deglutition. Occult difficulty with swallowing is frequently seen in OPMD. Patients may present with an unexplained cough or shortness of breath that occurs during or after meals. Unexplained weight loss and the need to mince food into smaller and smaller pieces are occasionally the only signs that patients are having trouble swallowing. Cricopharyngeal achelasia can be identified by radiography of swallowing (Figure 13–1). Patients with DM1 frequently deny swallowing problems even when they are present.[93]

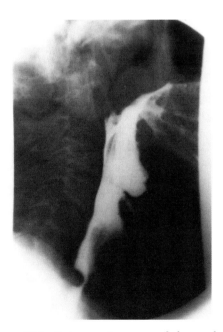

Figure 13–1. Barium roentgenogram of pharynx showing pooling of barium in the hypopharynx with constriction of hypopharyngeal outflow by the cricopharyngeus muscle: cricopharyngeal achalasia in an 80-year-old woman with oculopharyngeal muscular dystrophy.

Dysphagia has been associated with nutritional insufficiencies, aspiration pneumonia, decreased quality of life, and poor prognosis.[94]

Management

The primary treatment options for dysphagia are dietary adjustments or changes, teaching of safe swallowing techniques and exercises, surgical intervention, and enteral feeding.[95] There are no published randomized controlled trials that evaluate treatment for dysphagia in chronic muscle disease.[95] Published series are anecdotal or retrospective. A Cochrane report concluded that both cricopharyngeal myotomy and upper esophageal dilatation offer symptom relief in persons with dysphagia due to OPMD. Also, children with merosin-deficient congenital myopathy gained weight and had fewer respiratory infections following gastrostomy feeding.[95] There are case reports of botulinum toxin injection of the cricopharyngeus muscle to treat impaired swallowing.[96-98] Cricopharyngeal myotomy, dilatation, and botulinum injection all lose effectiveness over time as symptoms progress.

Severe weight loss or recurrent aspiration may necessitate an invasive procedure to provide adequate nutrition. Long-term enteral feeding is possible with percutaneous gastrostomy. Gastrostomy can be performed without general anesthesia and provides well-tolerated feeding access.

OTHER GASTROINTESTINAL COMPLICATIONS

Smooth muscle function is abnormal in many myopathies, including DM1, DM2, DMD, mitochondrial myopathy, and dermatomyositis. In DM1, gallbladder dysfunction and a variety of esophageal and intestinal disorders are frequent[99-101] and gastrointestinal symptoms are also frequent in DM2.[102] Patients with DMD have impaired gastric motility associated with dystrophin deficiency of smooth muscle and may present with severe gastric dilatation and intestinal pseudo-obstruction.[103,104] Electrolyte disturbances and aspiration may complicate gastric dilatation. Treatment consists of decompression of the dilated stomach with a nasogastric tube and the administration of appropriate fluids by a parenteral route.[103] In anecdotal experience, low-dose metoclopramide (10–20 mg/d) prevents this complication. Constipation is also a common symptom in DMD[90] and older boys may require daily laxatives such as lactulose in addition to increased fluid intake to avoid impaction.[52] However, any patient with muscle disease and decreased mobility, low fluid intake, and weak abdominal muscles is at an increased risk for developing constipation; those who also have hypomotility of the gastrointestinal tract requrie a regular bowel program.[105]

Abnormalities of the gastrointestinal tract are severe in certain mitochondrial disorders. In the mitochondrial neurogastrointestinal encephalopathy syndrome, intestinal involvement results in severe obstipation and episodes of intestinal pseudo-obstruction caused by severe visceral neuropathy.[106,107] (see chapter 8 for a more detailed discussion). Patients with childhood DM can have intestinal perforation resulting from the angiopathy that characterizes the illness.[108]

ORTHOPEDIC COMPLICATIONS

Scoliosis

The degree of scoliosisis directly related to the severity of truncal weakness and the age of the individual: the curve will progress more rapidly during growth spurts.[109] Consequently, any of the congenital myopathies can demonstrate severe scoliosis within the first decade. As the child's height increases, the curve may rapidly progress, as the weak trunk muscles must work harder against gravity and the elongated body mass. Boys with DMD untreated with corticosteroids and children with sarcoglycan-type LGMD, Ullrich's myopathy, and congenital muscular dystrophy with rigid spine syndrome can also develop progressive scoliosis by the teenage years.[110] The only proven prevention of scoliosis is corticosteroid treatment in DMD. Boys treated with daily prednisone or deflazacort did not develop significant (over 10°) scoliosis for at least 8 years.[64,111] Although the management of scoliosis by spinal fusion in neuromuscular diseases has improved in terms of decreased hospital days and recumbent

time,[112,113] there have been no randomized controlled trials to evaluate the benefits versus the risks of scoliosis surgery.[114] Specific spinal fusion methodology has evolved from the Harrington rod, Luque procedure, and pedicle screws, to combinations of all three.[115-117] Complications from any surgical method depend to a large degree on the severity of the curve and the respiratory and cardiac status of the patient.

Other Orthopedic Complications

Scapular winging can occur with any of the myopathies that present with proximal weakness, but is often severe in FSHD. Scapulothoracic fixation in carefully selected individuals can improve function by anchoring the scapula to the spine and providing the stability that the weak serratus anterior, middle, and lower trapezius muscles, and rhomboids cannot.[118-120] Pes planus, pes cavus, equinovarus, and congenital hip dislocation have all occured in the congenital myopathies. Surgical treatment generally is dependent on the child's ambulation potential or to reduce pain.[121] In boys with DMD who are no longer walking, there are mixed reports regarding the wisdom of surgical intervention to reduce or prevent foot deformities. One retrospective study concluded that there was no significant difference between patients who did or did not receive foot surgery in terms of shoe wear, hypersensitivity, or cosmesis, but equinus contracture was worse in those who declined surgery.[122] Another retrospective study concluded that 96% of boys who did undergo surgery were comfortable in any type shoe versus 60% of boys who declined surgery. This group did not compare equinus contractures between the two groups, but they reported that 94% of the operated group resulted in clinically satisfactory positioning.[123]

Soft tissue contractures are another familiar problem of most myopathies but the etiology remains speculative and likely is multifactorial. Certain disorders, such as EDMD, Ullrich and Bethlem myopathies, hereditary inclusion body myopathy type 3, and severe X-linked centronuclear myopathy have severe rigid joint contractures early in the disease process, but in addition, nearly all patients with myopathy suffer some loss of normal joint range of motion. Most experts feel that functional positioning plays an important role in contracture formation, observing that individuals who spend the majority of time sitting, for example, develop hip and knee flexion contractures.[124] Diverse types of muscle diseases display different patterns and severity of weakness, and the resulting unbalanced forces lead some muscles and tendons to shorten while their antagonists lengthen. For example, in DMD and certain other myopathies, the tibialis posterior and the gastrocnemius muscles are always stronger than their antagonists, the peroneus longus and brevis and tibialis anterior, and therefore result in the common equinovarus contracture. Sometimes muscle shortening develops as a way to preserve function. One example in DMD occurs when the gastrocnemius muscle initially shortens to function as a floor-reaction AFO (ankle foot orthosis). This occurs in young boys as both the gluteus maximus and quadriceps weaken to such an extent that the child can no longer maintain his center of gravity behind the hip joint and in front of the knee joint simultaneously. The boy must go up on his toes to continue standing and walking.[125] Last, muscle biopsies suggest that some myopathies have inherent connective tissue pathology.[126] Research in the mdx mouse (the murine model for DMD) has demonstrated increased fibrotic tissue in skeletal muscle, which may predispose these individuals toward joint contracture formation.[127,128]

Prevention of joint contractures remains elusive; there is no evidence that this goal is yet achievable. A 2011 review of passive stretch (defined as self-, therapist, or device administered and including positioning, splinting, and serial casting) concluded that "there is little or no effect of stretch on pain, spasticity, or active limitation in people with neurological conditions."[129] The effectiveness of stretch has been best studied for on DMD. A 2010 Cochrane review concluded that "there is limited evidence supporting any intervention for improving ankle flexibility in patients with Duchenne muscular dystrophy."[130] Still, most clinicians recommend regular stretching for individuals with muscle disease. The review of multidisciplinary care in DMD recommends stretching a minimum of 4 to 6 days per week for any specific joint.[52]

Osteoporosis is also a concern in the myopathies because the primary factor that determines bone density is the magnitude of muscle pull, or muscle strength. Virtually all individuals with muscle weakness (even if still ambulatory) have some degree of osteopenia. In progressive myopathies, osteoporosis can become severe and predisposes those affected to higher risk for fractures and medical complications such as hypercalciuria and kidney stones.[131]

Patients treated with corticosteroids, of course, are at an even higher risk of developing osteoporosis; the incidence of long bone fractures was 2.6 times greater in one series of DMD boys.[111] Some experts recommend a baseline dual-emission X-ray absorptiometry (DEXA) prior to initiating corticosteroid treatment and annually after. Unfortunately, there is no agreed-upon prophylactic treatment. Clinicians recommend calcium and vitamin D supplements,[52] but dosages vary.[132] Some also prescribe bisphosphonates, but there is not yet evidence to recommend bisphosphonates prophylactically to reduce fractures.[133] One retrospective study in DMD found that treatment with steroids and bisphosphonates was associated with significantly improved survival over steroid treatment alone.[134]

DMD boys treated with corticosteroids also are at higher risk of compression fractures.[133] Compression fractures, however, were rarely a cause for discontinuing steroid treatment; in fact, individuals were frequently unaware of their existence.[87]

A final complication of osteoporosis (at least in DMD) is fat emboli syndrome. In one series, eight boys with DMD who suffered unilateral or bilateral distal femoral fractures from low impact falls developed the syndrome within hours of the trauma. Six of the eight were on corticosteroid therapy. Final outcome ranged from full recovery to death.[135]

There are reports on orthognathic surgery in myopathy patients with facial weakness. These individuals have increased lower facial height and an open bite. One study reported excellent results at the 5-year follow up visit in a patient with congenital fiber-type disproportion.[136]

Last, cervical hyperextension as a fixed joint contracture can be a painful and debilitating orthopedic complication, particularly in children. Children with severe muscle weakness such as that found in the congenital myopathies may lack sufficient head control to keep their eyes focused horizontally. These children, almost invariably not walking, must routinely hyperextend their necks, and thus the cervical extensor muscles become restricted in length.

Along with cervical weakness, truncal weakness may mean the children assume a degree of trunk forward flexion, which also results in cervical hyperextension as the only means to view their world normally. A few case reports on surgical treatment for this problem have been published.[137, 138]

ORTHOTIC INTERVENTION

The majority of research reports on orthotic intervention in muscle disease focus on DMD. In the pre-steroid era, boys with DMD wore knee-ankle foot orthoses (KAFOs) to maintain short distance ambulation or functional standing starting at an average age of 10.3 years.[124] In later years, however, boys prescribed corticosteroids while still ambulating independently never progressed to orthoses, ambulating independently 2 to 5 years or longer on average by virtue of the corticosteroid treatment.[139] These boys ambulated without orthoses until they could no longer stand, thus bypassing KAFOs altogether. The evidence that KAFOs prolong functional ambulation in the steroid era is limited.[140]

Orthoses are often recommended for other muscular dystrophies, however. Ankle-foot orthoses for dorsiflexion weakness can decrease fatigue and prevent tripping in FSHD, DM1, scapuloperoneal muscular dystrophy, and the distal myopathies, for example.[141-145] There are many choices of style and materials from which to fabricate AFOs today, and the braces can be custom made or off the shelf. Carbon fiber–fabricated AFOs also provide plantar flexion assistance. One carbon fiber orthosis (ToeOFF) can function as a floor reaction AFO while providing quadriceps stability by virtue of its anterior shell. It may allow safe ambulation in selected patients with moderate quadriceps weakness (e.g., individuals with BMD, sIBM, and FSHD).

Another type of orthosis that can function well for myopathic patients is the stance control KAFO. This brace provides quadriceps stability by locking the knee during the weight bearing phase of gait, but releasing during swing phase. It can prolong ambulation in properly assessed individuals, but potential users must be screened carefully.[146]

Cervical orthoses are also commonly prescribed for individuals with weak neck extensors. Patients do not tolerate wearing these braces for long periods of time, however, and they can interfere with ambulation. Still, they are appropriate to recommend for at least part-time use when, for example, the patient is riding in a car or working on a computer.

Hand or wrist splints are prescribed both in an attempt to control joint contractures and to improve function. They typically work well initially, but if contractures or weakness progress they must be regularly adjusted or refitted.

MOBILITY AIDS AND ADAPTIVE EQUIPMENT

There are a variety of wheelchairs (manual, powered, or power assisted), motorized scooters, walkers, bath and toilet aids, ceiling lifts, and stair lifts. Economic considerations such as insurance coverage (in the United States) often determine equipment choices. These are practical considerations for their prescription, too. Ordering a walker for a patient, for example, could preclude him from receiving a wheelchair until a certain number of years have elapsed. Similarly, power-assist wheelchairs can provide a bridge between manual and full-power chairs, but they may be classified as a power wheelchair by the patient's insurance company. Occupational and physical therapists experienced in various neuromuscular diseases and their rate of progression, as well as in health care coverage, are essential as adaptive equipment consultants.

PREGNANCY

An increased rate of obstetric complications occur in individuals with myopathies. Pregnant women with LGMD and FSHD reported worsening of muscle weakness, and the same groups, in addition to women with DM1, had a higher rate of operative vaginal deliveries and Cesarean section than the general population,[147-149] as well as higher incidence of urinary tract infections, abnormal placentation, and pre- and postpartum hemorrhage. These same individuals are also at a higher risk for cardiac arrhythmias and respiratory complications. In addition, it has been suggested that gestation may cause a shift toward an earlier onset of symptoms in women with DM2 who give birth.[150] Pregnant individuals with myopathies that involve respiratory or abdominal muscle weakness or who are at risk for cardiac disease or anesthesia complications should be referred for high-risk obstetrical intervention. Women with DM1 are at especially high risk of maternal and fetal complications.

REFERENCES

1. Estenne M, Heilporn A, Delhez L: Chest wall stiffness in patients with chronic respiratory muscle weakness. Am Rev Respir Dis, 1983;128:1002–1007.
2. Perrin C, Unterborn JN, Ambrosio CD, Hill NS: Pulmonary complications of chronic neuromuscular diseases and their management. Muscle Nerve, 2004;29:5–27.
3. Black LF, Hyatt RE: Maximal static respiratory pressures in generalized neuromuscular disease. Am Rev Respir Dis, 1971;103:641–650.
4. Griggs RC, Donohoe KM, Utell MJ, Goldblatt D, Moxley RT 3rd: Evaluation of pulmonary function in neuromuscular disease. Arch Neurol,1981;38;9–12.
5. Bushby K, Finkel R, Birnkrant DJ, et al: Diagnosis and management of Duchenne muscular dystrophy, part 1: diagnosis, and pharmacological and psychosocial management. Lancet Neurol, 2010;9:77–93.
6. Newsom-Davis J, Goldman M, Loh L, Casson M: Diaphragm function and alveolar hypoventilation. Q J Med, 1976;45:87–100.
7. Shahrizaila T, Kinnear W: Recommendations for respiratory care of adults with muscle disorders. Neuromuscul Disord, 2007;17:13–15.
8. DePalo VA, McCool FD: Respiratory muscle evaluation of the patient with neuromuscular disease. Semin Respir Crit Care Med, 2002;23:201–209.
9. Fromageot C, Lofaso F, Annane D, et al: Supine fall in lung volumes in the assessment of diaphragmatic weakness in neuromuscular disorders. Arch Phys Med Rehabil, 2001;82;123–128.
10. Vincken WG, Elleker MG, Cosio MG: Flow-volume loop changes reflecting respiratory muscle weakness in chronic neuromuscular disorders. Am J Med, 1987;83:673–680.
11. Birnkrant D, Bushby KM, Amin RS: The respiratory management of patients with Duchenne muscular dystrophy: a DMD care considerations working group specialty article. Pediatr Pulmonol, 2010;45:739–748.
12. Steier J, Kaul S, Seymour JL: The value of multiple tests of respiratory muscle strength. Thorax 2007;62(11):975–80.
13. Advisory Committee for Immunization Practices (ACIP), Centers for Disease Control and Prevention. (2010). Recommendations 23-Valent Pneumococcal
14. Advisory Committee for Immunization Practices (ACIP), Centers for Disease Control and Prevention. (2011). Prevention and Control of Seasonal Influenza with Vaccines. Morbidity and Mortality Weekly Report, August 26, 2010; 60(33):1128–32.
15. Finder JD, Birnkrant D, Carl J et al:. Respiratory care of the patient with Duchenne muscular dystrophy: ATS consensus statement. Am J Respir Crit Care Med, 2004;170:456–465.
16. Tager I, Speizer FE: Role of infection in chronic bronchitis. N Engl J Med, 1975;292:563–571.
17. Kelly BJ, Luce JM: The diagnosis and management of neuromuscular diseases causing respiratory failure. Chest, 2991;99;1485–1494.
18. Garpestad E, Brennan J, Hill NS: Noninvasive ventilation for critical care. Chest, 2007;132:711–720.
19. Sancho J, Servera E: Noninvasive ventilation for patients with neuromuscular disease and acute respiratory failure. Chest. 2008;133:314–315 author reply 315.
20. Shneerson JM, Simonds AK: Noninvasive ventilation for chest wall and neuromuscular disorders. Eur Respir J, 2002;20:480–487.
21. Hill, N: Ventilator management for neuromuscular disease. Semin Respir Crit Care Med, 2002;23:293–305.
22. Hill N, Garpestad E: Author Reply. Noninvasive ventilation for patients with neuromuscular disease and acute respiratory failure. Chest, 2008;133:315.
23. Mehta S, Hill, NS:. Noninvasive Ventilation. Am J Respir Crit Care Med, 2001;163:540–577.
24. Hamada S, Ishikawa Y, Aoyagi T, et al: Indicators for ventilator use in Duchenne muscular dystrophy. Respir Med, 2011;105:625–629.
25. Bach, J: Mechanical insufflation-exsufflation. Comparison of peak expiratory flows with manually assisted and unassisted coughing techniques. Chest, 1993;104:1553–1562.
26. Allen, J: Pulmonary complications of neuromuscular disease: a respiratory mechanics perspective. Paediatr Respir Rev, 2010;11:18–23.
27. Eagle M, Baudouin SV, Chandler C, et al: Survival in Duchenne muscular dystrophy: improvements in life expectancy since 1967 and the impact of home nocturnal ventilation. Neuromuscul Disord, 2002;12:926–929.
28. Ishikawa, Y. Bach JR: Physical medicine respiratory muscle aids to avert respiratory complications of pediatric chest wall and vertebral deformity and muscle dysfunction. Eur J Phys Rehabil Med, 2010;46: 581–597.
29. Park JH, Kang SW, Lee SC et al: How respiratory muscle strength correlates with cough capacity in patients with respiratory muscle weakness. Yonsei Med J, 2010;51:392–397.
30. Vaszar LT, Weinacker AB, Henig NR, Raffin TA: Ethical issues in the long-term management of progressive degenerative neuromuscular diseases. Semin Respir Crit Care Med, 2002;23:307–314.
31. Perrin C, D'Ambrosio C, White A, Hill NS: Sleep in restrictive and neuromuscular respiratory disorders. Semin Respir Crit Care Med, 2005;26:117–130.
32. Labanowski M, Schmidt-Nowara W, Guilleminault C: Sleep and neuromuscular disease: frequency of sleep-disordered breathing in a neuromuscular disease clinic population. Neurology, 1996;47:1173–1180.

33. Cirignotta F, Mondini S, Zucconi M: Sleep-related breathing impairment in myotonic dystrophy. J Neurol, 1987;235: 80–85.

34. Piper, A: Sleep abnormalities associated with neuromuscular disease: pathophysiology and evaluation. Semin Respir Crit Care Med, 2002;23:211–219.

35. James J, Kinnett K, Wang Y, et al: Electrocardiographic abnormalities in very young Duchenne muscular dystrophy patients precede the onset of cardiac dysfunction. Neuromuscul Disord, 2011;21:462–467.

36. Silva MC, Meira ZM, Gurgel Giannetti J: Myocardial delayed enhancement by magnetic resonance imaging in patients with muscular dystrophy. J Am Coll Cardiol, 2007;49:1874–1879.

37. Finsterer J, Ramaciotti C, Wang CH, et al: Cardiac findings in congenital muscular dystrophies. Pediatrics, 2010;126:538–545.

38. Hermans MC, Pinto YM, Merkies IS, et al: Hereditary muscular dystrophies and the heart. Neuromuscul Disord, 2010;20:479–492.

39. Spurney, C: Cardiomyopathy of Duchenne muscular dystrophy: current understanding and future directions. Muscle Nerve, 2011;44:8–19.

40. Forgacs, P: The functional basis of pulmonary sounds. Chest, 1978;73:399–405.

41. Ehlers KH, Hagstrom JW, Lukas DS, et al: Glycogen-storage disease of the myocardium with obstruction to left ventricular outflow. Circulation, 1962;25;96–109.

42. Johnson RA, Palacios I: Dilated cardiomyopathies of the adult (first of two parts). N Engl J Med, 1982;307: 1051–1058.

43. Hor KN, Wansapura J, Markham LW, et al: Circumferential strain analysis identifies strata of cardiomyopathy in Duchenne muscular dystrophy: a cardiac magnetic resonance tagging study. J Am Coll Cardiol, 2009;53:1204–1210.

44. Hagenbuch SC, Gottliebson WM, Wansapura J, et al: Detection of progressive cardiac dysfunction by serial evaluation of circumferential strain in patients with Duchenne muscular dystrophy. Am J Cardiol, 2010;105:1451–1455.

45. Gaul C, Deschauer M, Tempelmann C, et al: Cardiac involvement in limb-girdle muscular dystrophy 2I: conventional cardiac diagnostic and cardiovascular magnetic resonance. J Neurol, 2006;253:1317–1322.

46. Schneider-Gold C, Beer M, Köstler H, et al: Cardiac and skeletal muscle involvement in myotonic dystrophy type 2 (DM2): a quantitative 31P-MRS and MRI study. Muscle Nerve, 2004;30:636–644.

47. Verhaert D, Richards K, Rafael-Fortney JA, Raman SV: Cardiac involvement in patients with muscular dystrophies: magnetic resonance imaging phenotype and genotypic considerations. Circ Cardiovasc Imaging, 2011;4: 67–76.

48. Mori K, Manabe T, Nii M, et al: Plasma levels of natriuretic peptide and echocardiographic parameters in patients with Duchenne's progressive muscular dystrophy. Pediatr Cardiol, 2002;23:160–166.

49. Mohyuddin T Jacobs IB, Bahler RC: B-type natriuretic peptide and cardiac dysfunction in Duchenne muscular dystrophy. Int J Cardiol, 2007;119:389–391.

50. Demachi J, Kagaya Y, Watanabe J, et al: Characteristics of the increase in plasma brain natriuretic peptide level in left ventricular systolic dysfunction, associated with muscular dystrophy in comparison with idiopathic dilated cardiomyopathy. Neuromuscul Disord, 2004; 14:732–739.

51. Cox FM, Delgado V, Verschuuren JJ, et al: The heart in sporadic inclusion body myositis: a study in 51 patients. J Neurol, 2010;257:447–451.

52. Bushby K, Finkel R, Birnkrant DJ, et al: Diagnosis and management of Duchenne muscular dystrophy, part 2: implementation of multidisciplinary care. Lancet Neurol, 2010;9:177–189.

53. Dellefave LM, McNally EM: Cardiomyopathy in neuromuscular disorders. Progress in Pediatric Cardiology, 2007;24:35–46.

54. Guglieri M, Bushby K: In: S. Venance, R. Tawil (eds), Neuromuscular Disorders (8 ed.). 2011, Oxford: John Wiley and Sons Ltd.

55. Calvo F, Teijeira S, Fernandez JM, et al: Evaluation of heart involvement in gamma-sarcoglycanopathy (LGMD2C). A study of ten patients. Neuromuscul Disord, 2000;10:560–566.

56. Epstein AE, DiMarco JP, Ellenbogen KA, et al: ACC/AHA/HRS 2008 Guidelines for Device-Based Therapy of Cardiac Rhythm Abnormalities: a report of the American College of Cardiology/American Heart Association Task Force on Practice Guidelines (Writing Committee to Revise the ACC/AHA/NASPE 2002 Guideline. Circulation, 2008;117:e350–e408.

57. Groh WJ, Groh MR, Saha C, et al: Electrocardiographic abnormalities and sudden death in myotonic dystrophy type 1. N Engl J Med, 2008;358:2688–2697.

58. Udd B, Meola G, Krahe R, et al: Myotonic dystrophy type 2 (DM2) and related disorders report of the 180th ENMC workshop including guidelines on diagnostics and management 3-5 December 2010, Naarden, The Netherlands. Neuromuscul Disord, 2011;21:443–450.

59. Lundberg, I. (2006). The heart in dermatomyositis and polymyositis. Rheumatology, 45 (Suppl 4), iv18–iv21.

60. Duboc D, Meune C, Pierre B, et al: Perindopril preventive treatment on mortality in Duchenne muscular dystrophy: 10 years' follow-up. Am Heart J, 2007;154:596–602.

61. Bushby K: 107th ENMC international workshop: the management of cardiac involvement in muscular dystrophy and myotonic dystrophy. 7th-9th June 2002, Naarden, the Netherlands. Neuromuscul Disord, 2003;13:166–172.

62. American Academy of Pediatrics: Cardiovascular health supervision for individuals affected by Duchenne or Becker muscular dystrophy. Pediatrics, 2005;116, 1569–1573.

63. Markham LW, Kinnett K, Wong BL, et al: Corticosteroid treatment retards development of ventricular dysfunction in Duchenne muscular dystrophy. Neuromuscul Disord, 2008;18:365–370.

64. Houde S, Filiatrault M, Fournier A, et al: Deflazacort use in Duchenne muscular dystrophy: an 8-year follow-up. Pediatr Neurol, 2008;38:200–206.

65. Allanore Y, Vignaux O, Arnaud L, et al: Effects of corticosteroids and immunosuppressors on idiopathic inflammatory myopathy related myocarditis evaluated by magnetic resonance imaging. Ann Rheum Dis, 2006;65:249–252.

66. Afzal A, Higgins RS, Philbin EF: Heart transplant for dilated cardiomyopathy associated with polymyositis. Heart. 1999;82:e4.

67. Wu RS, Gupta S, Brown RN, et al:. Clinical outcomes after cardiac transplantation in muscular dystrophy patients. J Heart Lung Transplant, 2010;29:432–438.

68. Nigro G, Politano L, Nigro V: Mutation of dystrophin gene and cardiomyopathy. Neuromuscul Disord, 1994;4:371–379.

69. Kaspar RW, Allen HD, Ray WC, et al: Analysis of dystrophin deletion mutations predicts age of cardiomyopathy onset in Becker muscular dystrophy. Circ Cardiovasc Genet, 2009;2:544–551.

70. Watkins H, Ashrafian H, Redwood C: Inherited cardiomyopathies. N Engl J Med, 2011;364: 1643–1656.

71. Ishikawa Y, Miura T, Ishikawa, et al: Duchenne muscular dystrophy: survival by cardio-respiratory interventions. Neuromuscul Disord, 2011 21, 47–51.

72. Larca LJ, Coppola JT, Honig S: Creatine kinase MB isoenzyme in dermatomyositis: a noncardiac source. Ann Intern Med, 1981;94:341–343.

73. Silverman LM, Mendell JR, Sahenk Z, et al. Significance of creatine phosphokinase isoenzymes in Duchenne dystrophy. Neurology, 1976;26, 561–564.

74. Gimenez-Muñoz A, Capablo JL, Alarcia R, et al: Intracardiac thrombus and cerebral infarction in a patient with duchenne muscular dystrophy. J Clin Neuromuscul Dis, 2009;11:79–80.

75. Tsakadze N, Katzin LW, Krishnan S, Behrouz R: Cerebral infarction in Duchenne muscular dystrophy. J Stroke Cerebrovasc Dis, 2011;20:264–265.

76. Abelmann, W: Treatment of congestive cardiomyopathy. Postgrad Med J, 1978;54:477–484.

77. Makabali C, Well MH, Henning RJ:. Dobutamine and other sympathomimetic drugs for the treatment of low cardiac output failure. Seminars in Anesthesia, 1982;1:63–69.

78. Blahd WH, Lederer M, Cassen B: The significance of decreased body potassium concentrations in patients with muscular dystrophy and nondystrophic relatives. N Engl J Med, 1967;276:1349–1352.

79. Moore-Ede MC, Meguid MM, Fitzpatrick GF, et al: Circadian variation in response to potassium infusion. Clin Pharmacol Ther, 1978;23:218–227.

80. Moxley, RT: Absence of major side effects of nifedipine following treatment of Duchenne dystrophy. Pediatrics, 1985;75:1168–1169.

81. Edwards RHT, Round JM, Jackson MJ, et al. Weight reduction in boys with muscular dystrophy. Dev Med Child Neurol, 1984;26, 384–90.

82. Griggs RC, Forbes G, Moxley RT, Herr BE: The assessment of muscle mass in progressive neuromuscular disease. Neurology, 1983;33:158–165.

83. Manzur AY, Kuntzer T, Pike M, Swan A: Glucocorticoid corticosteroids for Duchenne muscular dystrophy. Cochrane Database Syst Rev CD003725, 2008;23(1) doi: 10.1002/14651858.CD003725.pub3.

84. Bonifati MD, Ruzza G, Bonometto P, et al: A multicenter, double-blind, randomized trial of deflazacort versus prednisone in Duchenne muscular dystrophy. Muscle Nerve, 2000;23: 1344–1347.

85. Ciafaloni E, Moxley RT: Treatment options for Duchenne muscular dystrophy. Curr Treat Options Neurol, 2008;10:86–93.

86. Amato AA, Barohn RJ: Evaluation and treatment of inflammatory myopathies. J Neurol Neurosurg Psychiatry, 2009;80:1060–1068.

87. Bianchi ML, Biggar D, Bushby K, et al: Endocrine aspects of Duchenne muscular dystrophy. Neuromuscul Disord, 2011;21:298–303.

88. Casteels K, Fieuws S, van Helvoirt M: Metformin therapy to reduce weight gain and visceral adiposity in children and adolescents with neurogenic or myogenic motor deficit. Pediatr Diabetes. 2010;11:61–69.

89. Carter GT, Yudkowsky MP, Han JJ, McCrory MA: Topiramate for weight reduction in Duchenne muscular dystrophy. Muscle Nerve, 2005;31:788–789.

90. Pane M, Vasta I, Messina S: Feeding problems and weight gain in Duchenne muscular dystrophy. Eur J Paediatr Neurol, 2006;10.

91. Wohlgemuth M, deSwart BJ, Kalf JG, et al. Dysphagia in facioscapulohumeral muscular dystrophy. Neurology, 2006;66, 1926–1928.

92. King MK, Lee RR, Davis LE: Magnetic resonance imaging and computed tomography of skeletal muscles in oculopharyngeal muscular dystrophy. J Clin Neuromuscul Dis, 2005;6:103–108.

93. LaDonna KA, Koopman WJ, Venance SL: Myotonic dystrophy (DM1) and dysphagia: the need for dysphagia management guidelines and an assessment tool. Can J Neurosci Nurs, 2011;33:42–46.

94. Oh TH, Brumfield KA, Hoskin TL, et al:. Dysphagia in inflammatory myopathy: clinical characteristics, treatment strategies, and outcome in 62 patients. Mayo Clin Proc, 2007;82:441–447.

95. Hill M, Hughes T, Milford C: Treatment for swallowing difficulties (dysphagia) in chronic muscle disease. Cochrane Database Syst Rev (2), CD004303, 2004, DOI: 10.1002/14651858.CD004303.pub2.

96. Restivo DA, Marchese Ragona R, Staffieri A, de Grandis D: Successful botulinum toxin treatment of dysphagia in oculopharyngeal muscular dystrophy. Gastroenterology, 2000;119: 1416.

97. Restivo DA, Giuffrida S, Marchese Ragona R, Falsaperla R: Successful botulinum toxin treatment of dysphagia in a young child with nemaline myopathy. Dysphagia, 2001;16:228–229.

98. Liu LW, Tarnopolsky M, Armstrong D: Injection of botulinum toxin A to the upper esophageal sphincter for oropharyngeal dysphagia in two patients with inclusion body myositis. Can J Gastroenterol, 2004;18:397–399.

99. Bellini M, Biagi S, Stasi C, et al: Gastrointestinal manifestations in myotonic muscular dystrophy. World J Gastroenterol, 2006;12:1821–1828.

100. Chaudhry V, Umapathi T, Ravich WJ: Neuromuscular diseases and disorders of the alimentary system. Muscle Nerve, 2002;25:768–784.

101. Degraeuwe J, Van Laecke E, De Muynck M, et al: Faecal incontinence due to atrophy of the anal sphincter in myotonic dystrophy: a case report. Acta Gastroenterol Belg, 2011;74:88–90.

102. Tieleman AA, van Vliet J, Jansen JB, et al: Gastrointestinal involvement is frequent in myotonic dystrophy type 2. Neuromuscul Disord, 2008;18: 646–649.

103. Barohn RJ, Levine EJ, Olson JO, Mendell JR: Gastric hypomotility in Duchenne's muscular dystrophy. N Engl J Med, 1988;319:15–18.

104. Bensen ES, Jaffe KM, Tarr PI: Acute gastric dilatation in Duchenne muscular dystrophy: a case report and review of the literature. Arch Phys Med Rehabil, 1996;77:512–514.

105. Guandalini, S: Essential Pediatric Gastroenterology, Hepatology, and Nutrition. McGraw-Hill Medical Publishing Division, New York, 2004.

106. Hirano M, Silvestri G, Blake DM, et al: Mitochondrial neurogastrointestinal encephalomyopathy (MNGIE): clinical, biochemical, and genetic features of an autosomal recessive mitochondrial disorder. Neurology, 1994;44:721–727.

107. Bedlack RS, Vu T, Hammans S, et al: MNGIE neuropathy: five cases mimicking chronic inflammatory demyelinating polyneuropathy. Muscle Nerve, 2004;29:364–368.

108. Schullinger JN, Jacobs JC, Berdon WE: Diagnosis and management of gastrointestinal perforations in childhood dermatomyositis with particular reference to perforations of the duodenum. J Pediatr Surg, 1985;20:521–524.

109. Anderson M, Hwang SC, Green WT: Growth of the normal trunk in boys and girls during the second decade of life; related to age, maturity, and ossification of the iliac epiphyses. J Bone Joint Surg Am, 1965;47:1554–1564.

110. Amato, A. Russell JA Neuromuscular Disorders. New York: McGraw-Hill, 2008.

111. King WM, Ruttencutter R, Nagaraja HN, et al: Orthopedic outcomes of long-term daily corticosteroid treatment in Duchenne muscular dystrophy. Neurology, 2007;19:1607–1613.

112. Boachie-Adjei O, Lonstein JE, Winter RB, et al: Management of neuromuscular spinal deformities with Luque segmental instrumentation. J Bone Joint Surg Am,1989;71:548–562.

113. Takaso M, Nakazawa T, Imura T, et al: Two-year results for scoliosis secondary to Duchenne muscular dystrophy fused to lumbar 5 with segmental pedicle screw instrumentation. J Orthop Sci, 2010;15:171–177.

114. Cheuk DK, Wong V, Wraige E, et al: Surgery for scoliosis in Duchenne muscular dystrophy. Cochrane Database Syst Rev CD005375, 2007:(1). DOI: 10.1002/14651858.CD005375.pub2.).

115. Arun R, Srinivas S, Mehdian SM: Scoliosis in Duchenne's muscular dystrophy: a changing trend in surgical management: a historical surgical outcome study comparing sublaminar, hybrid and pedicle screw instrumentation systems. Eur Spine J, 2010;19: 376–383.

116. Modi HN, Suh SW, Hong JY, et al: Treatment and complications in flaccid neuromuscular scoliosis (Duchenne muscular dystrophy and spinal muscular atrophy) with posterior-only pedicle screw instrumentation. Eur Spine J, 2010;19:384–393.

117. Debnath UK, Mehdian SM, Webb JK: Spinal deformity correction in Duchenne muscular dystrophy (DMD): comparing the outcome of two instrumentation techniques. Asian Spine J, 2011;5:43–50.

118. DeFranco MJ, Nho S, Romeo AA: Scapulothoracic fusion. J Am Acad Orthop Surg, 2010;18:236–242.

119. Orrell RW, Copeland S, Rose MR: Scapular fixation in muscular dystrophy. Cochrane Database Syst Rev CD003278, 2010;20(1). DOI: 10.1002/14651858. CD003278.pub2.

120. Diab M, Darras BT, Shapiro F: Scapulothoracic fusion for facioscapulohumeral muscular dystrophy. J Bone Joint Surg Am, 2005;87:2267–2275.

121. Finsterer J, Strobl W: Orthopaedic abnormalities in primary myopathies. Acta Orthop Belg, 2011;77:563–582.

122. Leitch KK, Raza N, Biggar D, et al: Should foot surgery be performed for children with Duchenne muscular dystrophy? J Pediatr Orthop, 2005;25:95–97.

123. Scher DM, Mubarak SJ: Surgical prevention of foot deformity in patients with Duchenne muscular dystrophy. J Pediatr Orthop, 2002;22:384–391.

124. Brooke MH, Fenichel GM, Griggs RC, et al: Clinical investigation in Duchenne dystrophy: 2. Determination of the "power" of therapeutic trials based on the natural history. Muscle Nerve, 1983;6: 91–103.

125. Sutherland DH, Olshen R, Cooper L, et al: The pathomechanics of gait in Duchenne muscular dystrophy. Dev Med Child Neurol, 1981;23:3–22.

126. Duance VC, Stephens HR, Dunn M, et al: A role for collagen in the pathogenesis of muscular dystrophy? Nature, 1980;284:470–472.

127. Goldspink G, Fernandes K, Williams PE, Wells DJ. Age-related changes in collagen gene expression in the muscles of mdx dystrophic and normal mice. Neuromuscul Disord, 1994;4:183–191.

128. Alexakis C, Partridge T, Bou-Gharios G: Implication of the satellite cell in dystrophic muscle fibrosis: a self-perpetuating mechanism of collagen overproduction. Am J Physiol Cell Physiol, 2007;293:C661–C669.

129. Katalinic OM, Harvey LA, Herbert RD: Effectiveness of stretch for the treatment and prevention of contractures in people with neurological conditions: a systematic review. Phys Ther, 2011;91:11–24.

130. Rose KJ, Burns J, Wheeler DM, North KN: Interventions for increasing ankle range of motion in patients with neuromuscular disease. Cochrane Database Syst Rev (2), 2010CD006973. doi: 10.1002/14651858.CD006973.pub2.

131. Shumyatcher Y, Shah TA, Noritz GH, et al: Symptomatic nephrolithiasis in prolonged survivors of Duchenne muscular dystrophy. Neuromuscul Disord, 2008;18(7):561–4.

132. Bianchi ML, Morandi L, Andreucci E, et al: Low bone density and bone metabolism alterations in Duchenne muscular dystrophy: response to calcium and vitamin D treatment. Osteoporos Int, 2010;22:529–539.

133. Quinlivan R, Shaw N, Bushby K: 170th ENMC International Workshop: bone protection for corticosteroid treated Duchenne muscular dystrophy. 27-29 November 2009, Naarden, The Netherlands. Neuromuscul Disord, 2010;20:761–769.

134. Gordon KE, Dooley JM, Sheppard KM, et al: Impact of bisphosphonates on survival for patients with Duchenne muscular dystrophy. Pediatrics, 2011;127: e353–e358.

135. Medeiros MO, Behrend C, King W, et al: Fat embolism syndrome in patients with Duchenne muscular dystrophy. Neurology, 2013;80(14):1350–1352.

136. Lehman H, Harari D, Tarazi E, et al: Orthognathic surgery in primary myopathies: severe case of congenital fiber type disproportion with long-term follow-up and review of the literature. J Oral Maxillofac Surg 2011;70(7):1636–42.

137. Giannini S, Ceccarelli F, Faldini C, et al: Surgical treatment of neck hyperextension in myopathies. Clin Orthop Relat Res, 2005;434:151–156.

138. Giannini S, Faldini C, Pagkrati S, et al: Surgical treatment of neck hyperextension in Duchenne muscular dystrophy by posterior interspinous fusion. Spine, 2006;31:1805–1809.
139. Moxley RT 3rd, Pandya S, Ciafaloni E, et al: Change in natural history of Duchenne muscular dystrophy with long-term corticosteroid treatment: implications for management. J Child Neurol, 2010;25: 1116–1129.
140. Bakker JP, de Groot IJ, Beckerman H, et al: The effects of knee-ankle-foot orthoses in the treatment of Duchenne muscular dystrophy: review of the literature. Clin Rehabil, 2000;14:343–359.
141. Farmakidis C, Tawil, R: In: S. Venance, R. Tawil (eds), Neuromuscular Disorders. Oxford: John Wiley & Sons, Ltd., 2011.
142. Tawil R, van der Maarel S, Padberg GW, van Engelen BG: 171st ENMC international workshop: Standards of care and management of facioscapulohumeral muscular dystrophy. Neuromuscul Disord, 2010;20: 471–475.
143. Pandya S, King WM, Tawil R: Facioscapulohumeral dystrophy. Phys Ther, 2008;88:105–113.
144. Johnson N, Heatwole CR: In: S. Venance, R. Tawil (eds), Neuromuscular Disorders. Oxford: John Wiley & Sons, Ltd., 2011.
145. Udd, B: Neuromuscular Disorders. (V. S. Tawil RN, Ed.) Oxford: John Wiley & Sons, 2011.
146. Bernhardt K, Oh T, Kaufman K: Stance control orthosis trial in patients with inclusion body myositis. Prosthet Orthot Int, 2011;35:39–44.
147. Rudnik-Schöneborn S, Glauner B, Röhrig D, Zerres K: Obstetric aspects in women with facioscapulohumeral muscular dystrophy, limb-girdle muscular dystrophy, and congenital myopathies. Arch Neurol, 1997;54:888–894.
148. Ciafaloni E, Pressman EK, Loi AM, et al: Pregnancy and birth outcomes in women with facioscapulohumeral muscular dystrophy. Neurology, 2006;67: 1887–1889.
149. Rudnik-Schöneborn S, Zerres K: Outcome in pregnancies complicated by myotonic dystrophy: a study of 31 patients and review of the literature. Eur J Obstet Gynecol Reprod Biol, 2004;114:44–53.
150. Rudnik-Schöneborn S, Schneider-Gold C, Raabe U, et al: Outcome and effect of pregnancy in myotonic dystrophy type 2. Neurology, 2006;66:579–580.

Index

Page numbers followed by *b*, *t* and *f* indicate boxes, tables, and figures, respectively.